Social Attitudes in the Early 21st Century

Chau-kiu Cheung

Social Attitudes in the Early 21st Century

Springer

Chau-kiu Cheung
City University of Hong Kong
Hong Kong, China

ISBN 978-981-96-9704-5 ISBN 978-981-96-9705-2 (eBook)
https://doi.org/10.1007/978-981-96-9705-2

This Springer imprint is published by the registered company Springer Nature Singapore Pte Ltd.
The registered company address is: 152 Beach Road, #21-01/04 Gateway East, Singapore 189721, Singapore

Competing Interests The author has no competing interests to declare that are relevant to the content of this manuscript.

Contents

Chapter 1
Introduction

Social attitudes in the contemporary era are valuable and necessary for a better understanding through the analytical-functionalist framework (Parsons 1968; Munch 1987; J. Turner 2013). Such understanding means explaining, predicting, and evaluating social attitudes in a general person in the current world concerning their causes or predictors. This understanding is to clarify what influences and predicts social attitudes and why the influences and predictions occur, and as such, evaluate the goodness of social attitudes, notably their promotion or early intervention. Differentiating the influences and forecasts for China and the United States is crucial for the current bipolar world (Tunsjo 2018).

Social attitudes are a person's association of oneself with social objects (H. Cheng et al. 2012; Wegener and Carlston 2014). The association can be the maintenance of acceptance, confidence, favor, justification, or trust, whereas the objects can be intuitions, misdeeds, sexuality, religion, outsiders, deviants, and other people. These objects are socially relevant or visible, that is, among people or society. As such, social attitudes encompass confidence in institutions, justification for misdeeds, justification for unconventional sexuality, faith in religion, acceptance of outsiders, acceptance of deviants, and trust in other people. They are measurable or reportable worldwide, as exploited in World Values Surveys. Confidence in institutions includes confidence in banks, courts, television, government, and police. Such institutions are authoritative, longstanding, engaging, functional, and indispensable daily (Kozuch and Dobrowolski 2014). Justification for misdeeds includes justification for cheating, suicide, violence, and stealing. These misdeeds are prevalent and ineradicable among people (Vauclair and Fischer 2011). Justification for unconventional sexuality involves its components or concomitants in terms of abortion, divorce, and homosexuality. They are integral to life, notably its enjoyment and reproduction (Giddens 1992; Primoratz 1999). Faith in religion involves the church, religiosity, and the belief in hell. Religion provides axioms and ethics for life (Stavrova and Siegers 2014). Acceptance of outsiders includes accepting or liking foreign workers, people of a different religion, and people speaking a different language. Outsiders

C.-k. Cheung, *Social Attitudes in the Early 21st Century*,
https://doi.org/10.1007/978-981-96-9705-2_1

are common because of immigration, globalization, and multiculturalism (Jensen et al. 2017). Acceptance of deviants includes acceptance or liking of drug addicts, heavy drinkers, and people with acquired immunodeficiency syndrome (AIDS). Such deviants are common and lurking among people (Iacobucci and Frieh 2018; Patterson and Keefe 2008). Trust in other people includes trust in people who are known personally, of another religion, of another nationality and have met for the first time. These other people constitute members of contemporary society (Freitag and Bauer 2016; L. Cao et al. 2015).

Social attitudes are crucial because attitudes are functional (Aiken 2002; Kruglanski and Stroebe 2014; Riemer et al. 2014). The functions of attitude or associating oneself with an object include adjustment, appraisal, consistency, coping, defense, grouping, guidance, instrumentality, knowledge, self-expression, and uniqueness. Adjustment means meeting the demand from outside, notably the social environment. For instance, it represents acceptance of the social norm. Appraisal is necessary for taking further actions, such as approaching or avoiding. Consistency is the display of the basis for attitude on value (orientation). Coping is a reaction to a stimulus conditional on attitude. As such, the attitude steers the way of coping with the stimulus. Defense means defending, advertising, or externalizing the blame from oneself. It can involve blaming or scapegoating others with prejudice or a negative attitude. Moreover, acceptance of deviants can be defensive by presenting broad-mindedness. Grouping, affiliation, or association is viable for showing and sharing an attitude with others. Sharing the attitude defines comrades for commitment. Guidance means steps based on attitude toward behavior. These steps include behavioral intention or the conative component of attitude. Instrumentality or utilitarian function suggests that an attitude is helpful to secure an outcome. Herein, an attitude functions as an act to get a return. For instance, accepting and trusting others can invite others' acceptance and trust in return. Knowledge also rests on attitude. A positive attitude or trust in an object constitutes knowledge about its positive and more general properties. For example, trust in a person constitutes knowledge that the person has trustworthy properties. Self-expression means the use of attitude to express oneself. For instance, trust in others expresses kindness to people. Uniqueness means the use of attitude to anchor one's identity. For example, confidence in the national government manifests one's national identity. These various functions are better interpretable with the analytical-functionalist framework.

Analytical-Functionalist Framework

The analytical-functionalist framework identifies four key functions: goal attainment, adaptation, integration, and latency or pattern maintenance (Parsons 1968; Munch 1987). Goal attainment or fulfillment embraces the appraisal, coping, and guidance functions of attitude. Regarding attitude functions, goal attainment or fulfillment means setting or enabling the direction for further action or attitude. Adaptation subsumes attitude adjustment, defense, instrumentality, and knowledge functions.

Herein, adaptation means creating fitness with or benefits from the environment or others. Integration upholds the grouping function of attitude. Integration means learning from, conforming to, and affiliating with others. Latency or pattern maintenance involves attitude consistency, self-expression, and uniqueness functions. Herein, latency means maintaining personal consistency or identity.

The four functions of the analytical-functionalist framework set guidelines for understanding, including explanation, prediction, and evaluation. In addition to understanding the functions of social attitude for further action or attitude, understanding the causes or predictors of social attitude is viable through the framework. Accordingly, social attitudes function to fulfill the four requisite functions of goal attainment or fulfillment, adaptation, integration, and latency or pattern maintenance (Parsons 1968; Munch 1987). Function, in the first place, means that a part sustains the whole. That is, a function applies to a subsystem to uphold the whole system. For instance, organs function to maintain a person's entire body, and the education (sub)system functions to uphold society as a whole system. This is structural functionalism, which maintains the functions of structural parts to buttress the structural, enduring, constraining whole. The functions, in the beginning, originate from the crossing or interaction of two axes, intrinsic versus extrinsic and internal versus external functions. Intrinsic function means direct, consummatory value creation, whereas extrinsic function means indirect, instrumental value creation to create intrinsic value indirectly through extrinsic value. For instance, working can be intrinsically functional or valuable, and earning money can be an extrinsic function or value to satisfy an intrinsic need indirectly. Internal function means functional to the ingroup or oneself, whereas external function means functional interaction with others, outside, or the external environment. In other words, internal function represents harmony and consistency within, whereas external function indicates influence and acquisition from without. Crossing the two axes engenders the four functions of fulfillment, adaptation, integration, and latency. Specifically, fulfillment is applying an intrinsic function to the external environment. Adaptation is the application of an extrinsic function to an external environment. Integration is applying an intrinsic function to the internal environment. Latency is applying an extrinsic function to the internal environment.

With society as the whole system, the four functions identify four subsystems correspondingly. The subsystems are the political, legal, administrative, economic, communal, cultural, educational, or fiduciary, respectively, for the functions of fulfillment, adaptation, integration, and latency. These subsystems are essential objects in shaping social attitudes. As such, political and economic subsystems entail confidence in political and financial institutions, respectively. The communal subsystem concerns justification for misdeeds, justification for unconventional sexuality, acceptance of outsiders, acceptance of deviants, and trust in other people. Meanwhile, the cultural subsystem rests on faith in religion.

The latency function particularly sustains substantive, axiological, internal, intrinsic, or value (or value-based or oriented) rationality, as treasured in rationalism (Bolis et al. 2017; Rutgers and Schreurs 2006). Such rationality rests on values, which can prevail in society to constitute a culture, which in turn is adapted by the person through socialization and internalization (Reeskens and Vandecasteele 2017). Thus, substantive rationality means following cultural values to register the latency function for the cultural system of society. These cultural values can include altruism, ambition or achievement, democratism, dialecticism, dignity functionalism, hedonism, materialism, rationalism, relationalism, and traditionalism (Boudon 2008; de C. R. Araujo 2020; Diesing 1999; Maltseva 2016; Szakolczai and Fustos 1998). Notably, functionalism values perpetuating the whole system through goal attainment, adaptation, integration, and latency (de C. R. Araujo 2020). In other words, functionalism envisions the development of the structures of power, utility, norms, ideology, knowledge, or religion. Meanwhile, rationalism generally embraces logical thinking to achieve enlightenment (Szakolczai and Fustos 1998). Thinking to realize substantive rationality or accord with values is to fulfill rationalism. Particularly essential to the values or culture are ethical or moral values, which define what is right or wrong (R. Thomas 1997). Such values underlie moral principles whose application upholds deontological or formalist ethics (N. Duncan 2017; Rachels and Rachels 2015). Deontological ethics, values, or principles subsume the ethics of contracting, divine command, duty or obligation, natural law, and universalism (Darwall 2003; R. Hall et al. 2000). The ethics of contracting, contractualism, or contractarianism emphasizes that compliance with the social contract or contract made with society is ethical (Darwall 2003; de Jonge 2012). Such a contract can be hypothetical, based on rational consent, cooperation, and free choice. Natural law means the rules of the functioning of nature, including humanity (Darwall 2003). Meanwhile, universalism or universalistic ethics emphasizes the ethical good and right as universalizable, categorical, and imperative maxims to champion dignity and rationality (Boudon 2010; R. Hall et al. 2000). These values are criteria for evaluating social attitudes, considering the latency function.

As such, a function is analytical in terms of its four components requisite for any structural whole, which means the social environment to the person, the nation, or anything suprapersonal. To the person, personal factors function as voluntaristic factors to fulfill the four functions. Moreover, to the person, national, suprapersonal, or extrapersonal factors function as deterministic factors to fulfill the four functions. That is, the function works at two levels: personal or voluntaristic and extrapersonal or deterministic. The voluntaristic level means that personal experience underlies the function. In contrast, the deterministic level means that personal experience is not necessarily present, such that extrapersonal influence can occur without personal experience or free will.

At the voluntaristic level of analytical-functionalism, fulfilling the four functions operates with the four mechanisms of power realization, utility optimization, norm conformity, and ideal or idealistic consistency (Munch 1987). Power realization means realizing power, resources, strengths, goals, motivation, or dispositions to drive, steer, or set the direction. This mechanism is the fulfillment function of driving. It signifies that voluntaristic action or attitude ensues from power or planning for the action. The mechanism registers power, empowerment, conflict, (dialectical-) materialist, resource, capital (i.e., human, social, or cultural capital), need, drive, and personality explanations (Aiken 2002; DiMaggio 2015). Utility optimization holds utility or gain as the incentive to fulfill the adaptation function. At the personal or voluntaristic level, when something is gainful, gravitation toward the thing ensues. Thus, utility or gain is attractive to uphold gravitation. This mechanism reflects utilitarian or instrumental rationality, which rests on calculation to optimize the gain or benefit over cost (Bolis et al. 2017). This mechanism corresponds to exchange, rational (choice), rationalist, utilitarian, and functional (i.e., not functionalist) explanations (O'Keefe 2002; Wang and Liu 2019). Norm conformity incorporates learning, conforming, and assimilating with others or their norms. This mechanism is the assimilating mechanism to fulfill the function of integration. This mechanism accords with (social) learning, social-cognitive or sociocognitive, (social) norm, (social) comparison, and reference (group), and (symbolic or social) interactionist explanations (Aiken 2002; B. Johnson et al. 2014; Prislin and Wood 2014; Suls and Wheeler 2012). For instance, learning and persuasion are typical sources of social attitude (Prislin and Wood 2014). Ideal consistency builds on maintaining (cognitive or symbolic) consistency to generate the functional force. This mechanism fulfills the latency function by rationalizing to maintain cognitive consistency or suppress cognitive dissonance. Such rationalizing rests on substantive or value rationality to realize intrinsic value (Bolis et al. 2017). The rationalizing mechanism is consonant with (cognitive or symbolic) consistency or dissonance, (social) identity, (personal) constructivist, and phenomenological explanations (Aiken 2002; Fabrigar et al. 2014; Marsh and Wallace 2014; Read and Simon 2012; D. Simon et al. 2004). The mechanism finds its everyday use in holding faith in religion and endorsing ideology as causes or predictors of social attitude (Aiken 2002; Sears and Brown 2013).

At the deterministic level of analytical functionalism, personal function is fulfillable indirectly through extrapersonal influence on the person's voluntaristic level (J. Turner 2013). The latter means activating voluntaristic functioning through four deterministic mechanisms: empowering or coercing, incentivizing, normalizing or standardizing, and framing or signifying. That is, empowering external to the person increases power to facilitate power realization, or conversely, disempowering or restraining power to restrain power realization (Clark and Inglehart 1998; Peterson et al. 2005). The latter happens through domination, entrapping, or exploitation (Espelage et al. 2007; Winstock and Eisikovits 2003). Such happening derives from the conflict, materialist, or class perspective, which posits the dominance of structural force over personal consciousness and potential (Cheliotis and Xenukis 2017; Walsh 2014). Conversely, personal consciousness and potential benefit from empowerment or social support (Bystrov 2012; Shafir and LeBouef 2002). Typically, education, training, and institutional support are instances of empowerment (Stanton-Salazar 2011). Incentivizing means providing incentives from outside to induce personal attraction and gravitation to the gain according to the utility optimization mechanism (Haslam et al. 2011; N. Zhao 2008). Herein, the value of the incentive matters and the value increases or decreases with the scarcity or abundance of the incentive (Fennis and Stroebe 2016; Shao et al. 2021). Awards and punishment administered in society typically represent positive and negative incentivizing or reinforcements, respectively

(Bekkers 2010; Jaeger 2004; Kaplan et al. 2013). Normalizing or standardizing from outside refers to providing a norm or standard for the person to follow concerning the norm conformity mechanism (Leung and Koh 2018; Thomas and Lous 2013). The norm or standard builds on its popularity or moral prescriptiveness (Nakazato and Lim 2016; Skitka and Morgan 2014). Fads and ethics prevailing in society typically register norms (Freitas et al. 1997; Olsen et al. 2003). Framing or signifying refers to providing ideals, definitions, or meanings from outside (Fernandes-Jesus et al. 2020; Pineiro-Nval et al. 2018). The ideals, definitions, or meanings do not need to be normative, popular, or prescriptive to be distinguishable from norms. Such framing or signifying is influential through invoking the person's mechanism of ideal consistency to maintain consistency with the person's attitude and/or behavior. For instance, framing something as miserable instigates a kind person's mercy and helpfulness. Signifying or defining something as an illness raises concern for curing or avoidance. Framing or signifying is common in advertising and ritual, which describes the situations and procedures to follow (Coyne et al. 2018; Maryanski 2014).

The analytical-functionalist framework incorporates mechanisms in both voluntaristic and deterministic forms for understanding social attitudes. The mechanisms can combine for the understanding such that a social attitude can involve multiple mechanisms working jointly and complementarily. This combination is notable in the indirect path of deterministic mechanisms, which activate voluntaristic mechanisms to complete their functions. In addition, mechanisms can combine with more flexibility to fulfill their functions. For instance, the mechanisms of norm conformity and ideal consistency can combine in the function of learning to establish an attitude for maintaining consistency with another attitude. Moreover, an attitude favoring learning can facilitate learning through the ideal consistency mechanism to activate the norm conformity mechanism.

Understanding Social Attitudes

The seven social attitudes, defined as associations of oneself with social objects, are understandable with available empirical studies and data, notably those from the World Value Surveys. Each attitude is necessary for a better understanding because of its possible functions and controversies.

A better understanding of social attitudes is necessary because they are functional and/or dysfunctional in generating impacts on society or the social system. The functions and dysfunctions stem from the properties of social attitude as mental fuel to propel social action and, thus, impact. A social attitude represents an evaluation, knowledge, or even self-reported behavior regarding a social object (Aiken 2002; Fabrigar et al. 2014; Kaiser and Byrka 2015). This representation corresponds to the tripartite nature of attitude's affective, cognitive, and conative components. In its positive sense, the attitude is representable with favor or favorableness (Wyer and Abbarracin 2014). Moreover, more nuanced manifestations of attitude include acceptance, confidence, justification, and trust. Acceptance of something denotes being close to something. Confidence in something implies that something is functioning well. Justification for something means holding something right. Trust indicates an expectation that something is beneficial. Acceptance, confidence, favor, justification, and trust thus represent associations of oneself with a social object, including institutions, misdeeds, sexuality, religion, outsiders, deviants, and other people to constitute social attitudes. The functions of a social attitude then depend on the coupling of the association and social object. When the association is positive in valence, the functions hinge on the associated object. An object can be functional or dysfunctional for goal attainment, adaptation, integration, and latency or their corresponding political, economic, communal, and cultural subsystems, respectively. Whereas functional objects are strengthening, gainful, solidifying, and perpetuating, dysfunctional objects are weakening, depriving, dividing, and disrupting.

In the analytical-functionalist framework, the seven socially attitudinal objects perform social functions for fulfillment or goal attainment, adaptation, latency, and integration. Specifically, institutions generate power for fulfillment, goal attainment, or structuring. Misdeeds, misbehavior, or deviant behavior and sexuality perform adaptation to reap utility or disutility. Religion feeds ideals to sustain latency or pattern maintenance. Other people furnish the norm for integration, whereas deviants and outsiders represent anomalies for disintegration. Disutility and disintegration are dysfunctions, the flip side of function.

Confidence in Institutions

Confidence in institutions involves confidence in government, courts, banks, armed forces, and others. Herein, an institution means a stable and valuable establishment (Fountain 2009; Lista and Rojas 2018). An institution functions to set rules and norms and provide incentives (Mantzvavinos 2011). An institution delivers instrumental and ceremonial functions (Ziegler 1994). Instrumental functions enhance competence, courage, creativity, curiosity, experience, experimenting, forward-looking, imagination, innovativeness, potentiality, skill, and synthesizing. Ceremonial functions establish the equilibrium, face, stability, and status according to people's age, gender, nationality, and wealth. More specifically, institutional functions embrace administration, communication, education, nurturing, procreation, replenishment, policy-making, problem-solving, socialization, and support. According to the analytical-functionalist framework, the functions encompass goal attainment, such as policy-making; adaptation, such as problem-solving; integration, such as socialization; and latency, such as education. The instrumental functions represent the adaptation function, whereas the ceremonial functions integrate goal attainment, integration, and latency functions. As such, an institution functions to develop people's strengths or virtues. An institution is functional through voluntaristic rather than coercive mechanisms (Ziegler 1994). Nevertheless, an institution needs to establish its authority to dictate absolute truth and provide guidance hierarchically, thus fulfilling the conservation or latency function (Ziegler 1994). This function is the exercise of the framing or signifying mechanism at the deterministic level to facilitate ideal consistency at the voluntaristic level. Herein, an institution identifies an elite and creates a community (Ziegler 1994). In addition, an institution functions to satisfy people's desires and wants (Ziegler 1994). The good performance of the functions keeps an institution surviving in competition and struggle (Ziegler 1994). Nonetheless, all the political, economic, communal, and cultural institutions exercise similar or common functions, such that people are similarly confident in all of them, according to factor analysis.

Confidence in institutions reflects a judgment that institutions perform well. Such confidence also reflects a person's civic engagement, commitment, and consciousness (Kozuch and Dobrowolski 2014). Such confidence maintains an action orientation (Kozuch and Dobrowolski 2014). This maintenance registers the instrumental of the adaptation function of confidence.

Confidence in institutions is worth studying because it is a basis for such social
Confidence in institutions is worth studying because it is a basis for such social
functioning as civil society, democracy, institutional legitimacy, social capital, social justice, and social solidarity (Grimes 2006; Habibov 2014; Kozuch and Dobrowolski 2014; Marozzi 2015; Newton 2006; Paxton 1999). Civil society checks the state, integrated, mutualistic, protective, responsible, solidary, and characterized by the functioning of non-governmental organizations (Alexander 1997; Howell 2012; Powell 2007; Wnuk-Lipinski 2007). It is functional for democracy and socialization (Alexander 1997; Wnuk-Lipinski 2007). Civil society is thus a functionalist requisite (Alexander 1997). Meanwhile, democracy is a way to let the masses check and legitimize authority and its functions (Warren 2011). As such, democracy features popular and equal compromise, information sharing, inclusiveness, and participation (Fairfield 2008; Moller and Skaaning 2013; Saward 1998). Democracy as a form of operation is treasurable because it is adaptive, delightful, developmental, empowering, honoring people's agency, including consciousness, intentionality, and volition, and integrative (Fairfield 2008; Saward 1998). These represent the function of adaptation, integration, and latency in fulfilling people's nature and the political function of goal attainment. Institutional legitimacy means the acceptability of the institution (Gilley 2009; Holbig 2011). It is conducive to institutional efficiency (Tyler 2006). Thus, institutional legitimacy buttresses the adaptation function. Social capital means resources accessible through social relations (Flap and Volker 2013; Woolcock 1998). It underlies democracy, productivity, providing public goods, and social control (Aldridge and Halpern 2002; Coleman 1988; Holliday and Tam 2001; Woolcock and Narayan 2000). As such, social capital fulfills adaptation and integration functions. Social justice means justice found in society, including relationships among people and institutions (Campbell 2010). Justice, in turn, upholds institutional legitimacy and people's satisfaction (Campbell 2010; Tornblom and Vermunt 2007). Hence, social justice realizes integration and adaptation functions in securing norms and gains, respectively. Social solidarity means a good relationship within society, including affiliation with, attachment to, attraction to, belonging to, commitment to, cooperation with, contribution to, harmony with, identification with, inclusiveness in, mutuality in, responsibility to, sharing within, and trust within society (Dench 2006; Dickes et al. 2010; Gaffikin and Morriessey 2011; Helly 2003; Lawler and

Thye 2006; McGhee 2003; Miranti and Evans 2019; Wilson et al. 2018). Solidarity is conducive to economic growth, freedom, political stability, protection and safety, social capital, and social justice (Berger-Schmitt 2002; Dayton-Johnson 2003; Helly 2003; Hulse and Stone 2007; Lawler et al. 2009; Maloutas and Malouta 2004). Moreover, social solidarity facilitates socialization and social interaction according to the functionalist perspective (Karuppannan and Sivam 2011). Hence, social solidarity contributes to the functions of adaptation and integration.

Confidence in institutions is an evaluative issue for empirical investigation. The problem emerges from the contradiction between supporting and opposing values or ideologies. Supporting ideologies include communitarianism and liberalism, whereas opposing ideologies include anarchism and libertarianism (Etzioni 1996; Friedman 2011; Miller and Dagger 2003; Newey 2001). Communitarianism holds that institutions merit people's confidence and support for achieving the valuable collective good, fellowship, love, piety, and solidarity (Khatchadourian 1999; Selznick 2002). As such, institutions can secure the communitarian values of mutuality, responsibility, and solidarity (Frazer 1999). Meanwhile, communitarianism regards institutions as natural to realize people's solidarity, trust, and virtues (Etzioni 1996; Frazer 1999). Conversely, communitarianism reasons that the individual is precarious and needs to learn from institutions (Selznick 2002). Alternatively, liberalism supports institutions as building blocks of civil society (Newey 2001). The ideology also honors institutions for maintaining justice, pluralism, and rationality (Newey 2001). By contrast, anarchism prefers autonomy, thus detesting institutional constraints (Miller and Dagger 2003). Anarchism presupposes that people are capable to manage and serve themselves. Libertarianism also disfavors institutions with its preference for dignity, entitlement or ownership, liberty, and separateness of people (Friedman 2011).

Confidence in institutions, meanwhile, requires more understanding to sustain their functions (Lee-Treweek 2002). Herein, the confidence is declining and needs restoring or advancing (Marozzi 2015). The decline can signal a crisis (D. Kong 2014). The understanding is also necessary as the confidence is not unambiguously favorable. An instance of this confidence suggests that people passively rely on institutions rather than demonstrating their agency (Lee-Treweek 2002). This suggestion forges a social trap regarding people's dependency on institutions (Gilson 2003; Richey and Ikeda 2009). Worse consequences are institutional abuse, corruption, and exploitation (Gilson 2003; Richey and Ikeda 2009). These instances indicate that confidence in institutions is counterproductive to the functions of adaptation, integration, and latency regarding economic, interpersonal, and personal benefits, respectively. Moreover, confidence is situational and unstable (Kozuch and Dobrowolski 2014).

Justification for Misdeeds

Justification for misdeeds involves approval of wrongdoings such as cheating, fraud, stealing, suicide, and violence. The misdeeds cover illegal and unethical ones, such as crimes and vices, respectively. Alternatively, they signify antisocial, deviant, problem behavior, or conduct disorder (Vauclair and Fischer 2011; Waiton 2008; Weiner 2012). As revealed in factor analysis, these misdeeds are indistinguishable from people who justify them uniformly. That is, a person tends to justify all the misdeeds consistently. As such, misdeeds commonly breach rules, are punishable and are socially harmful (Costello 2013; Warr 2002; Wikstrom 2010).

Misdeeds are dysfunctional or impair the functions of goal attainment, adaptation, integration, and latency. In failing the function of goal attainment, misdeeds breach rules, defy control, generate cynicism, and impede compliance and obedience (Pulkkinen et al. 2009; Wikstrom 2010; Waiton 2008; Warr 2002). Misdeeds undermine social control or order (de Castro-Rodrigues and Sacau 2015). Misdeeds also jeopardize the function of adaptation by destroying property, fomenting discomfort and panic, and harming lives (Hoffman 2003; Kennedy et al. 1998; Waiton 2008). That is, misdeeds are costly (Piquero et al. 2013). In undermining the integration function, misdeeds are antisocial, isolating or separating from others, violating social norms, learning, and love, and asserting selfishness (Daneygier and Green 2010; Farrington 2010; Jones 2016; Pulkkinen et al. 2009). Thus, misdeeds mean the impairment of the community (Waiton 2008). Moreover, deviation from social norms is undesirable (de Motte and Gabriella 2019). Misdeeds impair the latency function by subverting ethics or morals, responsibilities, and socialization (Pulkkinen et al. 2009; Waiton 2008). They represent harm to morality or its conservation (Waiton 2008).

Suicide is also a social misdeed, not only harming or killing oneself. Like other misdeeds, suicide undermines the requisite social functions. Suicide jeopardizes the function of goal attainment by defying the authority, forbidding suicide, thus abandoning duties to the authority and raising oneself above the authority (Lewis 2001; W. Siu 2008). Therefore, suicide means the undermining of political order (Lewis 2001). Suicide undercuts the adaptation function by ending life and its contribution and production (Lewis 2001). It is thereby costly to society (Feldman 2006). Suicide ruins the integration function by removing oneself from the community (Brandt 1992). This removal registers a blow to social solidarity (Lewis 2001). Suicide impairs the latency function for adherence to the ethics of personal dignity, self-love and self-perpetuation, and character building for courage, endurance, patience, and tolerance (Cosculluela 1995; Lewis 2001). This impairment is antithetical to culture and religion (Brandt 1992).

Justification for misdeeds is problematic as it represents one's dehumanization, incivility, and problems in socialization (Douglas 2006; Matthews and Channon 2016; Montgomery et al. 2004). Dehumanization indicates treating the person as an object and discounting dignity in the person (Foy et al. 2014; Zurbriggen 2013). Incivility violates normative or virtuous character (Boyd 2006; P. Smith 2002). These indicate the harm of the justification to the functions of integration and latency in maintaining norms and ethics. Furthermore, the justification reflects resistance to social control or order (Javakhishvili and Jibladze 2018). This resistance violates the function of goal attainment in preserving authority and command.

Misdeeds and their justification can be controversial, considering divergent views predicated on ethical or other social values. Values or ideologies wronging misdeeds include communitarianism, conservatism, and securitization, while skepticism about the wronging arises from social constructionism, nominalism, and postmodernism. Communitarianism rejects misdeeds for their undermining of the community, even if they gratify actors' interests (Waiton 2008). Conservatism favors morality to stabilize society, thus denouncing misdeeds deviating from morality (Waiton 2008). The ideology or discourse of securitization treasures national security and, therefore, seeks to eradicate misdeeds disturbing the security (Runhovde 2017). By contrast, social constructionism casts doubt on the wrongness of misdeeds because misdeeds result from social construction or definition (Waiton 2008; Walsh 2014). Social constructionism indicates that misdeeds are not factual and thus not awful or harmful. Similarly, nominalism regards misdeeds as labels arbitrarily named or defined (Walsh 2014). This suspicious view also inheres in postmodernism, which emphasizes mediation by language, especially from the rich or powerful (Walsh 2014).

Justification for Unconventional Sexuality

Justification for unconventional sexuality, including homosexuality, or its concomitant issues of abortion, divorce, and premarital sex, is a controversial issue for better understanding. Justifications for abortion, divorce, homosexuality, and premarital sex represent a consistent social attitude because of the common sexual root. Notably, sexuality is a necessary condition for abortion, clearly present in homosexuality and premarital sex, and highly germane to divorce (Brines and Joyner 1999; Major et al. 2009). Abortion particularly means sexuality without childbirth and childrearing for the woman. Because of their everyday basis on sexuality, the justifications consistently happen in a person, according to factor analysis.

Sexuality facilitates such social functioning as engagement, love, marriage, passion, pleasure-seeking, romance, procreation, and realizing the sexual desire for people and, thus, society (Belliotti 1993; Conde Dias et al. 2012; Primoratz 1999; Shrage 1994). Hence, sexuality fulfills the functions of integration in building social relationships, adaptation to secure pleasure, latency to sustain the culture or society, and goal attainment to realize sexual desire. The woman's choice of abortion, particularly, is functional to upholding autonomy, feminism, freedom, liberalism, individualism, and relief of victimhood (Anitha and Gill 2018; Beynon-Jones 2017; Feltham-King and Macleod 2016; E. Lee 2017). Herein, autonomy is favorable according to universalistic ethics, which holds that autonomy is a universalizable good (Fagot-Largeault 2008). Feminism valorizes women's choices, goodness, rights, and self-determination to eliminate male oppression (Anitha and Gill 2018; Feltham-King and Macleod 2016). In support of abortion, liberalism assumes no conflict between the woman and others to constrain the woman's choice (Beynon-Jones 2017). That is, the woman as an individual can live independently from others. Victimhood, which means constraining or disturbing the woman with pregnancy, motherhood, and even raping, is removable by abortion (Feltham-King and Macleod 2016). As such, abortion is conducive to achieving the functions of adaptation to gain and latency to realize cultural values. Similarly, divorce is functional to individualization or individualism, which favors such personal performance as achievement, agency, autonomy, choice, emancipation, eroticism, gratification, independence, liberty, self-determination, and singleness (Bauman 2001; Beck and Beck-Gernsheim 2002; Krys et al. 2019; Krys et al. 2019; Yang and Yen 2012). Individualism stands on humanism, which holds that the person is capable independently and individually (Welzel 2013). As such, divorce champions the function of latency in promoting the individualized culture. In addition, homosexuality is functional in eliminating oppression, liberation, realizing autonomy, dignity, essentialism, human rights, individualism, liberalism, pluralism, romanticism, self-determination, recreation, and showing love (Ball 2003; Corvino 2008; Smith and Windes 2000). The functions rest on the premise that homosexuality is under control, oppression, and unfair treatment. Particularly, essentialism holds that homosexuality is ubiquitous and unchangeable, thus in need of normalization (Smith and Windes 2000; E. Stein 1999). Romanticism treasures ecstasy, equality, free expression, innovation, and wonder (TenHouten 2017). Romanticism is valuable in gratifying human desires and instincts (TenHouten 2017). Meanwhile, pluralism valorizes diversity, liberty, receptiveness, tolerance, and tradeoffs (Connolly 2005; Galston 2005). Homosexuality embodies cultural values countering oppression. This function means the achievement of the functions of adaptation and latency. In all, justification for unconventional sexuality reflects the cultural values of feminism, individualism, liberalism, pluralism, and romanticism.

Justification for unconventional sexuality, including homosexuality, is exceptionally functional to liberation and upholding feminism and queer theory (Kirsch 2000; Tsang and Ho 2007). Feminism maintains that the deprivation of women's sexuality by patriarchy makes women's sexual liberation justifiable (Tsang and Ho 2007). Queer theory emphasizes individuality, performativity, relativity, oneself, and self-expression, and downplays, deconstructs, or rejects the community, hegemony, identity, roles, and tradition regarding sexuality (Kirsch 2000). Hence, the justification fulfills the functions of adaptation and latency regarding women and the ideologies. In addition, justification for abortion is exceptionally functional to the maintenance of feminism and liberalism (Prusaczyk and Hodson 2018; Singer 2001). These ideologies prize women's rights, independence, and tolerance. Meanwhile, justification for homosexuality is functional in removing discrimination or unfairness, sexual revolution, social change, and upholding feminism (de la Ossa 2016; Gerhards 2010; Y. Hu 2016; Macmillan and Baiocchi 2010). According to feminism, homosexuality erases exploitation and violence in heterosexuality (de la Ossa 2016). Hence, justification for homosexuality fulfills the function of adaptation in improving society, particularly its female members' lives.

However, sexuality, in terms of abortion, divorce, homosexuality, and premarital sex, and its justification are nevertheless controversial. Such controversy arises from ideologies discouraging or regulating sexuality, such as Christianity, Confucianism, naturalism or natural law ethics, paternalism, socialism, and stoicism (Belliotti 1993; Primoratz 1999; Shim 2001). Christianity avers that sexuality needs to be fruitful, heterosexual, and monogamous for procreation (Primoratz 1999). Moreover, the Catholic Church of Christianity requires celibacy for priests. Similarly, Confucianism treasures female chastity and obedience and rejects feminism (Shim 2001). Naturalism or natural law ethics also prizes celibacy, love, and procreation and rejects fetishism, homosexuality, and libertinism (Belliotti 1993; Primoratz 1999). This ideology emphasizes the potency and pervasive influence of nature and thus abidance by its law (Hocksmann 2004; Moeller 2004). Paternalism argues for the need for protection from sexual risk and, as such, disapproves of choice and consent (Primoratz 1999). Socialism particularly faults the grounds of sexuality on capitalism or commodification for fabricating alienation and inequality (Belliotti 1993; Primoratz 1999). Stoicism valorizes asceticism and self-discipline instead of passion, characterizing sexuality (Belliotti 1993; Primoratz 1999). This contrast stems from stoic beliefs in rationality and self-containment (Holowchak 2008).

In addition, discourses against abortion refer to the fetal gift, life, and rights, physical and psychological harm and safety, post-abortion syndrome, and paternalism or protection (Eklund and Purewal 2017; Leask 2013; Pierson 2017; Saurette and Gordon 2013; Shrage 1994). Accordingly, abortion is harmful and dangerous to the woman, not to mention the fetus. Similarly, divorce is unjustifiable in Christianity as defying God's design (Hobbs 2020).

Likewise, discourses or ideologies against homosexuality are Christianity, communitarianism, conservatism, fundamentalism, hygiene, majoritarianism, natural law ethics, protection, socialism, and traditionalism (Ball 2003; Carlstrom 2020; Larsen 2015; Mole 2011; Robinson 2018; Smith and Windes 2000; Wong and Leung 2012). Accordingly, Christianity or particularly its Catholic Church, prizes heterosexuality or heteronormativity, naturalness, procreation, and the traditional family (Carlstrom 2020; Mole 2011; Norris 2001; Smith and Windes 2000). Christianity rests on faith in the divine (Jones and Yarhouse 2000). Communitarianism rejects feminism and its belief in the heterosexual oppression of women (Ball 2003). Instead, communitarianism favors cooperation as opposed to homosexual seclusion—similarly, conservatism treasures heterosexuality, normalcy, and procreation as opposed to hedonism (Ball 2003). Meanwhile, fundamentalism upholds social order, stability, and the traditional family (Smith and Windes 2000). This ideology holds a conviction in divine definition. Majoritarian discourse prefers the majority norm at the expense of the homosexual minority (Ball 2003). Natural law ethics also favors natural communion and procreation (Corvino 2008). Socialism opposes individualism underlying homosexuality (Mole 2011). Traditionalism treasures civilization, social order, and the traditional community and family, as opposed to freedom and hedonism (Smith and Windes 2000). This ideology presupposes homosexuality as a choice.

Controversy remains, considering discourses or ideologies justifying sexuality. They are contractualism, essentialism, feminism, hedonism, liberalism, libertarianism, queer theory, rights, romanticism, and social constructionism (Ball 2003; Belliotti 1993; Conde Dias et al. 2012; Kitzinger and Wilkinson 1995; Nixon 2008; Rodriguez 2013; Shrage 1994). Notably, contractualism or contractarianism accepts agreement, autonomy, consent, freedom, and negotiation in sexuality (Ball 2003; Belliotti 1993). Social constructionism maintains that heterosexuality is a social construction by the powerful and is thus reversible (Ball 2003; Kitzinger and Wilkinson 1995). Such a contradiction of discourses or ideologies necessitates an empirical investigation to evaluate the axiological basis for the justification of unconventional sexuality.

Faith in Religion

Faith in religions is prevalent and functional, thus worth better understanding. Such faith covers belief in hell, confidence in churches, and regarding oneself as a religious person. Religion is an established and shared way to define the divine (McDowell and Brown 2009). This faith is vital because it is axiomatic, ethical, ingrained, and practicable (Gay and Lynxwiler 2009; Stavrova and Siegers 2014; Wuthnow 2011). Such vitality magnifies the functions of the favor for acquiring meanings, affiliating, building character, disciplining, flourishing, and moralizing (Demerath 2002; Levin and Chatters 1998; Medvedovski and Allison 2017). These functions correspond to adaptation in acquiring utility, integration with people, and latency in perpetuating the culture. Specifically, the favor has contributed to the practices of civic activism, engagement, and participation, cohesion, compliance, coping, donation, forgiving, health behavior, political participation, prosocial behavior, protection of the environment, volunteering, and voting (Bekkers et al. 2008; Claassen and Povtak 2010; Fridberg and Kangas 2008b; Kim and Wilcox 2013; Marien and Hooghe 2001; Myers 2008; Norris 2002; Phalet et al. 2010; Ravanera et al. 2003; Saroglou and Anciaux 2004; Sherkat and Ellison 2007; Taniguichi and Thomas 2011; Wuthnow 2004), They represent contributions to or functions for society, including its administrative and communal subsystems. Conversely, the favor has dampened the practices of consumption or wastage, crime or deviant behavior, doping, gambling, protest, sexual behavior, and suicide (Andrews et al. 2015; Duberstein et al. 2004; Guo et al. 2008; Hatch 2007; Katz-Gerro and Shavit 1998; Skerkat and Ellison 1999; van de Werfhorst and Kraaykamp 2001), Such dampening is also functional to sustain the community, economy, and polity in society, as well as oneself. Similarly, religion also is functional in moralizing and organizing (McDowell and Brown 2009). It has been conducive to class consciousness, collectivism, fertility, and punishment, such as the death sentence in society (Abercrombie et al. 1980; Cotter et al. 1998; Jacobs and

Carmichael 2004; Realo et al. 2008). These influences demonstrate the integration function of faith in religion to maintain social norms, order, and longevity.

Particularly, faith in religion has contributed to the latency function by sustaining such cultural characteristics as authoritarianism, civility, conservatism, egalitarianism, familism, hawkishness, moralism, patriotism, pronatalism, racism, radicalism, and traditionalism (Diez-Nicolas 2002; D. Hall et al. 2010; Hooghe 2003; Ishio 2010; Jones and Brayfield 1997; Jost 2020; Keyes 2002; Kim and Wilcox 2013; Pedahzur and Canetti-Nisim 2004; Saunders and Wong 2012). In other words, the favor has buttressed support for or valuation of authority, equality, family, fertility, good manners, morality, militancy, nation, racial discrimination, radical action, and tradition. By contrast, the favor has weakened such cultural characteristics as hedonism, humanitarianism, individualism, leftism, liberalism, materialism, and postmaterialism (Barker and Tinnick 2006; Coffe and Geys 2007; Devos et al. 2002; Dy-Liacco et al. 2009; Flouri 2003; Gill 2004; Jou 2011). The faith has resisted fun-seeking, independence, kindness, liberty, redistribution of public resources, and both material and nonmaterial life, such as democracy and environmental protection.

Faith in religion is justifiable with cultural values and ideologies, showing its latency function of perpetuating the culture. In the first place, faith represents a functional requisite for latency or cultural maintenance, known as absorption (Haddorff 2000). Society requires faith to function, as religion is a structural part of society. More specifically, religion or its faith is functional in defining beauty (i.e., aestheticization), enlightening or promoting (religious) rationality, healing, moralizing, promoting solidarity, regulating, relaxing, and sustaining a community (i.e., communitarization) (Grayling 2013; Marks 2004; von Stuckrad 2013). These functions strengthen adaptation and integration, as well as latency in society. Moreover, faith strengthens people's existentialist values of affirmation of others, identity with others, love, meaning, awe, humility, reverence, surrendering, and wonder (Friedman 1992). The faith also sustains institutionalized individualism, such as Protestantism, which prizes choice, liberalism, and tradeoffs (Turner 2009).

However, faith in religion is questionable according to other discourses or ideologies, including behaviorism, humanism, materialism, psychoanalysis, and socialism (Ager and Ager 2011; Browning and Cooper 2004; Grayling 2013). Behaviorism holds that faith is unrealistic and thus unnecessary, as reinforcement from outside is decisive in people (Browning and Cooper 2004). Religious reward rather than faith is consequential and researchable in behaviorism. By denouncing the afterlife, myth, ritual, and Satanic threat, humanism demeans religious faith (Grayling 2013). Instead, humanism extols autonomy, curiosity, intelligence, reality, responsibility, and reasoning (Grayling 2013). Humanism also engages Confucianism and stoicism, emphasizing self-control and self-cultivation to oppose religion (Grayling 2013). Materialism downplays a spirit, such as religion and faith (Ager and Ager 2011). Psychoanalysis regards faith as an obsession and, thus, a psychic illness (Myers 2014). According to socialism, religion dominates and diverts one from working, which is valuable in socialism (Browning and Cooper 2004; Hjelm 2014). Thus, the value bases for the faith need empirical clarification.

Acceptance of Outsiders

Acceptance of outsiders, including immigrants and people of different races, religions, and languages, becomes a prominent issue (Young et al. 2019). This issue involves affirmative action or preferential treatment of underprivileged people, dehumanization, ethnocentrism, Islamophobia, multiculturalism, neophobia, racism, stereotyping, and xenophobia (Bobo and Massagli 2001; Dixon et al. 2010; Dunn et al. 2004; Falomir-Pichastor et al. 2013; H. Kim et al. 2016; Leong and Ward 2006; Meuleman et al. 2019; Pantti et al. 2019; Thornhill and Fincher 2014). There are issues regarding whether the acceptance is counterproductive to cohesion, freedom, and integration (Chiang 2010; Jensen et al. 2017). These issues imply a question of whether the acceptance fulfills or undermines the function of integration.

Acceptance of outsiders has demonstrated its function in reducing violence (Korostelina 2008). This reduction fulfills the integration function. In addition, the acceptance is justifiable with its ideological manifestations of civic virtue or civicism, emancipation, hospitality, liberalism, multiculturalism, neoliberalism, pluralism, and tolerance (Burchianti and Zapata-Barrero 2014; Capdevila and Callaghan 2007; Gotsbachner 2001; S. Kim 2012; Nishi et al. 2015; Zienkowski 2017). Similarly, discourse about protection and security for immigrants emphasizes providing them with social welfare (Rochel 2018). For the acceptance of immigrants particularly, supportive discourses are those about denaturalizing (i.e., not naturalizing immigrants), humanitarianism, neoliberalism, and universalism to denounce discrimination and prejudice against immigrants (Andreouli and Figgou 2019; Van Hootegem et al. 2000) These ideologies converge to underlie equal treatment, liberty, rationality, sympathy, tolerance, and thus acceptance of outsiders. This convergence registers the function of acceptance to realize latency or perpetuate cultural values.

However, acceptance of outsiders or immigrants, particularly, has also appeared to be dysfunctional. Notably, the acceptance has diminished cohesion, patriotism, and solidarity (Granzin and Olsen 1998; Wang and Chen 2004). This diminishment undercuts the function of integration. The acceptance is also justifiable with discourses about blame on outsiders' deviance, divisiveness, poverty, and terrorism, culturalism about outsiders' backwardness, government limitedness in subsisting outsiders, homogeneity, individualism to serve oneself, natives' superiority, nationalism and patriotism to maintain loyalty to the nation, and victimhood or victimization by outsiders (Banks and Valentino 2012; Blum 2008; Zienkowski 2017; Feinberg et al. 2012; Gotsbachner 2001; Hagren 2019; Zienkowski 2017). These discourses regard outsiders as undermining the functions of adaptation about harm, integration, and latency or cultural maintenance. In addition, some discriminatory discourses regard immigrants as anarchists, burdensome, criminals, dangerous, different, invaders, non-citizens or non-nationals, not morally obliged, stressful, terrorists, threatening, and violent (Del-Teso-Craviotto 2009; Jaworsky 2014; Kadianaki et al. 2018; Lopez-Sanders and Brown 2020; Park and Bhuyan 2012). The ideologies of nativism, patriotism, populism about citizens' say, and welfare chauvinism to minimize social welfare also oppose immigrants (Bloch 2016; Bloch et al. 2020; Krzyzanowski 2020). These discourses and ideologies indicate that immigrants subvert the functions of integration and latency to preserve some cultural values. Likewise, acceptance of immigrants is problematic, according to discourses or ideologies concerning conservatism about social integrity, essentialism about immigrants' unchangeability, populism or natives' rights, and securitization or safety (Andreouli and Figgou 2019; Davies 2009; Paterson 2018; Van Hootegem et al. 2000). As such, these discourses regard immigrants as a threat, vermin, and swarms. As such, these discourses or ideologies find accepting immigrants deleterious to the functions of adaptation, integration, and latency. These contradictory views necessitate the empirical evaluation of the acceptance of outsiders.

Acceptance of Deviants

Acceptance of deviants, including drug addicts, heavy drinkers, homosexuals, people with AIDS, and unmarried couples, as neighbors is a prominent concern. The acceptance reflects approval, tolerance, and inclusion of deviants (Coffe and Geys 2007; Eibach et al. 2009). Liberal democracy is a primary reason justifying the acceptance (Verkuyten and Yogeeswaran 2017). That is, the acceptance fulfills the political function of goal attainment for realizing liberal democracy. Such acceptance also reflects the values of diversity, nonjudgment, openness, and self-restraint (Verkuyten and Yogeeswaran 2017). This endorses the latency function for upholding such cultural values.

Acceptance of deviants, including drug addicts, heavy drinkers, homosexuals, people with AIDS, and unmarried couples, as neighbors is a prominent concern. The acceptance reflects approval, tolerance, and inclusion of deviants (Coffe and Geys 2007; Eibach et al. 2009). Liberal democracy is the primary reason for acceptance (Verkuyten and Yogeeswaran 2017). That is, acceptance fulfills the political function of attaining the goal of liberal democracy. Such acceptance reflects diversity, nonjudgment, openness, and self-restraint (Verkuyten and Yogeeswaran 2017). This reflection endorses the latency function for upholding such cultural values.

Acceptance of deviants is justifiable with discourses about equality, liberalism, and moralism, such as maintaining harmony, reciprocity, republicanism, and rights (Verkuyten and Yogeeswaran 2017). Notably, discourse about reciprocity anticipates that acceptance of deviants earns their acceptance in return. The discourses refer to some cultural values that the acceptance upholds. Herein, republicanism emphasizes adaptation, citizenship, the common good and value, enlightenment, equality, interdependence, publicity, responsibility, and solidarity instead of coercion, domination, interference, and subordination (Delanty 2009; Honohan 2002). Meanwhile, deviants are acceptable according to discourses about evolution, morality emphasizing caring and respect, normalization, and work such that they can cooperate, reciprocate, become normalized, and work well, respectively (Gazso 2020; Iacobucci and Frieh 2018; Vauclair and Fischer 2011). Herein, the value of cooperation is central to the discourse on evolution (Vauclair and Fischer 2011). Moreover, deviants are acceptable according to discourse against objectification or treating people as objects (Vauclair and Fischer 2011). These discourses reflect the cultural values of cooperation, dignity, education, rehabilitation, and work or production. Acceptance of deviants contributes to the latency function in upholding values.

However, accepting deviants is unjustifiable, especially with discourses or ideologies about culturalism, cultural superiority, and harm or offense (Verkuyten and Yogeeswaran 2017). As such, acceptance contradicts cultural values that favor culture and safety, and thus, the latency function is to uphold the culture. Moreover, accepting deviants has fomented protest and, thus, social disturbance (Lodewijkx et al. 2008). This fomenting undermines the function of integration to maintain social harmony. In addition, deviants are unacceptable according to discourses about discipline, fairness or justice in universalism, and self-control emphasized in neoliberalism (Iacobucci and Frieh 2018; Vauclair and Fischer 2011). These discourses contend that deviants deserve discipline and rejection for the values of fairness, responsibility, and universalism. As such, the acceptance contradicts the function of latency in sustaining these cultural values. Because of the antagonistic views, empirical evaluation of the acceptance is necessary.

Trust in Other People

Trust in other people, or social trust, involves trust in acquaintances, strangers, neighbors, and people of different nationalities and religions. Such trust reflects understanding people and social resources or capital (Paraskevopoulos 2010; B. Six 2014; Sundquist and Yang 2007). This reflection suggests the adaptation function of social trust in generating benefits. Meanwhile, social trust has contributed to donation, involvement, and volunteering (Uslaner 2000). This contribution affirms the integration function as well as the adaptation function of social trust. Furthermore, social trust sustains such social functioning as collectivity, cooperation, democracy, emancipation, exploration, fraternity, maturity, morality, organization, reciprocation, security, social order, and transaction (K. Brown et al. 2014; Falkenberg 1998; Fine and Holyfield 1996; Newton 1999; Olivera 2015; Pretsch and Ehrhardt-Madapathi 2018; Rahn 2008; B. Six 2014; Yamagishi et al. 1999). Accordingly, social trust fosters and reflects social connection, cooperation, coordination, exchange with people, mutual help, order, and security to emancipate oneself for exploration. Notably, trust in others is a precursor to maturity in living with others (K. Brown et al. 2014). They thus fulfill the adaptation function, generating benefits and integration and achieving social harmony. Social trust is further justifiable according to the ideologies of communitarianism, egalitarianism, and socialism, which emphasize community, equality, and social control, respectively (Abascal 2015; K. Brown et al. 2014; Volker and Flap 1997). As such, social trust embodies the function of latency in maintaining cultural values.

However, social trust is at odds with discourses or ideologies about individualization or individualism, risks of victimization, and social trapping or dependency

(Rothstein and Eek 2009; Taylor-Gooby 2005; van Swol 2003). These discourses or ideologies favor individualism or independence to develop a self-culture as opposed to victimization by others. Social trust thereby fails to accommodate the function of latency in maintaining the self-culture. The contradictory discourses about social trust necessitate its empirical evaluation.

Predicting Social Attitudes

Prediction of social attitudes is necessary to understand their causes or functional and/or dysfunctional bases for early intervention. Thus, such understanding includes explaining, predicting, intervening, and evaluating social attitudes. The evaluation concerns whether a social attitude results from a functional predictor, such as health, or a dysfunctional predictor, such as victimization. When the attitude results from a functional predictor, the attitude has a functional basis to be functional. This basis reflects functionalism, which holds that the functional basis or linkage happens because the linkage is functional (Turner and Maryanski 1979; J. Turner 2013). Conversely, when the attitude results from a dysfunctional predictor, the attitude has a dysfunctional basis to be dysfunctional. A functional predictor sustains a functional attitude, whereas a dysfunctional predictor sustains a dysfunctional attitude. A social attitude's functionality thus depends on its predictors' functionality. That means that the predictors' functionality helps evaluate the attitude's functionality.

A necessary condition for prediction is that predictors need to precede social attitudes empirically or logically (Antonakis et al. 2010; J. Davis 1985; Marini and Singer 1988). Whereas social attitudes are measurable as current states, their predictors need to have existed or happened in some years, months, or days before. Eligible predictors include personal and national experiences, personal and national characteristics, particularly the nations of China and the United States, and time. An experience refers to having or not having received or witnessed something. Thus, not receiving enough food, income, or medicine indicates the experience of economic hardship. Receiving interference or witnessing robberies in the neighborhood represents the experience of neighborhood nuisance. Receiving hurt as a victim refers to the experience of victimization. Experiencing safety or security registers the experience of security. In addition, the experiences of life and health constitute life satisfaction and self-assessed health, respectively. Aggregating by taking the averages of personal experiences in a nation reveals national experiences. Meanwhile, personal characteristics include gender, age, education, employment, earning status, religious affiliation, marital status, and immigration history. By contrast, national performance characteristics include the nation's population size, land area, phone rate, innovative technology rate, bank credit rate, gross domestic product, income inequality (Gini), globalization, government effectiveness, democracy, liberty, human development, human capital, and environmental disadvantage in terms carbon dioxide (CO_2)

emission. They tap the political, economic, communal, cultural, and ecological functioning. All the personal, national, and even time factors are potentially functional or dysfunctional as reasonable predictors of social attitudes.

Personal and National Experiences

An experience in the past precedes an attitude reported at the present. Personal experiences can aggregate to represent national experiences. A personal or national experience is likely to materialize functions or dysfunctions, notably regarding a social attitude. The experiences include economic hardship, neighborhood nuisance, security, victimization, health, and life satisfaction.

Economic hardship and its associated poverty, deprivation, economic or financial difficulty, inadequacy, pressure, strain, or stress are likely dysfunctional (Robinaugh et al. 2016; Robila 2006). The hardship denotes a dysfunction in providing finance, materials, utility, gains, and other resources and sinews to satisfy needs and thus fulfill the function of adaptation (Carle et al. 2009). Personally, economic hardship has dampened well-being (Gudmundsdottir 2013; Reeskens and Vandecasteele 2017). Economic hardship has impaired economic satisfaction, health, and even self-transcendence, which connects the self to nature and/or other people (Reeskens and Vandecasteele 2017). Conversely, the hardship has invoked depression, distress, economic strain, and a sense of normlessness (Ahnquist et al. 2012; Aytac and Rankin 2009; Ross and Mirowsky 2009). In addition, the hardship has generated the experience of victimization (Ross and Mirowsky 2009). Furthermore, the hardship has fomented suicide and impeded persistence in work (Economou et al. 2016; Mirowsky and Ross 2001). All these impacts of economic hardship undermine the function of adaptation to optimize utility for the person and society. Furthermore, economic hardship has constrained political and social trust and support for welfare spending (Blomberg and Kroll 1999; Reeskens and Vandecasteele 2017; Ross and Mirowsky 2009). These impacts interfere with the function of integration and goal attainment in government. Similarly, poverty as the root of economic hardship indicates economic incapability, material deprivation, malnutrition, social exclusion, and vulnerability (Ahnquist et al. 2012; Devereux 2002; Dowler 2002; Leu et al. 2016). They register the dysfunction in adaptation. Essentially, poverty means dissatisfaction of need and disutility due to the deficit of income (Phillips 2006). Poverty is crucial for social work (Rothwell et al. 2016). Poverty has also eroded well-being or quality of life (A. Clark et al. 2008; Lever et al. 2005). Poverty, particularly, has fomented strain (Walker et al. 2010). Moreover, poverty has underlain such adversity as family problems, financial pressure, illness, imprisonment, social disconnection, exclusion, and isolation experienced (Ahnquist et al. 2012; Dhal et al. 2008; Fischer et al. 1996; Stephens et al. 2014; Walker et al. 2010). In practice, poverty has fomented suicide and weakened civic participation, health service use, and volunteering (Caputo 2010; J. Chen et al. 2004; Swanson et al. 1992; R. Walker et al. 2010). Poverty has also discouraged support for government and trust in government and others (Jost et al.

2003; Stephens et al. 2014). All these impacts interfered with the functions of goat attainment, adaptation, and integration in society and the person.

Nuisance, deprivation, disorder, disorganization, incivility, problems, or inadequate quality experienced in the neighborhood are likely dysfunctional (G. Brown et al. 2004; Congdon 2010; Kanan and Pruitt 2002). The functions of adaptation and integration suffer in neighborhood nuisance. To the person, neighborhood nuisance has eroded well-being, notably in generating depression and a sense of normlessness (Pei and Kim 2017; Ross and Mirowsky 2009; van Praag et al. 1999). The nuisance has also engendered experiences of economic hardship, unsafe conditions, and victimization (Kanan and Pruitt 2002; Like 2011; Whelan and Maitre 2013). Furthermore, the nuisance has impeded social capital, including weak social ties (Congdon 2010; Ross and Mirowsky 2009). Neighborhood nuisance has impeded attachment to the neighborhood and social trust (G. Brown et al. 2004; Ross and Mirowsky 2009). These impacts, hence, undercut the functions of goal attainment concerning power realization, adaptation regarding utility optimization, and integration in the person and society. In addition, incivility experienced has impeded political trust (Mutz and Reeves 2005). This impedance hinders goal attainment and integration functions in the polity and community, respectively.

Security, safety, or even abundance or certainty experienced is functional (Coffe and Geys 2007; Sacks and Levi 2010; Taylor-Gooby 2001). It constitutes utility to uphold the function of adaptation or utility optimization. Security experience has been conducive to social capital, notably accessibility to resources through social relations (Curley 2010; Pena-Lopez and Sanchez-Santos 2016). Moreover, security experience has sustained well-being (Ackerman et al. 1997; Jones et al. 2014; Muffels and Fouarge 2004; M. Wen et al. 2010; Ziersch et al. 2005). Security experience, particularly, has sustained health, satisfaction with the country, neighborhood, and life, and a sense of neighborhood quality (D. Chen et al. 2008; Cummins et al. 2003; Frey et al. 2007; Olson et al. 2016; Parkes et al. 2002). Conversely, security experience has prevented fear of crime (Chiricos et al. 2000). Security experience has furthermore championed liking for the city, support for democracy, law, market, and youth development, and trust (Braithwaite 1998; Hraba et al. 2001; Schwartz et al. 2010; Zeldin 2002). Eventually, security experience has fostered social support provision (Pena-Lopez and Sanchez-Santos 2016). These impacts thereby buttress goal attainment, adaptation, and integration functions for the person and society.

Victimization, abuse, crime, offense, threat, or violence experienced manifests a dysfunction (Jacobs and Carmichael 2002; Pratt et al. 2010; Sedziafa and Tenkorang 2016; Wittebrood and Nieuwbeerta 2000; Yount and Carrera 2006). The nature of victimization in arousal, readjustment required, and scarring is upsetting (Russo and Roccato 2010; Shippee 2012). This upsetting is detrimental to the function of adaptation in utility optimization. Victimization has provoked experiences of conflict, problems, and unsafe conditions, notably in the neighborhood (Fernandes 2018; Gray et al. 2019; Kanan and Pruitt 2002; Bar-Tal and Halperin 2013). Similarly, victimization has heightened the perception of risk (McNeeley and Yuan 2017). As such, victimization has eroded well-being (Graham et al. 2010). Particularly, victimization has impeded intimacy and satisfaction with police (Hanson et al. 2010; Singer et al.

2019; Sun et al. 2013). Victimization, conversely, has engendered distress, fear of crime, posttraumatic stress, and a sense of normlessness and powerlessness (Krulichova 2019; Lineres 2004; Ross and Mirowsky 2009; Wager 2012). In addition, victimization has social trust (Olivera 2015; Ross and Mirowsky 2009). Victimization furthermore has cultivated cynicism and valuation of violence (Nabi and Horner 2001; Kirk and Papachristos 2011). Eventually, victimization has provoked the practices of doping and migration (Ramesh et al. 2019; Lineres 2004). Conversely, victimization has eroded performance or productivity (Hanson et al. 2010). These impacts exhibit impedance to the functions of goal attainment, adaptation, integration, and latency for society and the person.

Health self-assessed or experienced embodies personal functioning. As such, health embodies capability and utility (Lelli 2008; Zweifei and Breyer 1997). Health thus represents the functions of goal attainment and adaptation in the person. For personal capability, health has strengthened memory, resourcefulness, and wisdom (Friborg et al. 2002; Stevens et al. 2001; Webster 2003). Health has also underlain morality in the person (Pratt et al. 1996). For personal experiences, health has buttressed the securing of such social functioning as confidants, control, popularity, social integration, social networking, and social support received (Barrett 1999; Groot et al. 2007; Huxhold et al. 2014; Pena-Lopez and Sanchez-Santos 2016; Tomich and Helgeson 2002). Health has been conducive to other aspects of well-being (Jiang et al. 2011; Melzer 2011). For instance, health has enhanced well-being such as pleasure, satisfaction including that with the family, finance, life, and marriage, self-esteem, social well-being, and a sense of community and financial adequacy (Carr and Friedman 2005; Guo and Huang 2005; Hadjar and Samuel 2015; Jorgensen et al. 2010; Koromeckyj-Cox et al. 2007; Mroczek 2004; Plagnol 2011; Powdthavee 2009; Son and Wilson 2012; Zotti et al. 2016). Conversely, health has prevented such ill-being as anxiety, death, depression, and loneliness (Koromeckyj-Cox et al. 2007; Young et al. 2001; Yu and Chiu 2016). Health has also sustained such social attitudes as acceptance of others, evaluation of society, and trust in medicine and people (Ahern and Hendryx 2003; Hayes and Ross 1986; Tomich and Helgeson 2002; Yu and Chiu 2016). For practice, health has enabled such social functioning as cohesion, coping, cultural activities, religious attendance, search for meaning, self-enhancement, social activities, volunteering, and voting (Ben-Zur 2002; Goerres 2007; Kazarian and Martin 2006; Scherger 2009; Son and Wilson 2012; Tolsma et al. 2009). Overall, health contributes to the functions of goal attainment, adaptation, integration, and latency in the person and society, including its political, economic, communal, and cultural subsystems.

Life satisfaction is an experience of or reaction to life that is functional. Such satisfaction indicates the function of adaptation or utility optimization (Ambrey and Fleming 2014; Cummins et al. 2003). Furthermore, life satisfaction is conducive to a person's intelligence (Schaie 2013). Life satisfaction has contributed to the experiences of social networking and support received and prevented the experiences of loss (Luhmann et al. 2013; Pena-Lopez and Sanchez-Santos 2016; Yoo and Jeong 2017). Hence, life satisfaction contributes to other aspects of well-being, including health, satisfaction with democracy, and a sense of self-efficacy, including the political one (Celso et al. 2003; Corcoran et al. 2011; U. Kim et al. 2002; Nevitte and Kanji 2002; Rocke and Lachman 2008). Conversely, life satisfaction has prevented loneliness (Neto and Barros 2003). Life satisfaction has generated social attitudes such as political interest, support for democracy and foreign affairs, and trust in government and people (E. Chan 2014; Chen and Zhong 1998; Cheng and Smyth 2016; Rochelle 2015). In practice, life satisfaction has contributed to such social functioning as cohesion, political participation, volunteering, and voting (Bengtson et al. 1994; E. Chan 2014; Flavin and Keane 2011). These contributions manifest the functions of goal attainment, adaptation, and integration for the person and society.

National Performance

National performance transpires in political, economic, communal, cultural, and environmental aspects, representing functions or dysfunctions. Political performance involves democracy, liberty, and government effectiveness. Economic performance transpires in the phone rate, innovative technology rate, bank credit rate, globalization, gross domestic product, income inequality, and human capital. Communal, cultural, and environmental performance hinge on population size, human development, and environmental quality, respectively.

Political performance realizes authority and capacity for decision-making hierarchically by the elite, in partnership with the populace, independently of other nations (Chhotray and Stoker 2009; Grcic 2000; Rothstein 2005; Wallis and Dollery 2001). The performance is functional in addressing market failures and improving equity (Wallis and Dollery 2001). This function is to provide public goods, including defense, education, environmental protection, insurance, law, order rights, healthcare, relief, poverty alleviation, and utilities, and to prevent monopolies in the market. It works through coordinating, fostering, and redistributing. These functions cover goal attainment, adaptation, integration, and latency thoroughly. For the goal attainment function, political performance champions people's power in terms of agency, autonomy, capability, civil society dignity, independence, liberty, ownership, and rationality, as opposed to exploitation (Newey 2001; Friedman 2011). For the adaptation function, political performance enhances people's utility, including freedom, pleasure, and satisfaction (Gandjour and Lauterbach 2003; Riley 2008). For the function of integration, political performance sustains the community by promoting affection, attachment, civility, cleanliness, collective good, equality, family, fellowship, mutuality, participation, piety, responsibility, shamefulness, self-discipline, solidarity, sympathy, and volunteerism (Frazer 1999; Khatchadourian 1999; Selznick 2002). Political performance is noteworthy for the function of latency in perpetuating religions and virtues (Atkins 2008; Ney and Molenaars 1999; Selznick 2002).

Economic performance or prosperity embodies the adaptation function of utility optimization (Peet and Hatwick 2009). Herein, utility embraces or evolves from consumption, income, technology, trade, and wealth, as opposed to debt, hunger, inflation, mortality, and poverty (Hunt 1989; Peet and Hatwick 2009; Wolff and Resnick 2012). The performance is essential for realizing human dignity and modernization (Fukuyama 1995; Peet and Hatwick 2009). For the function of adaptation, economic performance has optimized well-being, including relational quality, satisfaction with democracy and life, and survival (Fridberg and Kangas 2008a; Helliwell et al. 2010; Inglehart 2010; Norris 2011; Williamson and Bochmer 1997). Conversely, economic performance has contributed to the adaptation function by preventing economic hardship, illnesses, risks, and threats (Fridberg and Kangas 2008a; Schneider 2007; Schwartz and Melech 2000). In addition, economic performance has contributed to the goal attainment function by empowering people's knowledge (Booth and Richard 1998; Norris 2011). Economic performance has also achieved the function of integration by sustaining collective and political participation, institutional and social trust, and volunteering (Corcoran et al. 2011; Inglehart 2003; Norris 1999a; Traunmuller 2011; van Oorschot and Arts 2005). For the function of latency, economic performance has strengthened education and the values of emancipation, imagination, and independence (Fjellvang 2011; Shu and Bian 2002; Welzel 2013).

Communal performance or community or social building or development embodies the integration function (Stevenson et al. 2010; Vajja and White 2008). This function embraces the contribution to such social functioning as community resilience, social cohesion, and social inclusion (Mannion 2003; Ungar 2011). Notably, communal performance has fulfilled the function of integration by enhancing civic engagement, favor for the community, helping, political participation, recourse, and trust in government and medicine (Ahern and Hendryx 2003; Z. Han et al. 2017; Mitrut and Wolff 2011; Palmer et al. 2011; Su and Feng 2013; Whitham 2012; Xu et al. 2010). Conversely, communal performance has buttressed the integration function by preventing violence (E. Wright et al. 2015). In addition, communal performance has achieved the function of adaptation by people's success and well-being, including health, neighborhood quality, and satisfaction with life and the neighborhood (Cramm et al. 2012; Fujisawa et al. 2009; Furstenberg and Hughes 1995; Olson et al. 2016; Sampson 1991; M. Wen et al. 2010). In addition, communal performance has raised such national qualities as national happiness, income, and prosperity (D. Lee et al. 2011; Semenova et al. 2020). Conversely, communal performance has prevented such dysfunction as depression, distress, illness, and victimization (Gary et al. 2007; Hansen-Nord et al. 2014; M. Wen et al. 2010; E. Wright et al. 2015). For the function of latency, communal performance has contributed to education (D. Lee et al. 2011). For the function of goal attainment, communal performance has sustained national regulation quality (D. Lee et al. 2011). In addition, communal performance has strengthened the polity by enhancing people's political participation and trust in government (Z. Han et al. 2017; Xu et al. 2010).

Cultural performance, such as educational performance, meets the function of latency. Essential to the function is strengthening national identity, especially under globalization, which can dissolve the identity (Maurer 2011; Olssen et al. 2004). Such performance preserves or sustains citizenship, conventions, ethics, loyalty, and the use of tools such as language (Corrigan et al. 2013; Olssen et al. 2004; Stevenson

2011; Toomela 2008). For the latency function, cultural performance has championed the value of emancipation and prevented lying (van Hemert et al. 2002; Welzel 2013). Meanwhile, cultural performance has facilitated the goal attainment function by fostering people's intelligence and social capital (Portes and Vickstrom 2011; Schaie 2013). Furthermore, cultural performance has benefited the adaptation function by sustaining health and income and preventing illnesses, obesity, poverty, and victimization (Goetz et al. 2011; Herian et al. 2014; A. Jones et al. 2015; Lipford and Yandle 2009; Poveda 2011). Cultural performance has furthermore strengthened the goal attainment function by contributing to the legitimacy and trustworthiness of the polity and discouraging the corruption of the polity (Cohen and Bolt 2005; Gilley 2009). In addition, cultural performance has realized the function of integration by facilitating civic engagement or participation, employment, trust in government and people, volunteering, and preventing violence (Cohen and Bolt 2005; Lipford and Yandle 2009; Poveda 2011; Robert and Bukodi 2005; Rupasingha et al. 2006; Uslaner and Brown 2005).

National Superpower

China and the United States are national superpowers that coordinate the bipolar world nowadays (Tunsjo 2018). They are likely to make a difference in functioning for goal attainment through empowering, which entails using power or resources. Such power includes cultural, economic, ideological, institutional, military, and political (Adler 2013; Domhoff 2017; Kroenig et al. 2010). The power is likely to magnify the functions of the national characteristics of the two superpowers. Both China and the United States have political, economic, communal, and cultural power to heighten their achievement of goal attainment, adaptation, integration, and latency functions. According to analytical functionalism, the deterministic mechanism of empowering can strengthen other mechanisms to maximize their influence.

China's political power transpires in the Chinese state's practices of advertising or propaganda, authoritarian governance, central planning, Confucian indoctrination, educational control, ideological control, indoctrination, military forces, nationalist and patriotist education or indoctrination, partisan monopoly or party state, repression, securitization, social control, and soft power capitalizing to sustain its stability and statism (L. Cao et al. 2016; Deng and Smith 2018; Fallman 2010; Gilley and Holbig 2009; Karmazin 2017; Landsberger 2009; Lee and Zhang 2013; Liu and Tsai 2021; Loh 2017; Meng 2011; Shambaugh 2007). Herein, authoritarian governance hinges on bureaucracy, censorship, legal control, publicity, and religion-like authority (Lagerwey 2010; Meng 2011). Central planning exerts control over migration, settlement, other social activities, and the economy (J. Hou 2011). The Confucian doctrines about hierarchy, nationalism, and paternalism, as opposed to Westernization, strengthen political power (Deng and Smith 2018; Moore 2017). Educational control prevails in ideological education, moral education, patriotic education, and political education to privilege state power (Hoffman 2006; Rosen 2009; Z. Wang

2008; Woronov 2007). Ideological control, including indoctrinating Confucianism, nationalism, and patriotism as opposed to Western ones, also pervades outside education to legitimize political control (Gilley and Holbig 2009; Rosen 2009). The ruling party's monopoly heightens state power by claiming its representation of all people in China (Lagerwey 2010; Meng 2011). Repressive readiness based on military forces for securitization or stability also actualizes political power (Lee and Zhang 2013; Liu and Tsai 2021; Weiss 2013; Zeng 2015). In addition, soft power capitalizes on Confucian doctrines and other Chinese cultural attractions, emphasizes foreign humiliation and victimization, and complements hard political power (Barabantseva 2012; Edney 2012; Loh 2017). Statism, highlighting the leadership and representation by the state to enforce laws, also accentuates political power (Liu and Tsai 2021; Xu and Chan 2011).

China's economic power rests on China's economic growth, global strategy, size of the economy, and statist orchestration (Ly and Boateng 2021; Ly and Meissner 2020, 2021; Liu and Tsai 2021; Sun et al. 2013). As such, China's unparalleled and uninterrupted economic growth provides surpluses to exercise and thus heighten power. This power is global because of China's global strategy to realize and stabilize its status as a superpower. The global strategy means that China is influencing the world rather than vice versa. In addition, the size of China's economy is powerful, especially leveraged by China's statist collective manipulation.

China's communal power derives from such social functioning as familialization, hierarchical structure, homogeneity, and networking, as well as population size (Wang and VanderWeele 2011; Xu et al. 2010). Familialization means power vested in the extended family, which extends and consolidates familial influences onto kin members. Similarly, a hierarchical structure legitimizes and safeguards communal influences, particularly on the masses. Homogeneity among Chinese people strengthens their interaction and mutual influence. Networking, known as *guanxi*, is pervasive when it connects people with nominal or minimal relationships to tighten communal influences. In addition, population size heightens the power of the scale effect.

China's cultural power builds on China's authoritarianism and submissiveness, collectivism, Confucianism, hierarchy, interdependence, learning, nationalism, patriotism, traditionalism, and resistance to Westernization (Chen and Martin 2007; Cheung and Pomerantz 2011; Heffernan et al. 2010; Lagerwey 2010; Meng 2011; Sun and Bitter 2012; Zhang with Stening 2010). Authoritarianism means the emphasis on authority, its control, and submissiveness. Collectivism suggests conformity and submissiveness to the group and its influence. Confucianism indoctrinates conformity to or respect for hierarchy, interdependency, learning for self-cultivation, loyalty, authoritarianism, and collectivism (Heffernan et al. 2010). Hierarchy, interdependence, learning, nationalism, and patriotism are all essential to or compatible with Confucianism. Confucianism gets reinforcement from traditionalism, which strives to distinguish China from others. Such cultural power has facilitated formalization and integration in China's social functioning (Schlevogt 2002). Herein, formalization or setting regulations is essential to maintain social order.

The United States demonstrates political power in its hegemony or even imperialism in the world and monetary policy regarding the US dollar (Law 2009; Steinmetz 2005; Tunsjo 2018). Such hegemonic or imperial power rests on unparalleled diplomatic and military advantages to marshal global alliances and even underlings or vassals (Kruse 2015; Steinmetz 2005; Pass 2019; Stokes 2018; Tunsjo 2018). In addition, the US dollar as a world standard currency heightens the political power of US monetary policy.

The economic power of the United States is evident in its economic competitiveness or even supremacy or superiority, the global currency of the US dollar, and the size of the economy (Shortall and Warner 2010). Such competitiveness rests on the autonomous, liberal, mobile, and private properties of the US economy to make it adaptive, flexible, and productive. The US dollar as a global currency helps sustain the US economy in economic crises (Liang 2010).

The cultural power of the United States stems from its aggressiveness, competitiveness or social Darwinism, success ideology, and valuation of power (Garrett et al. 2014; Kruse 2015). Herein, social Darwinism recognizes and adores competition, strength, and struggle (Cordes 2006; Hudson 2000; J. Turner et al. 2020). That is, emphasizing power heightens the development, exertion, and influence of power in the United States.

Time

Time as a factor helps indicate social changes worth examining and predicting (Harper and Leicht 2011). Social changes are understandable as denaturalization, globalization or universalization, individualization, modernization, and postmodernization (Adams 2007; Harper and Leicht 2011; Morody and Giza-Poleszczuk 2018). Denaturalization means reducing nature or the natural environment and forces due to the growth of the human population and its work (Morody and Giza-Poleszczuk 2018). The work characterizes civilization or humanization, which supersedes natural logic. Globalization or universalization builds on the free flow of people, materials, and information worldwide (Harper and Leicht 2011). It brings issues about cultural class, delegitimization of the nation, migration, and the race to the bottom or exploitation. Meanwhile, standardization is also a concomitant of globalization. Individualization means the growing importance of individual life and logic and the decline in the logic of social groups, norms, and stratification. Individualization thus centers on agency, autonomy, choice, competition, deregulation, discontinuity, disembeddedness, disintegration, disengagement, emancipation, heterogeneity, independence, liberty, self, singleness, and variation (Bauman 2001; Beck and Beck-Gernsheim 2002; Burgess 2018; Krys et al. 2019). Conversely, individualization erodes attachment, commitment, obligation, and ties. Modernization, industrialization, or Westernization means life improvement (Harper and Leicht 2011). It encompasses the complication and diversification of society. Postmodernization, in one sense nowadays, represents the deepening of modernization (Morody and

Giza-Poleszczuk 2018). Thus, whereas modernization features differentiation, postmodernization signifies hyperdifferentiation (Ashley 1997; Mouzelis 2012; Turner 2003). Nevertheless, whereas modernization upholds rationalization, postmodernization embraces arationality, irrationality, or romanticism (Mouzelis 2012; Ritzer 1997; Tester 2004; J. Turner 2003; Yeganeh 2017).

Social change overall is an uncertainty requiring expounding and evaluation. From conservative discourse, social change needs to uphold morality and social and professional societal norms (Fein 2015). By contrast, liberal discourse demands social change to promote societal equality and justice (Fein 2015). From populist discourse, social change desirably enriches material life in society (Harman 2009). Meanwhile, social democratic discourse expects social change to spread universal fairness and eliminate exploitation (Fein 2015). Whereas being functional, as expected in the discourses, social change can also be dysfunctional. This dysfunction accords with the conservative discourse that social change is unnecessary and disruptive (Fein 2015). Such discourse treasures the latency function of preserving the culture.

Denaturalization may be dysfunctional such that population size has provoked such societal disturbances as rates of conflict, crime, environmental degradation, punishment, revolution, and terrorism and reduced such societal quality as rates of cohesion, development, employment, health, innovation, investment, liberty, social capital, sustainable development, and trading (Abouharb and Cingranelli 2007; Alderson 2004; S. Cho et al. 2013; Coffe and Geys 2006; Collier and Hoeffler 2004; Cotter et al. 1998; Dreher et al. 2008; Foster et al. 2013; Havinga 2002; Kwan and Chiu 2018; Yagci 2017; R. York et al. 2003). Conflict and even crime, revolution, and terrorism arise from competition for benefits and resources demanded by people with their interests. Competition, in turn, springs from the shortage of benefits and resources people consume. Nevertheless, conflict, crime, revolution, and terrorism invite punishment. To acquire benefits and resources for subsistence, people change and degrade the natural environment through building, farming, and emitting waste from production. Conversely, cohesion suffers as people cannot be cohesive with numerous others under the time constraint. Likewise, people cannot help maintain social relations and thus social capital with numerous others. Health deteriorates due to people's congestion and contagion of disease. While people can trade with some others, they cannot deal with many or all others. When people consume or occupy scarce resources, resources left for employment, innovation, and investment can dwindle. Overall, people constrain the environments and resources available for development, particularly sustainable development. All these indicate dysfunctions in power or the polity, such as health and liberty; utility or the economy, such as employment and trading; and integration or the community, such as cohesion. Environmental degradation has, in turn, triggered migration and protest and diminished health, family functioning, social capital, and well-being (Black et al. 2011; Cummins et al. 2003; Scafuto and La Barbera 2016; Stafford et al. 2005; Van Haaften et al. 2004). Migration and protest can result from resource loss due to environmental degradation. Health deteriorates due to pollution and other forms of environmental degradation. The family also cannot function without decent housing and a surrounding environment. Environmental problems drain family efforts and resources and, thus, function—these manifest dysfunctions in or to the capability, utility, community, and polity.

Globalization has unfolded dysfunctions that have fomented confusion about identity, inequality, and stress, and it has shed the traditional culture in society (Arnett 2002; Dreher et al. 2008). As such, people's identities linked with a place become uncertain due to the flow, migration, and mix of people there. When globalization clusters or redistributes people worldwide, people find more inequality within and among places. Stress arises from diverse interactions with people and cultures flowing with globalization. For example, migrants experience stress from acculturation. The mass of migrants can also have their culture dilute or transform the host culture. These dysfunctions thus erode the community and culture. In addition, the dysfunctions of globalization transpire in the erosion of and threat to the nation and instigating discontent and resistance (O'Byrne and Hensby 2011; Timberlake et al. 2014). Hence, the polity also suffers.

Individualism is blameworthy for dysfunctions in invoking anomie or normlessness, anti-sociality, conflict, insecurity, risks, and societal uncertainty (Burgess 2018; Frank and Meyer 2002; Fuchs 2015). Anomie results from the collapse of traditional social categorization and stratification through individualization. As such, people lose their norms and ways to function in an individualized society. Without the norms, anti-sociality and conflict emerge with individualization. As such, personal interest preempts social interest, thus sparking conflict. Risks encompass those about the climate, culture, environment, exclusion, family, food, homicide, morality, nuclear energy, technology, victimization, and work or labor in society (Breakwell 2007; Lupton 2013; Nalla et al. 2011; Nowlin and Rabovsky 2020; Ojala 2005; Taylor-Gooby 2004; Welch et al. 2002; Wales and Mythen 2002; Zwick 2005). Risks arise from the collapse of norms and sociality when individualized people act according to their interests. Uncertainty also prevails under the collapse of social norms and the mushrooming of risks through individualization. The dysfunctions thus pervade the community, culture, and economy in undermining integration, latency, and utility, respectively.

Modernization has bred dysfunctions such as ageism or antipathy against elders, crises, environmental degradation, narcissism or self-love, and societal stress (Doale and Seda 2001; Quadagno 1987; Kick and McKinney 2014). Conversely, modernization has attenuated freedom and work centrality or value, which are dysfunctional to society (Moller and Skaaning 2013; Yeganeh 2017). Ageism arises from elders' declining expertise and, thus, status in the modernized society. Crises such as economic and fiscal ones emerge from massive, risky investments or leveraging in society (Benassy-Quere et al. 2010). Moreover, crises can ensue from industrial malpractice and disaster, heightened by modernization, such as technological trials and people's interrelationships (Castells 2000). Environmental degradation results from people's exploitation and intervention enabled by modernization. Socially divisive narcissism mounts following the increase of personal power with modernization. Stress accrues with new development and adjustment concomitant with modernization. These mark the dysfunctions of modernization in integration, latency, and utility, or the community, culture, and economy, respectively.

Postmodernization has eroded the culture and ethics of fairness and work (Yeganeh 2017). Moreover, postmodernization is blameworthy for dysfunctions in breeding alienation, disorientation, identity confusion, loneliness, schizophrenia, uncertainty, and vulnerability in society (Brand 1999; Goulding 2000). Alienation, which means the loss of identity, ownership, and relationship, looms as postmodernization overthrows traditional norms. Such an overthrow also deprives people of orientation and heightens their confusion, loneliness, uncertainty, and vulnerability. Confused and divided identity can culminate in schizophrenia. The dysfunctions thus undercut the functions of integration and latency.

Tracking Social Change

Predicting social attitudes with personal and national characteristics addresses knotty questions about social change. Social change includes denaturalization, globalization, individualization, industrialization, liberalization, rationalization, vitalization, and other ways of modernization (Harper and Leicht 2011; Morody and Giza-Poleszczuk 2018). Modernization, combining various social changes, evolves toward complexity, development, and progress (Harper and Leicht 2011). Denaturalization, meaning human displacement of nature, involves carbon dioxide emission and increased population to reduce land per capita nationally (Morody and Giza-Poleszczuk 2018). Globalization, meaning human, information, and material flows across nations, features immigration at the personal level and global connection and flow at the national level (Harper and Leicht 2011). Individualization, meaning personal self-sufficiency and social disconnection, transpires in marriage and living arrangements, self-employment, and independent work at the personal level (Morody and Giza-Poleszczuk 2018). Industrialization, meaning development in industry and work, emphasizes employment and work at the personal level and phone ownership, technology, government effectiveness, and bank credit at the national level (Harper and Leicht 2011). Liberalization, meaning the increase in deregulation and liberty, hinges on democracy, income inequality, and liberty at the national level (Abouharb and Cingranelli 2007; S. Smith 2011). Rationalization, meaning heightening rationality, transpires in education, irreligiousness, and creative and intellectual work at the personal level (Yeganeh 2017). Vitalization, meaning improvement in life quality, rests on health, life satisfaction, security, family income, and social status at the personal level and human capital and development or prosperity at the national level (Inglehart and Welzel 2005). The questions addressed are thus how social changes predict or impact social attitudes, which anticipate social actions, including social conflict, disturbance, exclusion, oppression, and strife among social institutions and groups (Alvarez and Brehm 2002; De Houwer et al. 2013; Kemmis and McTaggart 2005).

A critical, unsettled question is how social change, including modernization and its derivatives, impacts social attitudes to foment conflict among individuals, groups, and institutions (Bickel 2018). Such conflict arises from low acceptance, confidence, favor, justification, or trust regarding social institutions, deviants, outsiders, and others (Bar-Tal and Halperin 2013; Zhuang 2020). These social attitudes have responded differently to different social changes in different studies, posing a question for clarification in a globally holistic way. For instance, confidence in social institutions has risen and declined with personal education as a rationalization indicator in different studies in different places (S. Chi et al. 2021; van der Cruijsen et al. 2014). This confidence has also escalated and slid with personal employment as an industrialization indicator in different studies in different places (McAllister 1999; Elchardus and De Keere 2013). Furthermore, this confidence has increased and decreased with national prosperity as a vitalization indicator in different studies (McAllister 1999; van Oorschot and Arts 2005). At least, puzzles requiring clarification and verification have arisen from the adverse impacts of social changes. For example, denaturalization, globalization, and individualization have eroded confidence in national institutions (Gilley 2009; Joslyn and Haider-Markel 2002; Kunovich 2009). Industrialization is blameworthy for losing acceptance or tolerance for others (Fukuyama 2003). Liberalization, including democratization and marketization or neo-liberalization, has weakened confidence, favor, and trust in social institutions and others (Gelissen 2002; Geys 2012; Lundasen et al. 2013; Persson et al. 2017; van Oorschot and Arts 2005). Rationalization has shrunk the acceptance of outsiders (Boeri et al. 2002). Vitalization has impeded acceptance of outsiders and trust in others (Cheng and Smyth 2016; Sun and Wang 2012).

Besides effects on social attitudes, variations across countries' effects constitute an additional question to verify the impact obtained from a single country. Such single-country effects have predominantly applied to the United States and China, which are noteworthy superpowers (Q. Huang 2018; Pace 2015; Persson et al. 2017; Richey and Ikeda 2009). Variations due to these countries are thus vital for gauging the global ranges of the effects.

Guide to Subsequent Chapters

Subsequent chapters unfold the understanding of social attitudes based on the functioning of personal and national experiences, personal characteristics, national performance, national superpowers, and social change. Based on World Values Surveys, social attitudes are sevenfold, comprising confidence in institutions, justification for misdeeds, justification for unconventional sexuality, faith in religion, acceptance of outsiders, acceptance of deviants, and trust in other people. Their most proximate predictors are preceding experiences, based on World Values Surveys, comprising economic hardship, neighborhood nuisance, security, victimization, health, and life satisfaction. Aggregating or taking averages of personal experiences over the nation yields national experience. Personal characteristics, which precede personal experiences and social attitudes, include the person's gender, age, education, migration status, employment, marital status, and religious affiliation, based on World Values

Surveys. National performance, one year before social attitudes, includes national population size, land area, rates of phones, technological innovation, bank credit, gross domestic product, household income inequality, globalization, democracy, liberty, government effectiveness, human development, human capital, and carbon dioxide emission. They register in the World Bank database, the Quality of Government Basic Dataset (Dahlberg et al. 2018), and the Standardized World Income Inequality Database (Solt 2016). Alternatively, the national superpowers of China and the United States are national predictors possible to introduce main and interaction effects on social attitudes. A more fundamental predictor is time, which represents social changes, including denaturalization, globalization, individualization, and modernization or postmodernization.

The combined personal and national data based on the World Values Surveys, World Bank database, Quality of Government Basic Dataset, and Standardized World Income Inequality Databases matched 51,940 individual cases in the early 21st Century for analysis. These cases represent people worldwide, so those from countries with larger populations are more likely to appear. For instance, larger countries include Brazil, China, Ethiopia, Germany, India, Indonesia, Iran, Japan, Mexico, Nigeria, Pakistan, the Philippines, Russia, Turkey, the United States, and Vietnam. Factor analyses of these data identified seven social attitude factors, including confidence, justification, favor, acceptance, and trust in institutions, people, and practices from 47 survey items and four experience factors from 13. The experiences, health, life satisfaction, and 33 personal background characteristics are predictors of social attitudes at the personal level. Additional predictors are survey time and 14 national characteristics. Crucially, statistical analysis employed weighting for the data to make them representative of people, not countries, worldwide. As such, countries with larger populations are more representative of all people worldwide. This weighting aligns with treating the person as the unit of analysis. Such analysis seeks to understand the person, not the country. The functioning of these personal and national predictors unfolds in the following chapters.

Chapter 2 details the functioning bases and impacts of social attitudes on sociality. Specifically, confidence in institutions and trust in other people represent the constructive dimension of sociality, and faith in religion, justifications for misdeeds and unconventional sexuality, and acceptance of outsiders and deviants register the destructive dimension of sociality. The reverses of the destructive dimensions, namely, unfaith in religion, refutations against misdeeds and unconventional sexuality, and rejections of outsiders and deviants, characterize sociality. Hence, sociality differentiates the constructive inside and the destructive outside to set the boundary for acceptance and rejection. Analysis of World Value Survey data showed that seven social attitudes represented sociality. Among them, refutation against misdeeds was the most representative, and rejection of deviants was the least representative. Contrary to the expectation for the prosocial role of religious faith, this faith inversely loaded on the factor of sociality.

Chapter 3 exhibits the functioning of personal characteristics for social attitudes. A personal characteristic, such as education or educational attainment, exerts functions through enlightenment, learning, identity, interest, and social status (Wodtke 2012).

Enlightenment means capability building or development in intelligence, knowledge, skill, and wisdom. This development functions with the voluntaristic mechanism of power realization. Learning concerns social norms and knowledge—the former functions with the voluntaristic mechanism of norm conformity. Identity involves ideals or values shared with a group, such as one composed of college graduates. It functions with the voluntaristic mechanism of ideal consistency. Its functions work through the voluntaristic mechanisms of power realization and ideal calibration. Personal education has weakened confidence in institutions (Hakhverdian and Mayne 2012; Yang et al. 2014). This negative effect also appears in the analysis of World Values Surveys data. According to the function of enlightenment, education impacts the power to challenge and question institutions. Similarly, the function of learning suggests that education provides learning for the challenge and questioning. The function of identity or interest holds that education fosters ideals, beliefs, or values about challenge and questioning. In addition, the function of social status provides power and ideals for challenge and questioning. When challenge and questioning are conducive to improvement in institutions and their functioning, education realizes its function. The challenge and questioning of education also apply to the acceptance of outsiders. According to the analysis of World Values Surveys data, education displayed a significant negative effect on such acceptance. This effect suggests that outsiders or their acceptance are questionable to educated people. In addition, other social attitudes have their functional bases on various personal characteristics.

Chapter 4 reveals the functioning of personal experiences for social attitudes. An experience such as economic hardship displays its functions mainly through inability, material, and strain paths (Carle et al. 2009; Robinaugh et al. 2016). The inability means the deficiency of power, with the material path including the functions of resources such as money, durables, and services, and the strain path dealing with negative mental states. They are influential at a personal, voluntaristic level through the mechanisms of power realization, utility optimization, and ideal consistency. Power realization exerts its functions through ability or resources. Utility optimization maintains its functions through utility and its basis on resources. Ideal consistency demonstrates its functions or dysfunctions through strain. Such voluntaristic mechanisms underlie the negative effect of such an experience of economic hardship on such a social attitude as confidence in institutions. Poverty and unemployment have had a negative effect (Child and Nikolova 2020; Elchardus and De Keere 2013; Mishler and Rose 2001). A very weak but statistically significant negative effect of personal economic hardship on confidence in institutions also arises from the World Values Surveys data analysis. This effect shows the dysfunction of personal economic hardship in impeding the functions of institutions or confidence in them.

Chapter 5 reveals the functional impacts of national norms for social attitudes on the attitudes at the personal level. These national norms were the averages of the social attitudes in the country. At the extrapersonal or deterministic level, national inability, materials, and strain influence through voluntaristic mechanisms through the deterministic mechanisms of empowering, incentivizing, and framing. Herein, national inability, material deprivation, and strain are respectively disempowering, incentivizing, and framing the mental state of strain. By contrast, national economic hardship manifests a significantly weak effect on faith in religion, based on analysis of data from World Values Surveys. This effect implies a function of religion or its favor for relieving the dysfunction of national economic hardship. The function reflects the incentivizing mechanism of national economic hardship. Various personal and national experiences display their functional bases for various social attitudes.

Chapter 6 recites the functioning of national performance for social attitudes. National performance, such as national democracy, encompasses the functions of adaptation, cohesion or integration, compromise, deliberation, equalizing, and liberating (Fairfield 2008; Saward 1998; Warren 2011). The functions of adaptation and deliberation are to optimize utility, whereas the functions of integration, cohesion, compromise, equalizing, and liberating sustain social harmony. These functions can work through the deterministic mechanisms of incentivizing and normalizing concerning benefits versus costs and norms, respectively. Democracy has alleviated confidence in institutions (Dyck and Lascher Jr 2009; Persson et al. 2017). Such alleviation also transpires in the analysis of World Values Survey data. According to the deterministic mechanism of incentivizing, democracy functions to show the gain from improving institutions but fails to attract confidence. Meanwhile, the deterministic mechanism of normalizing functions in democracy to normalize people's equality and liberty represents grounds for reforming institutions. Hence, democracy is functional in improving the functions of institutions. In addition, various national performances generated diverse impacts on various social attitudes.

Chapter 7 highlights the functioning of national superpowers for social attitudes. A national superpower like China can exert its functions through deterrence, gaining consent, hegemony or leadership, and power or coercion (Ly and Boateng 2021; Ly and Meissner 2020). Whereas deterrence applies the deterministic mechanism of incentivizing by showing the cost or harm, gaining consent applies the deterministic mechanism of framing or persuasion, hegemony or leadership employs the deterministic mechanism of normalizing, and coercion applies the deterministic mechanism of empowering. China has generated more support for authority than other nations (Pinker 2011). In the analysis of World Values Survey data, China or its people indicate higher confidence in institutions than other nations. This indication reflects the deterministic mechanism of normalizing China's authoritarian, hegemonic norm. Moreover, education displays a more negative effect on confidence in institutions in China than in other nations. This surplus means that China strengthens the power realization function of education in challenging and questioning institutions according to the deterministic mechanism of empowering. By contrast, trust in other people is higher in the United States than other nations (Buchan et al. 2002). This surplus is also evident in the analysis of World Values Survey data. This evidence manifests the deterministic mechanism of normalizing liberalism or openness, which is conducive to social trust (Freitag and Bauer 2016). In addition, the effect of age is significantly more positive in the United States than in other countries, according to the analysis of World Values Survey data. This surplus indicates the enhancement of the age function through the deterministic mechanism of empowerment due to the power of the United States in maintaining healthy and productive aging. In all, China and the

United States are forceful in distinguishing their various social attitudes from other nations.

Chapter 8 outlines conclusions about the functional bases of social attitudes on personal and national experiences, personal characteristics, national performance, national superpowers, and time or social change. Confidence in institutions has functional bases on national security, national population size, national non-democracy, and China. As national security is functional, confidence in institutions is a functional product, particularly for a large, non-democratic nation such as China. Justification for misdeeds finds its basis in national income inequality. The justification may be a functional response to national inequality. Justification for unconventional sexuality, including abortion, homosexuality, divorce, and premarital sex, is based on national dissatisfaction with life and a nation with a small population. The justification may be functional for dissatisfied people. Faith in religion arises from national democracy and national economic hardship. The arising is probably functional for people with economic hardship. Acceptance of outsiders has a basis in national democracy. Conversely, rejecting outsiders is a function of national globalization, national health, and national life satisfaction in both China and the United States. Accepting outsiders is functional to democracy, and acceptance of unhealthy and dissatisfied people may be functional for people in a poor nation. Trust in other people is higher in the nation with higher government effectiveness but lower human development, and in the United States than in other countries. Hence, this trust is a functional product of government effectiveness and a superpower. This trust is also functional for people in nations that are low in human development.

Chapter 2
Functioning of Sociality for Social Attitudes

From the functionalist framework, sociality is social attitudes' functional basis and fruit. This framework maintains that sociality and attitudes are functional (Fowers 2015; Kruglanski and Stroebe 2014). The functioning of sociality builds on its components, social attitudes, to realize its function to sustain humanity and society (Fowers 2015). As such, social attitudes enable the functioning of sociality, humanity, and society (Kruglanski and Stroebe 2014). Essentially, the functionalist framework emphasizes components' functioning to buttress the whole's functioning. Social attitudes are components herein, and sociality, humanity, and society are the wholes. Sociality means social living involving the group or society (Tomasello 2014). Social attitudes encompass acceptance, confidence, faith, justification, and trust regarding society or its components, members, or behaviors. Specifically, confidence in institutions, faith in religion, justification for misdeeds or misbehavior or sexuality, acceptance of deviants or outsiders, and trust in others are seven independent social attitudes emerging from the World Values Surveys. To be functionally integral to sociality, these social attitudes become confidence in institutions, faith in religion, refutation against misdeeds or sexuality, rejection of deviants or outsiders, and trust in others. This functioning builds on ethics, goodness, morality, and humanity to characterize sociality (Fowers 2015). Moreover, the functioning strengthens community, relationships, and solidarity integral to sociality (T. Johnson et al. 2013; Matusov 2024). According to Judeo-Christianity and Catholicism, natural law ethics, Aristotelian teleological philosophy, and Kantian universalism, sexuality contradicts sociality (Soble 2008). Accordingly, sexuality underlies lechery, homosexuality, objectification, patriarchy, and prostitution denounced by the philosophies (Soble 2008). Sexuality also challenges sociality grounded in civilization (Soble 2008). Besides, sexuality is risky by instigating risking (Moran et al. 2021; Tsang and Ho 2007). The risks arise from abortion, divorce, homosexuality, infidelity, licentiousness, polygamy, promiscuity, and prostitution concomitant to sexuality (Markey and Markey 2007; Schafer 2011; Vauclair and Fischer 2011). Moreover, sexuality has eroded sociality by eroding attachment security and evoking aggression (Dunkel

C.-k. Cheung, *Social Attitudes in the Early 21st Century*,
https://doi.org/10.1007/978-981-96-9705-2_2

et al. 2016; Vrangalova and Bukberg 2015). Sociality builds on attachment security and non-aggression (Fowers 2015).

Hence, analytical-functionalism posits that social functioning generates power, utility, ideals, and norms to reinforce social functioning. Functioning means health, capability, performing, resilience, resourcefulness, strength, working, and success (Biggs and Lowenstein 2011; Corbin and Hall 2019; Follette et al. 2001; Huta 2014; K. John 2001; Zautra et al. 2010; Phillips 2006). It covers competence, flourishing, and fullness (Hahn et al. 2010; Huta 2017; K. John 2001). Social functioning then means functioning at the social aspect to encompass social cohesion, development, harmony, integration, legitimacy, normalcy or normality, order, power, predictability, productivity, resourcefulness, robustness, security, solidarity, stability, and sufficiency (Douds 2021; Fararo 2001; Joseph 2006; Kegley and Raymond 2021; S. Kim 2019; Nash and Calonico 2003; Srbljinovic and Bozic 2014; Swartz 2013). Furthermore, social functioning encompasses sociality and its manifestations in confidence in institutions, refutation against misdeeds and sexuality, rejection of deviants and outsiders, and trust in others personally. Moreover, social functioning operates in institutions at the societal level. As such, analytical-functionalism maintains that one form of social functioning emits power, utility, ideals, and norms to reinforce another form of social functioning within a level or across levels. Power derived from social functioning reinforces social functioning through its empowering or realization mechanism. Accordingly, power drives social functioning as it is workable. Utility from social functioning reinforces social functioning through its incentivizing or optimization mechanism. Accordingly, utility attracts social functioning as it is gainful. Ideals derived from social functioning reinforce social functioning through their framing or calibration mechanism. Accordingly, ideals rationalize social functioning as reasonable. Norms derived from social functioning reinforce social functioning through their normalizing or conformity mechanism. Accordingly, norms assimilate social functioning as it is popular.

Existing Knowledge

Sociality is the underlying factor of social attitudes. Specifically, sociality embraces elements to assimilate social attitudes, orienting them toward sociality. In addition, sociality engenders forces, including sociality-oriented power, utility, ideals, and norms, to sustain such assimilation. Attitudes are mental actions building on the forces (De Houwer et al. 2013). The positive side of attitude, favor, encompasses acceptance, confidence, faith, justification, and trust. Within sociality, attitudinal objects are institutions, religion, non-deviants, non-outsiders, non-misdeeds, non-sexuality, and others within society. As such, favor for these objects benefits from power, utility, ideals, and norms generated by sociality. Power drives attitudes by braking, controlling, coercion, dominating, enabling, pressing, and structuring (Clegg 2023; Dunbar and Abra 2021; Littlejohn et al. 2017; Pike and Galinsky 2020).

The bases of power include agency, arousal, authority, autonomy, coercion, commitment, community, conflict, connectivity, copresence, discipline, domination, education, entraining, health, income, knowledge, membership, material, order, protection, resistance, social integration, social support or assistance received status, and structure (Bruff 2009; Campos-Castillo and Hitlin 2013; Clegg 2023; Collins 2004; Dolinski 2016; Engelstad 2009; Haugaard 2003, 2020, 2021; Liu and Pratto 2018). Utility attracts attitudes through cost-benefit analysis, information processing, and reasoning or rational choice (J. Liu et al., 2023; L. Thompson et al., 2004). The bases of utility include achievement, care received, company, enjoyment, fun, gifting, help received, payment, praise, pride, satisfaction, savoring, security, sex, and well-being (Aberg 2000; Haller and Hadler 2006; Jau and Hodgson 2018; Isham et al. 2006; Kubayashi and Kerbo 2012; Pavani and Colombo 2024; Stavrova 2014; Zelizer 1996). Ideals calibrate attitudes through consistency maximizing, dissonance reduction, reasoning, reflection, and self-expression (Ajzen and Fishbein 2014; Crane et al. 2019; Fjellvang 2011; Wegener and Carlston 2014). The bases of ideals include evaluation, expectation, identity, intention, value, and worldviews (Fabrigar et al. 2014; Greenberg and Arndt 2012; Jennings and Russell 2019; Zunick et al. 2017; Wyer and Abbarracin 2014). Norms assimilate attitudes emanate from categorizing, communication, cultivation, enforcement, framing, instigation, institutionalization, labeling, mediatization, membership, modeling, narration, norming, nudging, partisanship, persuasion, sharing, social construction, social integration, social interaction, socialization, and typification (Arriaga et al. 2018; Dolch 2003; Harrington 2004; Heitmeyer and Reimund Anhut 2008; Klandermans and van Stekelenburg 2013; Kral 2019; Marcus et al. 2000; McPhail and Tucker 2003; Mizen 2015; O'Keefe 2002; Smith and Hamon 2012; Uzumceker and Akfirat 2024; S. Wong 2008). Further, norms assimilate attitude through adherence, attachment, compliance, conformity, depersonalization, discussion, exposure, identification, imitation, internalization, learning, matching, observation, participation, reasoning, and role-taking (Bjarnegard et al. 2019; Huddy 2013; Kolker 2004; Lahey and Waldman 2007; Markowitz 2001; Messner et al. 2013; Proctor and Niemeyer 2019; Stavrova 2014; Wahlstrom 2011; Zahnow et al. 2024). The bases of norms include appropriateness, culture, definitions, feedback, frames, media, myths, narrative, programs, regulations, rules, and rumors (Jensen 2007; Klandermans and van Stekelenburg 2013; Mahoney 2021; Navarra et al. 2018; Proctor and Niemeyer 2019; Therborn 2002; Van Ness and Summers-Effler 2016; Wahlstrom 2011; R. Ward 2002).

Sociality

Sociality means living in a group or society, thus involving related attitudes, behaviors, and personality (Cottrell et al. 2007; Tomasello 2014). Inherently, sociality realizes ethics, goodness, humanity, and morality for social living (Fowers 2015). They feature communality, eudaimonia or flourishing, and sacrifice. Principally, sociality displays construction and withdraws destruction to society (Hughes et al.

2017). Construction to society comprises cooperation, honoring, leadership, support, sympathy, and teaching. Destruction to society comprises autonomy, forfeiting, instalocking or non-cooperating and non-consulting, raging or aggression, stealing, and trolling. Similarly, sociality withdraws individualism, which features independence and self-interest (Fowers 2015). Besides, sociality takes assortative or discriminate, collective, embodied, and moral forms (Boer and Fischer 2013; Cottrell et al. 2007; Fowers 2015; Sunar 2009; Tomasello 2020). Accordingly, sociality favors similarity, collectivity, and morality. Notably, embodied sociality means body integrity, which keeps the body appropriate, healthy, or functioning (Sunar 2009). Embodied sociality thus necessitates good food and sexuality to optimize nutrition and avoid depletion, exhaustion, and risk (Cohen and Fromme 2002; Sunar 2009). Sociality also features second-personality, comprising accountability or responsibility, commitment, fairness, and respect (Tomasello 2019). According to the analytical-functionalist framework, these features engage the four requisite functions of fulfillment or goal attainment, adaptation, latency, and integration. The voluntaristic mechanisms of the framework specify power, utility, and norms for achieving the four functions, including maintaining social attitudes. Power rests on direction, energy, motivation, and structure to drive social attitudes through realization. Utility means benefit, gain, and reward to attract social attitudes through optimization. Ideals include beliefs, thoughts, and values to rationalize social attitudes through calibration. Norms signify collective or extrapersonal ideals to assimilate social attitudes through conformity.

Power provided by sociality for the fulfillment or goal attainment function grows from the sociality features of accountability or responsibility, assertiveness, attachment, bonding, collective identity, commitment, conscientiousness, emotional stability, extraversion, friendship, gregariousness, group membership, guilt, health, leadership, participation, punishment, relatedness, self-expansion, and shame (Boer and Fischer 2013; Capraro 2024; Cottrell et al 2007; Fowers 2015; Hughes et al. 2017; Koster 2013; Tomasello 2014). Conversely, power discouraged by sociality rests on autonomy and raging (Fowers 2015; Hughes et al. 2017). Accountability or responsibility secures power in adulthood, agency, control, courage, empowerment, and social cohesion (Cheng and Huang 2017; Hoare 2002; Lawler and Thye 2006; Wildemeersch 2014). With the power, accountability or responsibility has withdrawn acceptance of outsiders (Granzin and Olsen 1998). Conversely, accountability or responsibility can dismiss violence (Milner and Myers 2007). Thus, accountability or responsibility would diminish justification for misdeeds. Assertiveness exerts power in dissent, initiation, and refusal (Paluck et al. 2009; Santos-Iglesias et al. 2013). With such power, assertiveness has reduced risking (Morokoff et al. 2009). Hence, assertiveness would downplay the acceptance of deviants and justification for misdeeds and sexuality. Attachment secures power through social integration (Rippl et al. 2010). With such power, attachment has induced confidence in economic and political institutions, including its voting practice (Kentmen 2010; Mayda and Rodrik 2005; Straughn and Andriot 2011). Bonding expresses power in flourishing and resourcefulness as opposed to experienced oppression (Comstock et al. 2008; Pangallo et al. 2015). With such power, bonding has buttressed confidence and discouraged crime (Hoffmann 2023; Zheng and Gan 2018). Thus, bonding would also dismiss justification for misdeeds and acceptance of deviants. Collective identity provides power through emotional discharge, relating, and sharing (Rudd and Hughes 2020; Stets 2010). With such power, collective identity champions ingroup favoritism and outgroup or outsider rejection (Paquin and Keating 2017). Social commitment can display power through affection and aggression (Guerrero 2015; Lawler et al. 2016). With such power, social commitment has furnished morality (Van Kenhove et al. 2003). Hence, social commitment would refute misdeeds and reject deviants. Conscientiousness embodies integrity and maturity or adulthood (Caprara and Vecchione 2013; Sirgy 2012). The power displayed in conscientiousness rests on achievement orientation, competence, control, courage, industriousness, persistence, striving, and tenacity (Ackerman and Wolman 2007; Hannah et al. 2007; Roberts et al. 2009; Wright and DeLisi 2016). With such power, conscientiousness has diminished justification for unconventional sexuality (de Jong et al. 2012). Emotional stability entails emotional power (Village and Francis 2010). With such power, emotional stability has enabled social acceptance and withdrawal from crime or misdeeds (Mullet et al. 2005; Pulkkinen et al. 2009). Hence, emotional stability would prompt the rejection of deviants. Extraversion, which includes gregariousness, demonstrates power through activeness, ambition, assertiveness, boldness, enthusiasm, and liveliness (Foschi and Lauriola 2014; J. Sun et al. 2018; Witt and Revelle 2009). With such power, extraversion has supported confidence in civic and political institutions (Peterson and Maiden 1993). Friendship represents soft power, social capital, and social support (Greene 1991; Koerner 2018; Wuthnow 2002). Furthermore, friendship offers power through affection and companionship as support (Filip et al. 2006; Sharabany 1994). With such power, friendship has boosted social trust (Kende et al. 2022). Group membership represents collective power (Shah and Scheufele 2006). Furthermore, group membership delivers power through activeness, activation, competence, and expression (Andreouli and Figgou 2019; Bendek 2002; Mihailidis and Thevenin 2013; Shah and Scheufele 2006). Guilt raises emotional power to become normative and redress sin (Pinhey and Perez 2000; Stets et al. 2008; J. Turner 2015). Hence, guilt would prop refutation against misdeeds and rejection of deviants. Health maintains power in terms of capability (Lelli 2008). With this power, health has facilitated confidence in the medical institution and social trust (Ahern and Hendryx 2003; Yu and Chiu 2016). Leadership represents power for management (Fitch et al. 2011). Such power comprises coercion, expertise, information, legitimacy, respect or referral, and reward (Haslam et al. 2011). Hence, leadership can share power (Gordon 2011). With such power, leadership in a person has reduced the person's antisocial and risky attitudes (Reitan and Stenberg 2019). Hence, leadership would diminish justification for misdeeds and sexuality and acceptance of deviants. Social participation represents the power of social capital (Saegert and Winkel 2004). Such power transpires in social empowerment, helping, influence, maintenance, sharing, and support (Christens et al. 2011; Heckscher 2015; Yetim and Yetim 2014). With this power, social participation enables trust (Rochelle 2015). Punishment expresses power through coercion and exclusion (Corlett 2006; Molm 1997). With this power, punishing others represents education, moral development and responsibility, and protection to fight crime (Aiken 2002; Birkett 2014; Corlett 2006). As such, punishment would dismiss misdeeds and deviants and favor the educational institution. Relatedness registers the power of passion, empowerment, and social capital (Kipnis 2002; Lenz 2016). Moreover, relatedness features attachment, commitment, friendship, and security, which are power providers (Hample 2018; Koerner 2018). With such power, relatedness sustains social stability (Fingerman et al. 2011). As such, relatedness would stabilize confidence in institutions, which functions to maintain social stability. Self-expansion to integrate with others delivers power through friendship, inclusion, liking, love, and partnership (Aron et al. 2006; Sivami 2016; Stanton et al. 2020; R. Turner et al. 2007). With such power, self-expansion advances morality (Gino and Galinsky 2012). Hence, self-expansion would prompt refutation against misdeeds and rejection of deviants. Shame displays emotional power in repression and self-protection to maintain acceptability or likability (Cosic et al. 2018; Kekes 2006). With such power, shame has enhanced morality and prosocial behavior as opposed to stealing (Blackwell and Eschholz 2002; McCaffoee 2016). Therefore, shame would uphold refutation against misdeeds and rejection of deviants. Conversely, autonomy conveys power to oneself rather than others through individualizing (Regalia et al. 2013). As such, autonomy can reduce confidence in the political and welfare institutions through individualizing (Gilens 1999; Wang and You 2016). Raging represents exerting power against others (Petkanopoulou et al. 2019). With such power, raging has engendered acting out, dehumanizing, and hostility (Pacilli et al. 2018; Roeser et al. 2002; Vandervoort 2006). Hence, raging would sustain justification for misdeeds and mistrust of others.

Utility offered by sociality for the adaptation function transmits from altruism, caring, cooperation, fairness or justice, honesty, honoring or respect, investment, morality, reciprocity, sacrificing, sharing, support, sympathy, trust, and trustworthiness (Capraro 2024; Fowers 2015; Hughes et al. 2017; Tomasello 2019, 2020). Conversely, disutility imposed by sociality stems from aggression, destruction, forfeiting, and stealing (Fowers 2015; Hughes et al. 2017). Altruism means providing utility to others (Singer 2001). With such utility provision, altruism has upheld confidence in the welfare institution (Rasinski et al. 1994). Caring means providing utility through empowering, love, protection, support, volunteering, and working to maintain harmony (Fine 2007; P. Ip 2014; Tracy 2002; Wuthnow 2004). Such utility covers sympathy and warmth (Baldner et al. 2020; Fine 2007). With this utility provision, caring has strengthened faith in religion (Kramer and Lambert 1999). Cooperation reflects altruism (Batson and Moran 1999). Specifically, cooperation happens in giving, investing, and rewarding (Brewer 1996; Hilbig et al. 2013; Sanderson 2001). Cooperation has propped attachment to the community (Tak 2017). Hence, cooperation would maintain trust in others. Fairness or justice provides utility through caring, compassion, compensation, and harmony (Cohrs et al. 2013; Galvin et al. 2018; S. Li 2014; S. Williams 2008). With such utility provision, fairness or justice generates confidence in legal and political institutions (Chang et al. 2013). Besides, fairness or justice has boosted morality and prosocial behavior (Barber 2004; McCaffoee 2016). Hence, fairness or justice would sustain refutation against misdeeds and rejection of deviants. Honesty provides utility through prosocial behavior (Thielmann et al.

2020). With this utility provision, honesty has reduced sexuality and violence (Lee and Ashton 2012; Thielmann et al. 2020). Hence, honesty would dismiss justification for misdeeds and sexuality and acceptance of deviants. Honoring or respect can involve paying as utility giving (Radford and Bloch 2012). With this utility provision, honoring or respect has maintained the rejection of deformity or deviance (Swami et al. 2009). Investment means utility provision through funding (Croy et al. 2010). With such utility provision, investment has indicated confidence in the welfare institution (Kluegel and Miyano 1995). Morality provides utility through altruism, beneficence, benevolence, caring, charity, collaboration, cooperation, generosity, honesty, hospitality, justice, love, respect, and sacrifice (Carmeli et al. 2017; de Jonge 2012; Hookway 2019; Killen 2018; Mihailov 2023; Stavrova and Siegers 2014). With such utility provision, morality has raised confidence in the political institution (Alvarez and Brehm 2002). Moreover, morality has reduced violence (Piquero and Hickman 2002). Hence, morality would buttress refutation against misdeeds and rejection of deviants. Morality also dismisses lewdness and obscenity (McCaffoee 2016). Thus, morality would underpin refutation against unconventional sexuality. Reciprocity represents utility sharing based on justice and respect (Mason 2012; Moss 2014; Reininger et al. 2020). With such utility sharing, reciprocity has underlain prosocial behavior (Thielmann et al. 2020). Hence, reciprocity would diminish justification for misdeeds and acceptance of deviants. Sacrificing represents utility provision through rewarding and returning favors based on morality and prosociality (Antoni and Grimalda 2024; Gino and Galinsky 2012; Molm 1997; Stagnaro et al. 2017). Sacrificing has upheld faith in religion and prevented violence (Day 2010). The latter would dampen justification for misdeeds and acceptance of deviants. Sharing involves utility in economic and information forms (Kas et al. 2022; Labrecque 2014). Sharing represents prosocial behavior and virtue (H. Ding et al. 2021). Hence, sharing would uphold refutation against misdeeds and rejection of deviants. Support, involving caring, collaboration, contribution, cooperation, helping, and sharing, represents utility provision based on altruism (Luria et al. 2019; Matts et al. 2009; Premo et al. 2018; Stagnaro et al. 2017; K. Zhao et al. 2017). With such utility provision, support has enhanced confidence in the welfare institution and faith in religion (Marsh and Dik 2021; Rasinski et al. 1994). Sympathy provides utility through a desire to help (Peplak and Malti 2022). With this utility, sympathy has propelled prosocial behavior (Clobert et al. 2015). Hence, sympathy would sustain refutation against misdeeds and rejection of deviants. Trust offers utility covering resources through cooperativeness, favor, investment, and kindness (Bellemare and Kroger 2007; Lewicki and Polin 2013; B. Six 2014). With such utility provision, trust has maintained confidence in institutions (Delhey et al. 2011). Trustworthiness offers utility based on social capital (X. Chen et al. 2015). Moreover, trustworthiness has reflected cooperation (Gerbasi and Cook 2008). With this utility provision, trustworthiness has engendered fair or just behavior (Molm et al. 2003). Hence, trustworthiness would dispel justification for misdeeds. Conversely, aggression generates disutility through anger, antisocial behavior, crying, harming, hijacking, intransigence, and tension (Eatough et al. 2008; Emjaian et al. 2018; Nassauer 2019; Spitzberg 2013; Pulkkinen 2018). Aggression has also preceded crime (Tanner-Smith et al. 2013). With such disutility, aggression has maintained justification for misdeeds and acceptance of deviants (Markowitz 2001). Destruction represents disutility through antisocial influence and resistance (Dolinski 2016; Ewick and Silbey 2003). Such antisocial disutility provision justifies misdeeds and acceptance of deviants (S. Henry 2009). Forfeiting or stealing generates disutility in terms of property (J. Brown 2016). Forfeiting or stealing reflects justification for misdeeds (Ingram and Hinduja 2008).

Ideals promulgated by sociality for the latency function evolve from communication, conservation, group focus, open-mindedness, social interaction, teaching, and tolerance (Capraro 2024; Cottrell et al. 2007; Fenwick 2008; T. Johnson et al. 2013; Phithakkitnukoon and Smoreda 2016). Conversely, ideals opposed by sociality are individualism, misanthropy, and risking (Bissell 2010; Fowers 2015). Individualism emphasizes independence, individual identity, and self-interest (Fowers 2015). Communication embraces or reflects ideals for closeness, collaboration, communality, empathy, equality, openness, peacefulness, reconciling, regard, respect, sharing, togetherness, and transparency (Burgoon et al. 2010; Kelley et al. 2019; Klyukanov 2021; Mirivel 2014; Pressgrove et al. 2020; Reavy 2023; Sanders 2009; Stoker 2020; J. Wood 2015). Communality is prosocial and sharing (Dovidio et al. 2006; Kayabol et al. 2022). Empathy sustains prosocial behavior and faith in religion (Fraser et al. 2012; Ishii and Watanable 2023). Furthermore, empathy highlights boundaries, differentiation, and distinction (Manassis 2017). This highlight would activate the rejection of outsiders. Togetherness manifests friendship (R. Turner et al. 2007). The ideal for equality or egalitarianism has boosted confidence in political and welfare institutions (Faricy and Ellis 2014; Roosma et al. 2014). Accordingly, egalitarianism demonstrates welfarism or the preference for social welfare (Moss 2014). Peacefulness exhibits morality and legality as opposed to conflict (Arat and Kerelian 2019; G. Zhang 2006). Hence, peacefulness would maintain refutation against misdeeds and rejection of deviants. Transparency functions to uphold social integration and trust (Erkkila 2012). Notably, communication incorporates trust (Klyukanov 2021). With these ideals, communication has buttressed confidence in civic and political institutions and social trust (Miyata et al. 2008; Rothstein and Uslaner 2005). Conservation conveys ideals for conformity, continuity, security, and stability (Bender and Cnaiotis 2011; J. Parker et al. 2020). Essentially, conservation reflects the ideal of conservatism (M. Ma 2021). Conservatism has maintained confidence in institutions (Feinberg et al. 2019). Moreover, conservatism exhibits faith in religion and rejection of outsiders (Malka and Soto 2011; Rhodes-Purdy et al. 2023). With these ideals, conservation has fostered confidence in the civic institution and reduced violence (Pulkkinen et al. 2009; Wernet et al. 2005). Hence, conservation would discourage justification for misdeeds and acceptance of deviants. Group focus opposes the ideal of individualism (Fine 2012). Individualism rejects confidence in institutions (Lowndes and Roberts 2013). Hence, individualism has dampened confidence in the political institution and faith in religion (Pollack and Pickel 2007; Wang and You 2016). Furthermore, individualism can breed crime and violence (Stott et al. 2017; Vander Ven and Colvin 2013). Individualism thus would maintain acceptance of deviants and justification for misdeeds. Hence, group focus has reflected confidence in institutions (Greenwood 2008). Open-mindedness reflects the ideal of openness (Draper and Holman 2005). Openness has bred confidence in the civic institution and prosocial motivation (Howard and Alipour 2014). Hence, openness or open-mindedness would maintain refutation against misdeeds and rejection of deviants. Social interaction realizes the ideal of communitarianism (H. Lu et al. 2002). Communitarianism displays confidence in institutions and trust (Frazer 1999). Moreover, communitarianism emphasizes ethnicity (Delanty 2009). Communitarianism, thus, would support the rejection of outsiders. Hence, social interaction has fostered social trust (Guillen et al. 2011). Teaching champions ideals for loyalty and morality as opposed to violence (Bachkirova and Cox 2007; Sinha 2013). With these ideals, teaching would establish confidence in institutions, refutation against misdeeds, and rejection of deviants. Tolerance embraces faith in religion (Lubis and Sianipar 2022). With the ideal, tolerance has facilitated confidence in the welfare institution and social trust (Barker and Tinnick 2006; Uslaner 2002). Nonetheless, sociality underlies the ideals of ethnocentrism and xenophobia through the assortative strand (M. Ma 2021). Ethnocentrism or xenophobia exhibits the rejection of outsiders (Nijs et al. 2022). Conversely, misanthropy is mistrust, thus weakening trust in others (T. Smith 1997). Risking suffers from legalism (Y. Zhang 2005). Moreover, risking involves sexual risk (Tyson et al. 2014). Hence, risking would induce acceptance of deviants and justification for misdeeds and sexuality.

Norms highlighted by sociality for the integration function accrue from conformity, consulting, dependence, imitation, learning, normativity, and role-taking (Capraro 2024; Fowers 2015; Hughes et al. 2017). Conformity reflects norms for authority, citizenship, morality, order, and virtue (Kaurin 2020). With the norms, conformity emphasizes government, justice, and medicine (Belkin and Kong 2022; Klingle 2004; Skitka et al. 2915). Citizenship exhibits exclusivity, loyalty, morality, nationalism, piety, respect, and trust (Blanchard 2000; Edyvane 2017; Elliott 2003; Hudson 2023; Mason 2012; Williamson 2002). Conversely, citizenship opposes the antisocial norm (Bannister and O'Sullivan 2013). Hence, citizenship has maintained confidence in the political institution (Vera-Toscano et al. 2013). Citizenship would also buttress faith in religion, refutation against misdeeds, and rejection of deviants and outsiders. The norm for order has incubated confidence in the business institution (Costa et al. 2023). Hence, conformity has enhanced confidence in institutions and discouraged violence (Schwartz et al. 2014). Conformity thus would undermine the acceptance of deviants and justification for misdeeds. Consulting, imitation, or learning reflects norms for culturalism and institutionalism (R. Thomas 1997; Zurbriggen 2013). With the norms, learning has generated confidence in political and welfare institutions and faith in religion (Roosma et al. 2016; Immerzeel and van Tubergen 2013). Hence, learning would support confidence in institutions. Normativity displays norms for the elite, law, morality, nativism, and voting (Bolet 2023; Nilsson et al. 2020; Xia 2021; Zechmeister 2006). Nativism features the rejection of outsiders (Macedo 2021). With the norms, normativity has reflected the rejection of outsiders (Bolet 2023). Moreover, normativity would enhance confidence in the political institution, refutation against misdeeds, and rejection of deviants.

Sociality also directly or holistically generates power, utility, ideals, and norms to maintain social attitudes. This generation leverages the voluntaristic mechanisms of analytical functionalism to complete the functions of fulfillment, adaptation, latency, and integration. Power generated by sociality to enable sociality-oriented attitudes rests on morality and socializability (Sunar 2009). Morality means optimizing well-being for all (Lakoff 2009). As such, morality has nurtured faith in religion (Matsuba and Walker 2004). Socialization has fostered trust (K. Scott et al. 2012). Sociality also evolves from power derived from social intelligence and needs to tackle stress and uncertainty to facilitate sociality-oriented attitudes (Boer and Fischer 2013; Fowers 2015). Utility created by sociality to attract sociality-oriented attitudes involves pleasure, the satisfaction of needs, and well-being generally (Falk 2018; Spilka et al. 2003). Moreover, utility evolves from utility based on collaboration, exchange, and interdependence to attract sociality-oriented attitudes (Fowers 2015). Ideals raised by sociality to rationalize sociality-oriented attitudes characterize conservatism, religiosity, and solidarity (Fenwick 2008; M. Ma 2021; Spilka et al. 2003). Sociality also evolves from ideals for homophily, social categorization, and social interaction to rationalize sociality-oriented attitudes (Cottrell et al. 2007; Phithakkitnukoon and Smoreda 2016; Fowers 2015). Conversely, sociality erodes ideals for radicalism (Winter and Feixas 2019). In addition, norms reflected by sociality to assimilate sociality-oriented attitudes popularize or constitute caring and learning (Fowers 2015).

Morality and solidarity are the manifestations of sociality, which display sociality-oriented attitudes. Besides upholding all people's well-being, morality means culturally informed social conduct amid group or social living to regulate relationship quality (Cast and Stets 2016; Kesebir and Kesebir 2012). Such social emphasis is consonant with sociality (Tomasello 2014). Morality means the obverse of selfishness (Kesebir and Kesebir 2012). Solidarity means upholding common or communal interests to maintain social order (Alharbi and Rucker 2023; Lawler et al. 2009). This maintenance builds on affect, orientation, and resilience to unify the social entity (Lawler et al. 2009).

Morality reflects the power bases of attachment, cooperation need, security, and social connection to drive sociality-oriented attitudes (Koppel and Fondacaro 2017; Lucas and Livingston 2014; Narvaez 2014; R. Thompson 2020). Attachment features confidence, loyalty, maintenance, nationalism, and trust (Gillath et al. 2016; Shemmings 2006; Straughn and Andriot 2011). These features would constitute confidence in institutions and social trust. Hence, attachment has supported confidence in economic and political institutions (Kentmen 2010; Mayda and Rodrik 2005; Straughn and Andriot 2011). Cooperation favors the ingroup (Sidanius and Kurzban 2013). Conversely, cooperation dismisses crime, revolution, and violence (Sanderson 2001). These features would underpin refutation against misdeeds and rejection of deviants and outsiders. Moreover, cooperation has secured confidence in the community institution (Tak 2017). Security involves nationalism and patriotism (Raijman and Hochman 2011). Such involvement would strengthen confidence in institutions. As such, nationalism has underlain confidence in political, welfare, and other institutions and rejecting outsiders (N. Chen 2012; Huddy et al. 2021; Jost 2020; Sumino

2013). Similarly, patriotism has warranted confidence in political and welfare institutions and rejection of outsiders (Gross et al. 2004; Heinemann 2008; Ishii 2009). Social connection emphasizes the group, primarily family and friends (H. Li et al. 2006). This emphasis would discount the acceptance of outsiders.

Morality represents utility as relational quality to attract sociality-oriented attitudes (R. Thomas 1997). Similarly, morality evolves from utility derived from interdependence and social support received to attract sociality-oriented attitudes (Killen 2018). Relationship quality features attachment, closeness, friendship, security, and sharing (Hample 2018; Koerner 2018; Mikulincer and Shaver 2018; Van Lear et al. 2006). Conversely, relationship quality dismisses aggression and otherness or foreignness (Comstock et al. 2008; Littlejohn et al. 2017). These features would consolidate social trust, refutation against misdeeds, and rejecting deviants and outsiders. Interdependence implies caring, coordination, friendship, intimacy, and social interaction (Heckscher 2015; Lo and Bettinger 2009; Rokach 2019; Wickham and Knee 2012). These implications would secure social trust. Similarly, interdependence generates attachment, cohesion, compliance, conformity, cooperation, discrimination, group identification, and intimacy (Johnson and Johnson 2005; Levitt and Cici-Gokaltun 2011; Skitka et al. 2014; Z. Xin et al. 2017). Such generations would establish confidence in institutions, social trust, and rejection of outsiders. Likewise, interdependence features cooperation, coordination, exchange, harmony, and relatedness (Johnson and Johnson 2005). These features would consolidate social trust. Furthermore, interdependence has enhanced attachment (Z. Xin et al. 2017). Attachment has facilitated confidence in economic and political institutions (Herrmann et al. 2009; Mayda and Rodrik 2005). Social support reception reflects citizenship and social capital (Godoy et al. 2007; Tsai et al. 2018). Citizenship has underlain confidence in the political institution (Vera-Toscano et al. 2013). Social capital has enabled confidence in institutions and social trust (Chua et al. 2021; Narayan and Cassidy 2001). Social support reception engenders attachment, conformity, exchange, love, and togetherness (Feeney and Collins 2018; Filip et al. 2006; Tomlinson et al. 2018). Such engendering would safeguard confidence in institutions and social trust. Similarly, social support reception features attachment, caring provided and received, friendship, and networking (Baptista et al. 2021; Collins et al. 2011; Glendinning et al. 2003; Patulny and Morris 2012). With these features, social support received has bred social trust (Steinhardt 2012).

Morality represents such ideals as group living, regulation or self-regulation, and social conduct to rationalize sociality-oriented attitudes (Besser-Jones 2012; Boer and Fischer 2013; Kesebir and Kesebir 2012; R. Thomas 1997). Group living would heighten ingroup favoritism and rejection of outsiders (Fischer et al. 2007). Regulation has reduced risking, crime, and violence (Y. Cheung et al. 2014; Koegl and Day 2019; Welch et al. 2008). Hence, regulation would dampen justification for misdeeds and sexuality and acceptance of deviants. Social conduct has underlain social trust (Guillen et al. 2011). Moreover, morality stands on the ideals of communitarianism, evolutionism, institutionalism, and traditionalism to rationalize sociality-oriented attitudes (Gibbs 2014; R. Hall et al. 2000; Hookway 2017). Communitarianism features confidence in institutions, loyalty, and trust (Delanty 2009; Frazer

1999). Evolutionism supports confidence in institutions for distribution, education, production, regulation, and reproduction (J. Turner et al. 2020). Institutionalism highlights confidence in institutions, faith in religion, and law (A. Hu 2013; Lytkina and Reeskens 2025; Peters and Pierre 2020). Hence, institutionalism would denounce the acceptance of deviants and justification for misdeeds. Traditionalism has underlain confidence in economic and political institutions, refutation against unconventional sexuality, and rejection of outsiders (Costa et al. 2023; Meuleman et al. 2019; Schwartz et al. 2010; Wang and You 2016). Morality also features the ideals for citizenship, obedience, law, loyalty, piety, religion, the state or statism, solidarity, trust, and unity to rationalize sociality-oriented attitudes (N. Duncan 2017; Haidt 2012; Jagger 2000; McCaffoee 2016; Mott 2011; Skitka et al. 2014; Talaifar and Swann 2019; Welch 2000). These features would constitute confidence in institutions and faith in religion. Notably, statism emphasizes confidence in the state or political institution, covering the functions of bounding, development, servicing, taxing, and welfare provision (Biersteker 2013). The ideal for unity advances attachment, liking, love, and relating (Ledbetter et al. 2013; Sivami 2016; Tomlinson et al. 2018). Therefore, this ideal would underlain social trust. Morality also evolves from ideals for business, cooperation, group identity, group-mindedness, religiosity or religious faith, sharing, social interaction, and trust to strengthen sociality-oriented attitudes (N. Duncan 2017; Killen 2018; Lucas and Livingston 2014; Narvaez 2014; Patwardhan et al. 2012; Vitell et al. 2007). These ideals would hence foster confidence in institutions, faith in religion, social trust, and rejection of outsiders. Conversely, morality rationalizes sociality-oriented attitudes by rejecting the ideals of individualism, lewdness, lust, obscenity, and violence (McCaffoee 2016; Mott 2011; Pickard 2010; Rachels and Rachels 2015). By discounting these features, morality would erode acceptance of deviants and justification for misdeeds and sexuality. Therefore, morality has prevented violence (Piquero and Hickman 2002).

Morality stems from social norms for collectivism, generosity, morality or ethicality, and religiosity to dictate sociality-oriented attitudes (Gino and Galinsky 2012; Narvaez 2014). Collectivism has strengthened confidence in the political institution (J. Lu 2014). Moreover, collectivism features faith in religion and ingroup favoritism (Braun 2011; Triandis 1995). Hence, collectivism would breed rejection of the outsiders. As a social norm, collectivism has raised confidence in institutions (McAllister 1999). Generosity has sustained faith in religion and reduced violence (Day 2010; Messner et al. 2008). Hence, generosity would dampen justification for misdeeds and acceptance of deviants. The norm for religiosity has boosted faith in religion (Stavrova and Siegers 2014).

Solidarity represents power for driving sociality-oriented attitudes through communication, participation, and trust (Alharbi and Rucker 2023; Laurence 2011). Communication gathers power in terms of information or knowledge (Mcclurg 2006; Pressgrove et al. 2020). With such gathering, communication has enhanced social trust (Rothstein and Uslaner 2005). Participation has increased knowledge and induced empowerment experienced (Christens et al. 2011). Getting such power, participation has fostered trust (Rochelle 2015). Solidarity maintains power for driving sociality-oriented attitudes through attachment, belongingness, closeness, empowerment, neighboring, social capital, sympathy, and understanding (Duhaime et al. 2004; La Grange 2011; Woosnam et al. 2018; Robinson 2005; Schiefer and van der Noll 2017; Woosnam et al. 2018). Attachment has raised such power as social capital and stress reduction (Curley 2010; Gillath et al. 2016). With such power, attachment has consolidated confidence in economic and political institutions (Herrmann et al. 2009; Mayda and Rodrik 2005). Belongingness has enhanced power through friendship (Eberl 2020). As such, belongingness promotes prosocial behavior (Dovidio et al. 2006). Hence, belongingness would enhance refutation against misdeeds and rejection of deviants. Closeness underlies exclusiveness, loyalty, and trust (Sharabany 1994). Therefore, closeness would maintain power facilitating confidence in institutions, rejection of outsiders, and social trust. Empowerment experienced engages community involvement (Zimmerman 1995). As such, empowerment would raise confidence in the community institution. Social capital has elevated confidence in institutions and social trust (Chua et al. 2021; Narayan and Cassidy 2001). Sympathy has reflected faith in religion (Brown and Ferris 2007). Understanding has facilitated confidence in institutions, rejection of outsiders, and social trust (Barker and Tinnick 2006; Pattie et al. 2004; Rose and Pettersen 2000).

Solidarity offers utility for attracting sociality-oriented attitudes through community and life quality, entertainment, equality, pleasantness, similarity, and uniformity (Berger-Schmitt 2002; de Beer and Kostere 2009; Duhaime et al. 2004; Lawler and Thye 2006; Paez et al. 2015; Turner and Maryanski 2005). Life quality has attracted social trust and confidence in the political institution (A. Hu 2013; Masters 2001). Such attraction represents utility optimization, such as based on reciprocity. Equality experienced can reduce crime and illegal behavior (Kyriacou 2020). As such, equality experienced would dampen acceptance of deviants and justification for misdeeds. Entertainment or pleasantness has sustained confidence in the political institution (Hunt et al. 2019). Representing utility, similarity is likable and satisfactory (Launay and Dunbar 2015; Wortman and Lucas 2016). Similarity or uniformity experienced has bred general trust and social trust (Volker and Flap 1997). Hence, similarity or uniformity experienced would enhance confidence in institutions. Solidarity has utility through social support received. Social support reception has facilitated general and social trust (Livingstone et al. 2023; Steinhardt 2012). Hence, social support received would sustain confidence in institutions.

Solidarity stands on the ideals of Christianity, communitarianism, localism, social integration, multiculturalism, nationalism, particularism, patriotism, prioritarianism, redistribution, social kinship, social democracy, and welfarism to rationalize sociality-oriented attitudes (Husband and Alam 2011; Dench 2006; Husband and Alam 2011; Janmaat 2011; Kolers 2016; Lawler et al. 2009; Robinson 2005; Schiefer and van der Noll 2017; Wills 2016). Christianity peaches salvaging and treating others as family members (Wills 2016). Christianity treasures faith in Jesus, love, and peace and opposes violence (Collier 2001; Reynolds 2015). As such, Christianity would uphold faith in religion, social trust, refutation against misdeeds, and rejecting deviants. Communitarianism extols care and order for the community (Robinson 2005). Notably, communitarianism features institutionalism, loyalty, nationalism, patriotism, self-discipline, and trust (Delanty 2009; Frazer 1999; Moore 2010). As such, communitarianism would buttress confidence in institutions, social trust, and refutation against unconventional sexuality. Localism emphasizes society as opposed to greater collectivity (Hickson 2013). As such, localism manifests the rejection of outsiders (Macedo 2021). Particularism highlights cultural differences (Janmaat 2011). Notably, particularism favors social relationships within a context (Spicker 2019). As such, particularism would dictate the rejection of outsiders. Social democracy advocates equality, redistribution, and welfare (Green and Janmaat 2011; Larsen 2013). Hence, social democracy would favor confidence in the welfare institution and social trust.

Conversely, solidarity opposes the ideals of capitalism, individualism, liberalism, libertarianism, neoliberalism, postmodernism, and rationalism for maintaining sociality-oriented attitudes (Dench 2006; Larsen 2013; Lawler et al. 2009; Loewy 1993; Semino 2015; Weissman 2000). Capitalism treasures social inequality (Loewy 1993). Furthermore, capitalism denounces statism (Bernstein 2012). Hence, capitalism would dampen confidence in the political institution. Individualism prioritizes distrust, self-interest, and instrumentalizing others (Lawler et al. 2009). Notably, individualism has reduced confidence in political and welfare institutions and acceptance of outsiders (Gilens 1999; Leong 2008; Wang and You 2016). Liberalism prefers autonomy and standing up as opposed to deference (Kolers 2016). As such, liberalism has discouraged confidence in institutions (Feinberg et al. 2019). Liberalism also prizes diversity, minorities, multiculturalism, and sexuality and opposes religious faith, morality, and the state (Gaus 2003; Kekes 1997; Ramsay 1997; Wright and Tokunaga 2018; Yoos 2007). As such, liberalism would also enhance acceptance of deviants and justification for misdeeds and sexuality. Libertarianism hails minimizing the state (Ellis et al. 2006). As such, libertarianism has eroded confidence in the political institution (Grasso 2014). Meanwhile, libertarianism has raised tolerance for deviance (Flanagan and Lee 2003). Libertarianism thus would diminish the rejection of deviants and outsiders. Neoliberalism opposes social equality (Semino 2015). Neoliberalism disregards morality and the state (Narayan 2020; Smart 2003). Hence, neoliberalism would discourage confidence in the political institution, refutation against misdeeds, and rejection of deviants. Postmodernism hails self-creation (Weissman 2000). Rationalism presumes self-interest (Larsen 2013). Notably, postmodernism supports anarchism and populism and doubts or opposes moralism, the political institution (Bowring 2011; Rosenau 1992). Hence, postmodernism would discourage confidence in the political institution, refutation against misdeeds, and rejecting deviants. Solidarity upholds the ideals of collectivism or group orientation, republicanism, and volunteerism (de Beer and Kostere 2009; Phillips 2006; Sturm 1998). Collectivism has espoused confidence in the political institution (J. Lu 2014). Moreover, collectivism consolidates faith in religion (Braun 2011). Republicanism emphasizes fraternity (Green and Janmaat 2011). As such, republicanism champions confidence in political and welfare institutions (Green and Janmaat 2011). Volunteerism has championed moral responsibility, social trust, and confidence in the political institution (Chappell and Prince 1997; Richey 2010; Richey and Ikeda 2009). Hence, volunteerism would sustain refutation against misdeeds and rejection of deviants. Solidarity also extols ideals for caring, commonality, commonweal, compliance, cooperation, generosity, gifting, loyalty, morality, mutuality, normativity, participation, preservation, reciprocity, redistribution, responsibility, sacrifice, sharing, social contribution, social control, social order, stability, and submissiveness to rationalize sociality-oriented attitudes (Avery et al. 2021; Collins 2004; Friedkin 2004; Helly 2003; Hogg 2007; Kolers 2016; Loewy 1993; Miranti and Evans 2019; Robinson 2005; Schiefer and van der Noll 2017; Thijssen 2016; Tolsma et al. 2009; Uzzell et al. 2002; Wilde 2004; Wills 2016; Yuki 2003). Caring has consolidated faith in religion (Kramer and Lambert 1999). Moreover, caring represents prosocial behavior and virtue (Matts et al. 2009). Hence, caring would enhance refutation against misdeeds and rejection of deviants. Likewise, commonality, commonweal, generosity, gifting, sacrifice, or sharing represents prosocial behavior and virtue (H. Ding et al. 2021; M. Wang et al. 2014). Thus, this representation would uphold refutation against misdeeds and rejection of deviants. Compliance or submissiveness has supported confidence in the political institution and rejection of outsiders (Schwartz et al. 2014; Van Hootegem et al. 2000). Moreover, compliance represents virtue (Kaurin 2020). Hence, compliance would espouse refutation against misdeeds and rejection of deviants. Cooperation has maintained confidence in the community institution (Tak 2017). Loyalty upholds confidence in the political institution (J. Fan et al. 2022b). Morality has underlain confidence in the political institution (Alvarez and Brehm 2002). Mutuality or reciprocity has upheld prosocial behavior (Thielmann et al. 2020). Hence, mutuality or reciprocity would dampen justification for misdeeds and acceptance of deviants. Normativity has reflected the rejection of outsiders (Bolet 2023). Participation has increased knowledge and induced empowerment (Christens et al. 2011). Hence, participation has fostered trust (Rochelle 2015). Preservation or stability has sustained confidence in the civic institution and reduced violence (Pulkkinen et al. 2009; Wernet et al. 2005). Moreover, conservatism as the ideal for preservation or stability has secured confidence in institutions (Feinberg et al. 2019). The ideal for redistribution has reflected faith in religion and social trust (Nagayoshi and Sato 2014). Responsibility has eroded the acceptance of outsiders (Granzin and Olsen 1998). Social contribution involves trust (Stets et al. 2018). Thus, social contribution would sustain confidence in institutions and social trust. Social control experienced has fostered confidence in the political institution, refutation against misdeeds, and rejection of deviants (Overall et al. 2020). The ideal for social order has bred confidence in the business institution (Costa et al. 2023). Solidarity engages religious faith and trust (Green and Janmaat 2011; Moskalenko et al. 2007).

Conversely, solidarity dismisses ideals for aggression or violence, competition, and incivility to maintain sociality-oriented attitudes (Kolers 2016; Loewy 1993; McGhee 2003). Solidarity has dampened tolerance (Stafford et al. 2005). As such, solidarity would erode justification for misdeeds and acceptance of deviants and outsiders. Competition has raised individualism and diminished volunteering (Bobo and Hutchings 1996; Martinez and McMullin 2004). Individualism has eroded confidence in political and welfare institutions and faith in religion (Pollack and Pickel 2007; Wang and You 2016). Volunteering has championed social trust and confidence in the political institution and reduced tolerance (Richey 2010; Richey and Ikeda

2009; Woolley 2003). Incivility has impeded confidence in the welfare institution (Clemence 2001).

Solidarity conveys norms for Buddhism, Christianity, Confucianism, Islam, Judaism, and socialization to assimilate sociality-oriented attitudes (Green and Janmaat 2011; Karuppannan and Sivam 2011). Buddhism accentuates compassion (Sturm 1998). Furthermore, Buddhism prioritizes discipline and morality and opposes violence (Hocksmann 2004; Orjuela 2020). Hence, Buddhism would uphold faith in religion, refutation against misdeeds and sexuality, and rejecting deviants. Christianity hails love (Sturm 1998). Moreover, Christianity upholds peace and opposes violence (Collier 2001). Christianity has also opposed moral permissiveness (Hollinger 2017). Hence, Christianity would secure faith in religion, refutation against misdeeds, and rejecting deviants. Confucianism highlights peace, respect, and stability (Green and Janmaat 2011; Sturm 1998). Furthermore, Confucianism extols discipline, hierarchy, loyalty, moralism, righteousness, and the state and opposes violence (Hocksmann 2004; Le Monkhouse et al. 2013; Y. Lin et al. 2021; Peng 2003; Woo 2008). Hence, Confucianism would cultivate confidence in institutions, refutation against misdeeds and sexuality, and rejecting deviants. Islam advocates peace (Sturm 1998). Furthermore, Islam valorizes authoritarianism, brotherhood, discipline, and divinity and opposes tolerance (Braun 2011; Esposito 2002; Scruton 2014; Verkuyten 2014). Therefore, Islam would secure confidence in institutions, faith in religion, refutation against misdeeds and sexuality, rejection of deviants and outsiders, and trust in others. Judaism extols justice (Sturm 1998). Furthermore, Judaism emphasizes prayer, submission, and worship and opposes sexuality (S. May 2011; Richards 2012; H. Smith 1991). Thus, Judaism would espouse confidence in institutions, faith in religion, and refutation against unconventional sexuality. Socialization experience fosters political allegiance, trust, and self-control and rejects delinquency (McDevitt 2018; K. Scott et al. 2012; J. Taylor et al. 2000). Thereby, socialization would enhance confidence in institutions, social trust, and refutation against misdeeds and sexuality.

Confidence in Institutions

Confidence signifies confirmation, evaluation, morale, satisfaction, and support (Assiter 2003; Cheung and Leung 2011; Y. Wu et al. 2019; P. Yue et al. 2020). Essentially, confidence is anticipatory acceptance (TenHouten 2007). Alternatively, confidence combines authority ranking, equality matching, and market pricing (TenHouten 2007). Authority ranking means deference for authority; equality matching means equal sharing; and market pricing means fairness. Furthermore, confidence implies resolution and human capital (Castro and Murray 2010; Strozier and Heppner 1991). An institution is an artificial collective or social arrangement that is constraining, continuing or persistent, formal, immaterial, self-preserving, and stable (Jupille and Caporaso 2022; Menon 2011; de Souza et al. 2023). Furthermore, an institution has habits, rules, structure, and values (Jupille and Caporaso 2022; Lista and Rojas 2018). As such, an institution means rules, resources, and skills combined (Jupille and Caporaso 2022). The institutional structure is encompassing, permeating, and ubiquitous (Jupille and Caporaso, 2022). From the analytical-functionalist perspective, institutions fulfill political, economic, cultural, and communal or civic functions. The political institution encompasses law (J. Turner 2017). The economic institution includes media or communication, medicine, and science (Holdo 2022; J. Turner 2017). The cultural institution includes arts, education, religion, and sports (J. Turner 2017). The civic institution includes kinship (J. Turner 2017). Overall, confidence in institutions represents institutionalism, which idealizes institutions.

Confidence is functional in generating power, utility, and ideals for achieving the functions of fulfillment or goal attainment, adaptation, and latency. First, confidence generates power in adulthood or maturity, capacity, and control or regulation (Bright 2018; Cochrane 2018; de Courville Nicol 2011). Moreover, confidence implies power in ability, effectiveness, and hardiness. And human capital (Castro and Murray 2010; Perry et al. 2013; L. Turner 2008). Second, confidence signifies utility in morale, resolution, and satisfaction as opposed to anxiety and distress (Carver and Scheier 2012; Cheung and Leung 2011; de Courville Nicol 2011; Strozier and Heppner 1991; Y. Wu et al. 2019). Confidence also fosters utility in benefit experienced, intimacy, security, and well-being (Elfenbein 2013; Nofziger and Williams 2005; Petronio and Durham 2015; Reeskens and Vandecasteele 2017). Third, confidence espouses ideals for confirmation, prevention, protection, responsibility, support, and trust as opposed to protesting (Atkeson and Maestas 2012; Assiter 2003; Bierhoff 2002; Dominitz and Manski 1997; Pires 2022; Quaranta 2016; Warner et al. 2022).

Confidence is a function of power, utility, and ideals based on their power realization, utility optimization, and ideal calibration mechanisms. First, confidence has evolved from power in inspiration provided, spirituality, social capital, and training (Cotterill 2017; Creed and Gagliardi 2015; MacDonald 2000). Second, confidence has benefited from utility based on achievement, miracles, and validation experienced (Cotterill 2017; De Graaf 2013). Third, confidence has arisen from ideals for perspiration, preparation, self-evaluation, and self-regulation (Cotterill 2017; Creed and Gagliardi 2015).

The institution is functional to sociality by providing power, utility, ideals, and norms to achieve the functions of fulfillment, adaptation, latency, and integration. With such provision, the institution is integral to sociality, including connection and relationships (Jupille and Caporaso 2022). Notably, the institution is a social arrangement for the social function of sociality (Jupille and Caporaso 2022).

The institution offers power in centralization, formality, guiding, motivation, structure, and superadditivity to drive sociality (Amenta 2005; Jupille and Caporaso 2022; Kalu 2019; Menon 2011). Superadditivity means that the sum of two is three or more (Kalu 2019). Centralization consolidates authority and resources to enable organization (Baofu 2009; Morgan 1997). Formality has enhanced sociality by raising consensus experienced, political interest, trust in government, and volunteering (E. Chan 2014; Ketelaars et al. 2017; Li and Ferraro 2006). Guidance received has promoted sociality regarding relationship quality (Lapan et al. 2001). Motivation underlies morality to facilitate sociality (Bretz and Sun 2018). Structure represents power for securing harmony (Haugaard 2003; P. Ip 2014).

As a social arrangement, the institution displays utility in efficiency and profit to attract sociality (de Souza et al. 2023; Moroni 2010). Profit has exhibited such attraction to sociality, including social participation and trust, as opposed to nimbyism (Grimes 2006; Islam et al. 2006; Spie et al. 1998).

The institution hails ideals for continuity, coordination, interdependency, linkage, networking, participation, persistence, preservation, stability, and support for rationalizing sociality (Jupille and Caporaso 2022; Kalu 2019). Continuity, persistence, preservation, or stability has secured sociality, including civic engagement, cohesion, neighboring, and relational quality, as opposed to violence (Pulkkinen et al. 2009; C. C. Ross et al. 2000; Swaroop and Morenoff 2006; Villarreal and Silva 2006). Stability and conservation characterize sociality (Boer and Fischer 2013; Cottrell et al. 2007). Coordination or linking has enhanced sociality regarding morality, prosocial behavior, and social capital (Halevy et al. 2019; J. Michael et al. 2020). Interdependency has strengthened sociality regarding attachment, cohesion, compliance, cooperation, exchange, group identity, and prosocial behavior (Buechler 2011; Gaertner and Dovidio 2012; Levitt and Cici-Gokaltun 2011; Skitka et al. 2014; Z. Xin et al. 2017). Networking has fostered sociality regarding connectedness, friendship, giving, and social interaction (Eberl 2020; Liebler and Sandefur 2002; Nelson-Coffey et al. 2023; Phan et al. 2009). Participation has consolidated sociality regarding cooperation, networking, social capital, and trust (Groves et al. 2000; Molitor et al. 2011; Rochelle 2015). Support has raised sociality regarding civility, connectedness, cooperation, protection, responsibility, and volunteering as opposed to loneliness (Dinic and Bodroza 2021; Hample 2018; Musick and Wilson 2008; Nelson-Coffey et al. 2023; Shahzalal and Adnan 2022). Moreover, the institution fosters ideals for adaptation, cooperation, compatibility, social identity, and rationality (Ferrara 2022; Jupille and Caporaso 2022; Kalu 2019). Adaptation has secured sociality regarding partnership, social adjustment, and satisfaction as opposed to discord (Chow et al. 2014; Mitchell 2005). Cooperation has strengthened sociality regarding attachment and trustworthiness as opposed to argument (Gerbasi and Cook 2008; Hample 2018; Tak 2017). Compatibility or fitness has raised sociality regarding attachment, prosocial behavior, and sharing (Becker and Clement 2006; Brown and Brown 2006; Tsaur et al. 2014). Social identity has buttressed sociality regarding cohesion (Fischer et al. 2007). Rationality has championed sociality by dampening aggression and antisociality (DiGiuseppe et al. 2017). The institution also displays ideals for authenticity, communication, contracting, morality, and mutual understanding to rationalize sociality (de Souza et al., 2023; Holdo, 2022; Shook and Giordano, 2017). Authenticity has fostered sociality regarding relational quality (Kernis and Goldman 2006). Communication has weaved sociality regarding social cohesion, participation, and trust (Miyata et al. 2008; Rothstein and Uslaner 2005). Contracting enhances sociality by embracing attachment, civic engagement, civility, compliance, compromise, consent, cooperation, coordination, equality, fairness, morality, and trust (Bowker 2016; Dalbert 2001; Darwall 2003; de Jonge 2012; Ellis et al. 2006; Gardiner 2009; Irwin 2016; Jarvinen and Branders 2020; Kaurin 2020). Morality has championed sociality by boosting volunteering and inhibiting violence (Piquero and Hickman 2002; Whitford et al. 2006). Understanding has raised sociality regarding civic engagement, community involvement, compliance, cooperation, prosocial behavior, protection, volunteering, and social cohesion and trust (de Groot and Steg 2009; Bish and Michie 2010; Hunter et al. 2013; Lepkowski and Couper 2002; Pattie et al. 2004; Sarkheyli et al. 2012; Simon-Bemd and Steffens 2000; Volker et al. 2007; Wernet et al. 2005). Conversely, the institution minimizes ideals for disruption, freedom, nepotism, opportunism, and social movement to sustain sociality (de Souza et al. 2023; Ferrara 2022; Goldstone and Useem 2012; Jupille and Caporaso 2022; Kalu 2019). Disruption has impaired sociality by raising antisocial behavior and delinquency and reducing community participation and preference for peers (Currie and Stabile 2009; Khamis 2006; Leflot et al. 2011). Freedom has undermined sociality by fomenting crime (Costello 2013). Liberalism as the ideal for freedom has also impeded sociality regarding morality (Feinberg et al. 2019). Nepotism can impair sociality by breeding conflict (Y. Kim 2013). Opportunism has impaired sociality by dampening agreeableness and cooperation (Sakalaki and Fousiani 2012). Social movement participation has impeded sociality by eroding moral motivation and religious faith (Kutlaca et al. 2020).

The institution issues norms through enforcement, isomorphism or mimesis, laws, orders, and rules to assimilate sociality (Jupille and Caporaso 2022; Kalu 2019; Lista and Rojas 2018). Such norms have upheld sociality by prohibiting radicalism (Muthuswamy 2022). Radicalism has undermined sociality by raising violence and diminishing collective practice and confidence in government (Achilov 2016; Levi and Strker 2000).

The institution builds on empowerment, incentivizing, framing, and normalizing to strengthen power, utility, ideals, and norms to function, as predicated on deterministic mechanisms of analytical-functionalist theory. Power functions to maintain the institution's equilibrium, evolutional functions for living and reproduction (Eastwood 2015; Ferrara 2022). Collective bargaining and economic and military power are crucial (Ferrara 2022). Conversely, shock is power disrupting the equilibrium. The institution also rests on human capital, including education (de Souza et al. 2023). Utility offered by the institution lies in sustaining living and reproduction or minimizing risks. As such, survival threat invokes the utility of the institution to reduce the threat (Eastwood 2015). Moreover, realizing the institution's capability buttresses utility for underpinning the institution (Ferrara 2022; Jupille and Caporaso 2022). Ideals upholding the institution include democracy, legitimacy, public choice or interest, social identity, and system justification (de Souza et al. 2023; Ferrara 2022; Mantzvavinos 2011). Legitimacy stands on ideals for order and morality successively (Ferrara 2022). Such morality can build on Buddhist, Christian, Confucian, Hindu, and Islamic ethics, highlighting duty, obedience, respect, and unity as opposed to freedom (Ferrara 2022). Meanwhile, order underlying legitimacy can suffer from injustice and oppression (Ferrara 2022). Conversely, alternatives to social identity and the instability of social identity inhibit the institution (Ferrara 2022). Furthermore, the regime as the superordinate environment furnishes the norm for the institution to follow (de Souza et al. 2023).

The ideal or ideological bases of the institution are those for efficiency, experimentalism, idealism, pragmatism, or progressivism (Ziegler 1994). Idealism valorizes absolutism or eternal truth, authority or authoritarianism, conservation, puritanism, and salvation (Ziegler 1994). Authoritarianism hails superior guidance. Puritanism mandates the community, the elite, and redemption. Experimentalism, pragmatism, or progressivism foregrounds adjustment, functioning or functionalism, knowledge, moralizing, resolution, and skill (Ziegler 1994). Adjustment emphasizes commonality, feasibility, and interdependence as opposed to dislocation. Functioning comprises administration, communication, counseling, education, energization, nurturing, policymaking, procreation, resolution, and socialization. Furthermore, functions are ceremonial and instrumental. Ceremonial functions stabilize age, sex, face, finality, genealogy, religion, rationality, tradition, and wealth. Instrumental functions sustain competence, courage, creativity, curiosity, dynamics, evocation, experience, experimentation, forward-looking, imagination, innovativeness, skill, and synthesis. Functionalism prizes voluntariness rather than coercion in obedience. Pragmatism accentuates adaptation, capacitation, evolution, education, individuality rather than individualism, interaction, modification, means rather than ends, and testing or experimentation. Meanwhile, the institution stands on the ideal against realism, positivism, or evolutionism (Menon 2011; Ziegler 1994). Realism, positivism, or evolutionism prefers competition, individualism, laissez-faire, nature, and struggle over institutionalization.

The political institution, mainly the state, upholds sociality by providing power, utility, ideals, and norms to achieve the functions of fulfillment or goal attainment, adaptation, latency, and integration. Sociality features attachment, bonding, caring, cooperation, community, fairness, friendship, participation, punishment, relatedness, self-expansion, sharing, social interaction, trust, trustworthiness, and xenophobia (Capraro 2024; Cottrell et al. 2007; Fenwick 2008; Fowers 2015; Ratner et al. 2023; Tomasello 2019). Conversely, sociality rejects aggression, destruction, emotionality or neuroticism, risking, and violence (Cottrell et al. 2007; Fowers 2015; Hughes et al. 2017; Schinkel 2010). Meanwhile, the political institution functions to maintain authority, centralization, duty, law, norms, order, rules, and unity (Altman and Wellman 2009; Jessop 2016; Loo 2020; Prokhovnik 2007; Rasmussen 2023; Szondi 2010).

Power created by the political institution to enable sociality rests on community or collective involvement and control (Dryzek and Dunleavy 2009; Loo 2020). The community represents social capital to boost sociality (Saegert and Winkel 2004). Hence, community involvement has facilitated sociality regarding cooperation, networking, and trust (Groves et al. 2000; Molitor et al. 2011; Rochelle 2015). Control received has guided sociality regarding self-control and trust as opposed to violence (Gelfand and Lun 2013; Overall et al. 2020).

Utility afforded by the political institution to attract sociality stems from shared interests and benefits or welfare distribution or redistribution (Buckley 2009; Dryzek and Dunleavy 2009). Common interests constitute the self-expansion of sociality (Sivami 2016). Hence, common interests induce sociality regarding attachment, liking, love, morality, and relatedness (Ledbetter et al. 2013; Sivami 2016; Tomlinson et al. 2018; Z. Xin et al. 2017). Benefit or welfare distributed or redistributed has elevated sociality regarding social participation, preference for redistribution, and welfare support (Kriesi 1993; Reeskens and van Oorschot 2013; van Oorschot and Meuleman 2011).

Ideals cultivated by the political institution to rationalize sociality emphasize activeness, citizenship, communication, continuity, culture, deontology, discussion, duty, history, mutual understanding, networking, publicity, regularity, relatedness, sharing, social order, and trust (Dryzek and Dunleavy 2009; Jessop 2016; Moore 2001; Prokhovnik 2008; Szondi 2010). Activeness involves social capital to constitute sociality (Holland et al. 2007). Citizenship underlies sociality regarding confidence in public institutions (Vera-Toscano et al. 2013). Communication or publicity has incubated sociality regarding social cohesion, participation, and trust (Miyata et al. 2008; Rothstein and Uslaner 2005). Continuity or regularity has constituted sociality regarding civic engagement, cohesion, neighboring, and relational quality as opposed to violence (Pulkkinen et al. 2009; C. Ross et al. 2000; Swaroop and Morenoff 2006; Villarreal and Silva 2006). Cultural involvement has fostered sociality regarding organizational involvement and social trust (Freitag 2003b; Guillen et al. 2011). Deontological orientation as morality has buttressed sociality regarding volunteering as opposed to violence (Piquero and Hickman 2002; Whitford et al. 2006). Discussion has raised confidence in government (Hooghe et al. 2015). Dutifulness or responsibility has fostered sociality regarding compliance, morality, and xenophobia as opposed to violence (Bussey 2020; Granzin and Olsen 1998; Kaurin 2020; Milner and Myers 2007). Historicist orientation upholds sociality regarding collectivism and morality (B. Zhu 2007). Besides, nostalgia within historicist orientation has consolidated sociality regarding attachment and donation (Juhl et al. 2019). Understanding has brewed sociality regarding civic engagement, community involvement, compliance, cooperation, prosocial behavior, protection, volunteering, and social cohesion and trust (de Groot and Steg 2009; Bish and Michie 2010; Hunter et al. 2013; Lepkowski and Couper 2002; Pattie et al. 2004; Sarkheyli et al. 2012; Simon-Bemd and Steffens 2000; Volker et al. 2007; Wernet et al. 2005). Networking has constituted sociality regarding connectedness, friendship, giving, and social interaction (Eberl 2020; Liebler and Sandefur 2002; Nelson-Coffey et al. 2023; Phan et al. 2009). Relatedness has consolidated sociality by raising sharing, social interaction, and relationship satisfaction (Downie et al. 2008; Frazer 1999; Wickham and Knee 2012). Sharing represents prosocial behavior and virtue to strengthen sociality (H. Ding et al. 2021; M. Wang et al. 2014). The ideal for social order has bred sociality based on confidence in the business institution (Costa et al. 2023). Trust has constituted sociality through donation, involvement, and volunteering (Uslaner 2000). Conversely, the political institution repels ideals for conflict and resistance to sustain sociality (Prokhovnik 2008; Rasmussen 2023). Conflict has impeded sociality regarding donation and trust as opposed to violence (Farmer and Fedor 2001; Farrington 2018; Kunovich and Hodson 1999). Resistance has impaired sociality by eroding solidarity and fomenting deviance (Foy et al. 2014; J. Williams 2011).

Norms shared by the political institution to assimilate sociality popularize law and normativity (Dryzek and Dunleavy 2009; Jessop 2016). The norm for law has sustained sociality by resisting radicalism (Muthuswamy 2022). Normativity has countenanced sociality by raising civic engagement, donation, prosocial behavior, punishment, support for policy, volunteering, and voting, and eroding cheating, violence, and tolerance for violence (Brown and Ferris 2007; Hennessy et al. 2015; Huesmann 2018; B. Liu et al. 2023; Opp 2002; Pavlova and Silbereisen 2015; Wade-Benzoni and Tost 2009; Waterman et al. 2022; Wenzel 2004). Herein, punishment characterizes sociality (Fowers 2015). Notably, voting has enhanced sociality regarding civic engagement, community participation, and confidence in institutions (Djupe and Lewis 2015; Hakhverdian and Mayne 2012; McCabe 2014).

The political institution builds on power, utility, ideals, and norms generated through empowerment, incentivizing, framing, and normalizing in the deterministic mechanisms of analytical functionalism. Essentially, the political institution achieves the functions of centralization, control, criminalizing, cultivation, defense, development, legislation, modernization, normalizing, propaganda, sanctioning, securitizing, servicing, taxation, and warfare (Batta 2011; M. Berger 2003; Buckley 2009; Jessop 2016; Moore 2001, 2015; Prokhovnik 2007; Szondi 2010). Modernization covers industrialization, rationalization, and urbanization (M. Berger 2003).

Power for building the political institution evolves from bureaucracy, client politics, conflict from class and war, corporations, fiscal buoyancy, governmentality, industrialization, mobilization, productivity, taxation, and technological development (Hood 1991b; Kiser and Powers 2013; Sutherland 2005; J. Turner 2013). Productivity benefits from efficiency, resourcefulness, population, and technology (J. Turner 2013). The continuity and unity of the political institution also generate power for maintaining the institution (Rasmussen 2023). Conversely, identity politics has generated power against the political institution (Alumona and Azom 2018). Identity politics has resulted from power generated from elite manipulation (Alumona and Azom 2018).

Utility for attracting the political institution stems from needs or demands for collective action, competitiveness, differentiation or specialization, income, legitimacy, management, profit, redistribution, and trade, entitlement, risks, suitability for coordination, warfare, and wealth maximization (Barr 2012; Hood 1991b; Kiser and Powers 2013). Such management handles discrimination, isolation, losses, stigma or labeling, and other impressions (Rivera 2008). Risks anticipate the utility of risk management from the political institution. Entitlement consolidates benefits or utility from the political institution. Besides, income inequality has created utility or a desire for redistribution, which is expected from the political institution to consolidate the institution (Bjornskov 2005).

Ideals for rationalizing the political institution emerge from social construction, notably concerning feminism, historicism, nationalism, paternalism, perfectionism, republicanism, rightism, romanticism, social identity, and statism (Altman and Wellman 2009; Buckley 2009; Chahboun 2024; Hobson 2005; Negri and Emery 2022; Prokhovnik 2007). Feminism advocates strengthening female people and discounts masculinity by the political institution (Hobson 2005). Furthermore, feminism favors authority, equality, rights, and solidarity that the political institution can wield to advance sociality (Hutchings 2010; Sanderson et al. 2005; Zumbrunnen and Gangl 2008). Historicism mandates authoritarianism, civilization, collectivism, morality, nostalgia, sentimentalism, and succession as opposed to rationality to fit the political institution (B. Zhu 2007; Paez et al. 2016). Nationalism upholds sociality regarding attachment, belongingness, commonness, government, hierarchy, homogeneity, institutions, loyalty, morality, order, politics, purity, sacrifice, social harmony, socialization, xenophobia, and unity (Baldwin et al. 2018; Batto 2019; Fuchs 2020; Fukuyama 2018; Moore 2001; Ozkirimli 2005; A. Smith 2010; Sutherland 2012; E. Thomas 2002; Yack 2012). Specifically, nationalism has boosted confidence in government, intolerance, and prejudice (Blank and Schmidt 2003; N. Chen 2012; Li and Brewer 2004). Hence, nationalism would underlie confidence in the political institution and rejection of outsiders. Paternalism favors capability, expertise, and hierarchy, characterizing the political institution (Buckley 2009). Moreover, paternalism underlies sociality featuring morality (Kullgen 1995). Paternalism also features or builds on legalism or law value and overriding or interference with the individual to espouse the political institution (Arneson 2005; Kullgen 1995). Perfectionism valorizes morality for the political institution (Buckley 2009). Moreover, perfectionism espouses sociality regarding social adaptation, obligation, and concern for others (Grzegorek et al. 2004; Stoeber and Janssen 2011). Republicanism upholds sociality regarding citizenship, the commonweal, interdependence, morality, nationalism, publicity, responsibility, social adaptation, and solidarity (Delanty 2009; Honohan 2002). Romanticism treasures differentiation and dismisses revolution to secure the political institution (Negri and Emery 2022). Furthermore, romanticism treasures sociality regarding community (TenHouten 2017). Romanticism has also vindicated sociality by refuting sexuality (G. Li et al. 2023).

Conversely, ideals against the political institution are cosmopolitanism, humanism, internationalism or transnationalism, neoliberalism, populism, and postmodernism (Altman and Wellman 2009; Buckley 2009; du Gay 2012; Hobson 2005; Rasmussen 2023; Sutherland 2005). Cosmopolitanism, internationalism, or transnationalism espouses decentering, dispersal, and openness and dismisses the national political institution (Baildon and Alviar-Martin 2020; Gu and Schweisfurth 2015; Igarashi and Saito 2014). Hence, cosmopolitanism is antithetical to the political institution featuring centralization, order, and unity (Jessop 2016; Rasmussen 2023; Szondi 2010). Humanism hails diversity, freedom, and individuality as opposed to manipulation to counter the political institution (Browning and Cooper 2004; Doane 2017; Selznick 2008). Neoliberalism mandates atomization, deregulation, deterritorialization, globalization, liberalization, privatization, and silos as opposed to the state to subvert the political institution (Barthold et al. 2018; Kinchy et al. 2008; Lakoff 2009; Rhodes-Purdy et al. 2023; Zucker and Bay-Cheng 2021). Populism denounces the political institution or establishment, bureaucracy, constitution, elite, law or rules, loyalty, nation or state, nationalism, repression, sovereignty and favors anarchy, division, occupying, radicalism, resistance, revolution, and subversion (Barr 2009; Fahey 2022; Grattan 2016; S. Lo 2021; Norris and Inglehart 2019; Nowakowski 2021;

Pappas 2019; Yilmaz and Erturk 2021). Postmodernism rejects authoritarianism or domination, coercion, and moralism and valorizes decentering, fragmentation, radicalism, and resistance to downplay the political institution (Alvesson 2002; Antonio 2000; Bauman 2001; Beardsworth 2020; Bowring 2011; Ritzer and Goodman 2001).

Norms for assimilating the political institution stem from international and neighboring institutions (Rai 2020; Wallis and Dollery 2001). This assimilation relies on social construction by international institutions to legitimize or normalize grouping or collectivity (Dobbin et al. 2007; McLevey and Deschamps 2018; Steinacker 2006).

Confidence in the political institution or government represents sociality regarding sociotropy, stabilizing, support, and trust as opposed to alienation (Dabros et al. 2015; Kabashima et al. 2000; Kumlin et al. 2025; J. Lu 2014; Stoyan et al. 2016). Specifically, such confidence suggests that the political institution can share power, utility, and ideals to strengthen sociality by leveraging the voluntaristic mechanisms of analytical-functionalism. The political institution encompasses the armed force or military, cabinet or congress, chief, court, criminal justice system, defense, election, executive, legislature, official or officer, party, police, policy, and welfare (Fishkin 2018; Garb 2015; Kagotani 2015; Munro 2018; Power and Jamison 2005; Richardson et al. 2001; Singer et al. 2019; Sun et al. 2013; Tang and Cheng 2021; Tsfati et al. 2009; Zhou and Zeng 2024).

Power shared from confidence in the political institution resides in competence, effectiveness or efficacy, functionality, legitimacy, and responsiveness through empowering (Atkeson and Maestas 2012; Campbell and Wolbrecht 2020; Hawdon et al. 2000; Menahem 2001; Tsang et al. 2022; Tyler and Degoey 1995; Ulbig 2002; Wei et al. 2022). Such power shared or empowered can enhance sociality (Fowers 2015). Notably, institutional effectiveness has secured sociality regarding social harmony and trust (Guisan 2009; Wong and Shik 2011). Besides, personal effectiveness has buttressed sociality regarding love as opposed to radicalism (Louis et al. 2022; Nezlek et al. 2008). Competence or efficacy has buttressed sociality regarding civic engagement, discussion, donation, leadership, prosocial behavior, social interaction, social trust, and intolerance for violence (Bednall et al. 2013; Frye 2007; Gnambs and Batinic 2012; Mazziotta et al. 2011; Pei and Pan 2018; Rahn 2008; Tausch et al. 2011; Yao and Enright 2019). Functionality has fostered sociality through raising social capital (Cornwall 2009). Legitimacy perceived has induced sociality by eschewing crime and protesting (Buechler 2011; Lilly et al. 2011). Responsiveness perceived has enhanced sociality regarding trust (Brik et al. 2023).

Utility conveyed by confidence in the political institution covers exchange, freedom, goodwill, gratitude, justice or fairness, harmony, and transparency (Braithwaite 1998; Q. Huang 2018; D. Kong 2013; Tyler 2001). Conversely, disutility reduced by confidence in the political institution arises from corruption, error, and isolation (Cheng and Ngok 2020; Redlawsk and McCann 2005; Q. Huang 2018). Exchange has sustained sociality regarding compliance, cooperation, morality, social cohesion, social commitment, social integration, social interaction, social participation, trust, and volunteering (Bagherior et al. 2009; Carter 2016; Drollinger 2010; Lawler et al. 2016; Skopek et al. 2011; Yoon et al. 2013; Zhang and Zhou 2018).

Conversely, exchange has maintained sociality by dampening resistance and violence (Foy et al. 2014; Hattery and Smith 2012). Goodwill has expressed or fostered sociality regarding adaptation, intimacy, and social capital (X. Chen et al. 2015; Harvey and Wenzel 2006; Larsen 2018). Gratitude constitutes sociality through expressing or raising morality, social awareness, liking, and understanding, and reducing avoidance (Eibach et al. 2015; Tudge et al. 2022; Kloos et al. 2022). Justice or fairness perceived has uplifted sociality regarding civility, cooperation, community identification, political participation, and social trust as opposed to protesting (A. Hu 2013; Lawrence and Daniels 1997; Sunshine and Tyler 2003; Tyler and Degoey 1995; van Prooijen et al. 2008; Wenzel 2000). Harmony perceived has fostered sociality characterized by adjustment, attunement, civility, compromise, connectedness, interdependency, order, peace, relatedness, respect, sacrifice, selflessness, solidarity, and sympathy as opposed to competition and conflict (Arat and Kerelian 2019; Cheung and Ma 2011; P. Ip 2014; Kjell et al. 2016; Peck 2002; G. Zhang 2005). Transparency perceived has boosted sociality regarding social integration and trust (Erkkila 2012). Confidence in the political institution has advanced utility in neighborhood quality perceived, pride, and life as well as political satisfaction (Abbott et al. 2011; Greenberg 1999; van Ryzin et al. 2004; Vogl et al. 2019). Neighborhood quality has elevated sociality by building social capital, order, and cohesion (Rupp et al. 2020; Sampson and Raudenbush 2004). Pride has advanced sociality through raising attachment, prosociality, and political participation (Emler and Frazer 1999; Kitayama and Markus 2000; Tracy et al. 2009). Political participation has buttressed sociality regarding civility (Campbell 2003). Life satisfaction has incubated sociality regarding political participation, social cohesion, social trust, and volunteering (E. Chan 2014; Flavin and Keane 2011; Rochelle 2015).

Ideals implied in confidence in the political institution emphasize compliance, cooperation, ethicality or morality, honesty, integrity, legality, loyalty, normativity, rationality or deliberation, and regulation (Dean 2010; Hinds 2007; Hough 2012; Q. Huang 2018; Menahem 2001). Compliance has constituted sociality by raising patriotism and impeding violence and acceptance of deviants and outsiders (Pulkkinen et al. 2009; Schwartz et al. 2014; Van Hootegem et al. 2000; Yeo and Chu 2018). Patriotism has consolidated sociality by uplifting prosociality, social cohesion, volunteering, and xenophobia (Granzin and Olsen 1998; Ishii 2009; Straume and Odeen 2010; Vida and Reardon 2008; Y. Yang et al. 2010). Ethicality or morality encompasses honesty, integrity, and loyalty (N. Duncan 2017; McCaffoee 2016; Talaifar and Swann 2019). As such, ethicality has advanced sociality by raising volunteering and inhibiting violence (Piquero and Hickman 2002; Whitford et al. 2006). Honesty has built sociality by increasing compliance and prosocial behavior and eschewing crime (Jolley et al. 2019; Thielmann et al. 2020; Twardawski et al. 2021). Legality has buttressed sociality by dismissing radicalism (Muthuswamy 2022). Normativity has underpinned sociality by fostering civic engagement, donation, prosocial behavior, punishment, support for policy, volunteering, and voting, and diminishing cheating, violence, and tolerance for violence (Brown and Ferris 2007; Hennessy et al. 2015; Huesmann 2018; B. Liu et al. 2023; Opp 2002; Pavlova and Silbereisen 2015;

Wade-Benzoni and Tost 2009; Waterman et al. 2022; Wenzel 2004). Herein, punishment characterizes sociality (Fowers 2015). Rationality has championed sociality by dampening aggression and antisociality (DiGiuseppe et al. 2017). Regulation has fostered sociality by eschewing risking, crime, and violence (Y. Cheung et al. 2014; Koegl and Day 2019; Welch et al. 2008). Confidence in the political institution has raised the ideal for conformity (Ulbig 2002). The ideal for conformity has built sociality regarding xenophobia or rejection of outsiders (Costa et al. 2023).

Confidence in the political institution develops from power, utility, ideals, and norms to activate the voluntaristic mechanisms of analytical-functionalism. Such activation can also engender sociality. Sociality represents ethicality, friendship, and humanity (de Vries and Megathlin 2009; Fowers 2015). Besides, sociality features altruism, attachment, bonding, caring, collective identity, conscientiousness, conservation, cooperation, extraversion, fairness, gifting, gregariousness, honesty, learning, normativity, reciprocity, sharing, socializing, social interaction, social participation, trust, trustworthiness, and xenophobia (Boer and Fischer 2013; Capraro 2024; Cottrell et al 2007; Fenwick 2008; Fowers 2015; Koster 2013; M. Ma 2021; Ratner et al. 2023). Conversely, sociality dismisses aggression, destruction, individualism, misanthropy, risking, and violence (Bissell 2010; Fowers 2015; Hughes et al. 2017; Schinkel 2010).

Power driving confidence in the political institution stems from justification or defense and motivation (van der Toorn et al. 2010). This justification evolved from disadvantaged status and need (Huang and Gao 2018; Jost et al. 2003). Such motivation originates from epistemic, existential, and relational motives and pessimism (Mutz 1998; van der Toorn et al. 2010). Power driving confidence in the political institution has evolved from well-being (Sun et al. 2013). Such well-being includes adequacy in finance, affect or mood, confidence, sense of community, need, pride, satisfaction, and self-efficacy (M. Anderson 2010; Atkeson and Maestas 2012; Li and Mayraz 2017; Mangum 2012; Xiang and Hmielowski 2017). Satisfaction has covered democracy, the economy, finance, gathering, income, life, municipality, policy, politics, rights, and services (Catterberg and Moreno 2005; E. Chi and Kwon 2016; Hooghe and Kern 2015; Huang and Gao 2018; Kabashima et al. 2000; U. Kim et al. 2002; Kumlin et al. 2025; F. Lee 2022; Menahem 2001; Ulbig 2002; J. Yang et al. 2021). Conversely, power dispelling confidence in the political institution rests on education, social capital, and union membership (Norris 2011). Social capital features association, community, cooperation, networking or relatedness, sharing, and support (Norris 2011). Power for dampening that confidence has stemmed from anger, anxiety, discontent, and fear (Atkeson and Maestas 2012; F. Lee 2022b; Singer et al. 2019),

Utility attracting confidence in the political institution arises from calculation or reasoning and institutional implementation or performance, including communication, outcomes, and processes (Cairney 2012; Chanley et al. 2001; Mishler and Willerton 2003; Suh et al. 2012). Such utility rests on the institution's benevolence, competence, compliance, control, customer orientation, democracy, expansion, fairness, inclusiveness, legitimacy, rationality or rationalism, scale, sharing power, skill, simplicity, support reception, welfare provision, workability (Cairney 2012; Hjerm

2010; D. Kong 2014; Lubell 2003; Nunkoo 2015; Papadopoulos and Warin 2007; Reddick et al. 2022; Rose and Pettersen 2000; Sunshine and Tyler 2003; Wallner 2008; Yuan 2002; Zmerli and Castillo 2015). The institution's expansion heightens the expectation for and thus confidence in the institution (Rose and Pettersen 2000). Legitimacy includes alignment or resonance, appropriateness, emotional appeal, education, engagement, incubation, and justness (Wallner 2008). This utility also arises from deprivation, exchange, risk, welfare received, and reward as opposed to cost (Huang and Gao 2018; Nunkoo 2015; Sunshine and Tyler 2003; Zmerli and Castillo 2015). Utility has also arisen from benefits, drug problems, economic or political evaluation, educational aspiration, political expectancy or expectation, political efficacy perceived, political responsibility perceived, and quality assessment (Belle et al. 2024; Su, Lee, and Borah 2021; Kumlin et al. 2025; Marien 2017; Nunkoo 2015; Wirtz et al. 2019; Y. Zhou 2024). The evaluation has covered political accessibility, benevolence, civility, competence, democracy, effectiveness or efficacy, legitimacy, meritocracy, and neutrality (Gibson and Caldeira 2003; Jeong and Han 2020; B. Johnson 2004; D. Kong 2014; Mutz and Reeves 2005; Rieger and Wang 2021; Zimmerman and Reyna 2013). Effectiveness or efficacy has concerned corruption, crime, the economy, the group, and rights (Kim and Voorhees 2011; Mangum 2012). Notably, effectiveness found has raised sociality regarding prosociality (J. Li et al. 2020). Legitimacy perceived has enhanced sociality by preventing crime and protesting (Buechler 2011; Lilly et al. 2011). Fairness perceived has elevated sociality regarding civility, cooperation, community identification, political participation, and social trust as opposed to protesting (A. Hu 2013; Lawrence and Daniels 1997; Sunshine and Tyler 2003; Tyler and Degoey 1995; van Prooijen et al. 2008; Wenzel 2000). Neutrality is also a component of fairness (Hegtvedt and Scheuerman 2010). Thus, meritocracy and neutrality perceived would raise sociality. Besides, performance assessment covers the community, economy, government, and living (Cohen and Bolt 2005; D. Kong 2014; Stoyan et al. 2016; Tyler 2001; Uslaner 2002). Government has included its services and standards (Stoyan et al. 2016). Expectancy covers political collaboration, ease, participation, transparency, and usefulness (Wirtz et al. 2019).

Conversely, disutility against confidence in the political institution stems from the institution's bureaucracy, monopoly, rent-seeking, and uncontrollability (Cairney 2012). Bureaucracy is a feature of modernity (Marotta 2017). Modernity has eroded sociality by raising autonomy (Delhey 2010). Monopoly characterizes capitalism (Meszaros 2015). Capitalism dismisses sociality by prioritizing alienation, autonomy, freedom, and individualism (Meszaros 2015; Parker 2009; Rindermann 2018). Rent-seeking constitutes corruption (Abegaz 2013). Corruption perceived has impaired sociality regarding civic relatedness and social trust (Seligson 2005). Uncontrollability perceived has worsened sociality regarding social trust (Burke and Stets 1999). Moreover, disutility against confidence in the political institution has concerned corruption, deprivation, and favoritism (Fishkin 2018; Redlawsk and McCann 2005). Deprivation experienced erodes sociality by breeding conflict (J. Turner 2013b). Favoritism constitutes corruption (Inglehart and Welzel 2005). Hence, favoritism experienced would diminish sociality.

Ideals rationalizing confidence in the political institution need to be accessible or salient, bounded, cognitive, credible, congruent or fitting, involved, legitimate, representative, and truthful as knowledge (Niederberger 2005; Norris 2011; Pfau et al. 2001; Schnaudt 2019). Such rationalizing reflects ideal calibration, consistency maintenance, or dissonance reduction, and processing (Jost et al. 2003; Maule and Goidel 2003; Sears 2001). These ideals include confirmation as opposed to disconfirmation, community or its sense, contracting, expectation, identity, interest, involvement, liking, and participation (M. Anderson 2010; N. Chen 2012; A. He and Ma 2021; Hjerm 2010; Hjortskov 2019; Norris 2011; M. Li 2023; Schnaudt 2019; Wroe 2014). Moreover, ideals rationalizing confidence in the political institution have concerned acceptance of politics, approval regarding politics, attribution of satisfaction to politics, closeness to politics, deservingness perceived, gender stereotyping, identification with parties, interest in politics, justification for the system, preference of ideology, respect for authority or physicians, support for politics, trust, and willingness to vote (Craig et al. 2005; Citrin and Luks 2001; Hooghe and Kern 2015; B. Johnson 200; Maule and Goidel 2003; McGraw 2001; Rose and Pettersen 2000; Taylor-Gooby 2006; van der Toorn et al. 2010; Xiang and Hmielowski 2017; J. Yang et al. 2021). Supported politics has covered the system, volunteering, and political contribution, policy, reform, and welfare provision (Kelly 2009; Kwak et al. 2010; Tyler 2001). These ideals represent political interest or value. Political interest has elevated sociality by raising civic engagement, civic and social motivation, civility, and discussion as opposed to protesting (Gil de Zuniga et al. 2017; Lee and Chan 2011; Pattie et al. 2004). Moreover, gender stereotyping represents traditionalism (Yeh et al. 2013). Traditionalism has buttressed sociality by enhancing patriotism and faith in religion and discouraging protesting and accepting deviants and outsiders (Costa et al. 2023; Datler et al. 2013; Meuleman et al. 2019; Schwartz et al. 2014). System justification has propped sociality by preventing protesting (Jost 2020). Support for authority, representing authoritarianism, would constitute sociality by raising altruism, attachment, intolerance, nationalism, networking, obedience, patriotism, relatedness, and religiosity (Dunwoody and Funke 2016; Mallinas et al. 2020; MuBotter 2024; Sinn and Hayes 2018). Voting has engendered sociality by boosting civic and community participation and neighboring (Djupe and Lewis 2015; Dorff 2017; Hays and Kogl 2007). Trust has covered the media, nongovernmental organizations, parties, police, religion, unions, and people (Beldad et al. 2012; Cacciatore et al. 2018; Hassan 2000; Jeong and Han 2020; D. Kong 2014; Li and Mayraz 2017; Mahmud 2021).

Ideals rationalizing confidence in the political institution have favored socialism, impartiality, redistribution, and national security (Garb 2015; D. Ho et al. 2003; H. Li et al. 2016; Persson et al. 2017). Favor for socialism embodies sociality regarding harmony, love, morality, relationality, responsibility, and togetherness (Collier 2001; D. Lin 2017; Z. Liu 2008; Scruton 2014; Sturm 1998). Furthermore, favoring socialism has enhanced sociality regarding cooperation and discussion, as opposed to crime (Collier 2001; Lilly et al. 2011; Sanderson 2001). Favor for socialism also embraces sociality regarding caring, commonality, communication, community, cooperation, equality, patriotism, publicness, reciprocity, social interaction, spreading benefits, trust, and unity (Collier 2001; Frazer 1999; Fuchs 2020; Lalander and Merimaa 2018; Panitch 2008; Scruton 2014; Sherman 1995; Sturm 1998; Volker and Flap 1997). Conversely, favor for socialism champions sociality by dismissing alienation, autonomy, competition, deviance, division, exploitation, individualism, liberalism, narcissism, oppression, psychologism, and voluntarism (Collier 2001; de Vos 2013; Fuchs 2020; Lasch 1984; Mole 2011; Panitch 2008; Sherman 1995; Satgar and Williams 2017; Sturm 1998). Psychologism signifies distress and disconnection or separation as opposed to conscientiousness (Al-krenawi et al. 2011; Parker 2002; Village and Francis 2010). Moreover, psychologism disrupts sociality by dampening civility and cooperation and engendering crime, impulsivity, and violence (Hample 2018; Pulkkinen et al. 2009; Sammons and Putwain 2019). The ideal for national security has furnished sociality by reducing liberalism, deviance, and its tolerance for deviance (Gibson 2013; Wright and DeLisi 2016). Liberalism has impeded sociality regarding morality, normativity, and social order (Feinberg et al. 2019). The ideal for impartiality has fostered sociality by raising empathy and dampening radicalism (Lauriola et al. 2015; Lucas and Kteily 2018). The ideal for redistribution has reflected sociality regarding faith in religion and social trust (Nagayoshi and Sato 2014).

Conversely, ideals dispelling confidence in the political institution have rested on blaming politics, concern about social problems, identification with democrats, interest in democracy, suspicion, tolerance for corruption and risk, and support for rebellion (Atkeson and Maestas 2012; Catterberg and Moreno 2005; R. Chan 2012; Funk 2001; McGraw et al. 2002; Su, Lee, and Borah 2021; Tang and Cheng 2021). Concern for social problems has eroded sociality by reducing civility, political participation, and social trust and fermenting deviance (Backman and Nilsson 2011; Fahmy 2006; Marschall and Stolle 2004; Tyler and Degoey 1995). Identification of or interest in liberal democracy stands on liberalism and self-interest (Caplan 2002; Tang et al. 2009). Liberalism has dismissed sociality regarding morality, normativity, and social order (Feinberg et al. 2019). Self-interest impairs sociality by weakening deontology or duty and strengthening egocentrism (Beauregard and Dunning 1998; Rocha and Ghoshal 2006). Tolerance for risk or risking has disrupted sociality by generating crime, hate, and violence (Farrington 2018; Hawdon et al. 2019; Merdian et al. 2017). Rebellion has impaired sociality by raising deviance and eroding solidarity (Foy et al. 2014; J. Williams 2011). Moreover, rebellion opposes sociality regarding civility as opposed to autonomy, militancy, and protesting (Chenoweth 2021; D. Lin 2017; Sexton and Benson 2006; Ewick and Silbey 2003).

Norms assimilating confidence in the political institution pass through agenda setting, coercion or enforcement, conformity, culture or enculturation, cultural compatibility, framing, group identification, journalism, mediatization, propaganda, socialization, and trickling down from the elite (Hjerm 2010; X. Fu 2018; Maule and Goidel 2003; Mishler and Willerton 2003; Norris 2011; Rose and Pettersen 2000; Tsfati et al. 2009; Wallner 2008; Xiang and Hmielowski 2017). Such norms popularize altruism, civic engagement, collectivism, Confucianism, expectation, social capital, and social trust (Belle et al. 2024; Hjerm 2010; D. Kong 2014; Norris

2011; Wang and You 2016). These norms constitute sociality (Capraro 2024; Fowers 2015; Koster 2013). Thus, civic engagement has propped sociality by strengthening attachment, civility, collective behavior, discussion, donation, neighboring, patriotism, prosociality, social capital, socialism, trust, and volunteering and impeding cheating and individualism (Coffe and Geys 2007; Gilberbloom and Markham 1995; Kerrissey and Schofer 2013; Mata and Pendakur 2014; Ozbay 2008; Pattie et al. 2004; Pena-Lopez and Sanchez-Santos 2016; Rahn 2008; Richey 2011; Tak 2017; M. Tang 2011; Taniguchi 2013; Yip et al. 2007). Confucianism braces socialism with awe or reverence, benevolence, caring, charity, collectivism or groupness, empathy, fraternity, harmony, humaneness, love, loyalty, morality, normativity, peace, relationality, respect, sacrifice, socialization or cultivation, trustworthiness, and unity as opposed to freedom, individualism, isolation, self-interest, selfishness, and violence (Curzer 2012; Fang 2003; Hocksmann 2004; Y. Lin et al. 2021; Peng 2003; Shin 2012; Song 2002; Woo 2008). With these emphases, Confucianism has championed sociality regarding association, civility, and collectivism as opposed to violence (Y. Lin et al. 2021; Shin 2012; Stotzer 2014). Collectivism has constituted sociality by securing civility, cooperation, prosocial behavior, and religiousness and preventing extremism (Hample 2018; Harzing 2006; Oyserman et al. 1998; Saucier and Skrzypinska 2006; Thielmann et al. 2020). Social capital constitutes sociality by registering collectivity, community, cooperation, networking, reciprocity, responsibility, social integration, social interaction, trust, and trustworthiness (Caballero-Dominguez et al. 2021; X. Chen et al. 2015; Frank et al. 2014; Lofors and Sundquist 2007; Nahapiet 2011; Robison and Ritchie 2010; Sabet and Khaksar 2025; Williams and Pocock 2010). Moreover, social capital sustains sociality by featuring association, civic engagement, closeness, communitarianism, connection, cooperation, embeddedness, exchange, friendship, helping or helpfulness, networking, organizational membership, reciprocity, sharing, sociability, social cohesion, social interaction, social participation, solidarity, sympathy, talking, togetherness, trust, and volunteering (Carlson 2004; Child and Nikolova 2020; Coleman et al. 2022; Curley 2010; Harpham et al. 2002; Kirkby-Geddes et al. 2013; Kleinhans et al. 2007; Murayama et al. 2019; Narayan and Cassidy 2001; Onyx and Bullen 2000; Ostrom 2009; Paraskevopoulos 2010; Poortinga 2012; X. Qi 2013; Robison et al. 2002; J. Son 2013; Wuthnow 2002). Social capital has consolidated sociality by raising civic engagement, community involvement, donation, political involvement, social trust, and volunteering (Bekkers et al. 2008; Broadbent and Papadopoulos 2011; Brown and Ferris 2007; Chua et al. 2021; Narayan and Cassidy 2001). Conversely, social capital has strengthened sociality by erasing violence (Pulkkinen et al. 2009). Meanwhile, norms against confidence in the political institution favor cosmopolitanism, democracy, individualism, leftism, libertarianism, postmaterialism, populism, progressivism, and self-expression (Norris 2011; Power and Jamison 2005; Wang and You 2016). These norms discourage sociality (Fowers 2015). Cosmopolitanism opposes sociality by downplaying attachment, collective identity, communality, localism, nationalism, and patriotism (Baildon and Alviar-Martin 2020; Bray 2013; Caruana 2014; Delanty 2009; Sorge 2008). Conversely, cosmopolitanism contradicts sociality by hailing autonomy, diversity, foreignness, fusion, individualism, and liberalism (Corstange and York 2018; Delanty 2009; Held 2010; Herrmann 2023). As such, cosmopolitanism has eroded sociality by discounting religiosity and raising liberalism and acceptance of deviants and outsiders (Costa et al. 2023; Motschenbacher 2013; Norris and Inglehart 2009). Individualism opposes sociality by representing liberalism as opposed to collectivism, communitarianism, and institutionalism (Lowndes and Roberts 2013; Sayer 2011; Myers 2020; Welzel 2013). Furthermore, individualism downplays sociality by devaluing the community and embeddedness (Davis and Robinson 1999; Krys et al. 2019). Conversely, individualism opposes sociality by hailing autonomy, competition, independence, privacy, and self-interest (Oyserman et al. 2002; Steffensmeier et al. 2017). As such, individualism has weakened sociality by reducing civic engagement, religiousness, social cohesion, and volunteering (Church 2010; Green and Janmaat 2011; J. He et al. 2014; Hener et al. 2016; Leong 2008; Pollack and Pickel 2007; Whitford et al. 2006). Conversely, individualism has impeded sociality by bolstering acceptance of outsiders, competition, crime, extremity, self-enhancement, protesting, and violence (Church 2010; J. He et al. 2014; Karstedt 2010; Leong 2008; Li and Song 1992; Pollack and Pickel 2007; Whitford et al. 2006). Leftism has diminished sociality by reducing donation, patriotism, religiousness, and value on loyalty (Filho and Modesto 2019; Flanagan and Lee 2003; Sandovici and Davis 2010; Yuchtman-Yaar 2002). Conversely, leftism has weakened sociality by bolstering acceptance of deviants, liberalism, protesting, and radicalism (Bystrov 2012; Filho and Modesto 2019; Jonsson and Jakobsson 2017; Rudig and Karyotis 2014). Liberalism challenges socialism by hailing distrust (Elliott 2014). As such, libertarianism has dampened sociality by weakening cooperation and patriotism and championing cynicism, protesting, and tolerance for deviance (Eggert and Giugni 2015; Flanagan and Lee 2003; Kertzer et al. 2014). Postmaterialism, which downplays material value, embraces environmentalism and self-expression (Norris 2011). With these, postmaterialism faults socialism by upholding tolerance for deviance and unconventionality (Aguila et al. 2008). Populism, which condemns the elite, questions sociality by representing antagonism, conflict, harm, hostility, polarization, radicalism, struggle (de la Torre 2018; Norris and Inglehart 2019; Pappas 2019; Rhodes-Purdy et al. 2021; van Prooijen et al. 2022). Furthermore, populism opposes sociality by espousing agonism, alienation, anarchism, autonomy, bellicosity, cynicism, enmity, exclusion, extremism, hatred, misogyny, occupying, radicalism, rebelliousness, resistance, and revolution (Aslanidis 2018; de la Torre 2018; Grattan 2016; Hameleers 2019; Jagers and Walgrave 2007; S. Lo 2021; Norris and Inglehart 2019; Nyenhuis 2020; Papaioannou et al. 2023; Pappas 2019; Sandel 2020). Conversely, populism disrupts sociality by dismissing compromise, institutionalization, loyalty, and nationalism (Barr 2009; Grattan 2016; S. Lo 2021; Pappas 2019). Progressivism downplays sociality by disfavoring the community, obedience, and socialism and elevating tolerance for deviance (Box 2008; Lakoff 2006; Sandel 2020; G. Wilson 2001).

Confidence in the economic institution involves the economy, business, and market. The economy focuses on income, property, and wealth (Deller and Maher 2009; Wilkinson and Pickett 2017; Wolff and Resnick 2012). Essentially, the economy represents or favors efficiency and modernity (Deller and Maher 2009;

Peet and Hatwick 2009). Business, including corporations and enterprises, operates in the market to register voluntary competition in repeated exchange using standardized monetary terms (W. Jackson 2019). The market functions to achieve efficiency, fairness, incentivization, innovation, simplicity, and productivity (W. Jackson 2019). Simplicity embodies openness, permanence, security, and standardization (W. Jackson 2019).

The market fosters sociality by providing power, utility, ideas, and norms for achieving the requisite functions of analytical functionalism. Sociality registers ethicality, friendship, and humanity (de Vries and Megathlin 2009). Furthermore, sociality features attachment, bonding, cooperation, ethnocentrism, sharing, and trust (Boer and Fischer 2013; Cottrell et al. 2007; Fowers 2015; Koster 2013; M. Ma 2021). Conversely, sociality eschews aggression, destruction, individualism, risking, and violence (Fowers 2015; Hughes et al. 2017; Schinkel 2010).

Power offered by the market to drive sociality rests on rationality (Zelizer 2011). Rationality sustains sociality as a virtue (Schafer 2015). Morality has underlain sociality by boosting volunteering and inhibiting violence (Piquero and Hickman 2002; Whitford et al. 2006). Moreover, rationality enhances sociality by supporting communication, deontological or moral understanding, discussion, expression, and social acceptability (Bolis et al. 2017; Bouwmeester 2017; Lambie 2008; Royzman et al. 2015). Communication has forged sociality regarding social cohesion, participation, and trust (Miyata et al. 2008; Rothstein and Uslaner 2005). Deontological understanding has buttressed sociality regarding volunteering as opposed to violence (Piquero and Hickman 2002; Whitford et al. 2006). Discussion has incubated sociality by facilitating civic engagement, political participation, and trust (Gil de Zuniga et al. 2017; Hooghe et al. 2015; Huber et al. 2022). Social acceptability has strengthened sociality by engendering communication, compliance, cooperation, donation, prosocial behavior, and volunteering and diminishing protesting and violence (Babrow and Striley 2015; Buechler 2011; Heitmeyer and Anhut 2008; Lepkowski and Couper 2002; Li and Ferraro 2006; Wiepking and Maas 2009). Conversely, rationality has safeguarded sociality by avoiding terrorism (Zezelj and Lazarevic 2019). Terrorism has ruined sociality by raising violence and diminishing collective practice and confidence in government (Achilov 2016; Levi and Strker 2000). Hence, rationality has buttressed sociality by impeding aggression, antisociality, and avoidance (DiGiuseppe et al. 2017).

Utility indicated by the market for attracting sociality reveals interdependency (Munch 2012). Interdependency has constituted sociality regarding attachment, cohesion, compliance, cooperation, exchange, group identity, and prosocial behavior (Buechler 2011; Gaertner and Dovidio 2012; Levitt and Cici-Gokaltun 2011; Skitka et al. 2014; Z. Xin et al. 2017). Ideals unfolded by the market to rationalize sociality favor contracting, coordination, exchange, humanism, integrity, mediation, networking, and order (Biggart and Beanish 2003; de Souza et al. 2023; W. Jackson 2019). Contracting enhances sociality by embracing attachment, civic engagement, civility, compliance, compromise, consent, cooperation, coordination, equality, fairness, morality, and trust (Bowker 2016; Dalbert 2001; Darwall 2003; de Jonge 2012; Ellis et al. 2006; Gardiner 2009; Irwin 2016; Jarvinen and Branders 2020; Kaurin

2020). As such, contracting has buttressed sociality by raising patriotism, prosocial behavior, and relatedness (Dovidio et al. 2006; Gilbert 2006; Hudson 2023; Segrin and Flora 2019). Coordination or mediation has constituted sociality regarding morality, prosocial behavior, and social capital (Halevy et al. 2019; J. Michael et al. 2020). Exchange has enabled sociality regarding compliance, cooperation, morality, social cohesion, social commitment, social integration, social interaction, social participation, trust, and volunteering (Bagherior et al. 2009; Carter 2016; Drollinger 2010; Lawler et al. 2016; Skopek et al. 2011; Yoon et al. 2013; Zhang and Zhou 2018). Humanism bolsters sociality by highlighting attachment, caring, collectivity, community, cooperation, friendship, helpfulness, institutions, loving, order, respect, relatedness, responsibility, and sharing (Browning and Cooper 2004; Fuchs 2020; Selznick 2008; Stefanski and Jach 2022; Visher 1997; Waterman 2013). Conversely, humanism sustains sociality by rejecting alienation, conflict, and individualization (Fuchs 2020; Selznick 2008). Integrity is thick morality (McCaffoee 2016). As such, integrity has buttressed sociality by boosting volunteering and inhibiting violence (Piquero and Hickman 2002; Whitford et al. 2006). Networking has constituted sociality regarding connectedness, friendship, giving, and social interaction (Eberl 2020; Liebler and Sandefur 2002; Nelson-Coffey et al. 2023; Phan et al. 2009). The ideal for order fosters sociality by signifying cohesion, community, harmony, propriety or ritualism, and security or protection (C. Chung 2000; Heckscher 2015; P. Ip 2014; McGhee 2003; Peng 2003). Furthermore, the ideal for order constitutes sociality by espousing civility, cohesion, commitment, compliance, cooperation, harmony, protection, social interaction, and solidarity (Arat and Kerelian 2019; Kaurin 2020; Lawler et al. 2009; McGhee 2003; Mondak and Hurwitz 2012; Qin 2013). As such, the order ideal has upheld sociality by dampening deviance and its tolerance (Gibson 2013; Wright and DeLisi 2016). Furthermore, ideals reflected by the market to rationalize sociality evolve from agreement, enterprising, social fitness, and trust (Biggart and Beanish 2003; Fligstein and Dauter 2007; W. Jackson 2019). Agreement has enhanced sociality by fostering cohesion, compliance, engagement, and rejection of outsiders (Fasel et al. 2016; Guan et al. 2021; Heshmati and Oravecz 2022; Yoon et al. 2013). Enterprising upholds sociality by treasuring communication, cooperation, empathy, networking, and trust (S. Lin 2018; Praszkier and Nowak 2012). Social fitness has advanced society by raising attachment, nationalism, prosocial behavior, and sharing (Becker and Clement 2006; Brown and Brown 2006; Gharaei et al. 2018; Tsaur et al. 2014).

Norms supporting the market to assimilate sociality concern stability and urbanization (de Souza et al. 2023; Welzel 2013). The norm for stability has propped sociality, including civic engagement, cohesion, neighboring, and relational quality, as opposed to violence (Pulkkinen et al. 2009; C. Ross et al. 2000; Swaroop and Morenoff 2006; Villarreal and Silva 2006). Urbanity stemming from urbanization has championed sociality by raising bonding and giving (Apinunmahakul and Devlin 2008; Degenne et al. 2004).

Confidence in the market achieves sociality by gathering power, utility, ideals, and norms to leverage the voluntaristic mechanisms of analytical functionalism. Such gathering drives, attracts, rationalizes, and assimilates market confidence.

Power underlying confidence in the market has arisen from community size (Hayo 2004). This size facilitates social capital (Williams and Pocock 2010). Hence, community size would maintain sociality by raising civic engagement, community involvement, donation, political involvement, social trust, and volunteering (Bekkers et al. 2008; Broadbent and Papadopoulos 2011; Brown and Ferris 2007; Chua et al. 2021; Narayan and Cassidy 2001).

Utility underlying confidence in the market to attract sociality has covered security (Hraba et al. 2001). Security upholds sociality by avoiding conflict, hostility, and rejection experience (Bina et al. 2020). As such, security has buttressed sociality regarding civility, social capital, and trust (Curley 2010; Watson et al. 2021; Williamson 2002).

Ideals underlying confidence in the market to rationalize sociality have valorized religion and tradition (Hayo 2004; Schwartz et al. 2010). The ideal for religion or religiosity has sustained sociality by fostering civic engagement, civility, cohesion, compliance, donation, empathy, morality, patriotism, prejudice against deviants and outsiders, prosocial behavior, social trust, and volunteering (Apinunmahakul and Devlin 2008; Corcoran et al. 2011; Ishio 2010; Keyes 2002; Kim and Wilcox 2013; Ravanera et al. 2003; van Tienen et al. 2011; Weisberg 2005; Wuthnow 2004). Conversely, religiosity has secured sociality by reducing crime, deviance, individualism, protesting, and sexuality (Andrews et al. 2015; Coffe and Geys 2007; Guo et al. 2008; Skerkat and Ellison 1999; Spilka et al. 2003). Moreover, religiosity realizes sociality regarding altruism, community, ethicality, groupism, sharing, and solidarity (Franks et al. 2013; Lichterman 2012; Peifer 2010; Spilka et al. 2003; Stavrova and Siegers 2014). Religiosity also upholds sociality by featuring altruism, attachment, caring, community, compassion, harmony, hospitality, love, morality, obedience, other-centeredness, peace, trust, unity, xenophobia (Ager and Ager 2011; Fontana 2003; Harris et al. 2018; Horell 2014; Paterson 2018; Shorey et al. 2018; Simpson et al. 2008; Spilka et al. 2003; Tenorio and Lo 2011; Werbner 2010). Conversely, religiosity maintains sociality by dismissing individualism, oppression, sexuality, and violence (Fontana 2003; Horell 2014; Spilka et al. 2003). The ideal for tradition or traditionalism has underlain confidence in economic and political institutions, refutation against unconventional sexuality, and rejection of outsiders (Costa et al. 2023; Meuleman et al. 2019; Schwartz et al. 2010; Wang and You 2016). Moreover, traditionalism upholds sociality regarding morality and patriotism (Maltseva 2016; Schwartz et al. 2014).

Norms underlying confidence in the market for assimilating sociality have publicized fairness (Mishler and Rose 1997; Zanin 2017). The norm of fairness has upheld sociality by elevating morality and prosocial behavior (Barber 2004; McCaffoee 2016).

Business, involving companies, corporations, and enterprises, maintains sociality by offering or reflecting power and ideals to achieve the requisite social functions of fulfillment or goal attainment and latency. Such achievement realizes the deterministic mechanisms of analytical functionalism. These mechanisms are societally influential even without personal voluntarism. Notably, ideals at the societal level mean norms at the personal level.

Power generated by business to empower sociality rests on societal cohesion, community, and social integration (Coffe and Geys 2006; Milner 2002). Cohesion, community, and social integration at the societal level construct social capital at the personal level (Inglehart and Welzel 2005). Societal cohesion has empowered personal sociality by enhancing personal civic engagement, favor for community, political participation, and trust (Z. Han et al. 2017; F. Lee 2012; Palmer et al. 2011; Whitham 2012). Conversely, societal cohesion has strengthened personal sociality by preventing personal violence (E. Wright et al. 2015). Business has also reflected power based on societal education, social capital, and urbanization to empower sociality (Kilburn and Maume 2000; Peng 2004). Societal education has empowered personal sociality by enhancing personal civic participation, social capital, trust, volunteering, and xenophobia or disfavor against immigrants (Boeri et al. 2002; Portes and Vickstrom 2011; Rupasingha et al. 2006; Uslaner and Brown 2005). Conversely, societal education has sustained personal sociality by dampening personal violence (Poveda 2011). Societal urbanization has empowered personal sociality by facilitating attachment, citizenship, civility, cohesion, collaboration, communication, and social capital and reducing conflict and crime (Cochrane 2007; Cushing and Miller 2020; Glaeser and Gottlieb 2006; Grant 2006; Kelly and Becker 2000; Sternberg 2000). Societal conflict involves societal violence (J. Turner 2013b). Societal violence has impaired sociality by fomenting personal tolerance for violence (Douglas 2006). Societal crime has impeded personal sociality by reducing personal community practice, prosocial behavior, and trust (Broadbent and Papadopoulos 2011; Zanin 2017; Zhong 2010). Conversely, business has declined due to societal poverty and vacant housing, which disempower sociality (Kilburn and Maume 2000). Such societal maldevelopment has undermined personal sociality by impairing personal donation, obedience, and trust and raising personal protesting (Fridberg and Kangas 2008b; Norris 2002).

Ideals hailed by business to frame sociality have highlighted societal communitarianism, conservatism, employment, humanism, reciprocity, sharing, solidarity, and trust (Chandler 2023; Fives 2008; Pargal et al. 2002; Peng 2004; Powell 2007). Communitarianism constitutes sociality by espousing caring, civility, collective identity, commonweal orientation, community, dutifulness or responsibility, education or socialization, equality, interdependence, loyalty, mentoring, patriotism, reciprocity, relatedness, self-discipline, servicing including volunteering, settlement, social construction, social participation, solidarity, and trust (Delanty 2009; Frazer 1999; Moore 2010; Speth 2012). Community encompasses attachment, identification, networking, and sharing (Frazer 1999). Relatedness includes attachment and sharing (Speth 2012). Social construction involves discourse, negotiation, and socialization (Frazer 1999). Conservatism sustains sociality by nurturing empathy, loyalty, prosocial behavior, religiousness, and sacrifice (Dutton and Rayner-Hilles 2022). Moreover, conservatism underpins sociality by maintaining allegiance or loyalty, attachment, civility, community, conformity, cooperation, discipline, ethnocentrism, honesty, humility, intimacy, legality, morality, nationalism, obedience, order, partnership, patriotism, peace, responsibility, sharing, trust, and xenophobia (Dutton and Rayner-Hilles 2022; Heilman and Kusev 2020; Hickson 2013; Lakoff 2009;

Rhodes-Purdy et al. 2023; Scruton 2014; Yoos 2007; Zuk and Zuk 2020). Conversely, conservatism upholds sociality by condemning dehumanizing, evilness, revolution, sexuality, terrorism, and transgression (Dutton and Rayner-Hilles 2022; Malka and Soto 2011; Scruton 2014; Suhay 2015). Societal employment stands on societal social democracy (De Deken 2002). Societal social democracy sustains sociality by championing equality and solidarity (Andersson 2006). Humanism favors sociality by highlighting attachment, caring, collectivity, community, cooperation, friendship, helpfulness, institutions, loving, order, respect, relatedness, responsibility, and sharing (Browning and Cooper 2004; Fuchs 2020; Selznick 2008; Stefanski and Jach 2022; Visher 1997; Waterman 2013). Conversely, humanism encourages sociality by rejecting alienation, conflict, and individualization (Fuchs 2020; Selznick 2008). Reciprocity has constituted sociality by fostering prosocial behavior (Thielmann et al. 2020). Furthermore, reciprocity, sharing, solidarity, and trust characterize sociality (Capraro 2024; Cottrell et al. 2007; Fenwick 2008; Koster 2013).

Confidence in business constitutes sociality by providing ideals to achieve the requisite functions of analytical functionalism. Such confidence has strengthened ideals for institutionalism and morality to constitute sociality (Farwell et al. 2019; Patwardhan et al. 2012). Institutionalism and morality characterize sociality (Rogers et al. 2014; Tomasello 2020).

Confidence in business benefits from sociality by providing ideals to secure functioning. Ideals for maintaining sociality have rested on conservatism and the ideal for business (Pace 2015; Zumbrunnen and Gangl 2008). Conservatism constitutes sociality by nurturing empathy, loyalty, prosocial behavior, religiousness, and sacrifice (Dutton and Rayner-Hilles 2022). Moreover, conservatism underlies sociality by maintaining allegiance or loyalty, attachment, civility, community, conformity, cooperation, discipline, ethnocentrism, honesty, humility, intimacy, legality, morality, nationalism, obedience, order, partnership, patriotism, peace, responsibility, sharing, trust, and xenophobia (Dutton and Rayner-Hilles 2022; Heilman and Kusev 2020; Hickson 2013; Lakoff 2009; Rhodes-Purdy et al. 2023; Scruton 2014; Yoos 2007; Zuk and Zuk 2020).

The cultural institution, exemplified by educational and religious institutions, represents or signifies civilization cooperation, idealism, ideology or superstructure, information, the lifeworld, sharing, soft power, and value structure (Inglis 2004; Kroenig et al. 2010; Luthar 2009; Mesoudi 2011; Minkov 2011; D. Rose 2019; Tumino 2011; J. Turner 2017). This institution publicizes achievement, art, dignity or esteem, harmony, honor, identity, joy, morality, normativity, personality, stability, and uniformity (Aslani et al. 2013); Basanez 2016; McCrae 2009; D. Rose 2019; Saha 2018). Achievement involves efficiency, egalitarianism, empowerment, frugality, individualism, masculinity, productivity, Protestantism, punctuality, saving, and wealth (Basanez 2016). Dignity conveys confrontation, dynamism, expressionism, independence, law, rationality, and self-regulation (Aslani et al. 2013). Honor rests on aggression, altruism, community, discipline, dominance, dynamism, expression, hierarchy, hospitality, loyalty, orthodoxy, toughness, and trustworthiness (Aslani et al. 2013; Basanez 2016). Joy resides in friendship, generosity, grandeur, leisure, rights, and skillfulness (Basanez 2016). Personality comprises agreeableness, conscientiousness, extraversion, openness, and emotional stability (McCrae 2009).

The cultural institution upholds sociality by offering power, utility, ideals, and norms to achieve the requisite function of analytical functionalism. Such offering works through cultivation, institutionalization, mediatization, normalization, social construction, and socialization (Guenther et al. 2016; Lizardo 2016; J. Turner 2017; Venn 2007). This work also hinges on evolution involving adaptation and selection between the person and society (Oyserman and Uskul 2008). Eventually, this work establishes the culture, habitus, language, lifeworld, religion, meanings, symbols, tastes, and values (Bennardo and De Munck 2014; Chhotray and Stoker 2009; Minkov 2011; Inglis 2004; Jasper 2005; J. Turner 2017). Notably, power, utility, and ideals at the societal level become norms at the personal level.

Power generated by the cultural institution to drive sociality resides in knowledge about history, language proficiency, morality, and social cohesion (Aslani et al. 2013; Oyserman and Uskul 2008; Munch 2012; D. Rose 2019). Generally, knowledge has raised sociality by enhancing cooperation, prosocial behavior, social cohesion, social trust, and volunteering (de Groot and Steg 2009; Lepkowski and Couper 2002; Pattie et al. 2004; Simon-Bemd and Steffens 2000; Volker et al. 2007). More specifically, history knowledge based on history education has enhanced sociality by consolidating citizenship, responsibility, and social trust (Geboers et al. 2013; Kahne et al. 2006). Citizenship raised by history education covers the commonweal, governance, identity, justice, membership, participation, and social cohesion (Geboers et al. 2013). Language proficiency has enabled sociality by elevating nationalism and social trust (Cai et al. 2022; Lancee and Dronkers 2011). Morality has constituted sociality by establishing volunteering and inhibiting violence (Piquero and Hickman 2002; Whitford et al. 2006). Social cohesion has constituted sociality by enhancing attachment and dampening tolerance for deviance (Stafford et al. 2005; Woosnam et al. 2018).

Utility offered by the cultural institution to attract sociality rests on harmony experienced (Jones-Smith 2014). Harmony experienced has induced sociality characterized by adjustment, attunement, civility, compromise, connectedness, interdependency, order, peace, relatedness, respect, sacrifice, selflessness, solidarity, and sympathy as opposed to competition and conflict (Arat and Kerelian 2019; Cheung and Ma 2011; P. Ip 2014; Kjell et al. 2016; Peck 2002; G. Zhang 2006).

Ideals preached by the cultural institution to rationalize sociality accentuate agreeableness, Catholicism, collectivism, communication, community, Confucianism, conscientiousness, coordination, discipline, egalitarianism, extraversion, friendship, generosity, honesty, hospitality, interdependence, legality, loyalty, nationalism, normativity, protection, rationality, relatedness, religiosity, responsibility, social interaction, tradition, trust, trustworthiness, warmth, and xenophobia (Aslani et al. 2013; Basanez 2016; Bennardo and De Munck 2014; Craig and Douglas 2012; McCrae 2009; Minkov 2011; Moore 2015; Oyserman and Uskul 2008; D. Rose 2019). Agreeableness has fostered sociality by enhancing attachment (Fraley et al. 2011). Moreover, agreeableness constitutes sociality by featuring communion, compliance, cooperation, empathy, helping, intimacy, morality, politeness, prosociality, respect, solidarity, sympathy, understanding, warmth, and unity (Dinic and

Bodroza 2021; Graziano and Tobin 2009; J. Sun et al. 2018). Catholicism promulgated by the cultural institution fosters sociality by emphasizing consensus, groupness, obedience, and teamwork (Basanez 2016). Moreover, Catholicism has enhanced sociality by raising conformity value and volunteering and dampening independence value and radicalism (Bekkers 2010; Devos et al. 2002; Fjellvang 2011). Catholicism has also safeguarded sociality by inculcating cooperation and interdependence (Bellah et al. 1991). Collectivism has constituted sociality by securing civility, cooperation, prosocial behavior, and religiousness and preventing extremism (Hample 2018; Harzing 2006; Oyserman et al. 1998; Saucier and Skrzypinska 2006; Thielmann et al. 2020). Communication has enabled sociality regarding social cohesion, participation, and trust (Miyata et al. 2008; Rothstein and Uslaner 2005). Community involvement has underlain sociality regarding cooperation, networking, and trust (Groves et al. 2000; Molitor et al. 2011; Rochelle 2015). Confucianism has championed sociality regarding association, civility, and collectivism as opposed to violence (Y. Lin et al. 2021; Shin 2012; Stotzer 2014). Conscientiousness has elevated sociality by consolidating attachment, compliance, order value, responsibility, social desirability, and volunteering and reducing deviance, violence, and justification for unconventional sexuality (Bekkers 2005; de Jong et al. 2012; Fraley et al. 2011; Gotzsche-Astrup 2020; Mondak and Hurwitz 2012; Mullet et al. 2005; Saucier and Skrzypinska 2006; Twardawski et al. 2021; Wright and DeLisi 2016). Coordination has constituted sociality by strengthening agreeableness, empathy, morality, and social capital (Halevy et al. 2019). Discipline has buttressed sociality by raising generativity and diminishing crime and violence (Y. Cheung et al. 2014; Welch et al. 2008; Peterson and Klohnen 1995). Generativity means caring and concern for others (Cote 2000; Peterson and Klohnen 1995). As such, generativity has enhanced sociality by raising helping value and political participation (Peterson and Klohnen 1995). Egalitarianism has underpinned sociality by enhancing empathy, support for welfare, and trust in government and impeding radicalism (Faricy and Ellis 2014; Lauriola et al. 2015; Lucas and Kteily 2018; Roosma et al. 2014). Extraversion has buttressed sociality by fostering attachment, civic engagement, civility, donation, humor, nationalism, political participation, social capital, socializing, volunteering, and favor for civic and political participation (Bekkers 2010; C. Cheng et al. 2019; Fraley et al. 2011; Gotzsche-Astrup 2020; Hample 2018; Omoto et al. 2010; Schbley and McCauley 2005; Vernon et al. 2008; Ward and Forney 2020). Friendship has constituted sociality by enhancing community attachment, compliance, donation, gratitude, political participation, social cohesion, social desirability, social integration, and social trust (Corcoran 2013; Fahmy 2006; Gundert and Hohendanner 2015; Keillor et al. 2001; Kende et al. 2022; Opp 2001; Rotkirch 2014). Moreover, the norm for friendship has consolidated sociality by reducing protesting (Sampson et al. 2005). Generosity has raised sociality by facilitating donation (Piferi et al. 2006). Moreover, generosity maintains sociality by involving social closeness, commitment, contribution, and gifting (Godoy et al. 2007; Murray and Holmes 2008). Honesty has built sociality by raising compliance and prosocial behavior and eschewing crime (Jolley et al. 2019; Thielmann et al. 2020; Twardawski et al. 2021). Hospitality has constituted sociality by enhancing trust (Vera-Toscano et al. 2013). Interdependence has buttressed sociality by securing attachment, donation, prosocial behavior, social inclusion, and social interaction (Feeney and Collins 2001; Uskul et al. 2004; Z. Xin et al. 2017). Legality has safeguarded sociality by dismissing radicalism (Muthuswamy 2022). Loyalty has constituted sociality by fostering collaboration, empathy, generosity, leadership, and morality (Lawler et al. 2016; Lee and Chan 2016; Wilcox and Dew 2016). Nationalism has underpinned sociality by fostering attachment, intolerance against deviance, patriotism, political participation, religiousness, social inclusion, trust in government, and xenophobia, and diminishing protesting (N. Chen 2012; Flanagan and Lee 2000; Huddy et al. 2021; Li and Brewer 2004; Osborne et al. 2017; Pinto et al. 2020; Rippl et al. 2010). Normativity has established sociality by uplifting civic engagement, donation, prosocial behavior, punishment, support for policy, volunteering, and voting, and eroding cheating, violence, and tolerance for violence (Brown and Ferris 2007; Hennessy et al. 2015; Huesmann 2018; B. Liu et al. 2023; Opp 2002; Pavlova and Silbereisen 2015; Wade-Benzoni and Tost 2009; Waterman et al. 2022; Wenzel 2004). Protection has bolstered sociality by enhancing affiliative humor and attenuating aggressive humor (Erickson and Feldstein 2007). Rationality has facilitated sociality by preventing aggression and antisociality (DiGiuseppe et al. 2017). Relatedness has consolidated sociality by consolidating sharing, social interaction, and relationship satisfaction (Downie et al. 2008; Frazer 1999; Wickham and Knee 2012). Religiosity has sustained sociality by fostering civic engagement, civility, cohesion, compliance, donation, empathy, morality, patriotism, prejudice against deviants and outsiders, prosocial behavior, social trust, and volunteering (Apinunmahakul and Devlin 2008; Corcoran et al. 2011; Ishio 2010; Keyes 2002; Kim and Wilcox 2013; Ravanera et al. 2003; van Tienen et al. 2011; Weisberg 2005; Wuthnow 2004). Conversely, religiosity has secured sociality by reducing crime, deviance, individualism, protesting, and sexuality (Andrews et al. 2015; Coffe and Geys 2007; Guo et al. 2008; Skerkat and Ellison 1999; Spilka et al. 2003). Moreover, religiosity realizes sociality regarding altruism, community, ethicality, groupism, sharing, and solidarity (Franks et al. 2013; Lichterman 2012; Peifer 2010; Spilka et al. 2003; Stavrova and Siegers 2014). Religiosity also upholds sociality by featuring altruism, attachment, caring, community, compassion, harmony, hospitality, love, morality, obedience, other-centeredness, peace, trust, unity, xenophobia (Ager and Ager 2011; Fontana 2003; Harris et al. 2018; Horell 2014; Paterson 2018; Shorey et al. 2018; Simpson et al. 2008; Spilka et al. 2003; Tenorio and Lo 2011; Werbner 2010). Conversely, religiosity maintains sociality by dismissing individualism, oppression, sexuality, and violence (Fontana 2003; Horell 2014; Spilka et al. 2003). Responsibility has sustained sociality regarding compliance, morality, and xenophobia as opposed to violence (Bussey 2020; Granzin and Olsen 1998; Kaurin 2020; Milner and Myers 2007). Social interaction has realized sociality by consolidating altruism, compliance, cooperation, donation, morality, political participation, reciprocity, social trust, and volunteering (Guillen et al. 2011; Dixon and McKeown 2021; Lucas and Livingston 2014; Musick 2000; Rodrigo-Gonzalez et al. 2019; Rubin and Step 2000). The ideal for tradition or traditionalism has underlain confidence in economic and political institutions, refutation against unconventional sexuality, and rejection of outsiders (Costa et al. 2023; Meuleman et al. 2019; Schwartz et al. 2010; Wang and You 2016). Moreover, traditionalism upholds sociality regarding morality and patriotism (Maltseva 2016; Schwartz et al. 2014). Trust has constituted sociality through donation, involvement, and volunteering (Uslaner 2000). Trustworthiness underlies sociality by establishing attachment, intimacy, social capital, and trust (X. Chen et al. 2015; Harvey and Wenzel 2006). As part of agreeableness, warmth has fostered sociality by enhancing attachment (Fraley et al. 2011; J. Sun et al. 2018). Xenophobia has constituted sociality by boosting patriotism and social cohesion (Granzin and Olsen 1998; Wang and Chen 2004). Moreover, xenophobia represents sociality by upholding nationalism (Biggs and Knauss 2012).

Conversely, the cultural institution strengthens sociality by discounting individualism (Minkov 2011). Individualism has weakened sociality by reducing civic engagement, religiousness, social cohesion, and volunteering (Church 2010; Green and Janmaat 2011; J. He et al. 2014; Hener et al. 2016; Leong 2008; Pollack and Pickel 2007; Whitford et al. 2006). Conversely, individualism has impeded sociality by bolstering acceptance of outsiders, competition, crime, extremity, self-enhancement, protesting, and violence (Church 2010; J. He et al. 2014; Karstedt 2010; Leong 2008; Li and Song 1992; Pollack and Pickel 2007; Whitford et al. 2006).

The cultural institution also rests on power, utility, ideals, and norms constituting or evolving from sociality. Sociality represents friendship, humanity, and morality (de Vries and Megathlin 2009; Fowers 2015). Specifically, sociality features altruism, attachment, caring, cooperation, fairness, friendship, groupness, openness, reciprocity, relatedness, sharing, social interaction, trust, and trustworthiness (Capraro 2024; Cottrell et al. 2007; Fenwick 2008; Fowers 2015; Koster 2013; Ratner et al. 2023). Conversely, sociality denounces aggression, individualism, risking, and violence (Fowers 2015; Schinkel 2010).

Power empowering the cultural institution to establish sociality rests on dialogue or negotiation, religion, sharing or transmission, and soft power (Holliday 2011; Minkov 2011; Kroenig et al. 2010; D. Rose 2019; M. Smith 2000). Dialogue or negotiation has buttressed sociality by fostering social trust (Barrera 2007). Besides, dialogue or negotiation sustains sociality by representing commonality, flexibility, and interdependency (Carrell and Heavrin 2008). Dialogue or negotiation also maintains sociality by espousing adaptation, agreement or consensus building, assimilation, collaboration, communality, concession, cooperativeness, empathy, equality, fairness, interdependence, logrolling, patience, reciprocity, relatedness, and soft power (Carrell and Heavrin 2008; Koning and van Dijk 2013; Kono and Ito 2021; Rudd and Hughes 2020; Stuhlmacher and Linnabery 2017). Soft power for negotiation includes charisma, cooperation, friendliness, gentleness, humility or humbleness, openness, patience, proactiveness, rapport building, self-discipline, supportiveness, trust, warmth, and win-win benefiting (Greene 1991). Conversely, dialogue or negotiation upholds sociality by dismissing disputing and irritating (Aslani et al. 2013; Carrell and Heavrin 2008). Societal religion has enhanced sociality by raising societal collectivism (Realo et al. 2008). Besides, societal religion maintains sociality directly and by establishing morality (Pelters and Wijma 2016; Rindermann 2018).

Morality has constituted sociality by boosting volunteering and inhibiting violence (Piquero and Hickman 2002; Whitford et al. 2006). Moreover, rationality enhances sociality by supporting communication, deontological or moral understanding, discussion, expression, and social acceptability (Bolis et al. 2017; Bouwmeester 2017; Lambie 2008; Royzman et al. 2015). Societal collectivism has secured sociality by boosting institutional trust and mentalizing or perspective-taking (Aival-Naveh et al. 2019; McAllister 1999). Sharing has raised sociality by facilitating donating (Piferi et al. 2006). Moreover, sharing maintains sociality by involving social closeness, commitment, contribution, and gifting (Godoy et al. 2007; Murray and Holmes 2008). Conversely, power empowering the cultural institution suffers from alienation and exploitation experienced (M. Smith 2000; Tumino 2011). Alienation experienced has eroded sociality regarding attachment (Bishop et al. 2002). Exploitation experienced impaired sociality by provoking conflict and confrontation (J. Turner 2013b).

Ideals framing the cultural institution to achieve sociality highlight communitarianism, cooperation, groupness, and republicanism (Minkov 2011; Oishi 2012; D. Rose 2019; Spicker 2019). Communitarianism constitutes sociality by espousing caring, civility, collective identity, commonweal orientation, community, dutifulness or responsibility, education or socialization, equality, interdependence, loyalty, mentoring, patriotism, reciprocity, relatedness, self-discipline, servicing including volunteering, settlement, social construction, social participation, solidarity, and trust (Delanty 2009; Frazer 1999; Moore 2010; Speth 2012). Cooperation has strengthened sociality regarding attachment and trustworthiness as opposed to argument (Gerbasi and Cook 2008; Hample 2018; Tak 2017). Groupness has fostered sociality regarding cohesion, common identity, and identification (Fischer et al. 2007). Republicanism upholds sociality regarding citizenship, the commonweal, interdependence, morality, nationalism, publicity, responsibility, social adaptation, and solidarity (Delanty 2009; Honohan 2002).

Confidence in the cultural institution transpires in cultural engagement featuring consumption, familiarity, lifestyle, passion, practice, and wisdom (de Vries and de Graaf 2008; Silva 2005; Walton 2012). Cultural engagement champions sociality by generating power, utility, ideals, and norms to achieve the requisite functions of analytical functionalism.

Power generated by cultural engagement to drive sociality rests on mobilization and solidarity (Gillham et al. 2019; Van Ness and Summers-Effler 2016). Mobilization has fostered sociality by enhancing civic engagement, consensus, political participation, and volunteering and reducing conflict (Djupe and Lewis 2015; Pattie et al. 2004; Sexton and Benson 2006). Moreover, mobilization registers sociality regarding consent, institutionalism, and social capital (Brunie 2009; Gilley 2009; Lowndes and Roberts 2013). Solidarity has empowered personal sociality by enhancing personal civic engagement, favor for community, political participation, and trust (Z. Han et al. 2017; F. Lee 2012; Palmer et al. 2011; Whitham 2012).

Utility created by confidence in cultural engagement to attract sociality has resided in resilience, satisfaction, and well-being generally (Corbin and Hall 2019; Grossi et al. 2013; Kuper et al. 2023). Resilience has attracted sociality by raising bonding and inhibiting crime and violence (Fields and McNamara 2003; Hoffman 2003; Solomon and Roloff 2018). Furthermore, resilience sustains sociality by embodying or fostering adaptation and legality (Hoffman 2003; Ungar 2012). Resilience also underlies sociality by demonstrating altruism, attractiveness, communication or conversation, community, compassion, empathy or perspective-taking, negotiation, peacefulness, relationality, relatedness, social capital or resourcefulness, social cohesion, and social competence (Elfers et al. 2024; Hjemdal et al. 2015; Jones and d'Errico 2019; Kelley et al. 2019; Kent and Davis 2010; Ungar 2010; Zautra 2014). Satisfaction has advanced sociality by strengthening political participation, social cohesion, social and government trust, and volunteering (E. Chan 2014; Flavin and Keane 2011; Rochelle 2015). Well-being has uplifted sociality by consolidating altruism, conformism, cooperation, donation, liking for people, prosociality, sociability, and trust and social trust (Fetvadjiev and He 2019; A. Hu 2013; Lyubomirsky et al. 2006; Y. Pan et al. 2023; Wang and Graddy 2008). Additionally, well-being sustains sociality by enabling civilization, fairness, forgiveness, intimacy, kindness, love, loyalty, modesty, morality, open-mindedness, social intelligence, and societal functioning (Cummins 2016; D'raven and Pasha-Zaidi 2016; Meadows 2014). Moreover, utility offered by cultural engagement to attract sociality evolves from sublimation (Walton 2012). Sublimation upholds sociality by securing morality and religiosity and dampening evilness (Aragno 2014; Forsyth 2003).

Ideals nurtured by cultural engagement to rationalize sociality have covered political interest, religiosity, and social trust (Freitag 2003b; Prior 2019; Wuthnow 2004). Political interest has elevated sociality by raising civic engagement, civic and social motivation, civility, and discussion as opposed to protesting (Gil de Zuniga et al. 2017; Lee and Chan 2011; Pattie et al. 2004). Religiosity has sustained sociality by fostering civic engagement, civility, cohesion, compliance, donation, empathy, morality, patriotism, prejudice against deviants and outsiders, prosocial behavior, social trust, and volunteering (Apinunmahakul and Devlin 2008; Corcoran et al. 2011; Ishio 2010; Keyes 2002; Kim and Wilcox 2013; Ravanera et al. 2003; van Tienen et al. 2011; Weisberg 2005; Wuthnow 2004). Conversely, religiosity has secured sociality by reducing crime, deviance, individualism, protesting, and sexuality (Andrews et al. 2015; Coffe and Geys 2007; Guo et al. 2008; Skerkat and Ellison 1999; Spilka et al. 2003). Moreover, religiosity realizes sociality regarding altruism, community, ethicality, groupism, sharing, and solidarity (Franks et al. 2013; Lichterman 2012; Peifer 2010; Spilka et al. 2003; Stavrova and Siegers 2014). Religiosity also upholds sociality by featuring altruism, attachment, caring, community, compassion, harmony, hospitality, love, morality, obedience, other-centeredness, peace, trust, unity, xenophobia (Ager and Ager 2011; Fontana 2003; Harris et al. 2018; Horell 2014; Paterson 2018; Shorey et al. 2018; Simpson et al. 2008; Spilka et al. 2003; Tenorio and Lo 2011; Werbner 2010). Conversely, religiosity maintains sociality by dismissing individualism, oppression, sexuality, and violence (Fontana 2003; Horell 2014; Spilka et al. 2003). Social trust has constituted sociality through donation, involvement, and volunteering (Uslaner 2000). Moreover, ideals espoused by cultural engagement to sustain sociality valorize consensus, popularity, rationality, and sympathy (Walton 2012; Watson 2019). Consensus has enhanced sociality by fostering cohesion, compliance, engagement, and rejection of outsiders (Fasel et al. 2016; Guan et al. 2021; Heshmati and Oravecz 2022; Yoon et al. 2013). Popularity has facilitated sociality by raising belongingness (Reich et al. 2018). Relationality has consolidated sociality by consolidating sharing, social interaction, and relationship satisfaction (Downie et al. 2008; Frazer 1999; Wickham and Knee 2012). Sympathy has constituted sociality by securing religiosity and volunteering (Barr et al. 2005).

Cultural engagement also stands on power based on friendliness to drive sociality (Kraaykamp and van Eijck 2005). Friendliness has enabled sociality regarding prosocial behavior (Foschi and Lauriola 2014).

The educational institution as a cultural institution manifests its functioning in societal education or educational attainment. Societal education means capability building or capacitation (Kelly 2020). It works through accreditation, balancing liberalization and regulation, and ranking (Dakka 2020; Komotar 2020). Societal education propels sociality by securing power, utility, ideals, and norms for empowering, incentivizing, framing, and normalizing to achieve the requisite functions of analytical functionalism. Notably, power, utility, and ideals at the societal level constitute norms at the personal level.

Power maintained by the educational institution to empower sociality has rested on health, intelligence, and social capital (Herian et al. 2014; Portes and Vickstrom 2011; Schaie 2013). Health has uplifted sociality by boosting community sense, morality, popularity, social activity, social cohesion, social integration, social trust, social well-being, and volunteering (Huxhold et al. 2014; Jorgensen et al. 2010; Son and Wilson 2012; Tolsma et al. 2009; Yu and Chiu 2016). Conversely, health has sustained sociality by preventing loneliness (Koromeckyj-Cox et al. 2007). Intelligence has raised sociality by facilitating donation and social capital and reducing criminality and protesting (Cornwall 2009; Feinstein and Bynner 2006; Paterson 2008; Piferi et al. 2006). Social capital has consolidated sociality by raising civic engagement, community involvement, donation, political involvement, social trust, and volunteering (Bekkers et al. 2008; Broadbent and Papadopoulos 2011; Brown and Ferris 2007; Chua et al. 2021; Narayan and Cassidy 2001). Conversely, social capital has strengthened sociality by erasing violence (Pulkkinen et al. 2009). Moreover, the educational institution elevates power or competence in coping, deliberation, mindfulness, productivity, rationality or reasoning, and self-control or self-regulation to facilitate sociality (Bowker 2016; Corrigan et al. 2013; A. Miller 2022; Olssen et al. 2004; Stevenson 2011). Coping has enabled sociality by facilitating compliance, intimacy, and relatedness (Chow et al. 2014; Gattino et al. 2015; Twardawski et al. 2021). Deliberation, rationality, or reasoning has facilitated sociality by preventing aggression and antisociality (DiGiuseppe et al. 2017). Mindfulness has facilitated sociality by raising affiliating, intimacy, and prosocial behavior (D. Berry et al. 2020; Flett 2018; Karremans et al. 2017). Productivity has enabled sociality by preventing crime (Tanner-Smith et al. 2013). Self-control or self-regulation has buttressed sociality by enhancing generativity and impeding crime, risking, and violence (Y. Cheung et al. 2014; Koegl and Day 2019; Peterson and Klohnen 1995; Welch et al. 2008).

Utility forged by the educational institution to incentivize sociality lies in achievement, meaningfulness, self-creation, and self-realization (Corrigan et al. 2013; A.

Miller 2022; Shan 2017). Achievement has induced sociality by enhancing love and trust (Nezlek et al. 2008; Rieger and Wang 2021). Meaningfulness has underlain sociality by boosting civic practice, responsibility, and volunteering and reducing rejection experience (Duffy and Raque-Bogdan 2010; Summers and Falco 2020; Twenge et al. 2003). Self-creation maintains sociality by espousing attachment (Raeff 2010). Self-realization can uphold sociality by raising political evaluation, which rests on communitarianism and republicanism (Caprara and Vecchione 2013). Political evaluation constitutes sociality by unfolding communitarianism and republicanism, which espouse community and solidarity (Pattie et al. 2004). Conversely, the educational institution mitigates oppression experienced (Stevenson 2011). Oppression experienced erodes sociality by fomenting violence (White et al. 2015).

Ideals created by the educational institution to frame sociality have valorized civic engagement, honesty, social and government trust, volunteering, and xenophobia (Boeri et al. 2002; Cohen and Bolt 2005; Lipford and Yandle 2009; Poveda 2011; Rupasingha et al. 2006; Uslaner and Brown 2005; van Hemert et al. 2002). Civic engagement has propped sociality by strengthening attachment, civility, collective behavior, discussion, donation, neighboring, patriotism, prosociality, social capital, socialism, trust, and volunteering and impeding cheating and individualism (Coffe and Geys 2007; Gilberbloom and Markham 1995; Kerrissey and Schofer 2013; Mata and Pendakur 2014; Ozbay 2008; Pattie et al. 2004; Pena-Lopez and Sanchez-Santos 2016; Rahn 2008; Richey 2011; Tak 2017; M. Tang 2011; Taniguchi 2013; Yip et al. 2007). Honesty has built sociality by raising compliance and prosocial behavior and eschewing crime (Jolley et al. 2019; Thielmann et al. 2020; Twardawski et al. 2021). Trust has constituted sociality through donation, involvement, and volunteering (Uslaner 2000). Volunteering has constituted sociality by raising altruism, charity orientation, civic motivation, donation, helping, moral responsibility, political participation, social integration, and social and government trust (Foster et al. 2001; Isham et al. 2006; Richey 2010; Richey and Ikeda 2009; Wiepking and Maas 2009). Conversely, volunteering has safeguarded sociality by preventing deviance and its tolerance, delinquency, and loneliness (Gillath et al. 2005; J. Wilson 2000; Woolley 2003). Xenophobia has constituted sociality by boosting patriotism and social cohesion (Granzin and Olsen 1998; Wang and Chen 2004). Moreover, xenophobia represents sociality by upholding nationalism (Biggs and Knauss 2012). Moreover, the educational institution fosters sociality by preaching caring, citizenship, communitarianism, compassion or sympathy, Confucianism, cohesion, collaboration or cooperation, collectivity, communality, communitarianism, equality, exchange, grouping, interdependence, loyalty, networking, partnership, prosociality, republicanism, respect, responsibility or accountability, responsiveness, social engagement, and solidarity (Aidnik 2024; Bowker 2016; Corrigan et al. 2013; Gewirtz and Cribb 2009; A. Miller 2022; Olssen et al. 2004; Shan 2017; Stevenson 2011). Caring, compassion, or sympathy has constituted sociality by securing religiosity and volunteering (Barr et al. 2005). Confucianism preached by the educational institution to boost sociality treasures loving, moderation, and unity (Shan 2017). Additionally, Confucianism has championed sociality regarding association, civility, and collectivism as opposed to violence (Y. Lin et al. 2021; Shin 2012; Stotzer 2014). Social cohesion has constituted sociality by enhancing attachment and dampening tolerance for deviance (Stafford et al. 2005; Woosnam et al. 2018). Collaboration or cooperation has strengthened sociality regarding attachment and trustworthiness as opposed to argument (Gerbasi and Cook 2008; Hample 2018; Tak 2017). Collectivism or communality has constituted sociality by securing civility, cooperation, prosocial behavior, and religiousness and preventing extremism (Hample 2018; Harzing 2006; Oyserman et al. 1998; Saucier and Skrzypinska 2006; Thielmann et al. 2020). Communitarianism taught in the educational institution valorizes the commonweal, equality, community, and negotiation to uplift sociality (Olssen et al. 2004). Besides, communitarianism constitutes sociality by espousing caring, civility, collective identity, commonweal orientation, community, dutifulness or responsibility, education or socialization, equality, interdependence, loyalty, mentoring, patriotism, reciprocity, relatedness, self-discipline, servicing including volunteering, settlement, social construction, social participation, solidarity, and trust (Delanty 2009; Frazer 1999; Moore 2010; Speth 2012). The ideal for equality or egalitarianism has underpinned sociality by enhancing empathy, support for welfare, and trust in government and impeding radicalism (Faricy and Ellis 2014; Lauriola et al. 2015; Lucas and Kteily 2018; Roosma et al. 2014). Exchange has sustained sociality regarding compliance, cooperation, morality, social cohesion, social commitment, social integration, social interaction, social participation, trust, and volunteering (Bagherior et al. 2009; Carter 2016; Drollinger 2010; Lawler et al. 2016; Skopek et al. 2011; Yoon et al. 2013; Zhang and Zhou 2018). Conversely, exchange has maintained sociality by dampening resistance and violence (Foy et al. 2014; Hattery and Smith 2012). Grouping has fostered sociality regarding cohesion, common identity, and identification (Fischer et al. 2007). Interdependence has buttressed sociality by securing attachment, donation, prosocial behavior, social inclusion, and social interaction (Feeney and Collins 2001; Uskul et al. 2004; Z. Xin et al. 2017). Loyalty has constituted sociality by fostering collaboration, empathy, generosity, leadership, and morality (Lawler et al. 2016; Lee and Chan 2016; Wilcox and Dew 2016). Networking has fostered sociality regarding connectedness, friendship, giving, and social interaction (Eberl 2020; Liebler and Sandefur 2002; Nelson-Coffey et al. 2023; Phan et al. 2009). Partnership constitutes sociality by realizing equality and responsibility and opposing conflict (Harvie and Manzis 2011; Mills and Taht 2010; Waiton 2008). Prosociality has constituted sociality by civility, consolidating connectedness, cooperation, religiosity, responsibility, and volunteering (Hample 2018; Marsh and Dik 2021; Musick and Wilson 2008; Nelson-Coffey et al. 2023; Shahzalal and Adnan 2022). Moreover, prosociality underlies sociality by enhancing citizenship, loyalty, social cohesion, socializing, and trust and diminishing self-interest (Dovidio et al. 2006; Hawley 2014; Kisliuk and WeiBmuller 2023; Music 2014). Republicanism enhances sociality regarding equalization and participation (Olssen et al. 2004). Furthermore, republicanism upholds sociality regarding citizenship, commonweal, interdependence, morality, nationalism, publicity, responsibility, social adaptation, and solidarity (Delanty 2009; Honohan 2002). Respect constitutes sociality regarding caring and equality (Renger and Reese 2017). Responsibility or accountability has sustained sociality regarding compliance, morality, and xenophobia as opposed to violence (Bussey 2020; Granzin and Olsen 1998; Kaurin 2020; Milner and Myers 2007). Responsiveness has uplifted sociality regarding prosocial behavior (Clobert et al. 2015). Social engagement has realized sociality by consolidating altruism, compliance, cooperation, donation, morality, political participation, reciprocity, social trust, and volunteering (Guillen et al. 2011; Dixon and McKeown 2021; Lucas and Livingston 2014; Musick 2000; Rodrigo-Gonzalez et al. 2019; Rubin and Step 2000). Solidarity has constituted sociality by enhancing attachment and dampening tolerance for deviance (Stafford et al. 2005; Woosnam et al. 2018).

Conversely, the educational institution sustains sociality by downplaying ideals for individualism, subversion, and violence (A. Miller 2022; Stevenson 2011). Individualism has weakened sociality by reducing civic engagement, religiousness, social cohesion, and volunteering (Church 2010; Green and Janmaat 2011; J. He et al. 2014; Hener et al. 2016; Leong 2008; Pollack and Pickel 2007; Whitford et al. 2006). Conversely, individualism has impeded sociality by bolstering acceptance of outsiders, competition, crime, extremity, self-enhancement, protesting, and violence (Church 2010; J. He et al. 2014; Karstedt 2010; Leong 2008; Li and Song 1992; Pollack and Pickel 2007; Whitford et al. 2006). Subversion features violence. (Hagan et al. 2016). As such, subversion or violence has undermined sociality by fomenting crime and tolerance for violence (Markowitz 2001; Tanner-Smith et al. 2013).

The community institution embodies civil society (Edwards 2004). This institution contrasts the political institution, social capital, and social integration (Linquiti 2023; Novak 2001; Wnuk-Lipinski 2007). Organizationally, the community institution features interest groups, public spheres, and voluntary associations (Edwards 2004; Fukuyama 2001). Functionally, the community institution features enforcing, including legitimizing, negotiation, networking, shaming, sharing, soliciting, and synergy (Akman 2012; Edwards 2004; Nickel 2012; Powell 2007; Teets 2014). Instrumentally, the community features association, charity, citizenship, civility, compassion, cooperation, equality, donation, harmony, mutuality or mutualism, partnership, respect, responsibility, self-discipline, social capital, social engagement or participation, social interaction, solidarity, togetherness or we-ness, and volunteering (Adloff 2018; Akman 2012; Choi 2004; DeLue and Dale 2009; Edwards 2004; Nickel 2012; O'Mahony 2013; Powell 2007). Civility comprises compromise, compliance as opposed to intransigence, responsibility, and self-limitation (Akman 2012). As such, the community institution functions to buttress sociality by generating and drawing power, utility, ideals, and norms to achieve the requisite functions dictated by analytical functionalism. Notably, power, utility, and ideals advanced at the societal level become norms at the personal level.

Power generated by the community institution to empower sociality rests on caring, coalitions, collaboration, and social capital (Edwards 2004). Cared received has consolidated sociality by raising civic engagement, community involvement, forgiveness, morality, prosocial behavior, recourse, relatedness, relationship value, social cohesion, social integration, social well-being, and trust (Bishop et al. 2002; E. Chan 2014; Garcia and Herrero 2004; C. Hui et al. 2013; Livingstone et al. 2023; Mata and Pendakur 2014; Palmer et al. 2011; Williams and Galliher 2006). Social capital has consolidated sociality by raising civic engagement, community involvement, donation, political involvement, social trust, and volunteering (Bekkers et al. 2008; Broadbent and Papadopoulos 2011; Brown and Ferris 2007; Chua et al. 2021; Narayan and Cassidy 2001). Coalitions or collaboration have strengthened sociality regarding attachment and trustworthiness as opposed to argument (Gerbasi and Cook 2008; Hample 2018; Tak 2017). The community institution can also raise power regarding support to empower sociality (Edwards 2004). Support received has strengthened sociality by enhancing attachment, gratitude, political participation, prosocial behavior, recourse, respect, responsibility, social integration, and social well-being (Boezeman and Ellemers 2008; Fahmy 2006; Phipps 2003; Williams and Galliher 2006; R. Wright et al. 2009; Zeldin et al. 2016; Zeng et al. 2024). Conversely, support received has boosted sociality by preventing aggression, conflict, delinquency, doping, externalizing, hyperactivity, loneliness, runaway, sexuality, suicide, and violence (Bernardon et al. 2011; Browning et al. 2005; Hayslip et al. 2000; Nieuwenhuis et al. 2017; Pearson and Wilkinson 2013; Terzi-Unsal and Karei 2005; Wight et al. 2006; R. Wright et al. 2009).

Utility offered by the community institution to incentivize sociality evolves from happiness, pleasure, and public goods (Kallhoff 2011; Kaurin 2020). Happiness has uplifted sociality by consolidating altruism, conformism, cooperation, donation, liking for people, prosociality, sociability, and trust and social trust (Fetvadjiev and He 2019; A. Hu 2013; Lyubomirsky et al. 2006; Y. Pan et al. 2023; Wang and Graddy 2008). Pleasure has maintained sociality by raising government trust and patriotism (Hunt et al. 2019; Turner and Stets 2005). The community institution can also boost utility in well-being to incentivize sociality (Scambler 2002). Well-being has buttressed sociality by securing intimacy, moral behavior, popularity, social cohesion, social well-being, and sociability, and preventing rejection experience, victimization experience, and violence (Dougherty 2006; Gallagher and Lopez 2007; Kayser et al. 2010; Lambert et al. 2009; Twenge et al. 2003; Yip and Martin 2006). Conversely, the community institution can dampen disutility in conflict to retain sociality (Langman 2005). Conflict has impeded sociality regarding donation and trust, as opposed to violence (Farmer and Fedor 2001; Farrington 2018; Kunovich and Hodson 1999).

Ideals generated by the community institution to frame sociality hail accountability or transparency, citizenship, consensus, humanizing, loyalty, reciprocity, sharing, social progress, and trust (Edwards 2004). Accountability has sustained sociality regarding compliance, morality, and xenophobia as opposed to violence (Bussey 2020; Granzin and Olsen 1998; Kaurin 2020; Milner and Myers 2007). Citizenship has constituted sociality by inducing fairness and trust (Vera-Toscano et al. 2013). Consensus has enhanced sociality by fostering cohesion, compliance, engagement, and rejection of outsiders (Fasel et al. 2016; Guan et al. 2021; Heshmati and Oravecz 2022; Yoon et al. 2013). Humanizing constitutes sociality regarding caring and equality (Renger and Reese 2017). Loyalty has constituted sociality by fostering collaboration, empathy, generosity, leadership, and morality (Lawler et al. 2016; Lee and Chan 2016; Wilcox and Dew 2016). Reciprocity has constituted sociality by fostering prosocial behavior (Thielmann et al. 2020). Sharing has constituted sociality by strengthening leadership and neighboring (Dubois et al. 2020; Grannis 2009).

Moreover, sharing constitutes sociality regarding friendship (Launay and Dunbar 2015). Sharing can also underlie sociality by boosting morality, punishment, and social cohesion (N. Duncan 2017; Delton and Krasnow 2017). The ideal for social progress espouses sociality regarding accountability or responsibility, collectivity, the commonweal, community, compassion, cooperation, empathy, equality, fairness or justice, humanitarianism, nurturance, partnership, peace, publicness, punishment, and redistribution as opposed to harm and violence (Box 2008; Fukuyama 2018b; Lakoff 2009; Mahoney 2004; Sandel 2020; Speth 2012). Trust has constituted sociality through donation, involvement, and volunteering (Uslaner 2000). Moreover, ideals embraced by the community institution to frame sociality prioritize Christianity, civility, communication, communitarianism, conservatism, donation, humanism, justice, networking, participation, respect, republicanism, social democracy, social interaction, social orientation, socialism, and solidarity or togetherness (Adloff 2018; Akman 2012; Choi 2004; Edwards 2004; DeLue and Dale 2009; O'Mahony 2013; Powell 2007). Christianity maintained in the community institution to foster sociality emphasizes charity and redemption (Powell 2007). Communitarianism upheld in the community institution to frame sociality accentuates charity, social capital, and volunteering (Powell 2007). Besides, Christianity has buttressed sociality by securing conformity, donation, and morality and impeding cosmopolitanism (Hollinger 2017; Phillips and Smith 2008). Civility has constituted sociality by inducing fairness and trust (Vera-Toscano et al. 2013). Communitarianism constitutes sociality by espousing caring, civility, collective identity, commonweal orientation, community, dutifulness or responsibility, education or socialization, equality, interdependence, loyalty, mentoring, patriotism, reciprocity, relatedness, self-discipline, servicing including volunteering, settlement, social construction, social participation, solidarity, and trust (Delanty 2009; Frazer 1999; Moore 2010; Speth 2012). Conservatism bolstered by the community institution to frame sociality valorizes charity, compassion, mutuality, religiosity, self-discipline, and social capital (DeLue and Dale 2009; Powell 2007). Besides, conservatism sustains sociality by nurturing empathy, loyalty, prosocial behavior, religiousness, and sacrifice (Dutton and Rayner-Hilles 2022). Moreover, conservatism underpins sociality by maintaining allegiance or loyalty, attachment, civility, community, conformity, cooperation, discipline, ethnocentrism, honesty, humility, intimacy, legality, morality, nationalism, obedience, order, partnership, patriotism, peace, responsibility, sharing, trust, and xenophobia (Dutton and Rayner-Hilles 2022; Heilman and Kusev 2020; Hickson 2013; Lakoff 2009; Rhodes-Purdy et al. 2023; Scruton 2014; Yoos 2007; Zuk and Zuk 2020). Conversely, conservatism upholds sociality by condemning dehumanizing, evilness, revolution, sexuality, terrorism, and transgression (Dutton and Rayner-Hilles 2022; Malka and Soto 2011; Scruton 2014; Suhay 2015). Societal employment stands on societal social democracy (De Deken 2002). Donation has constituted sociality by consolidating charity, service value, social capital, social trust, and volunteering (Bekkers 2010; Chang 2009; Foster et al. 2001; Uslaner 2000). Humanism cherished in the community institution to frame sociality highlights association, cooperation, and responsibility (Powell 2007). Besides, humanism bolsters sociality by highlighting attachment, caring, collectivity, community, cooperation, friendship, helpfulness, institutions, loving, order, respect, relatedness, responsibility, and sharing (Browning and Cooper 2004; Fuchs 2020; Selznick 2008; Stefanski and Jach 2022; Visher 1997; Waterman 2013). Conversely, humanism sustains sociality by rejecting alienation, conflict, and individualization (Fuchs 2020; Selznick 2008). The ideal for justice has championed sociality by raising cooperation, egalitarianism, reciprocity, and support for redistribution (Kertzer et al. 2014; Rodrigo-Gonzalez et al. 2019; X. Wu 2009). Networking has fostered sociality regarding connectedness, friendship, giving, and social interaction (Eberl 2020; Liebler and Sandefur 2002; Nelson-Coffey et al. 2023; Phan et al. 2009). Participation has consolidated sociality regarding cooperation, networking, social capital, and trust (Groves et al. 2000; Molitor et al. 2011; Rochelle 2015). Respect constitutes sociality regarding caring and equality (Renger and Reese 2017). Republicanism upholds sociality regarding citizenship, the commonweal, interdependence, morality, nationalism, publicity, responsibility, social adaptation, and solidarity (Delanty 2009; Honohan 2002). Social democracy evolving from the community institution expands citizenship, cooperation, and partnership to frame sociality (Powell 2007). Besides, the societal ideal or personal norm of social democracy sustains sociality by championing equality and solidarity (Andersson 2006). Social interaction has realized sociality by consolidating altruism, compliance, cooperation, donation, morality, political participation, reciprocity, social trust, and volunteering (Guillen et al. 2011; Dixon and McKeown 2021; Lucas and Livingston 2014; Musick 2000; Rodrigo-Gonzalez et al. 2019; Rubin and Step 2000). Social orientation derived from the community institution treasures compliance, compromise, responsibility, and self-limitation and discourages risking (Akman 2012). Risking hurting sociality comprises attacking, hating, insulting, and violence (Akman 2012). Besides, social orientation has constituted sociality by elevating compliance (Pool and Schwegler 2007). Socialism maintained in the community institution to frame sociality anticipates association, cooperation, equality, harmony, and mutuality as opposed to conflict (Powell 2007). Besides, socialism has enhanced sociality regarding cooperation and discussion as opposed to crime (Collier 2001; Lilly et al. 2011; Sanderson 2001). Solidarity or togetherness has constituted sociality by enhancing attachment and dampening tolerance for deviance (Stafford et al. 2005; Woosnam et al. 2018). The community institution also buttresses the ideal for commonness to frame sociality (Edwards 2004). Commonness has constituted sociality by strengthening leadership and neighboring (Dubois et al. 2020; Grannis 2009).

Conversely, the community institution inhibits ideals for competition, opportunism, and violence to withhold sociality (Edwards 2004). Competition has impeded sociality by eroding volunteering (Martinez and McMullin 2004). Opportunism has impaired sociality by dampening agreeableness and cooperation (Sakalaki and Fousiani 2012). Violence has undermined sociality by breeding antisociality, crime and recidivism, blaming, conflict, hostility, rejecting others, and impairing agreeableness, morality, and responsibility (Asendorpf et al. 2008; Del Bove et al. 2008; Morrison 2006; Scholte et al. 2009; Vitaro et al. 2007).

Power registered by the community institution to empower sociality stems from education, social capital, social integration, and solidarity (Naftali 2021; Wnuk-Lipinski 2007). Education has fostered sociality by raising civic engagement, civility, conformism, crime disapproval, equality support, morality, political discussion, political interest, political participation, socialism, and trust (Bullock 2021; E. Chan 2014; Djupe and Lewis 2015; Gilberbloom and Markham 1995; Kerrissey and Schofer 2013; Miyata et al. 2008; Norris 2011; Norris and Inglehart 2009; Ulbig 2002; Wilson and Dunham 2001). Conversely, education has sustained sociality by reducing political alienation, deviance, prostitution, resistance, and violence and its tolerance (Backman and Nilsson 2011; Coffe and Geys 2007; Lubbers et al. 2006; Michalski 2005; Simon et al. 2001; Swader and Vorobeva 2015). Social capital has consolidated sociality by raising civic engagement, community involvement, donation, political involvement, social trust, and volunteering (Bekkers et al. 2008; Broadbent and Papadopoulos 2011; Brown and Ferris 2007; Chua et al. 2021; Narayan and Cassidy 2001). Social integration has constituted sociality by strengthening cooperation and preventing suicide (Duberstein et al. 2004; Lepkowski and Couper 2002). Solidarity has constituted sociality by enhancing attachment and dampening tolerance for deviance (Stafford et al. 2005; Woosnam et al. 2018).

Ideals registered by the community institution for framing sociality favor compassion, compromise, humanity, legality, love, responsibility, and socialization (Alexander 1997; Brint 2005; Edwards 2004; Wnuk-Lipinski 2007). Compromise constitutes sociality by representing harmony (G. Zhang 2006). Conversely, compromise maintains sociality by espousing reconciliation and dismissing conflict and radicalism (Auerbach 2009; J. Berger 2018). Compassion has underlain sociality by securing religiosity and volunteering (Barr et al. 2005). The ideal for humanity or humanitarianism has enhanced sociality by activating political participation (Foschi and Lauriola 2014). Besides, humanitarianism upholds sociality by embracing altruism, caring, coalitions, empathy, justice, other orientation, pity, prosociality, responsibility, and solidarity (Angelis and Pensini 2024; Bendixsen 2018; Brigg 2018; Chouliaraki 2013; Hoekstra 2021). Legality has buttressed sociality by dismissing radicalism (Muthuswamy 2022). Love sustains sociality by enhancing adaptation and dampening aloneness, conflict, and loneliness (Jeffries 2000; Rokach 2019; Sanderson 2001; Soble 2008). Responsibility has fostered sociality regarding compliance, morality, and xenophobia as opposed to violence (Bussey 2020; Granzin and Olsen 1998; Kaurin 2020; Milner and Myers 2007). Socialization has constituted sociality by impeding violence (Pulkkinen et al. 2009). Furthermore, socialization can advance sociality by fostering family cohesion and role-taking and preventing crime, doping, and violence (Dolch 2003; L. Ray 2017; Steel et al. 2012; Sussman and Ames 2001). Moreover, the community institution adduces ideals for association, caring, Christianity, civility, communitarianism, Confucianism, conservatism, contractarianism, criticalness, empathy, equality, feminism, functionalism, Islam, Judaism, and republicanism to frame sociality (Christians et el. 2009; DeLue and Dale 2009; Frerichs and Munch 2010; Fyfe 2005; Held 2008; Madsen 2002; Mosher 2002; Novak 2001; Pakaluk 2002; Powell 2007; S. Stone 2002; Weldon 2004). Association has fostered sociality regarding connectedness, friendship, giving, and social interaction (Eberl 2020; Liebler and Sandefur 2002; Nelson-Coffey et al. 2023; Phan et al. 2009). Caring has constituted sociality by securing religiosity and volunteering (Barr et al. 2005). Christianity has buttressed sociality by securing conformity, donation, and morality and impeding cosmopolitanism (Hollinger 2017; Phillips and Smith 2008). Civility has constituted sociality by inducing fairness and trust (Vera-Toscano et al. 2013). Communitarianism constitutes sociality by espousing caring, civility, collective identity, commonweal orientation, community, dutifulness or responsibility, education or socialization, equality, interdependence, loyalty, mentoring, patriotism, reciprocity, relatedness, self-discipline, servicing including volunteering, settlement, social construction, social participation, solidarity, and trust (Delanty 2009; Frazer 1999; Moore 2010; Speth 2012). Confucianism, adduced by the community institution to frame sociality, emphasizes civility, consensus, conciliation, cultivation, discussion, interdependence, loyalty, responsibility, relatedness, synthesis, and transmission as opposed to freedom (Madsen 2002). Besides, Confucianism has championed sociality regarding association, civility, and collectivism as opposed to violence (Y. Lin et al. 2021; Shin 2012; Stotzer 2014). Conservatism sustains sociality by nurturing empathy, loyalty, prosocial behavior, religiousness, and sacrifice (Dutton and Rayner-Hilles 2022). Contractarianism enhances sociality by embracing attachment, civic engagement, civility, compliance, compromise, consent, cooperation, coordination, equality, fairness, morality, and trust (Bowker 2016; Dalbert 2001; Darwall 2003; de Jonge 2012; Ellis et al. 2006; Gardiner 2009; Irwin 2016; Jarvinen and Branders 2020; Kaurin 2020). Criticalness adduced by the community institution to frame sociality extols participation, publicness, social interaction, and sharing as opposed to colonization (Chambers 2002). Empathy has elevated sociality by facilitating prosocial behavior (Fraser et al. 2012). The ideal for equality or egalitarianism has underpinned sociality by enhancing empathy, support for welfare, and trust in government and impeding radicalism (Faricy and Ellis 2014; Lauriola et al. 2015; Lucas and Kteily 2018; Roosma et al. 2014). Feminism, as introduced by the community institution to frame sociality, idealizes philanthropy and social interaction (Phillips 2002). Besides, feminism upholds sociality by embracing caring, closeness, cooperation, empathy, equality, justice, and solidarity (Hutchings 2010; Sanderson et al. 2005). Feminism has also buttressed sociality regarding solidarity (van Breen et al. 2017). Caring in feminism comprises dialogue, mediation, particularism, and sympathy as opposed to violence (Hutchings 2010). Functionalism adduced by the community institution to frame sociality prioritizes civility or civilizing, cohesion, consensus, equality, integration, normativity, and reciprocity, as opposed to conflict (Ashworth 2013; Boyd 2006; Frerichs and Munch 2010; Izquierdo and Minguez 2003; Rojek 1995; Vanderstraeten 2003). Islam, adduced by the community institution to frame sociality, dictates brotherhood, equality, nationalization, publicness, and unity (Hanafi 2002). Besides, Islam champions sociality by cherishing brotherhood, communality, conformity, and discipline and rejecting doping, enslavement, freedom, individualism, suicide, and terrorism (Braun 2011;

Esposito 2002; Scruton 2014; Verkuyten 2014). Judaism, adduced by the community institution to frame sociality, favors caring, education, humanitarianism, particularism, and social inclusion (Qian 2018; S. Stone 2002). Besides, Judaism safeguards sociality by upholding humanitarianism (H. Smith 1991). Republicanism upholds sociality regarding citizenship, the commonweal, interdependence, morality, nationalism, publicity.

Conversely, the community institution registers ideals against social exclusion and violence to frame sociality (Edwards 2004; Marotta 2017). Social exclusion has impeded sociality by fueling crime, doping, and violence (Barry and Hullett 1998). Moreover, social exclusion experience has disturbed sociality by eroding closeness and prosocial behavior (Bockler et al. 2021; K. Lin et al. 2013). Violence has undermined sociality by breeding antisociality, crime and recidivism, blaming, conflict, hostility, rejecting others, and impairing agreeableness, morality, and responsibility (Asendorpf et al. 2008; Del Bove et al. 2008; Morrison 2006; Scholte et al. 2009; Vitaro et al. 2007). Moreover, violence experienced has impaired sociality by fomenting antisocial behavior and violence (L. Berger 2005; Krahe 2013). Furthermore, community institutions add ideals against terrorism to frame sociality (Held 2008). Terrorism has undermined sociality by raising violence and diminishing collective practice and confidence in government (Achilov 2016; Levi and Strker 2000).

Norms registered by the community institution for standardizing sociality institutionalize civility (Edwards 2004). The norm for civility has constituted sociality by enhancing political trust (Mutz and Reeves 2005). Furthermore, civility has constituted sociality by inducing fairness and trust (Vera-Toscano et al. 2013).

Confidence in the community institution transpires in community involvement. Such involvement represents sharing and social capital (Huberman 2022; Saegert and Winkel 2004). The need for or deficiency in community involvement arises from stigmatization and neoliberalism, which impede community involvement (Notter et al. 2008; Farmer et al. 2015). Community involvement offers and draws power, utility, ideals, and norms to build sociality with the voluntaristic mechanisms of analytical functionalism.

Power generated by community involvement to drive sociality has rested on political (self-) efficacy and social networking or capital (Molitor et al. 2011; Ohmer 2007). Self-efficacy has sustained sociality by raising civic engagement, donation, government and social trust, leadership, political participation, prosocial behavior, and social activity (Bednall et al. 2013; Frye 2007; Gnambs and Batinic 2012; Huber et al. 2022; Mangum 2012; Rahn 2008; Pei and Pan 2018; Yao and Enright 2019). Community involvement manifests power in terms of influence and social integration to drive sociality (Yetim and Yetim 2014). Influence has enhanced sociality by boosting attachment, empathy, giving, punishment, and xenophobia (Campos-Castillo and Hitlin 2013; Molm 1997; Schwartz et al. 2014). Social integration has constituted sociality by strengthening cooperation and preventing suicide (Duberstein et al. 2004; Lepkowski and Couper 2002).

Utility delivered by community involvement to attract sociality has resided in collective efficacy belief (Ohmer 2007). Collective efficacy has constituted sociality by raising political participation and trust in government and mitigating violence (Caprara and Vecchione 2017; Stolle and Micheletti 2013; E. Wright et al. 2015). Besides, collective efficacy represents sociality regarding social capital and cohesion (Ferretti et al. 2024; Harpham et al. 2002). Community involvement displays utility in fulfillment and morale to attract sociality (Tsutsumi et al. 1998; Yetim and Yetim 2014). Fulfillment has sustained sociality by raising relationship satisfaction and social capital and reducing conflict and its defense (Patrick et al. 2007; Yetim and Yetim 2014). Morale has enhanced sociality by impeding suicide and unrest (O. Chen et al. 2025).

Ideals nurtured by community involvement to rationalize sociality have embraced cooperation and trust (Groves et al. 2000; Rochelle 2015). Cooperation has strengthened sociality regarding attachment and trustworthiness as opposed to argument (Gerbasi and Cook 2008; Hample 2018; Tak 2017). Trust has constituted sociality through donation, involvement, and volunteering (Uslaner 2000). Community involvement exhibits ideals for civility, collaboration, connectedness, contracting, integrity, meeting, membership, mutualism, order, religiosity, self-discipline, sharing, social interaction, and traditionalism to rationalize sociality (Heckscher 2015; Kerrissey and Schofer 2013; Saegert and Winkel 2004; Yetim and Yetim 2014). Civility has constituted sociality by inducing fairness and trust (Vera-Toscano et al. 2013). Additionally, civility maintains sociality by enhancing the commonweal, community, equality, friendship, reciprocity, and social capital (Hudson 2023). Collaboration has strengthened sociality regarding attachment and trustworthiness as opposed to argument (Gerbasi and Cook 2008; Hample 2018; Tak 2017). Connected or membership has constituted sociality by strengthening institutional commitment and conformity (Vartanian and Hopkinson 2010). Moreover, connectedness represents sociality regarding acceptance experienced, conflict resolution, social capital, and interaction as opposed to social exclusion (Campbell and Eggerling-Boeck 2006; Lim 2009; Mannan 2007; Raffo and Reeves 2000). Contracting has buttressed sociality by raising patriotism, prosocial behavior, and relatedness (Dovidio et al. 2006; Gilbert 2006; Hudson 2023; Segrin and Flora 2019). Integrity has buttressed sociality by boosting volunteering and inhibiting violence (Piquero and Hickman 2002; Whitford et al. 2006). Meeting or social interaction has realized sociality by consolidating altruism, compliance, cooperation, donation, morality, political participation, reciprocity, social trust, and volunteering (Guillen et al. 2011; Dixon and McKeown 2021; Lucas and Livingston 2014; Musick 2000; Rodrigo-Gonzalez et al. 2019; Rubin and Step 2000). Social interaction in community involvement comprises collaboration, commitment, contribution, helping, interdependence, networking, relatedness, sharing, supporting, and understanding to buttress sociality (Heckscher 2015). Mutualism has constituted sociality by fostering prosocial behavior (Thielmann et al. 2020). The ideal for order has bred confidence in the business institution (Costa et al. 2023). Religiosity has sustained sociality by fostering civic engagement, civility, cohesion, compliance, donation, empathy, morality, patriotism, prejudice against deviants and outsiders, prosocial behavior, social trust, and volunteering (Apinunmahakul and Devlin 2008; Corcoran et al. 2011; Ishio 2010; Keyes 2002; Kim and Wilcox 2013; Ravanera et al. 2003;

van Tienen et al. 2011; Weisberg 2005; Wuthnow 2004). Conversely, religiosity has secured sociality by reducing crime, deviance, individualism, protesting, and sexuality (Andrews et al. 2015; Coffe and Geys 2007; Guo et al. 2008; Skerkat and Ellison 1999; Spilka et al. 2003). Moreover, religiosity realizes sociality regarding altruism, community, ethicality, groupism, sharing, and solidarity (Franks et al. 2013; Lichterman 2012; Peifer 2010; Spilka et al. 2003; Stavrova and Siegers 2014). Religiosity also upholds sociality by featuring altruism, attachment, caring, community, compassion, harmony, hospitality, love, morality, obedience, other-centeredness, peace, trust, unity, xenophobia (Ager and Ager 2011; Fontana 2003; Harris et al. 2018; Horell 2014; Paterson 2018; Shorey et al. 2018; Simpson et al. 2008; Spilka et al. 2003; Tenorio and Lo 2011; Werbner 2010). Conversely, religiosity maintains sociality by dismissing individualism, oppression, sexuality, and violence (Fontana 2003; Horell 2014; Spilka et al. 2003). Self-discipline has buttressed sociality by enhancing generativity and impeding crime, risking, and violence (Y. Cheung et al. 2014; Koegl and Day 2019; Peterson and Klohnen 1995; Welch et al. 2008). Traditionalism in community involvement upholds dependency, dutifulness, groupness, loyalty, obedience, order, and religiosity to foster sociality (Heckscher 2015). Additionally, traditionalism has buttressed sociality by enhancing patriotism and faith in religion and discouraging protesting and accepting deviants and outsiders (Costa et al. 2023; Datler et al. 2013; Meuleman et al. 2019; Schwartz et al. 2014).

Power drawn from community involvement to drive sociality has stemmed from empowerment experienced and social capital (Broadbent and Papadopoulos 2011; Hunter et al. 2013). Empowerment has facilitated sociality by strengthening civility, collectivism, and donation (Bond and Lun 2014; Klucarova and He 2021; Y. Lin et al. 2021). Moreover, empowerment sustains sociality by highlighting bridging, caring, gratitude, political participation, and responsibility (Kaczmarek et al. 2014; Phillips 2006; Praszkier 2018; Tracy 2002; Wildemeersch 2014). Social capital has consolidated sociality by raising civic engagement, community involvement, donation, political involvement, social trust, and volunteering (Bekkers et al. 2008; Broadbent and Papadopoulos 2011; Brown and Ferris 2007; Chua et al. 2021; Narayan and Cassidy 2001). Conversely, social capital has strengthened sociality by erasing violence (Pulkkinen et al. 2009).

Utility drawn from community involvement to attract sociality has evolved from satisfaction with the community (Xu 2007). Community satisfaction has buttressed sociality by fostering attachment, social capital, and volunteering (Cummins et al. 2003; Xu 2007).

Ideals drawn from community involvement to rationalize sociality have realized community service, neighboring, and organizational involvement (Matarrita-Cascante and Luloff 2008; Palmer et al. 2011; Xu 2007). Community service has constituted sociality by raising altruism, charity orientation, civic motivation, donation, helping, moral responsibility, political participation, social integration, and social and government trust (Foster et al. 2001; Isham et al. 2006; Richey 2010; Richey and Ikeda 2009; Wiepking and Maas 2009). Conversely, community service has safeguarded sociality by preventing deviance and its tolerance, delinquency, and loneliness (Gillath et al. 2005; J. Wilson 2000; Woolley 2003). Neighboring has elevated sociality by raising consulting and influencing (Hays and Kogl 2007). Organizational involvement has fostered sociality by enhancing attachment, civility, political participation, social integration, socialism (favor), and trust (Geys 2012; Guillen et al. 2011; Pattie et al. 2004; Tak 2017). Socialism has enhanced sociality regarding cooperation and discussion as opposed to crime (Collier 2001; Lilly et al. 2011; Sanderson 2001). Moreover, community involvement can constitute sociality by enhancing the ideal for social interaction (Matarrita-Cascante and Luloff 2008). Social interaction has realized sociality by consolidating altruism, compliance, cooperation, donation, morality, political participation, reciprocity, social trust, and volunteering (Guillen et al. 2011; Dixon and McKeown 2021; Lucas and Livingston 2014; Musick 2000; Rodrigo-Gonzalez et al. 2019; Rubin and Step 2000). Community involvement also stands on ideals for communitarianism, conservatism, localism, and romanticism to build sociality (Heckscher 2015). Communitarianism underlying community involvement to elevate sociality valorizes association, contact, loyalty, and religion as opposed to competition, individualism, narcissism or self-indulgence, and privacy (Heckscher 2015). Besides, communitarianism constitutes sociality by espousing caring, civility, collective identity, commonweal orientation, community, dutifulness or responsibility, education or socialization, equality, interdependence, loyalty, mentoring, patriotism, reciprocity, relatedness, self-discipline, servicing including volunteering, settlement, social construction, social participation, solidarity, and trust (Delanty 2009; Frazer 1999; Moore 2010; Speth 2012). Conservatism sustains sociality by nurturing empathy, loyalty, prosocial behavior, religiousness, and sacrifice (Dutton and Rayner-Hilles 2022). Moreover, conservatism underpins sociality by maintaining allegiance or loyalty, attachment, civility, community, conformity, cooperation, discipline, ethnocentrism, honesty, humility, intimacy, legality, morality, nationalism, obedience, order, partnership, patriotism, peace, responsibility, sharing, trust, and xenophobia (Dutton and Rayner-Hilles 2022; Heilman and Kusev 2020; Hickson 2013; Lakoff 2009; Rhodes-Purdy et al. 2023; Scruton 2014; Yoos 2007; Zuk and Zuk 2020). Conversely, conservatism upholds sociality by condemning dehumanizing, evilness, revolution, sexuality, terrorism, and transgression (Dutton and Rayner-Hilles 2022; Malka and Soto 2011; Scruton 2014; Suhay 2015). Localism constitutes sociality by espousing communitarianism and community, cooperation, familiarity, harmony, nationalism, patriotism, reciprocity, social participation, and xenophobia (Gregg 2003; Macedo 2021; Ng and Kennedy 2019; Zhang and Gu 2022). Romanticism treasures sociality regarding community (TenHouten 2017). Romanticism has also vindicated sociality by refuting sexuality (G. Li et al. 2023). Moreover, community involvement reflects the ideal for sharing to uphold sociality (Huberman 2022). Sharing has raised sociality by facilitating donating (Piferi et al. 2006). Moreover, sharing maintains sociality by involving social closeness, commitment, contribution, and gifting (Godoy et al. 2007; Murray and Holmes 2008).

Norms drawn from community involvement to assimilate sociality have popularized social interaction and participation (Palmer et al. 2011; Saegert and Winkel 2004). Conversely, community involvement has drawn norms against crime and violence to champion sociality (Saegert and Winkel 2004). Social interaction or participation has realized sociality by consolidating altruism, compliance, cooperation, donation, morality, political participation, reciprocity, social trust, and volunteering (Guillen et al. 2011; Dixon and McKeown 2021; Lucas and Livingston 2014; Musick 2000; Rodrigo-Gonzalez et al. 2019; Rubin and Step 2000).

Confidence in institutions registers civic engagement (Kozuch and Dobrowolski 2014). This confidence stands on beliefs in institutional adaptability, constraint or shaping, efficacy, regulation, reproduction, sedimentation or building on the past, sociocultural integration, and stability or stickiness (Alasuutari 2015; Farrell and Newman 2010; Abrutyn and Turner 2011; Nee 2005; Peters 1999; Zuckerman 2021). Inherently, such confidence or institutionalism embraces corporatism, elitism, legalism, professionalism, and religiosity (Abrutyn and Turner 2011; A. Hu 2013; Lowndes and Roberts 2013; Lopez-Concepcion et al. 2023; Peters and Pierre 2020). Corporatism blends bureaucracy, centralization, concertation, consensus, coordination, harmony, integration, intermediation, and solidarity (Beccaro 2003; Molina and Rhodes 2002). Elitism treasures expertise and inequality as opposed to pluralism (A. Moore 2017). Legalism valorizes adaptation, certainty, enforcement, equality, ethicality, punishment, regulation, repression, uniformity, and unity (Clubb and O'Connor 2019; Edwards and Arnon 2021; Feldman 2018; Timberlake et al. 2003). Professionalism registers autonomy, competency, control, discipline, expertise, knowledge, monopoly, morality, privilege, service, status, and success (Carollo and Solari 2019; Evetts 2013; M. Simons et al. 2017; Svensson 2006). Inherently, professionalism embraces altruism, calling, continuance, dominance, dutifulness or accountability, efficiency, excellence, honesty or integrity, individuation, normativity, self-awareness, and self-regulation (Chisholm et al. 2006; Evetts 2003; McAulay et al. 2006; Svensson 2006; Vestergaard 2013; Wiseman and Shefler 2001). Religiosity represents altruism, authoritarianism, community, ethicality or morality, groupism or sharing, sacrifice, solidarity, spirituality, and transcendence (Franks et al. 2013; Kalkstein and Tower 2009; Lichterman 2012; Lloyd et al. 2022; Peifer 2010; Petrovic et al. 2020; Spilka et al. 2003; Stavrova and Siegers 2014). As such, confidence in institutions constitutes sociality by generating power, utility, ideals, and norms to achieve the requisite functions of fulfillment, adaptation, latency, and integration maintained in analytical functionalism. Such generation capitalizes on the institutional force embedded in confidence in institutions (Mewes et al. 2021). This force hinges on the empowering mechanism of institutional administration, bureaucracy, capacity, centralization, constraint, empowerment, enforcement, institutionalization, law or constitution, legislation, regulation, replication, sanctioning, and structuring (Amenta 2005; Edlund 2006; Lowndes and Roberts 2013; Peters 1999; Peters and Pierre 2020; W. Scott 2008; Yang and Tang 2010). Institutionalization proceeds with habitualization and routinization to secure consensus (W. Scott 2008). Besides, the force rests on the incentivizing mechanism of institutional finance and legitimacy (Alesina and La Ferrara 2002; W. Scott 2008). The force also relies on the framing mechanism of discourse, meaning-making, and narrative (Lowndes and Roberts 2013; Peters 1999; Peters and Pierre 2020). Furthermore, the force demonstrates the normalizing mechanism of isomorphism and norming (Alasuutari 2015; Peters and Pierre 2020).

Power generated by confidence in institutions to drive sociality has rested on health (Mayer 2017). Health has uplifted sociality by boosting community sense, morality, popularity, social activity, social cohesion, social integration, social trust, social well-being, and volunteering (Huxhold et al. 2014; Jorgensen et al. 2010; Son and Wilson 2012; Tolsma et al. 2009; Yu and Chiu 2016). Conversely, health has sustained sociality by preventing loneliness (Koromeckyj-Cox et al. 2007). Confidence in institutions also drives sociality by forming power regarding empowerment and social capital (Lowndes and Roberts 2013; Woolcock 1998). Empowerment has facilitated sociality by strengthening civility, collectivism, and donation (Bond and Lun 2014; Klucarova and He 2021; Y. Lin et al. 2021).

Utility offered by confidence in institutions to attract sociality has sprung from life satisfaction (Klein 2013). Life satisfaction has incubated sociality regarding political participation, social cohesion, social trust, and volunteering (E. Chan 2014; Flavin and Keane 2011; Rochelle 2015).

Ideals disseminated by confidence in institutions to rationalize sociality have valorized civility, compliance, political participation, prosocial behavior, responsibility, and social trust (Coffe and van der Lippe 2010; Jakobsen 2010; Grimes 2006; Seifert 2018; Stagnaro et al. 2017; Stolle and Micheletti 2013). Civility has constituted sociality by inducing fairness and trust (Vera-Toscano et al. 2013). Additionally, civility maintains sociality by enhancing the commonweal, community, equality, friendship, reciprocity, and social capital (Hudson 2023). Compliance, conformity, or conformism has constituted sociality by raising patriotism and impeding violence and acceptance of deviants and outsiders (Pulkkinen et al. 2009; Schwartz et al. 2014; Van Hootegem et al. 2000; Yeo and Chu 2018). Political participation has buttressed sociality regarding civility (Campbell 2003). Prosocial behavior has constituted sociality by civility, consolidating connectedness, cooperation, religiosity, responsibility, and volunteering (Hample 2018; Marsh and Dik 2021; Musick and Wilson 2008; Nelson-Coffey et al. 2023; Shahzalal and Adnan 2022). Moreover, prosocial behavior underlies sociality by enhancing citizenship, loyalty, social cohesion, socializing, and trust and diminishing self-interest (Dovidio et al. 2006; Hawley 2014; Kisliuk and WeiBmuller 2023; Music 2014). Responsibility has fostered sociality regarding compliance, morality, and xenophobia as opposed to violence (Bussey 2020; Granzin and Olsen 1998; Kaurin 2020; Milner and Myers 2007). Social trust has constituted sociality through donation, involvement, and volunteering (Uslaner 2000). Confidence in institutions also buttresses sociality by espousing ideals for agreement, civic engagement, charity, collectivism, communication, consensus, corporatism, embeddedness, honesty or integrity, order, religiosity, and social orientation (Amenta 2005; Farwell et al. 2019; A. Hu 2013; Lowndes and Roberts 2013; Kozuch and Dobrowolski 2014; Nee 2005; Peters and Pierre 2020; W. Scott 2008; Yang and Tang 2010). Agreement or consensus has enhanced sociality by fostering cohesion, compliance, engagement, and rejection of outsiders (Fasel et al. 2016; Guan et al. 2021; Heshmati and Oravecz 2022; Yoon et al. 2013). Civic engagement has propped sociality by strengthening attachment, civility, collective behavior, discussion, donation, neighboring, patriotism, prosociality, social capital, socialism, trust, and volunteering and impeding cheating and individualism (Coffe and Geys 2007; Gilberbloom and Markham 1995; Kerrissey and Schofer 2013; Mata and Pendakur 2014; Ozbay 2008; Pattie et al. 2004; Pena-Lopez and Sanchez-Santos 2016; Rahn 2008; Richey 2011; Tak 2017; M. Tang 2011; Taniguchi 2013; Yip et al. 2007). Corporatism upholds sociality by espousing community, concertation, consensus, coordination, exchange, guidance or tutelage, harmony, integration, intermediation, and solidarity (Beccaro 2003; Molina and Rhodes 2002). Embeddedness has fostered sociality regarding connectedness, friendship, giving, and social interaction (Eberl 2020; Liebler and Sandefur 2002; Nelson-Coffey et al. 2023; Phan et al. 2009). Honesty or integrity has built sociality by raising compliance and prosocial behavior and eschewing crime (Jolley et al. 2019; Thielmann et al. 2020; Twardawski et al. 2021). The ideal for order has bred confidence in the business institution (Costa et al. 2023). Religiosity has sustained sociality by fostering civic engagement, civility, cohesion, compliance, donation, empathy, morality, patriotism, prejudice against deviants and outsiders, prosocial behavior, social trust, and volunteering (Apinunmahakul and Devlin 2008; Corcoran et al. 2011; Ishio 2010; Keyes 2002; Kim and Wilcox 2013; Ravanera et al. 2003; van Tienen et al. 2011; Weisberg 2005; Wuthnow 2004). Conversely, religiosity has secured sociality by reducing crime, deviance, individualism, protesting, and sexuality (Andrews et al. 2015; Coffe and Geys 2007; Guo et al. 2008; Skerkat and Ellison 1999; Spilka et al. 2003). Moreover, religiosity realizes sociality regarding altruism, community, ethicality, groupism, sharing, and solidarity (Franks et al. 2013; Lichterman 2012; Peifer 2010; Spilka et al. 2003; Stavrova and Siegers 2014). Religiosity also upholds sociality by featuring altruism, attachment, caring, community, compassion, harmony, hospitality, love, morality, obedience, other-centeredness, peace, trust, unity, xenophobia (Ager and Ager 2011; Fontana 2003; Harris et al. 2018; Horell 2014; Paterson 2018; Shorey et al. 2018; Simpson et al. 2008; Spilka et al. 2003; Tenorio and Lo 2011; Werbner 2010). Conversely, religiosity maintains sociality by dismissing individualism, oppression, sexuality, and violence (Fontana 2003; Horell 2014; Spilka et al. 2003). Social orientation derived from the community institution treasures compliance, compromise, responsibility, and self-limitation and discourages risking (Akman 2012). Besides, social orientation has constituted sociality by elevating compliance (Pool and Schwegler 2007).

Conversely, confidence in institutions has sustained sociality by preventing the ideal for risking (Ehrke et al. 2023). The ideal for risking has disrupted sociality by generating crime, hate, and violence (Farrington 2018; Hawdon et al. 2019; Merdian et al. 2017). Confidence in institutions also upholds sociality by dispelling the ideal of individualism (Lowndes and Roberts 2013). Individualism has weakened sociality by reducing civic engagement, religiousness, social cohesion, and volunteering (Church 2010; Green and Janmaat 2011; J. He et al. 2014; Hener et al. 2016; Leong 2008; Pollack and Pickel 2007; Whitford et al. 2006). Conversely, individualism has impeded sociality by bolstering acceptance of outsiders, competition, crime, extremity, self-enhancement, protesting, and violence (Church 2010; J. He et al. 2014; Karstedt 2010; Leong 2008; Li and Song 1992; Pollack and Pickel 2007; Whitford et al. 2006).

Norms consolidated by confidence in institutions to assimilate sociality popularize social commitment and socializing (Peters and Pierre 2020). Social commitment has constituted sociality by enhancing attachment and dampening tolerance for deviance (Stafford et al. 2005; Woosnam et al. 2018). Socializing has fostered sociality regarding connectedness, friendship, giving, and social interaction (Eberl 2020; Liebler and Sandefur 2002; Nelson-Coffey et al. 2023; Phan et al. 2009).

Confidence in institutions can also draw power, utility, ideals, and norms to build sociality by achieving the requisite functions of analytical functionalism. These functions build on the four mechanisms of power realization, utility optimization, ideal calibration, and norm conformity. Power drives confidence in institutions through the power realization mechanism of arranging and capitalizing (Newton 2006; Norris 1999a). Utility attracts confidence in institutions through the utility optimization mechanism of stakeholding or stake or ownership building (Kozuch and Dobrowolski 2014). Ideals rationalize confidence in institutions through the ideal calibration mechanism of cultivation or socialization, mobilization or rallying, and modernization (Elchardus and De Keere 2013; Holdo 2022; Yang and Tang 2010). Modernization encompasses rationalization, secularization, and urbanization (Elchardus and De Keere 2013; Yang and Tang 2010). Norms assimilate confidence in institutions through the norm conformity mechanism of ritualization and normativizing (Cox 2016; Holdo 2022).

Power drawn for confidence in institutions to drive sociality has evolved from health and social capital (S. Chi et al. 2021; Lee-Treweek 2002). Health has uplifted sociality by boosting community sense, morality, popularity, social activity, social cohesion, social integration, social trust, social well-being, and volunteering (Huxhold et al. 2014; Jorgensen et al. 2010; Son and Wilson 2012; Tolsma et al. 2009; Yu and Chiu 2016). Conversely, health has sustained sociality by preventing loneliness (Koromeckyj-Cox et al. 2007). Social capital has consolidated sociality by raising civic engagement, community involvement, donation, political involvement, social trust, and volunteering (Bekkers et al. 2008; Broadbent and Papadopoulos 2011; Brown and Ferris 2007; Chua et al. 2021; Narayan and Cassidy 2001). Conversely, social capital has strengthened sociality by erasing violence (Pulkkinen et al. 2009). Confidence in institutions also stands on power stemming from social solidarity to drive sociality (Habibov 2014). Solidarity has constituted sociality by enhancing attachment and dampening tolerance for deviance (Stafford et al. 2005; Woosnam et al. 2018).

Utility drawn for confidence in institutions to attract sociality has resided in hope and satisfaction (Lytkina and Reeskens 2025; Mingo and Faggiano 2020). Hope has buttressed sociality by preventing migration and suicide (Adnanes 2004). Satisfaction has advanced sociality by strengthening political participation, social cohesion, social and government trust, and volunteering (E. Chan 2014; Flavin and Keane 2011; Rochelle 2015). Confidence in institutions also stems from institutional interactional legitimacy or utility from social interaction to induce sociality (Grimes 2006). Institutional legitimacy has championed sociality regarding trust as opposed to crime, discrimination, and protesting (Buechler 2011; Crandall and Beasley 2001; Gibson and Caldeira 2003; Lilly et al. 2011). Conversely, confidence in institutions has drawn utility from reducing anger and distress to sustain sociality (Lytkina and Reeskens 2025; Rhodes-Purdy et al. 2023). Anger has jeopardized sociality by eroding social integration and fomenting protesting and violence and its tolerance (Krahe 2013; Molm 2008; Passini 2019; Tausch et al. 2011). Moreover, anger can dampen sociality by breeding crime and radicalism (Brant 2019; Larson et al. 2020). Distress has undermined sociality by fomenting resistance and impeding social capital and trust (Pulkkinen et al. 2009; Webber and Huxley 2007).

Ideals drawn for confidence in institutions to rationalize sociality have accentuated collectivism, conservatism, political participation, religiosity, trust, and unification (Bolger et al. 2020; Elchardus and De Keere 2013; S. Chi et al. 2021; Hakhverdian and Mayne 2012; McAllister 1999; Mingo and Faggiano 2020; van Oorschot and Arts 2005). Collectivism has constituted sociality by securing civility, cooperation, prosocial behavior, and religiousness and preventing extremism (Hample 2018; Harzing 2006; Oyserman et al. 1998; Saucier and Skrzypinska 2006; Thielmann et al. 2020). Conservatism sustains sociality by nurturing empathy, loyalty, prosocial behavior, religiousness, and sacrifice (Dutton and Rayner-Hilles 2022). Moreover, conservatism underpins sociality by maintaining allegiance or loyalty, attachment, civility, community, conformity, cooperation, discipline, ethnocentrism, honesty, humility, intimacy, legality, morality, nationalism, obedience, order, partnership, patriotism, peace, responsibility, sharing, trust, and xenophobia (Dutton and Rayner-Hilles 2022; Heilman and Kusev 2020; Hickson 2013; Lakoff 2009; Rhodes-Purdy et al. 2023; Scruton 2014; Yoos 2007; Zuk and Zuk 2020). Conversely, conservatism upholds sociality by condemning dehumanizing, evilness, revolution, sexuality, terrorism, and transgression (Dutton and Rayner-Hilles 2022; Malka and Soto 2011; Scruton 2014; Suhay 2015). Political participation has buttressed sociality regarding civility (Campbell 2003). Trust has constituted sociality through donation, involvement, and volunteering (Uslaner 2000). The ideal for unification has upheld sociality regarding assimilation and trust (Guinjoan and Rico 2018; Wolsko et al. 2006). Confidence in institutions can also draw ideals for political interest to rationalize sociality (Yang and Tang 2010). Political interest has elevated sociality by raising civic engagement, civic and social motivation, civility, and discussion as opposed to protesting (Gil de Zuniga et al. 2017; Lee and Chan 2011; Pattie et al. 2004).

Conversely, confidence in institutions has built on the ideal against protesting to rationalize sociality (Tung et al. 2021). Protesting has impaired sociality by escalating distancing and radicalism and dampening moral motivation (Kutlaca et al. 2020; Vestergren et al. 2017). Besides, protesting impedes sociality by embracing antisociality, conflict, extremism, hostility, incivility, illegality, rioting, social exclusion, terrorism, and violence (Renger et al. 2020; Kaplan and Liu 2000; S. Lo 2021; McCright and Dunlap 2008; Morselli and Passini 2018; Smidt 2020; Stewart et al. 2012; Swart et al. 2020; Tan and Snow 2015).

Norms drawn for confidence in institutions to assimilate sociality have popularized accountability, fairness, and political participation (S. Chi et al. 2021; Elchardus and De Keere 2013; Farwell et al. 2019). Accountability has sustained sociality regarding compliance, morality, and xenophobia as opposed to violence (Bussey 2020; Granzin and Olsen 1998; Kaurin 2020; Milner and Myers 2007). The norm of fairness has upheld sociality by elevating morality and prosocial behavior (Barber 2004; McCaffoee 2016). Political participation has buttressed sociality regarding civility (Campbell 2003).

Confidence in institutions also stands on norms concerning civil society, justice, and support to assimilate sociality (Habibov 2014; Kozuch and Dobrowolski 2014). Civil society can maintain sociality by consolidating social capital and preventing conflict (Edwards 2004; Langman 2005). Besides, civil society constitutes sociality by championing association, civility, communitarianism, community, conservatism, donation, humanism, justice, networking, participation, philanthropy, responsibility, shaming, social democracy, social orientation, socialism, and solidarity (Adloff 2013; Choi 2004; DeLue and Dale 2009; Edwards 2004; O'Mahony 2013; Powell 2007). Communitarism held in civil society emphasizes charity, social capital, and volunteering (Powell 2007). Conservativism secured by civil society prioritizes charity, compassion, mutuality, self-discipline, and social capital (DeLue and Dale 2009; Powell 2007; Teets 2014). Humanism emphasized in civil society valorizes association, cooperation, and mutuality (Powell 2007). Social democracy enacted in civil society accentuates citizenship, cooperation, contracting, and partnership (Powell 2007). Socialism highlighted in civil society foregrounds association, cooperation, equality, harmony, and mutuality as opposed to competition and conflict (Powell 2007). The norm for justice has upheld sociality by elevating morality and prosocial behavior (Barber 2004; McCaffoee 2016). The norm for social support has elevated sociality by enhancing association, civic engagement, political participation, and recourse (Kampen 2010; F. Lee 2012; Palmer et al. 2011; Su and Feng 2013). Conversely, the norm of social support has secured sociality by preventing victimization and violence (E. Wright et al. 2015).

Faith in Religion

Religion as an institution hinges on awe or wonder, deity or god, divinity, meaning-making, and ritual or ceremony (Garrod and Jones 2009; McDowell and Brown 2009; van Uden and Zondag 2016). Inherently, religion features beliefs of convictions, especially moralized ones, collective memory, community, controlling, doctrines, gospels, identity, liberation, magic, modeling, morality, ritual, sacredness, salvation, social practice, tradition, worldviews (H. Campbell et al. 2018; Pelters and Wijma 2016; Rindermann 2018; J. Turner et al. 2018). Conversely, religion downplays freedom (Djupe 2018). Herein, social practice characterizes sociality (Featherstone and Morris 2012; Rindermann 2018). Religion also buttresses sociality by offering power, utility, ideals, and norms to achieve the requisite functions of analytical functionalism. Such religious offering engages discipline, doctrines, forbidding, leadership, legitimizing, magic, manipulation, messaging, modeling, protection, ritual, sharing, symbols, and therapy (Garrod and Jones 2009; McDowell and Brown 2009; Pelters and Wijma 2016; Rindermann 2018; J. Turner et al. 2018). Notably, power, utility, and ideals at the societal level become norms at the personal level.

Power maintained by religion to empower sociality rests on identity and meaningfulness (Garrod and Jones 2009). Identity facilitates sociality by raising belongingness (Reese et al. 2019). Meaningfulness has underlain sociality by boosting civic practice, responsibility, and volunteering and reducing rejection experience (Duffy and Raque-Bogdan 2010; Summers and Falco 2020; Twenge et al. 2003).

Utility offered by religion to incentivize sociality arises from fairness after death and salvation (Garrod and Jones 2009; Pelters and Wijma 2016; J. Turner et al. 2018). Fairness experienced has uplifted sociality regarding civility, cooperation, community identification, political participation, and social trust as opposed to protesting (A. Hu 2013; Lawrence and Daniels 1997; Sunshine and Tyler 2003; Tyler and Degoey 1995; van Prooijen et al. 2008; Wenzel 2000). Salvation has buttressed sociality regarding civility, social capital, and trust (Curley 2010; Watson et al. 2021; Williamson 2002). Conversely, religion induces sociality by dampening disutility in craving or desire and suffering (Garrod and Jones 2009; McDowell and Brown 2009). Craving or desire had provoked dissatisfaction (Nickerson et al. 2007). Satisfaction has eroded sociality by strengthening political participation, social cohesion, social and government trust, and volunteering (E. Chan 2014; Flavin and Keane 2011; Rochelle 2015). Suffering has impeded sociality by lowering social capital and social trust and escalating resistance (Pulkkinen et al. 2009; Webber and Huxley 2007).

Ideals set by religion to frame sociality have valorized cohesion, consensus, extraversion, and order (Garrod and Jones 2009; van Hemert et al. 2002). Social cohesion has constituted sociality by enhancing attachment and dampening tolerance for deviance (Stafford et al. 2005; Woosnam et al. 2018). Consensus has enhanced sociality by fostering cohesion, compliance, engagement, and rejection of outsiders (Fasel et al. 2016; Guan et al. 2021; Heshmati and Oravecz 2022; Yoon et al. 2013). Extraversion has buttressed sociality by fostering attachment, civic engagement, civility, donation, humor, nationalism, political participation, social capital, socializing, volunteering, and favor for civic and political participation (Bekkers 2010; C. Cheng et al. 2019; Fraley et al. 2011; Gotzsche-Astrup 2020; Hample 2018; Omoto et al. 2010; Schbley and McCauley 2005; Vernon et al. 2008; Ward and Forney 2020). The ideal for social order has bred sociality based on confidence in the business institution (Costa et al. 2023). Moreover, religion frames sociality by prioritizing ideals for allegiance, assistance, balance, cleanliness, community, discipline, egalitarianism, faith, humanity, morality or virtue, nationalism, propriety, selflessness, social practice, tradition, and utopianism (H. Campbell et al. 2018; Garrod and Jones 2009; McDowell and Brown 2009; Pelters and Wijma 2016; B. Turner 2005b; J. Turner et al. 2018). Allegiance or faith has constituted sociality by fostering collaboration, empathy, generosity, leadership, and morality (Lawler et al. 2016; Lee and Chan 2016; Wilcox and Dew 2016). Assistance has constituted sociality by civility, consolidating connectedness, cooperation, religiosity, responsibility, and volunteering (Hample 2018; Marsh and Dik 2021; Musick and Wilson 2008; Nelson-Coffey et al. 2023; Shahzalal and Adnan 2022). Moreover, assistance underlies sociality by enhancing citizenship, loyalty, social cohesion, socializing, and trust and diminishing self-interest (Dovidio et al. 2006; Hawley 2014; Kisliuk and

WeiBmuller 2023; Music 2014). Balancing has sustained sociality by enabling relatedness and social cohesion (Hornsey and Jetten 2004; SunWolf 2008). Cleanliness upholds sociality by characterizing communitarianism (Frazer 1999). The community represents social capital to boost sociality (Saegert and Winkel 2004). Hence, community involvement has facilitated sociality regarding cooperation, networking, and trust (Groves et al. 2000; Molitor et al. 2011; Rochelle 2015). Discipline has buttressed sociality by raising generativity and diminishing crime and violence (Y. Cheung et al. 2014; Welch et al. 2008; Peterson and Klohnen 1995). Egalitarianism has underpinned sociality by enhancing empathy, support for welfare, and trust in government and impeding radicalism (Faricy and Ellis 2014; Lauriola et al. 2015; Lucas and Kteily 2018; Roosma et al. 2014). Humanity in religion comprises compassion, kindness, love, reciprocity, and universalism or treating others as oneself (McDowell and Brown 2009). Compassion or kindness has constituted sociality by securing religiosity and volunteering (Barr et al. 2005). Love sustains sociality by enhancing adaptation and dampening aloneness, conflict, and loneliness (Jeffries 2000; Rokach 2019; Sanderson 2001; Soble 2008). Reciprocity has constituted sociality by fostering prosocial behavior (Thielmann et al. 2020). Universalism constitutes sociality by embodying morality (Mihailov 2023). Morality or virtue has constituted sociality by installing volunteering and inhibiting violence (Piquero and Hickman 2002; Whitford et al. 2006). Nationalism has underpinned sociality by fostering attachment, intolerance against deviance, patriotism, political participation, religiousness, social inclusion, trust in government, and xenophobia, and diminishing protesting (N. Chen 2012; Flanagan and Lee 2000; Huddy et al. 2021; Li and Brewer 2004; Osborne et al. 2017; Pinto et al. 2020; Rippl et al. 2010). Propriety underpins sociality by demonstrating benevolence, coordination, harmonizing, modesty, politeness, reciprocity, solidarity, and virtue (Z. Jiang 2012; Qin 2013). Selflessness embodies sociality by opposing egoism or egocentrism, individualism, and self-interest (Kitts 2003; Rocha and Ghoshal 2006). Social practice embodies sociality (Fenwick 2008). The ideal for tradition or traditionalism has underlain confidence in economic and political institutions, refutation against unconventional sexuality, and rejection of outsiders (Costa et al. 2023; Meuleman et al. 2019; Schwartz et al. 2010; Wang and You 2016). Utopianism bolsters sociality by hailing conservatism and egalitarianism as opposed to individualism (Castillo 2011). Conservatism sustains sociality by nurturing empathy, loyalty, prosocial behavior, religiousness, and sacrifice (Dutton and Rayner-Hilles 2022). Moreover, conservatism underpins sociality by maintaining allegiance or loyalty, attachment, civility, community, conformity, cooperation, discipline, ethnocentrism, honesty, humility, intimacy, legality, morality, nationalism, obedience, order, partnership, patriotism, peace, responsibility, sharing, trust, and xenophobia (Dutton and Rayner-Hilles 2022; Heilman and Kusev 2020; Hickson 2013; Lakoff 2009; Rhodes-Purdy et al. 2023; Scruton 2014; Yoos 2007; Zuk and Zuk 2020). Conversely, conservatism upholds sociality by condemning dehumanizing, evilness, revolution, sexuality, terrorism, and transgression (Dutton and Rayner-Hilles 2022; Malka and Soto 2011; Scruton 2014; Suhay 2015).

Conversely, religion secures sociality by inhibiting ideals for challenging, destruction, enslavement, freedom, harm, and hatred (Djupe 2018; Garrod and Jones 2009;

McDowell and Brown 2009). Challenging experienced has reduced sociality by impeding love, prosocial behavior, social capital, social interaction, and fomenting conflict, protesting, radicalism, and resistance (Lemay et al. 2023; Lubbers et al. 2006; Nezlek et al. 2008; Pfundmair and Mahr 2023; B. Rick et al. 2006; Savelkoul et al. 2011, 2014, 2015; Selvanathan and Lickel 2019). Destruction or harm undermines sociality by representing resistance (Ewick and Silbey 2003). Enslavement experienced impaired sociality by provoking conflict and confrontation (J. Turner 2013b). Freedom has inhibited sociality by fomenting crime (Costello 2013). Hatred impairs sociality by escalating radicalism, terrorism, and violence (Larson et al. 2020; Sternberg and Sternberg 2008; J. Turner 2007).

Norms popularized by religion to standardize sociality have emphasized collectivism and fertility (Cotter et al. 1998; Realo et al. 2008). Collectivism has constituted sociality by securing civility, cooperation, prosocial behavior, and religiousness and preventing extremism (Hample 2018; Harzing 2006; Oyserman et al. 1998; Saucier and Skrzypinska 2006; Thielmann et al. 2020). Fertility has raised sociality by enhancing civic engagement, community involvement, conformism, donation, social capital, social cohesion, social integration, social interaction, social support received, and volunteering (Apinunmahakul and Devlin 2008; Bjornberg and Ekbrand 2008; Frei et al. 2009; Ghimire 2021a; Kleinhans et al. 2007; Magdol and Bessel 2003; Taniguichi and Thomas 2011; Wilkinson 2008; Xiao 2000; Xu and Lai 2002). Conversely, fertility has advanced sociality by reducing social distance and violence (Broom et al. 2013; Tsai 2006).

Religion also builds on power in gathering to embody or sustain sociality (Turner and Maryanski 2008). Gathering characterizes sociality (Marres 2017). Moreover, gathering has empowered personal sociality by enhancing personal civic engagement, favor for community, political participation, and trust (Z. Han et al. 2017; F. Lee 2012; Palmer et al. 2011; Whitham 2012).

Faith in religion as an institution exemplifies religiosity, religiousness, or religious faith (Harris et al. 2018). Religious faith holds power, utility, ideals, and norms to bolster sociality in achieving its requisite functions dictated by analytical functionalism. Such holding engages religious adherence or affiliation, assertion, attachment, attendance or participation, attribution, awe or reverence, commitment, congregation, coping, enlightenment, identification, inculcation, learning, meditation, obedience, praying, reliance, sacrifice, service, tutoring, and worshipping (Ager and Ager 2011; Fontana 2003; Gay and Lynxwiler 2009; Ghimire 2021a; Hoffman and Bagdanov 2020; Lloyd et al. 2022; Rivera 2018; Maliepaard and Phalet 2012; Shorey et al. 2018; Spilka et al. 2003; Tenorio and Lo 2011; Upenieks 2022; Wollschleger 2012; Wuthnow 2004; Ysseldyk et al. 2012).

Power generated by religiosity to drive sociality has stemmed from empathy, health as opposed to illness, morality, responsibility, and social capital (W. Chang 2009; Helliwell and Putnam 2005; Keyes 2002; Muennig et al. 2013). Empathy has elevated sociality by facilitating prosocial behavior (Fraser et al. 2012). Health has uplifted sociality by boosting community sense, morality, popularity, social activity, social cohesion, social integration, social trust, social well-being, and volunteering (Huxhold et al. 2014; Jorgensen et al. 2010; Son and Wilson 2012; Tolsma et al.

2009; Yu and Chiu 2016). Conversely, health has sustained sociality by preventing loneliness (Koromeckyj-Cox et al. 2007). Meanwhile, illness has eroded sociality by impeding volunteering (Wuthnow 2004). Morality has constituted sociality by boosting volunteering and inhibiting violence (Piquero and Hickman 2002; Whitford et al. 2006). Responsibility has fostered sociality regarding compliance, morality, and xenophobia as opposed to violence (Bussey 2020; Granzin and Olsen 1998; Kaurin 2020; Milner and Myers 2007). Social capital has consolidated sociality by raising civic engagement, community involvement, donation, political involvement, social trust, and volunteering (Bekkers et al. 2008; Broadbent and Papadopoulos 2011; Brown and Ferris 2007; Chua et al. 2021; Narayan and Cassidy 2001). Conversely, social capital has strengthened sociality by erasing violence (Pulkkinen et al. 2009).

Utility offered by religiosity to attract sociality has rested on well-being, including adjustment, flourishing as opposed to depression, fear, loneliness, mastery, pleasure, relatedness, satisfaction, and self-esteem (Dy-Liacco et al. 2009; Ellison et al. 2001; Flouri and Buchanan 2002; V. Hui et al. 2007; Lauder et al. 2006; Meulemann 2010; Moschis and Ong 2011; Ng and Fisher 2016; Schieman 2001). Well-being uplifts sociality by consolidating altruism, conformism, cooperation, donation, liking for people, prosociality, sociability, and trust and social trust (Fetvadjiev and He 2019; A. Hu 2013; Lyubomirsky et al. 2006; Y. Pan et al. 2023; Wang and Graddy 2008). Additionally, well-being sustains sociality by enabling civilization, fairness, forgiveness, intimacy, kindness, love, loyalty, modesty, morality, open-mindedness, social intelligence, and societal functioning (Cummins 2016; D'raven and Pasha-Zaidi 2016; Meadows 2014). Moreover, religiosity raises perceived institutional efficacy or responsiveness (W. Tang 2014). Efficacy or responsiveness perceived has raised sociality by enhancing adaptation, forgiveness, and trust (Algoe and Zhaoyang 2016; Brik et al. 2023).

Religiosity uplifts sociality by inducing utility in blessedness, bliss, certainty, clarity, enlightenment, meaningfulness, peace, and warmth received (Fontana 2003; Spilka et al. 2003). Blessedness has upheld sociality by raising civic engagement, compliance, institutional trust, and political participation and dampened nimbyism (Grimes 2006; Islam et al. 2006; Kirchler and Maciejovsky 2001; Pattie et al. 2004; Spie et al. 1998). Bliss has maintained sociality by raising government trust and patriotism (Hunt et al. 2019; Turner and Stets 2005). Certainty or clarity has elevated sociality by reducing risking (Van Tongeren et al. 2023). Enlightenment felt has advanced sociality by enhancing attachment, generativity, and values on friendship and social engagement (Webster 2010). Meaningfulness has underlain sociality by boosting civic practice, responsibility, and volunteering and reducing rejection experience (Duffy and Raque-Bogdan 2010; Summers and Falco 2020; Twenge et al. 2003). Peace has fostered sociality characterized by adjustment, attunement, civility, compromise, connectedness, interdependency, order, peace, relatedness, respect, sacrifice, selflessness, solidarity, and sympathy as opposed to competition and conflict (Arat and Kerelian 2019; Cheung and Ma 2011; P. Ip 2014; Kjell et al. 2016; Peck 2002; G. Zhang 2006). Warmth received has consolidated sociality by raising civic engagement, community involvement, forgiveness, morality, prosocial behavior, recourse, relatedness, relationship value, social cohesion, social integration, social well-being, and trust (Bishop et al. 2002; E. Chan 2014; Garcia and Herrero 2004; C. Hui et al. 2013; Livingstone et al. 2023; Mata and Pendakur 2014; Palmer et al. 2011; Williams and Galliher 2006).

Ideals sustained by religiosity to rationalize sociality have emphasized benevolence, charity, civicness, civility, compliance, conformity or conformism, conservatism, donation, egalitarianism, forgiveness, generativity, helping, hospitality, hygiene, kindness, patriotism, political participation, punishment, redistribution, republicanism, tradition or traditionalism, social cohesion, social trust, and volunteering (Brown and Ferris 2007; Diez-Nicolas 2002; Horell 2014; Jost 2020; Kim and Wilcox 2013; Letki 2006; Myers 2008; Paterson 2018; Phalet et al. 2010; Ravanera et al. 2003; Marien and Hooghe 2001; Saunders and Wong 2012; Simpson et al. 2008; Spilka et al. 2003; Taniguichi and Thomas 2011; Werbner 2010; Wiepking and Maas 2009; Wuthnow 2004). Benevolence has upheld sociality by enhancing government trust and likability (Patricio et al. 2022). Charity embodies sociality regarding compassion, giving, mercy, and volunteering (Apinunmahakul and Devlin 2008; Eggemeier and Fritz 2020; Pommier et al. 2020). Mercy flows in comforting, counseling, and instructing (Eggemeier and Fritz 2020). Civicness has propped sociality by strengthening attachment, civility, collective behavior, discussion, donation, neighboring, patriotism, prosociality, social capital, socialism, trust, and volunteering and impeding cheating and individualism (Coffe and Geys 2007; Gilberbloom and Markham 1995; Kerrissey and Schofer 2013; Mata and Pendakur 2014; Ozbay 2008; Pattie et al. 2004; Pena-Lopez and Sanchez-Santos 2016; Rahn 2008; Richey 2011; Tak 2017; M. Tang 2011; Taniguchi 2013; Yip et al. 2007). Civility has constituted sociality by inducing fairness and trust (Vera-Toscano et al. 2013). Additionally, civility maintains sociality by enhancing the commonweal, community, equality, friendship, reciprocity, and social capital (Hudson 2023). Compliance, conformity, or conformism has constituted sociality by raising patriotism and impeding violence and acceptance of deviants and outsiders (Pulkkinen et al. 2009; Schwartz et al. 2014; Van Hootegem et al. 2000; Yeo and Chu 2018). Conservatism sustains sociality by nurturing empathy, loyalty, prosocial behavior, religiousness, and sacrifice (Dutton and Rayner-Hilles 2022). Moreover, conservatism underpins sociality by maintaining allegiance or loyalty, attachment, civility, community, conformity, cooperation, discipline, ethnocentrism, honesty, humility, intimacy, legality, morality, nationalism, obedience, order, partnership, patriotism, peace, responsibility, sharing, trust, and xenophobia (Dutton and Rayner-Hilles 2022; Heilman and Kusev 2020; Hickson 2013; Lakoff 2009; Rhodes-Purdy et al. 2023; Scruton 2014; Yoos 2007; Zuk and Zuk 2020). Conversely, conservatism upholds sociality by condemning dehumanizing, evilness, revolution, sexuality, terrorism, and transgression (Dutton and Rayner-Hilles 2022; Malka and Soto 2011; Scruton 2014; Suhay 2015). Donation has constituted sociality by consolidating charity, service value, social capital, social trust, and volunteering (Bekkers 2010; Chang 2009; Foster et al. 2001; Uslaner 2000). Egalitarianism has underpinned sociality by enhancing empathy, support for welfare, and trust in government and impeding radicalism (Faricy and Ellis 2014; Lauriola et al. 2015; Lucas and Kteily 2018; Roosma et al. 2014). Forgiveness has consolidated sociality by raising government trust (Choi and David 2012). Generativity has enhanced sociality by raising helping value and political participation (Peterson and Klohnen 1995). Helping has constituted sociality through civility, consolidating connectedness, cooperation, religiosity, responsibility, and volunteering (Hample 2018; Marsh and Dik 2021; Musick and Wilson 2008; Nelson-Coffey et al. 2023; Shahzalal and Adnan 2022). Moreover, helping underlies sociality by enhancing citizenship, loyalty, social cohesion, socializing, and trust and diminishing self-interest (Dovidio et al. 2006; Hawley 2014; Kisliuk and WeiBmuller 2023; Music 2014). Hospitality has constituted sociality by enhancing trust (Vera-Toscano et al. 2013). Hygiene upholds sociality by featuring prosociality (Motta and Goren 2021). Kindness has constituted sociality by securing religiosity and volunteering (Barr et al. 2005). Patriotism has constituted sociality by raising government trust, nationalism, prosocial behavior or prosociality, social cohesion, volunteering, and xenophobia (Beyerlein and Sikkink 2008; Gross et al. 2004; Ishii 2009; Straume and Odeen 2010). Political participation has buttressed sociality regarding civility (Campbell 2003). Punishment characterizes sociality (Fowers 2015). The ideal for redistribution has reflected sociality regarding faith in religion and social trust (Nagayoshi and Sato 2014). Republicanism upholds sociality regarding citizenship, the commonweal, interdependence, morality, nationalism, publicity, responsibility, social adaptation, and solidarity (Delanty 2009; Honohan 2002). The ideal for tradition or traditionalism has buttressed sociality by enhancing patriotism and faith in religion and discouraging protesting and accepting deviants and outsiders (Costa et al. 2023; Datler et al. 2013; Meuleman et al. 2019; Schwartz et al. 2014). Social cohesion has constituted sociality by enhancing attachment and dampening tolerance for deviance (Stafford et al. 2005; Woosnam et al. 2018). Social trust has constituted sociality through donation, involvement, and volunteering (Uslaner 2000). Volunteering has constituted sociality by raising altruism, charity orientation, civic motivation, donation, helping, moral responsibility, political participation, social integration, and social and government trust (Foster et al. 2001; Isham et al. 2006; Richey 2010; Richey and Ikeda 2009; Wiepking and Maas 2009).

Moreover, religiosity has buttressed sociality by valorizing ideals for altruism, caring, collaboration, compassion, humanitarianism, love, other-centeredness, recourse, and xenophobia (Devos et al. 2002; Newman et al. 2015; Spilka et al. 2003; Weisberg 2005; Wink and Dillon 2003; Zanin 2017). Altruism has constituted sociality by boosting attachment, civic engagement, friendship quality, likability, moral behavior, popularity, relatedness and diminishing loneliness and violence (Bond and Kwan 2000; W. Chen et al. 2022; Layous et al. 2012; Markiewicz et al. 2001; Martela and Ryan 2016; Mesch 2009; Na and Paternoster 2019; L. Taylor et al. 2018; Wright and Li 2011). Caring or compassion has underlain sociality by securing religiosity and volunteering (Barr et al. 2005). Collaboration has strengthened sociality regarding attachment and trustworthiness as opposed to argument (Gerbasi and Cook 2008; Hample 2018; Tak 2017). Love sustains sociality by enhancing adaptation and dampening aloneness, conflict, and loneliness (Jeffries 2000; Rokach

2019; Sanderson 2001; Soble 2008). Humanitarianism has enhanced sociality by activating political participation (Foschi and Lauriola 2014). Moreover, humanitarianism sustains sociality by favoring altruism, caring, civility, empathy, groupness, other orientation, pity, prosociality, and solidarity (Angelis and Pensini 2024; Bendixsen 2018; Chouliaraki 2013; Regilme 2020). Other-centeredness characterizes sociality (Marres 2017). Moreover, other-centeredness has fostered sociality by elevating compliance (Pool and Schwegler 2007). Recourse reflects sociality regarding affiliation and social support received (Ledbetter et al. 2013; Sullivan 2001). Other-centeredness can also enhance sociality by boosting forgiveness (Worthington 2006). Xenophobia has constituted sociality by promoting patriotism and social cohesion (Granzin and Olsen 1998; Wang and Chen 2004).

Conversely, religiosity has advanced sociality by rejecting ideals or tolerance for crime, deviance, individualism, oppression, protesting, sexuality, and violence (Andrews et al. 2015; Coffe and Geys 2007; Fontana 2003; Gaines and Garand 2010; Guo et al. 2008; Horell 2014; Saucier and Skrzypinska 2006). Tolerance for crime or violence has provoked violence (van Hiel et al. 2007). Violence has undermined sociality by breeding antisociality, crime and recidivism, blaming, conflict, hostility, rejecting others, and impairing agreeableness, morality, and responsibility (Asendorpf et al. 2008; Del Bove et al. 2008; Morrison 2006; Scholte et al. 2009; Vitaro et al. 2007). Deviance has ruined sociality by provoking social exclusion experienced (Backman and Nilsson 2011). Individualism has weakened sociality by reducing civic engagement, religiousness, social cohesion, and volunteering (Church 2010; Green and Janmaat 2011; J. He et al. 2014; Hener et al. 2016; Leong 2008; Pollack and Pickel 2007; Whitford et al. 2006). Conversely, individualism has impeded sociality by bolstering acceptance of outsiders, competition, crime, extremity, self-enhancement, protesting, and violence (Church 2010; J. He et al. 2014; Karstedt 2010; Leong 2008; Li and Song 1992; Pollack and Pickel 2007; Whitford et al. 2006). Oppressing can impede sociality by engendering violence (White et al. 2015). Protesting has impaired sociality by escalating distancing and radicalism and dampening moral motivation (Kutlaca et al. 2020; Vestergren et al. 2017). Besides, protesting impedes sociality by embracing antisociality, conflict, extremism, hostility, incivility, illegality, rioting, social exclusion, terrorism, and violence (Renger et al. 2020; Kaplan and Liu 2000; S. Lo 2021; McCright and Dunlap 2008; Morselli and Passini 2018; Smidt 2020; Stewart et al. 2012; Swart et al. 2020; Tan and Snow 2015). The ideal for sexuality has disrupted sociality by breeding risking (Moran et al. 2021). Sexuality or its ideal has also hurt sociality by fomenting aggression and isolation experience (Vrangalova and Bukberg 2015).

Norms sensitized by religiosity to assimilate sociality have popularized friendship, harmony, security, and volunteering (Clemence 2001; Musick 2000; Urbatsch 2014; Wuthnow 2002). Friendship has constituted sociality by enhancing community attachment, compliance, donation, gratitude, political participation, social cohesion, social desirability, social integration, and social trust (Corcoran 2013; Fahmy 2006; Gundert and Hohendanner 2015; Keillor et al. 2001; Kende et al. 2022; Opp 2001; Rotkirch 2014). Moreover, the norm for friendship has consolidated sociality by reducing protesting (Sampson et al. 2005). Security has buttressed sociality regarding civility, social capital, and trust (Curley 2010; Watson et al. 2021; Williamson 2002). Furthermore, the norm for security has enhanced sociality by maintaining neighboring, social cohesion, and trust and reducing aggression and opposition (Barbarin and Richter 2001; Grannis 2009; Rochelle 2015). Volunteering has constituted sociality by raising altruism, charity orientation, civic motivation, donation, helping, moral responsibility, political participation, social integration, and social and government trust (Foster et al. 2001; Isham et al. 2006; Richey 2010; Richey and Ikeda 2009; Wiepking and Maas 2009).

Religiosity also sustains sociality by drawing power, utility, ideals, and norms to achieve the requisite functions of analytical functionalism. These functions to consolidate religiosity transpire in attachment, attribution, compensation, familiarization, habituation, modeling, narrative, ritual, social construction, terror management, and tradeoff (Day 2011; Gorsuch 1994; Kay et al. 2008; Medvedovski and Allison 2017; Rose and Exline 2012; Shorey et al. 2018; Wollschleger 2012). This consolidation warrants that religiosity is feasible, gainful, ideal, and normative.

Power drawn for religiosity to drive sociality has rested on agreeableness, prosociality, social capital, and social desirability (Rivera 2018; Saucier and Skrzypinska 2006; Sedikides and Gebauer 2010). Agreeableness has fostered sociality by enhancing attachment (Fraley et al. 2011). Prosociality has constituted sociality by civility, consolidating connectedness, cooperation, religiosity, responsibility, and volunteering (Hample 2018; Marsh and Dik 2021; Musick and Wilson 2008; Nelson-Coffey et al. 2023; Shahzalal and Adnan 2022). Moreover, prosociality underlies sociality by enhancing citizenship, loyalty, social cohesion, socializing, and trust and diminishing self-interest (Dovidio et al. 2006; Hawley 2014; Kisliuk and Weißmuller 2023; Music 2014). Social capital has consolidated sociality by raising civic engagement, community involvement, donation, political involvement, social trust, and volunteering (Bekkers et al. 2008; Broadbent and Papadopoulos 2011; Brown and Ferris 2007; Chua et al. 2021; Narayan and Cassidy 2001). Social desirability has buttressed sociality by raising altruism, benevolence value, and empathy and perspective-taking and suppressing violence and its tolerance (Douglas 2006; Fisher and Katz 2000; Krumrei-Mancuso 2017; Pulkkinen et al. 2009). Moreover, religiosity draws power from morality and sympathy to enable sociality (Skerkat and Ellison 1999; Wollschleger 2012). Morality has championed sociality by boosting volunteering and inhibiting violence (Piquero and Hickman 2002; Whitford et al. 2006). Sympathy has constituted sociality by securing religiosity and volunteering (Barr et al. 2005). Religiosity also reflects power resting on community and solidarity to drive sociality (Kay et al. 2008; Spilka et al. 2003). The community represents social capital to boost sociality (Saegert and Winkel 2004). Hence, community involvement has facilitated sociality regarding cooperation, networking, and trust (Groves et al. 2000; Molitor et al. 2011; Rochelle 2015). Solidarity has constituted sociality by enhancing attachment and dampening tolerance for deviance (Stafford et al. 2005; Woosnam et al. 2018).

Utility drawn for religiosity to attract sociality originates from dependency (Spilka et al. 2003). Dependency can heighten received benefits (Adongo et al. 2019). Benefits received have buttressed sociality by boosting compliance, institutional trust, political participation, prosocial behavior, and recourse (Davis-Lipman et al. 2007; Grimes 2006; Kirchler and Maciejovsky 2001; Pattie et al. 2004; Premo et al. 2018).

Ideals drawn for religiosity to rationalize sociality have emphasized collectivism, empathizing, group involvement, nationalism, social concern, and traditionalism (Ishii and Watanable 2023; Kunovich and Hodson 1999; Saucier and Skrzypinska 2006; Wuthnow 2004). Collectivism has constituted sociality by securing civility, cooperation, prosocial behavior, and religiousness and preventing extremism (Hample 2018; Harzing 2006; Oyserman et al. 1998; Saucier and Skrzypinska 2006; Thielmann et al. 2020). Group involvement has fostered sociality regarding cohesion, common identity, and identification (Fischer et al. 2007). Nationalism has underpinned sociality by fostering attachment, intolerance against deviance, patriotism, political participation, religiousness, social inclusion, trust in government, and xenophobia, and diminishing protesting (N. Chen 2012; Flanagan and Lee 2000; Huddy et al. 2021; Li and Brewer 2004; Osborne et al. 2017; Pinto et al. 2020; Rippl et al. 2010). Social concern characterizes sociality (Marres 2017). Traditionalism has underlain confidence in economic and political institutions, refutation against unconventional sexuality, and rejection of outsiders (Costa et al. 2023; Meuleman et al. 2019; Schwartz et al. 2010; Wang and You 2016). Moreover, religiosity draws ideals for the afterlife, salvation, and belonging to rationalize sociality (Day 2011; A. Miller 1995). Against materialism, the ideal for the afterlife would sustain sociality by impeding risking (Kasser 2016). Salvation has buttressed sociality regarding civility, social capital, and trust (Curley 2010; Watson et al. 2021; Williamson 2002). Belongingness constitutes sociality (Fowers 2015). Religiosity also reflects ideals for altruism, groupism or sharing, and nationalism to rationalize sociality (Franks et al. 2013; Lichterman 2012; Requena and Stanek 2014). Sharing has constituted sociality by strengthening leadership and neighboring (Dubois et al. 2020; Grannis 2009). Moreover, sharing constitutes sociality regarding friendship (Launay and Dunbar 2015). Sharing can also underlie sociality by boosting morality, punishment, and social cohesion (N. Duncan 2017; Delton and Krasnow 2017). Furthermore, religiosity stands on ideals for binding and communitarianism to rationalize sociality (Haidt 2012; von Stuckrad 2013). Binding has constituted sociality by enhancing attachment and dampening tolerance for deviance (Stafford et al. 2005; Woosnam et al. 2018). Communitarianism constitutes sociality by espousing caring, civility, collective identity, commonweal orientation, community, dutifulness or responsibility, education or socialization, equality, interdependence, loyalty, mentoring, patriotism, reciprocity, relatedness, self-discipline, servicing including volunteering, settlement, social construction, social participation, solidarity, and trust (Delanty 2009; Frazer 1999; Moore 2010; Speth 2012).

Conversely, religiosity has rationalized sociality by drawing ideals against individualism and protesting (Saucier and Skrzypinska 2006; Skerkat 1998). Individualism has weakened sociality by reducing civic engagement, religiousness, social cohesion, and volunteering (Church 2010; Green and Janmaat 2011; J. He et al. 2014; Hener et al. 2016; Leong 2008; Pollack and Pickel 2007; Whitford et al. 2006). Conversely, individualism has impeded sociality by bolstering acceptance of outsiders, competition, crime, extremity, self-enhancement, protesting, and violence

(Church 2010; J. He et al. 2014; Karstedt 2010; Leong 2008; Li and Song 1992; Pollack and Pickel 2007; Whitford et al. 2006). Protesting has impaired sociality by escalating distancing and radicalism and dampening moral motivation (Kutlaca et al. 2020; Vestergren et al. 2017). Besides, protesting impedes sociality by embracing antisociality, conflict, extremism, hostility, incivility, illegality, rioting, social exclusion, terrorism, and violence (Renger et al. 2020; Kaplan and Liu 2000; S. Lo 2021; McCright and Dunlap 2008; Morselli and Passini 2018; Smidt 2020; Stewart et al. 2012; Swart et al. 2020; Tan and Snow 2015).

Norms drawn for religiosity to assimilate sociality have popularized religiosity and similarity and rejected cosmopolitanism (Baker and Smith 2009; Cheadle and Schwadel 2012; Norris and Inglehart 2009). Similarity has upheld sociality by enhancing social cohesion, social interaction, and trust and social trust (Stokman et al. 2013; Xiang et al. 2016). Cosmopolitanism contradicts sociality by hailing autonomy, diversity, foreignness, fusion, individualism, and liberalism (Corstange and York 2018; Delanty 2009; Held 2010; Herrmann 2023). Cosmopolitanism has eroded sociality by discounting religiosity and raising liberalism and acceptance of deviants and outsiders (Costa et al. 2023; Motschenbacher 2013; Norris and Inglehart 2009).

Justification for Misdeeds

Justification for misdeeds embraces acceptance, approval, endorsement, entitlement, evaluation, legitimation, neutralization, tolerance, and willingness regarding anger, antisocial behavior, crime, delinquency, doping, incivility, misbehavior, offense, risking, vice, and violence (Forsyth and Ward 2022; Mededovic and Kovacevic 2021; Matthews and Channon 2016; Montgomery et al. 2004; Rosselli and Jeglic 2017; Schumpe et al. 2020). Neutralization comprises dehumanization and separation from reality or responsibility (Matthews and Channon 2016). Such justification is justifiable by progressivism, which dismisses obedience and repentance (Garland et al. 2017). Furthermore, the justification is praiseworthy for inhibiting discrimination (Denver and Pickett 2022). This justification also stands on socialization (Luft 2015). Nonetheless, the justification is condemnable and necessary for reduction by policymaking (Denver and Pickett 2022; Javakhishvili and Jibladze 2018). Functionally, such justification has bred practice for misdeeds (van Hiel et al. 2007). At least, this breeding follows the voluntaristic mechanism of ideal calibration to achieve the latency function in analytical functionalism. That is, the justification represents an ideal to calibrate misdeed practice, including antisocial behavior, crime or offense, delinquency, doping, risking, and violence. These misdeeds undermine sociality through the voluntaristic mechanisms of power realization, utility optimization, ideal calibration, and norm conformity to hinder power, utility, ideals, and norms for sociality.

Antisocial behavior represents norm violation (S. Henry 2009). Such behavior covers addiction, callousness, dishonesty, hostility, illegality, immorality, impulsivity, and narcissism (Allen et al. 2005; Z. Guo et al. 2023; Iacobucci and Frieh 2018; Vauclair and Fischer 2011; M. Wang et al. 2015). Antisocial behavior undermines sociality by reducing power, utility, ideals, and norms for sociality to achieve its requisite functions. Notably, such reduction can apply to social reward or utility underlying sociality (Kaplan et al. 2013). Instead, antisocial behavior can create stress to diminish power for driving sociality (E. Smith et al. 2023).

Power for driving sociality reduced by antisocial behavior has resided in health (Backman and Nilsson 2011; Spohn and Kaplan 2000). Antisocial behavior can also reduce power for driving sociality by fomenting stress (E. Smith et al. 2023).

Disutility discouraging sociality created by antisocial behavior has originated from social exclusion experienced (Backman and Nilsson 2011). Conversely, antisocial behavior can lower utility in social reward for inducing sociality (Kaplan et al. 2013).

Ideals against sociality bred by antisocial behavior have favored egoism, lying, and violence (Kitts 2003; Kornienko et al. 2018; M. Wang et al. 2015). Egoism has hampered sociality by eroding intimacy, consensus, and prosocial behavior (Reykowski 2006; Wade-Benzoni and Tost 2009). Lying has undermined sociality by eroding honesty (O'Connor et al. 2022). Violence has undermined sociality by fomenting crime and tolerance for violence (Markowitz 2001; Tanner-Smith et al. 2013).

Antisocial behavior also draws power, utility, ideals, and norms against sociality, thus subverting its requisite functions dictated in analytical functionalism. Such subversion ensues from conflict, constraint, labeling, and self-categorization, and disrupted association, attachment, bonding, construction, containment, control and self-control, deterrence, interaction, and learning in antisocial behavior (S. Henry 2009; Herman-Kinney 2003; Kaplan et al. 2013; Seddig 2020).

Power for driving sociality has reduced due to neuroticism, which has underlain antisocial behavior (Wright and DeLisi 2016). Neuroticism underlying antisocial behavior has engaged depression, hostility, and impulsiveness (Wright and DeLisi 2016). Essentially, neuroticism has impaired sociality by reducing attachment security, civic engagement, coordination, forgiveness, nationalism, relatedness, and socializing and generating crime and hostility (Bekkers 2005; Fraley et al. 2011; Hounkpatin et al. 2015; Kalish 2008; Marks 1996; Mullet et al. 2005; Pulkkinen et al. 2009; Schbley and McCauley 2005; Ward and Forney 2020). Antisocial behavior can also reflect inadequate empathy or perspective-taking, guardianship received, parenting received, social bonding or control, and social integration to provide power to drive sociality (Kaplan et al. 2013; Y. Yau 2014). Empathy has buttressed sociality by safeguarding intimacy, prosocial behavior, and relational adjustment (Fraser et al. 2012; Redmond 2018; Rosen et al. 2017). Guardianship received reflects attachment to constitute sociality (Gillath et al. 2016). Essentially, guardianship represents social support. Social support received has strengthened sociality by enhancing attachment, gratitude, political participation, prosocial behavior, recourse, respect, responsibility, social integration, and social well-being (Boezeman and Ellemers

2008; Fahmy 2006; Phipps 2003; Williams and Galliher 2006; R. Wright et al. 2009; Zeldin et al. 2016; Zeng et al. 2024). Conversely, social support received has boosted sociality by preventing aggression, conflict, delinquency, doping, externalizing, hyperactivity, loneliness, runaway, sexuality, suicide, and violence (Bernardon et al. 2011; Browning et al. 2005; Hayslip et al. 2000; Nieuwenhuis et al. 2017; Pearson and Wilkinson 2013; Terzi-Unsal and Karei 2005; Wight et al. 2006; R. Wright et al. 2009). Parenting received has upheld sociality by encouraging recourse and preventing relationship breakdown (Cobb-Clark and Gorgens 2014). Social bonding comprises conventional attachment, belief, commitment, and involvement (Kaplan et al. 2013). Functionally, social bonding has constituted sociality regarding connectedness, friendship, giving, and social interaction (Eberl 2020; Liebler and Sandefur 2002; Nelson-Coffey et al. 2023; Phan et al. 2009). Social integration has constituted sociality by strengthening cooperation and preventing suicide (Duberstein et al. 2004; Lepkowski and Couper 2002). Conversely, antisocial behavior has emerged from disrupted power in agreeableness, empathy, and extraversion to maintain sociality (Rosenfield et al. 2000). Agreeableness impeding antisocial behavior embraces altruism, compliance, modesty, tender-mindedness, and trust (Wright and DeLisi 2016). With these features, agreeableness has fostered sociality by enhancing attachment (Fraley et al. 2011). Extraversion has buttressed sociality by fostering attachment, civic engagement, civility, donation, humor, nationalism, political participation, social capital, socializing, volunteering, and favor for civic and political participation (Bekkers 2010; C. Cheng et al. 2019; Fraley et al. 2011; Gotzsche-Astrup 2020; Hample 2018; Omoto et al. 2010; Schbley and McCauley 2005; Vernon et al. 2008; Ward and Forney 2020). Antisocial behavior can also reflect inadequate power, such as powerlessness and disorganization, to drive sociality (Herman-Kinney 2003; Kaplan et al. 2013; Konty 2007). Powerlessness has eroded sociality by dampening attachment and giving (Campos-Castillo and Hitlin 2013; Molm 1997). Social disorganization has undermined sociality by impeding attachment, social capital, and social trust (G. Brown et al. 2004; Congdon 2010; Ross and Mirowsky 2009).

Utility given by satisfaction and security for attracting sociality can be inadequate, as reflected by antisocial behavior (S. Henry 2009; Kaplan et al. 2013). Satisfaction has eroded sociality by strengthening political participation, social cohesion, social and government trust, and volunteering (E. Chan 2014; Flavin and Keane 2011; Rochelle 2015). Security has buttressed sociality regarding civility, social capital, and trust (Curley 2010; Watson et al. 2021; Williamson 2002). Conversely, antisocial behavior can reflect inferiorization and stigmatization received and strain as disutility to impede sociality (Dotter 2004; Kaplan et al. 2013). Stigmatization received has eroded sociality by damping social cohesion (Walton and Cohen 2007). Strain can emerge from blocked achievement and means, disjuncture between desire and means, failure, negative stimuli, and removed value (Kaplan et al. 2013). As such, strain has undermined sociality by fomenting resistance and impeding social capital and trust (Pulkkinen et al. 2009; Webber and Huxley 2007). Inferiority can diminish sociality by breeding migration and impeding cooperation (Mummendey et al. 1999; Van Lange et al. 2014).

Ideals against rationalizing sociality have favored pornography and sexuality (Lynxwiler and Gay 2000). Sexuality or lechery has eroded sociality by eroding attachment security and evoking aggression (Dunkel et al. 2016; Vrangalova and Bukberg 2015). The ideal for pornography has disrupted sociality by engendering the ideal for violence (Hald and Malamuth 2015). Moreover, the ideal for pornography can impede sociality by raising delinquency (Stevens et al. 2011). Antisocial behavior can also reflect ideals for anomie and law violation to impede sociality (Featherstone and Deflem 2003; Herman-Kinney 2003). Anomie means using deinstitutionalized means to achieve exaggerated or overemphasized goals for success (Featherstone and Deflem 2003). The ideal for law violation has impeded sociality by fomenting violence (van Hiel et al. 2007). Violence has undermined sociality by breeding anti-sociality, crime and recidivism, blaming, conflict, hostility, rejecting others, and impairing agreeableness, morality, and responsibility (Asendorpf et al. 2008; Del Bove et al. 2008; Morrison 2006; Scholte et al. 2009; Vitaro et al. 2007). Antisocial behavior can also reflect ideals for broken windows or disorder, deviance, neutralization, normlessness or social dysregulation, and resistance to impair sociality. (S. Henry 2009; Herman-Kinney 2003; Kaplan et al. 2013). Neutralization of antisocial behavior encompasses its acceptability, desert, loyalty, normality, and reward rather than its injury, intent, responsibility, and victimization (S. Henry 2009). Essentially, neutralizing antisocial behavior represents the approval of crime and violence (Matthews and Channon 2016). Normlessness has impeded sociality by raising radicalism and support for violence (Troian et al. 2019). Moreover, normlessness inhibits sociality by disregarding consensus and foregrounding isolation (Troian et al. 2019; Zhao and Cao 2010). Resistance has impaired sociality by eroding solidarity and fomenting deviance (Foy et al. 2014; J. Williams 2011). Conversely, antisocial behavior has originated from ideals against community or communitarianism, religiosity, and self-control to undermine sociality (Kaplan et al. 2013; Vauclair and Fischer 2011; Wright and DeLisi 2016; Y. Yau 2014). Communitarianism constitutes sociality by espousing caring, civility, collective identity, commonweal orientation, community, dutifulness or responsibility, education or socialization, equality, interdependence, loyalty, mentoring, patriotism, reciprocity, relatedness, self-discipline, servicing including volunteering, settlement, social construction, social participation, solidarity, and trust (Delanty 2009; Frazer 1999; Moore 2010; Speth 2012). Religiosity has sustained sociality by fostering civic engagement, civility, cohesion, compliance, donation, empathy, morality, patriotism, prejudice against deviants and outsiders, prosocial behavior, social trust, and volunteering (Apinunmahakul and Devlin 2008; Corcoran et al. 2011; Ishio 2010; Keyes 2002; Kim and Wilcox 2013; Ravanera et al. 2003; van Tienen et al. 2011; Weisberg 2005; Wuthnow 2004). Conversely, religiosity has secured sociality by reducing crime, deviance, individualism, protesting, and sexuality (Andrews et al. 2015; Coffe and Geys 2007; Guo et al. 2008; Skerkat and Ellison 1999; Spilka et al. 2003). Moreover, religiosity realizes sociality regarding altruism, community, ethicality, groupism, sharing, and solidarity (Franks et al. 2013; Lichterman 2012; Peifer 2010; Spilka et al. 2003; Stavrova and Siegers 2014). Religiosity also upholds sociality by featuring altruism, attachment, caring, community, compassion, harmony, hospitality, love, morality, obedience, other-centeredness, peace, trust, unity, xenophobia (Ager and Ager 2011; Fontana 2003; Harris et al. 2018; Horell 2014; Paterson 2018; Shorey et al. 2018; Simpson et al. 2008; Spilka et al. 2003; Tenorio and Lo 2011; Werbner 2010). Conversely, religiosity maintains sociality by dismissing individualism, oppression, sexuality, and violence (Fontana 2003; Horell 2014; Spilka et al. 2003). Responsibility has sustained sociality regarding compliance, morality, and xenophobia as opposed to violence (Bussey 2020; Granzin and Olsen 1998; Kaurin 2020; Milner and Myers 2007). Self-control has buttressed sociality by enhancing generativity and impeding crime, risking, and violence (Y. Cheung et al. 2014; Koegl and Day 2019; Peterson and Klohnen 1995; Welch et al. 2008).

Norms popularizing communality for assimilating sociality can be inadequate, as reflected by antisocial behavior (Kaplan et al. 2013). Communality has constituted sociality by securing civility, cooperation, prosocial behavior, and religiousness and preventing extremism (Hample 2018; Harzing 2006; Oyserman et al. 1998; Saucier and Skrzypinska 2006; Thielmann et al. 2020). Conversely, antisocial behavior can result from norms for antisociality or deviance, consumerism, competition, and sexuality, which contradict sociality (Dotter 2004; Kaplan et al. 2013; Seddig 2020). Consumerism has weakened sociality by boosting migration (Adnanes 2004). Competition has impeded sociality by eroding volunteering (Martinez and McMullin 2004). Sexuality has eroded sociality by eroding attachment security and evoking aggression (Dunkel et al. 2016; Vrangalova and Bukberg 2015).

Crime, delinquency, illegality, offense, or sin represents antisociality, deviance, evilness, normlessness, and law or rule breaching (Reiner 2016; Silver et al. 2025; Wikstrom 2010). Inherently, crime features extremism and immorality (D. Jones 2016; Kirkpatrick 2020). Extremism includes disrespect and intolerance (Kirkpatrick 2020). Immorality covers aggressiveness, antisociality, callousness, cunning, deceitfulness, egocentrism, glibness, grandiosity, hostility, impulsivity, manipulativeness, irresponsibility, irritability, lying, nervousness, normlessness, parasitism, recklessness, remorselessness, sexuality, shamelessness, unreliability, unresponsiveness, and untruthfulness (D. Jones 2016). Crime undermines sociality by weakening power, utility, ideals, and norms to achieve their requisite functions to maintain sociality under analytical functionalism. Such weakening sabotages the voluntaristic mechanisms of power realization, utility optimization, ideal calibration, and norm conformity. Furthermore, Hence, crime has impaired sociality by reducing community involvement, prosocial behavior, and social trust and fomenting avoidance, protesting, risking, victimization, and violence (Brayne 2014; McNeeley and Yuan 2017; Broadbent and Papadopoulos 2011; Sun and Wang 2012; Wittebrood and Nieuwbeerta 2000; Zhong 2010).

Power weakening due to crime to hinder sociality results from poverty and unemployment (Reiner 2016). Poverty has undermined sociality by reducing civic participation, trust, social connection, and volunteering (Caputo 2010; Stephens et al. 2014; R. Walker et al. 2010). Conversely, poverty has disrupted sociality by creating isolation, relationship problems, and social exclusion experienced (Dhal et al. 2008; Stephens et al. 2014; R. Walker et al. 2010). Unemployment has impeded sociality by dissolving social capital, social cohesion, and trust (Espvall and Dellgren

2008; Manturuk et al. 2010; Reeskens and Vandecasteele 2017). Conversely, unemployment has hurt sociality by breeding conflict experienced, moving, protesting, threats experienced, and victimization (Bramley and Morgan 2003; Kaukinen 2004; Lewin-Epstein et al. 2003; Schneider 2007; Su and Feng 2013).

Utility impaired by crime to inhibit sociality results from disorders, panic, and victimization (Deegan 2021; Waiton 2008; Wittebrood and Nieuwbeerta 2000). Disorders have obstructed sociality by diminishing community attachment, social capital, and social trust (G. Brown et al. 2004; Congdon 2010; Ross and Mirowsky 2009). Panic has undermined sociality by activating avoidance (Lee-Baggley et al. 2004). Conversely, panic has dampened sociality by reducing donation, friendship, political participation, and prosocial behavior (Best and Krueger 2010; Hewstone et al. 2005; Piliavin and Callero 1991; Zhong 2010). Victimization experienced has impaired sociality by eroding social trust (Olivera 2015). Conversely, victimization experienced has hurt sociality by activating conflict and migration (Bar-Tal and Halperin 2013; Ramesh et al. 2019). Crime also reduces utility based on confidence and security to attract sociality (Reiner 2016). Confidence has buttressed sociality by raising responsibility and trust and reducing protesting (Atkeson and Maestas 2012; Bierhoff 2002; Quaranta 2016). Security has buttressed sociality regarding civility, social capital, and trust (Curley 2010; Watson et al. 2021; Williamson 2002).

Ideals enhanced by crime to weaken sociality accentuate consumerism, cynicism, egoism or egocentrism, greed, impulsivity and recklessness, incivility, individualism, sexuality, and terrorism (Deegan 2021; D. Jones 2016; Reiner 2016; Sammons and Putwain 2019; Waiton 2008). Consumerism has weakened sociality by boosting migration (Adnanes 2004). Egoism or egocentrism has hampered sociality by eroding intimacy, consensus, and prosocial behavior (Reykowski 2006; Wade-Benzoni and Tost 2009). Greed has hindered sociality by dampening prosocial behavior (Thielmann et al. 2020). Impulsivity has impeded sociality by diminishing prosocial behavior and engendering protesting, radicalism, and violence (Breakwell 2007; Koehler and Fiebig 2019; Thielmann et al. 2020; Wright and DeLisi 2016). Incivility has harmed sociality by reducing fairness and trust (Vera-Toscano et al. 2013). Individualism has weakened sociality by reducing civic engagement, religiousness, social cohesion, and volunteering (Church 2010; Green and Janmaat 2011; J. He et al. 2014; Hener et al. 2016; Leong 2008; Pollack and Pickel 2007; Whitford et al. 2006). Conversely, individualism has impeded sociality by bolstering acceptance of outsiders, competition, crime, extremity, self-enhancement, protesting, and violence (Church 2010; J. He et al. 2014; Karstedt 2010; Leong 2008; Li and Song 1992; Pollack and Pickel 2007; Whitford et al. 2006). The ideal for sexuality has disrupted sociality by breeding risking (Moran et al. 2021). Sexuality or its ideal has also hurt sociality by fomenting isolation experienced and aggression (Vrangalova and Bukberg 2015). Terrorism has ruined sociality by raising violence and diminishing collective practice and confidence in government (Achilov 2016; Levi and Strker 2000). Moreover, crime has disrupted sociality by engendering avoidance (Brayne 2014). Avoidance has hindered sociality by diminishing communication and prosociality and provoking radicalism (Collins and Feeney 2004; Makhanova and Shepherd 2020; Soliman et al. 2016).

Conversely, crime impedes sociality by discounting ideals for love, normativity, reliability, respect, responsibility, responsiveness, and social integration (D. Jones 2016; Kirkpatrick 2020; Reiner 2016). Love sustains sociality by enhancing adaptation and dampening aloneness, conflict, and loneliness (Jeffries 2000; Rokach 2019; Sanderson 2001; Soble 2008). Normativity has countenanced sociality by raising civic engagement, donation, prosocial behavior, punishment, support for policy, volunteering, and voting and eroding cheating, violence, and tolerance for violence (Brown and Ferris 2007; Hennessy et al. 2015; Huesmann 2018; B. Liu et al. 2023; Opp 2002; Pavlova and Silbereisen 2015; Wade-Benzoni and Tost 2009; Waterman et al. 2022; Wenzel 2004). Reliability can sustain sociality by boosting or maintaining cooperation, intimacy, and social capital (X. Chen et al. 2015; Harvey and Wenzel 2006; Yamagishi et al. 2005). Respect constitutes sociality regarding caring and equality (Renger and Reese 2017). Responsibility has sustained sociality regarding compliance, morality, and xenophobia as opposed to violence (Bussey 2020; Granzin and Olsen 1998; Kaurin 2020; Milner and Myers 2007). Responsiveness has uplifted sociality regarding prosocial behavior (Clobert et al. 2015). Social integration has constituted sociality by strengthening cooperation and preventing suicide (Duberstein et al. 2004; Lepkowski and Couper 2002).

Crime also reflects inadequate power, utility, ideals, and norms to achieve sociality through the voluntaristic mechanisms of power realization, utility optimization, ideal calibration, and norm conformity stipulated in analytical functionalism. Conversely, crime builds on power, disutility, ideals, and norms against sociality. The power realization mechanism underlying crime engages conflict, facilitation, and structuring (Merdian et al. 2017; Reiner 2016; Sammons and Putwain 2019). That is, this mechanism generates power for crime and against sociality. Specifically, conflict counterposes and activates power, facilitation applies power, and structuring imposes power. The utility optimization mechanism underlying crime engages deterrence, rational choice, and reinforcement (Reiner 2016; Sammons and Putwain 2019). That is, this mechanism determines utility for crime and against sociality. Specifically, deterrence highlights disutility, rational choice calculates and clarifies utility, and reinforcement provides utility. The ideal calibration mechanism underlying crime engages attribution, cognition, neutralization, self-fulfillment, and self-verification (Brant 2019; Lilly et al. 2011; Swann 2012; Weiner 2012). That is, this mechanism determines ideals for crime and against sociality. Specifically, attribution and cognition activate ideals and neutralization, self-fulfillment, and self-verification apply ideals. The norm conformity mechanism underlying crime engages association, attachment or bonding, coercion, containment or control, cultivation, emancipation, labeling, learning, shaming, and social construction (Lilly et al. 2011; Maass et al. 2013; Reiner 2016; Salisbury 2013; Walsh 2011). That is, this mechanism determines norms for crime and against sociality. Specifically, association, attachment, bonding, and learning accept norms, coercion, containment, cultivation, labeling, shaming, and social construction provide norms, and emancipation removes norms.

Power for crime and against sociality has stemmed from anomie, externalizing behavior, impulsivity, hyperactivity, inattention, and internalizing behavior (Jolley et al. 2019; Karstedt and Farrall 2006; Piquero et al. 2007; Tanner-Smith et al.

2013). Anomie has impeded sociality by raising radicalism and support for violence (Troian et al. 2019). Externalizing behavior has blocked sociality by raising antisocial behavior and conflict and dampening community participation and social support receipt (Crockett et al. 2018; Khamis 2006). Hyperactivity has ruined sociality by hurting social well-being (Bennett et al. 2020). Inattention has impaired sociality by worsening peer relationship quality and fueling the oppositional-defiant disorder, peer aversion, and peer rejection experienced (del Mar Bernad et al. 2016; Tevis et al. 2021). Impulsivity has impeded sociality by raising protesting, radicalism, and violence and dampening prosocial behavior (Breakwell 2007; Thielmann et al. 2020; Koehler and Fiebig 2019; Wright and DeLisi 2016). Internalizing behavior has weakened sociality by breeding blaming, externalizing behavior, suicide, and victimization, and reducing moral behavior and popularity (Abrutyna and Mueller 2014; Dougherty 2006; Schreck et al. 2007; Wayment et al. 2010; Wentzel et al. 2004). Moreover, power for crime and against sociality can arise from alcoholism, anger, callousness, carefreeness, deviance, dominating strength, emotionality, freedom, masculinity, sadomasochism, self-centeredness, and sexual drive (Brezina and Agnew 2013; Crewe and Lippens 2009; Doerner and Lab 2012; Farrington 2010; Lilly et al. 2011; Reiner 2016; Renel and Segev 2014; Salisbury 2013; Walsh 2014). Alcoholism has impaired sociality by raising risking, victimization, and violence (Eakins et al. 2022; Krahe 2013; Zavala and Guadalupe-Diaz 2019). Anger has jeopardized sociality by eroding social integration and fomenting protesting and violence and its tolerance (Krahe 2013; Molm 2008; Passini 2019; Tausch et al. 2011). Moreover, anger can dampen sociality by breeding crime and radicalism (Brant 2019; Larson et al. 2020). Callousness has impaired sociality by breeding aggression, antisocial behavior, deviance, and violence and impeding empathy (Camara et al. 2025; Stulhofer 2021; M. Wang et al. 2015). Sadomasochism has undermined sociality by breeding violence (Semerikova et al. 2019). Carefreeness or freedom has undermined sociality by fomenting crime (Costello 2013). Dominating has impaired sociality by weakening social cohesion (E. Chan 2014). Emotionality has impaired sociality by reducing attachment security, civic engagement, coordination, forgiveness, nationalism, relatedness, and socializing and generating crime and hostility (Bekkers 2005; Fraley et al. 2011; Hounkpatin et al. 2015; Kalish 2008; Marks 1996; Mullet et al. 2005; Pulkkinen et al. 2009; Schbley and McCauley 2005; Ward and Forney 2020). Masculinity has hindered sociality by weakening regard (Bond et al. 2000). Self-centeredness has hampered sociality by eroding intimacy, consensus, and prosocial behavior (Reykowski 2006; Wade-Benzoni and Tost 2009). Sexual drive has eroded sociality by eroding attachment security and evoking aggression (Dunkel et al. 2016; Vrangalova and Bukberg 2015). By contrast, power deficient for sociality and crime prevention can arise from autism, depression, infantility, inferiority, neuroticism, pathology, psychopathy, and psychoticism (Addad 1987; Lilly et al. 2011; Sammons and Putwain 2019; Shoham et al. 1999). Autism has ruined sociality by fomenting hate (White et al. 2012). Moreover, autism embraces aggression and social anxiety and dismisses communication and social interaction to obstruct sociality (Tevis et al. 2021; White et al. 2012). Depression has eroded sociality by breeding conflict, hate, hostility perceived, loneliness, revenge, risking, suicide, and violence (Cacioppo and Hawkley 2009; Economou et al. 2016; Haner et al. 2020; Morokoff et al. 2009; Mullet et al. 2005; Proulx et al. 2004; H. Smith et al. 2016; E. Wright et al. 2015). Conversely, depression has attenuated sociality by impeding benevolence, closeness experienced, fairness, forgiveness, gratitude, honesty, leadership, love, social integration, teamwork, and volunteering (Blanchard et al. 2021; Cornwall 2009; Holzel et al. 2011; Mancini et al. 2011; Mullet et al. 2005; Thoits and Hewitt 2001). Infantility has obstructed sociality by hindering conformism and prosocial valuation (Fetvadjiev and He 2019). Inferiority can diminish sociality by breeding migration and impeding cooperation (Mummendey et al. 1999; Van Lange et al. 2014). Neuroticism has impaired sociality by reducing attachment security, civic engagement, coordination, forgiveness, nationalism, relatedness, and socializing and generating crime and hostility (Bekkers 2005; Fraley et al. 2011; Hounkpatin et al. 2015; Kalish 2008; Marks 1996; Mullet et al. 2005; Pulkkinen et al. 2009; Schbley and McCauley 2005; Ward and Forney 2020). Pathology has eroded sociality by impeding volunteering (Wuthnow 2004). Psychopathy has undermined sociality by withdrawing prosocial behavior and breeding radicalism, victimization, and violence (Ehrensuft et al. 2003; Krahe 2013; Soliman et al. 2016; Thielmann et al. 2020). Psychoticism features disorders and lacks agreeableness, conscientiousness, and openness (Village and Francis 2010). As such, psychoticism has disturbed sociality by eroding civility and cooperation and provoking violence (Hample 2018; Pulkkinen et al. 2009). Conversely, power for sociality and against crime has been academic motivation, agreeableness, honesty or humility, intelligence, openness, and self-control (Jolley et al. 2019; Jolliffe and Farrington 2010; Tanner-Smith et al. 2013). Moreover, power for sociality and against crime can evolve from compassion, considerateness, coping ability, empathy and perspective-taking, guardianship received, mindfulness, normalcy, problem-solving skill, rationality, reliability, self-efficacy, self-help grouping, social support received, spirituality, structuredness, and superiority (Benson and Simpson 2018; Gottfredson 2018; Hoffmann 2023; Lilly et al. 2011; Makarios and Sams 2013; Proctor and Niemeyer 2019); Renel and Segev 2014; Salisbury 2013; Shoham et al. 1999; Vander Ven and Colvin 2013; Walsh 2014). Compassion has underlain sociality by securing religiosity and volunteering (Barr et al. 2005). Considerateness has constituted sociality by enhancing attachment and dampening tolerance for deviance (Stafford et al. 2005; Woosnam et al. 2018). Coping has enabled sociality by facilitating compliance, intimacy, and relatedness (Chow et al. 2014; Gattino et al. 2015; Twardawski et al. 2021). Empathy has elevated sociality by facilitating prosocial behavior (Fraser et al. 2012). Guardianship as social support would strengthen sociality by enhancing attachment, gratitude, political participation, prosocial behavior, recourse, respect, responsibility, social integration, and social well-being (Boezeman and Ellemers 2008; Fahmy 2006; Phipps 2003; Williams and Galliher 2006; R. Wright et al. 2009; Zeldin et al. 2016; Zeng et al. 2024). Mindfulness has facilitated sociality by raising affiliating, intimacy, and prosocial behavior (D. Berry et al. 2020; Flett 2018; Karremans et al. 2017). Normalcy upholds sociality by dispelling radicalism (Koehler and Fiebig 2019).

Problem-solving has maintained sociality by lessening violence (Krahe 2013). Moreover, problem-solving can secure sociality by engendering social competence (Ting-Toomey 2004). Rationality has championed sociality by dampening aggression and antisociality (DiGiuseppe et al. 2017). Reliability maintains sociality by embracing social capital (X. Chen et al. 2015). Moreover, reliability can uphold sociality by securing intimacy (Harvey and Wenzel 2006). Self-efficacy has sustained sociality by raising civic engagement, donation, government and social trust, leadership, political participation, prosocial behavior, and social activity (Bednall et al. 2013; Frye 2007; Gnambs and Batinic 2012; Huber et al. 2022; Mangum 2012; Rahn 2008; Pei and Pan 2018; Yao and Enright 2019). Self-help grouping has constituted sociality by raising group satisfaction and social skills and preventing loneliness (Anderson-Butcher et al. 2004; Cameron 2002; Schiff and Bargal 2000). Social support received has strengthened sociality by enhancing attachment, gratitude, political participation, prosocial behavior, recourse, respect, responsibility, social integration, and social well-being (Boezeman and Ellemers 2008; Fahmy 2006; Phipps 2003; Williams and Galliher 2006; R. Wright et al. 2009; Zeldin et al. 2016; Zeng et al. 2024). Conversely, social support received has boosted sociality by preventing aggression, conflict, delinquency, doping, externalizing, hyperactivity, loneliness, runaway, sexuality, suicide, and violence (Bernardon et al. 2011; Browning et al. 2005; Hayslip et al. 2000; Nieuwenhuis et al. 2017; Pearson and Wilkinson 2013; Terzi-Unsal and Karei 2005; Wight et al. 2006; R. Wright et al. 2009). Spirituality means faith in the afterlife and incarnation and search for the sacred (Harris et al. 2018; Schwartz 2012). Inherently, spirituality features asceticism, calmness or serenity, compassion, forbearance, forgiveness, grandiosity, gratitude, meaning-making, mindfulness, irrationality, and transcendence (Day 2010; Hall and Edwards 2002; Harris et al. 2018; Kelly 2012; Patch 2012; Richards 2012). As such, spirituality has bolstered sociality by raising communitarianism and volunteering and preventing dominance and hostility (Bore et al. 2005; Saucier and Skrzypinska 2006; Seidlitz et al. 2002; van Tienen et al. 2011). Structuredness has buttressed sociality regarding civility, social capital, and trust (Curley 2010; Watson et al. 2021; Williamson 2002). Superiority can uphold sociality by facilitating communication (Keeting 2016).

Utility attracting sociality and impeding crime has rested on academic achievement, housing quality, neighborhood quality, relatedness with peers, and social integration (Hoffmann 2023; Piquero et al. 2007; Tanner-Smith et al. 2013; Welch et al. 2008). Academic achievement has boosted sociality by raising civic participation, leadership, morality, national identification, parental attachment and engagement, patriotism, social support received, and volunteering (Gault-Sherman 2012; Hsiao 2004; Mackinnon 2012; Murray 2009; Niemi et al. 2000; Zaff et al. 2003). Housing quality has buttressed sociality by preventing violence (Farrington 2007). Neighborhood quality has elevated sociality by building social capital, order, and cohesion (Rupp et al. 2020; Sampson and Raudenbush 2004). Relatedness has consolidated sociality by consolidating sharing, social interaction, and relationship satisfaction (Downie et al. 2008; Frazer 1999; Wickham and Knee 2012). Social integration has constituted sociality by strengthening cooperation and preventing suicide (Duberstein et al. 2004; Lepkowski and Couper 2002). Furthermore, utility for sociality and against crime can arise from acceptance, hope, justice, parenting quality, Respect, security, social integration, and success (Brezina and Agnew 2013; Kirkpatrick 2020; Lilly et al. 2011; Reiner 2016; Renel and Segev 2014; Sherman 2010). Acceptance experienced constitutes sociality regarding social capital and inclusion (Secker et al. 2009). Hope has maintained sociality by preventing migration and suicide (Adnanes 2004). Justice experienced has warranted sociality regarding civility, cooperation, community identification, political participation, and social trust as opposed to protesting (A. Hu 2013; Lawrence and Daniels 1997; Sunshine and Tyler 2003; Tyler and Degoey 1995; van Prooijen et al. 2008; Wenzel 2000). Parenting quality has sustained the offspring's sociality by preventing the offspring's delinquency and externalizing behavior (Mistry and Lowe 2006). Respect received has consolidated sociality by raising sharing, social interaction, and relationship satisfaction (Downie et al. 2008; Frazer 1999; Wickham and Knee 2012). Security upholds sociality by avoiding conflict, hostility, and rejection experience (Bina et al. 2020). As such, security has buttressed sociality regarding civility, social capital, and trust (Curley 2010; Watson et al. 2021; Williamson 2002). Success has induced sociality by enhancing love and trust (Nezlek et al. 2008; Rieger and Wang 2021).

Conversely, disutility impairing sociality and engendering crime has arisen from adversity, community disadvantage and inequality, national inequality, penalties, and stress (Hoffmann 2023; Kennedy et al. 1998; K. Land et al. 1996; Nguyen and McGloin 2013; Ousey and Lee 2013; Savolainen 2009; J. Wo et al. 2016). Adversity or stress has undermined sociality by eroding civility, forgiveness, generativity, relationship quality and satisfaction, social integration, social support received, and trust and heightening conflict, maltreatment, substance abuse, suicide, and violence (Atkinson et al. 2005; Dutton et al. 2016; Gelles 2007; Grzywacz and Almeida 2008; Jackson et al. 2006; Sobeck et al. 2020; Toussaint et al. 2016). Community disadvantage has hindered sociality by raising victimization and eroding community attachment, social capital, and social trust (Congdon 2010; Hughes 2001; Like 2011; Ross and Mirowsky 2009). National inequality has impeded sociality by eroding social capital, support for redistribution and welfare, sympathy, trust, and volunteering (Busemeyer 2013; Hitlin and Harkness 2018; Lipford and Yandle 2009; Oishi et al. 2011; Portes and Vickstrom 2011). Conversely, national inequality has impaired sociality by provoking crime and violence (Ousey and Lee 2013; van Wilsem 2007). Penalties or punishment received have deterred sociality by raising resistance (Shank 2012). Moreover, disutility impeding sociality to sustain crime can stem from adversity, anger, boredom, challenge, control, cost or loss, crowding, deterrence, deprivation, disadvantage or underprivilege, discontent, discrimination, dislocation, failure, frustration, guilt, harm, harshness or toughness, incarceration, punishment, risk, scarcity, social exclusion, stigmatization, strain, stress, tension, threat, unfairness, and victimization experienced (Blanchette and Brown 2006; Brant 2019; Brezina and Agnew 2013; Cohn et al. 2004; Daneygier and Green 2010; Farrington 2010; Frost and Clear 2013; Kirkpatrick 2020; Lilly et al. 2011; Proctor and Niemeyer 2019; Renel and Segev 2014; Sherman 2010; Swann 2012; Vander Ven and Colvin 2013; Welch et al. 2008). Strain can arise from adversity, blockage, and loss (Proctor and Niemeyer 2019). Stress can include deprivation, homelessness, rejection, unemployment, and victimization experienced (Agnew and Brezina 2010). Adversity, stress, or other negative experiences have eroded sociality by impairing civility, generativity, relatedness, social integration, social support receipt, and trust and provoking conflict, deviance, suicide, and violence (Backman and Nilsson 2011; Cano and Vivian 2003; Dutton et al. 2016; Garcia and Herrero 2004; Jackson et al. 2006; Sobeck et al. 2020). Besides, anger has jeopardized sociality by eroding social integration and fomenting protesting and violence and its tolerance (Krahe 2013; Molm 2008; Passini 2019; Tausch et al. 2011). Control experienced has worsened sociality by breeding violence (Felson and Outlaw 2007). Cost or loss experienced has hindered sociality by eroding compliance and government trust and fomenting suicide (Kirchler and Maciejovsky 2001; Nicholls and Picou 2012). Crowding experienced has weakened sociality by triggering migration (Crowder et al. 2006). Deprivation experienced erodes sociality by breeding conflict (J. Turner 2013b). Frustration has hampered sociality by eroding constructive communication and breeding avoidance (Vanhee et al. 2018). Rejection experienced has disturbed sociality by eroding closeness and prosocial behavior (Bockler et al. 2021; K. Lin et al. 2013). Unemployment has impeded sociality by dissolving social capital, social cohesion, and trust (Espvall and Dellgren 2008; Manturuk et al. 2010; Reeskens and Vandecasteele 2017). Conversely, unemployment has hurt sociality by breeding conflict experienced, moving, protesting, threats experienced, and victimization (Bramley and Morgan 2003; Kaukinen 2004; Lewin-Epstein et al. 2003; Schneider 2007; Su and Feng 2013). Victimization experienced has impaired sociality by eroding social trust (Olivera 2015). Conversely, victimization experienced has hurt sociality by activating conflict and migration (Bar-Tal and Halperin 2013; Ramesh et al. 2019).

Ideals for crime and against sociality have valorized conspiracy belief, excitement, sensation, and risking (Jolley et al. 2019; Nguyen and McGloin 2013). The ideal of conspiracy belief has eroded sociality by dampening compliance and trust (Freeman et al. 2022). The ideal for excitement or sensation has diminished sociality by dampening civic engagement and raising doping and approval of violence (Schumpe et al. 2020; Foschi and Lauriola 2014). The ideal for risking has disrupted sociality by generating crime, hate, and violence (Farrington 2018; Hawdon et al. 2019; Merdian et al. 2017). Ideals justifying crime to impede sociality espouse entitlement, individualism, and liberalism (Waiton 2008; Wright and DeLisi 2016). Entitlement has impaired sociality by eroding compliance and relatedness and provoking narcissism and hostility (Moeller et al. 2009; Piff 2014; Zitek and Jordan 2019). Individualism has weakened sociality by reducing civic engagement, religiousness, social cohesion, and volunteering (Church 2010; Green and Janmaat 2011; J. He et al. 2014; Hener et al. 2016; Leong 2008; Pollack and Pickel 2007; Whitford et al. 2006). Conversely, individualism has impeded sociality by bolstering acceptance of outsiders, competition, crime, extremity, self-enhancement, protesting, and violence (Church 2010; J. He et al. 2014; Karstedt 2010; Leong 2008; Li and Song 1992; Pollack and Pickel 2007; Whitford et al. 2006). Liberalism has impeded sociality regarding morality, normativity, and social order (Feinberg et al. 2019). Moreover, ideals for crime and against sociality can favor consumerism or consumption, creativity, defiance, dominance, escape, frustration, gang involvement, hedonism, migrating, mobility or residential instability, opposition, permissiveness, promiscuity, pleasure, protesting, and subculture (Agnew and Brezina 2010; Brant 2019; Brezina and Agnew 2013; Hallsworth and Young 2010; B. Hunter 2009; Lilly et al. 2011; Salisbury 2013; Sidanius and Pratto 1999; Walsh 2014; Reiner 2016; Walsh 2014). The ideal for consumption or consumerism has weakened sociality by boosting migration (Adnanes 2004). The ideal for dominance prioritizes force use, inequality, and stepping (Brant 2019). Creativity has impeded sociality by reducing volunteering or community service (Milgram and Hong 1994). Defiance has impaired sociality by eroding solidarity and fomenting deviance (Foy et al. 2014; J. Williams 2011). Domination has impaired sociality by weakening social cohesion (E. Chan 2014). Escapism can undermine sociality by fomenting radicalism and suicide (McCauley and Moskalenko 2017; Van Orden et al. 2010). Frustration has hampered sociality by eroding constructive communication and breeding avoidance (Vanhee et al. 2018). Hedonism, or the ideal for pleasure, has disrupted sociality by dampening communitarianism, legalism, and patriotism (Bore et al. 2005; Schwartz et al. 2014). Migration has impeded sociality by diminishing social integration (Kearns and Whitley 2015). Opposition has impaired sociality by eroding solidarity and fomenting deviance (Foy et al. 2014; J. Williams 2011). Permissiveness has disrupted sociality by eroding institutional trust and provoking protesting (Lodewijkx et al. 2008; Morris and Klesner 2010). Promiscuity can breed crime to hinder sociality (Walsh 2011). Protesting has impaired sociality by escalating distancing and radicalism and dampening moral motivation (Kutlaca et al. 2020; Vestergren et al. 2017). Besides, protesting impedes sociality by embracing antisociality, conflict, extremism, hostility, incivility, illegality, rioting, social exclusion, terrorism, and violence (Renger et al. 2020; Kaplan and Liu 2000; S. Lo 2021; McCright and Dunlap 2008; Morselli and Passini 2018; Smidt 2020; Stewart et al. 2012; Swart et al. 2020; Tan and Snow 2015). The ideal of subculture has ruined sociality by provoking social exclusion experienced (Backman and Nilsson 2011).

Conversely, crime has reflected ideals against the establishment, family involvement, and place identity to hinder sociality (Hernandez et al. 2010; Hoffmann 2023; Tanner-Smith et al. 2013). The ideal against the establishment, or populism, opposes sociality by espousing agonism, alienation, anarchism, autonomy, bellicosity, cynicism, enmity, exclusion, extremism, hatred, misogyny, occupying, radicalism, rebelliousness, resistance, and revolution (Aslanidis 2018; de la Torre 2018; Grattan 2016; Hameleers 2019; Jagers and Walgrave 2007; S. Lo 2021; Norris and Inglehart 2019; Nyenhuis 2020; Papaioannou et al. 2023; Pappas 2019; Sandel 2020). Conversely, populism disrupts sociality by dismissing compromise, institutionalization, loyalty, and nationalism (Barr 2009; Grattan 2016; S. Lo 2021; Pappas 2019). Family involvement has constituted sociality by enhancing cohesion and social support receipt (Espvall and Dellgren 2008; Rook and Ituarte 1999). Place identity has established sociality by boosting civic engagement, community attachment, neighborhood and relational quality, neighborhood satisfaction, and social capital (Bernardo and Palma-Oliveira 2016; Long and Perkins 2007; Pavlova et al. 2015; Rochelle and Shardlow 2013). Furthermore, ideals refuting crime to rationalize sociality favor communitarianism, consensus or collective conscience, conservativism, containment, moralism, and solidarity (de Castro-Rodrigues and Sacau 2015; Reiner 2016; Waiton 2008). Communitarianism constitutes sociality by espousing caring, civility, collective identity, commonweal orientation, community, dutifulness or responsibility, education or socialization, equality, interdependence, loyalty, mentoring, patriotism, reciprocity, relatedness, self-discipline, servicing including volunteering, settlement, social construction, social participation, solidarity, and trust (Delanty 2009; Frazer 1999; Moore 2010; Speth 2012). Consensus has enhanced sociality by fostering cohesion, compliance, engagement, and rejection of outsiders (Fasel et al. 2016; Guan et al. 2021; Heshmati and Oravecz 2022; Yoon et al. 2013). Conservatism against crime to sustain sociality upholds agreement, charity, Christianity, community, justice, legality, morality, punishment, respect, responsibility, social order and stability, and tradition and rejects divorce, risking, and social disorganization (Costello 2013; Wright and DeLisi 2016). Conservatism has maintained confidence in institutions (Feinberg et al. 2019). Moreover, conservatism exhibits faith in religion and rejection of outsiders (Malka and Soto 2011; Rhodes-Purdy et al. 2023). With these ideals, conservation has fostered confidence in the civic institution and reduced violence (Pulkkinen et al. 2009; Wernet et al. 2005). Hence, conservation would discourage justification for misdeeds and acceptance of deviants. Conservatism sustains sociality by nurturing empathy, loyalty, prosocial behavior, religiousness, and sacrifice (Dutton and Rayner-Hilles 2022). Moreover, conservatism underpins sociality by maintaining allegiance or loyalty, attachment, civility, community, conformity, cooperation, discipline, ethnocentrism, honesty, humility, intimacy, legality, morality, nationalism, obedience, order, partnership, patriotism, peace, responsibility, sharing, trust, and xenophobia (Dutton and Rayner-Hilles 2022; Heilman and Kusev 2020; Hickson 2013; Lakoff 2009; Rhodes-Purdy et al. 2023; Scruton 2014; Yoos 2007; Zuk and Zuk 2020). Conversely, conservatism upholds sociality by condemning dehumanizing, evilness, revolution, sexuality, terrorism, and transgression (Dutton and Rayner-Hilles 2022; Malka and Soto 2011; Scruton 2014; Suhay 2015). The ideal for containment has buttressed sociality by enhancing generativity and impeding crime, risking, and violence (Y. Cheung et al. 2014; Koegl and Day 2019; Peterson and Klohnen 1995; Welch et al. 2008). Moralism has sustained sociality by boosting gratitude (Pohling et al. 2010). Moreover, moralism can enhance sociality regarding social trust (Bersot and Arrigo 2015; Steinhardt 2012). Inherently, moralism embraces altruism, consensus, legality, obligation, and virtue to maintain sociality (R. Brown 2018). Solidarity has empowered personal sociality by enhancing personal civic engagement, favor for community, political participation, and trust (Z. Han et al. 2017; F. Lee 2012; Palmer et al. 2011; Whitham 2012). Besides, ideals against crime and for sociality can espouse attachment or bonding, commonality, community participation, compliance, conformity, containment, contracting, coping, discussing, frustration tolerance, goal orientation, normativity, parenting, pity, probity, redemption, religiosity, role-taking, sharing, and social orientation (Barak 2010; Brezina and Agnew 2013; Lilly et al. 2011; Lyng et al. 2009; Paternoster and Bachman 2010; Proctor and Niemeyer 2019; Walsh 2014; Warner and Clubb 2013; Wikstrom 2010). Attachment or bonding has constituted sociality regarding connectedness, friendship, giving, and social interaction (Eberl 2020; Liebler and Sandefur 2002; Nelson-Coffey et al. 2023; Phan et al. 2009). Commonality has raised sociality by facilitating donating (Piferi et al. 2006). Moreover, commonality maintains sociality by involving social closeness, commitment, contribution, and gifting (Godoy et al. 2007; Murray and Holmes 2008). Community participation has facilitated sociality regarding cooperation, networking, and trust (Groves et al. 2000; Molitor et al. 2011; Rochelle 2015). Compliance has constituted sociality by raising patriotism and impeding violence and acceptance of deviants and outsiders (Pulkkinen et al. 2009; Schwartz et al. 2014; Van Hootegem et al. 2000; Yeo and Chu 2018). The ideal for conformity has built sociality regarding xenophobia or rejection of outsiders (Costa et al. 2023). Contracting has buttressed sociality by raising patriotism, prosocial behavior, and relatedness (Dovidio et al. 2006; Gilbert 2006; Hudson 2023; Segrin and Flora 2019). Coping has enabled sociality by facilitating compliance, intimacy, and relatedness (Chow et al. 2014; Gattino et al. 2015; Twardawski et al. 2021). Discussion has incubated sociality by facilitating civic engagement, political participation, and trust (Gil de Zuniga et al. 2017; Hooghe et al. 2015; Huber et al. 2022). Frustration tolerance represents resilience (Connor et al. 2003). Resilience has attracted sociality by raising bonding and inhibiting crime and violence (Fields and McNamara 2003; Hoffman 2003; Solomon and Roloff 2018). Furthermore, resilience sustains sociality by embodying or fostering adaptation and legality (Hoffman 2003; Ungar 2012). Resilience also underlies sociality by demonstrating altruism, attractiveness, communication or conversation, community, compassion, empathy or perspective-taking, negotiation, peacefulness, relationality, relatedness, social capital or resourcefulness, social cohesion, and social competence (Elfers et al. 2024; Hjemdal et al. 2015; Jones and d'Errico 2019; Kelley et al. 2019; Kent and Davis 2010; Ungar 2010; Zautra 2014). Goal orientation has underlain sociality by boosting social trust (Uslaner 2002).

Norms against crime and for sociality have evolved from community parochialism and partnership, family cohesion, national social capital, and parent monitoring (Carr 2003; Hoffmann 2023; Kennedy et al. 1998; Tanner-Smith et al. 2013). Parochialism constitutes sociality by espousing communitarianism and community, cooperation, familiarity, harmony, nationalism, patriotism, reciprocity, social participation, and xenophobia (Gregg 2003; Macedo 2021; Ng and Kennedy 2019; Zhang and Gu 2022). Partnership has constituted sociality by preventing victimization (Jones and Ferguson 2009). Moreover, partnership establishes sociality by maintaining equality and responsibility (Harvie and Manzis 2011; Waiton 2008). Family cohesion has constituted sociality by boosting social cohesion and social support receipt (Espvall and Dellgren 2008). National social capital has normalized sociality by boosting civic engagement, community favor, political participation, institutional trust, and recourse (Z. Han et al. 2017; F. Lee 2012; Palmer et al. 2011; Whitham 2012). Conversely, national social capital has sustained sociality by preventing victimization and violence (Hansen-Nord et al. 2014; E. Wright et al. 2015). Parent monitoring has safeguarded sociality by enhancing compliance and dampening conflict and the ideal for risking (De Bruyn et al. 2003; Kilian et al. 2013). Besides, norms against crime and for sociality can stem from civilizing, parenting, social control, social support, socialization, and supervision received to popularize accommodation, caring, civility, communication, communitarianism, compliance, conventionality, egalitarianism, interrelatedness, legal responsiveness, prosociality, rule enforcement, social control, solidarity, subordination, and temperance (Costello 2013; Hoffman 2003; Lilly et al. 2011; Messner et al. 2013; Rocque et al. 2016; Salisbury 2013; Sidanius and Pratto 1999; Walsh 2014; Wikstrom 2010). Civilizing upholds sociality by embracing brotherhood, compassion, coordination, relatedness, religiousness, and social quality as opposed to violence (Dutton and Rayner-Hilles 2022; Hudson 2023; Phillips 2006; Rindermann 2018; Szakolczai 2001). Social quality comprises social cohesion, empowerment, inclusion, and security (Phillips 2006). Social cohesion covers equality and social capital (Phillips 2006). Parenting received has upheld sociality by encouraging recourse and preventing relationship breakdown (Cobb-Clark and Gorgens 2014). The experience of rule enforcement has sustained sociality by reducing delinquency, violence, and relational problems (Levitt and Lochner 2001; Sweeten et al. 2013; Woodward and Fergusson 1999). Social control receipt has sustained sociality by boosting community well-being and institutional trust (Overall et al. 2020). Socialization has constituted sociality by impeding violence (Pulkkinen et al. 2009). Furthermore, socialization can advance sociality by fostering family cohesion and role-taking and preventing crime, doping, and violence (Dolch 2003; L. Ray 2017; Steel et al. 2012; Sussman and Ames 2001). Accommodation can sustain sociality by raising loving (Aron et al. 2006). Moreover, accommodation experienced has constituted sociality by strengthening cooperation and preventing suicide (Duberstein et al. 2004; Lepkowski and Couper 2002). Caring has constituted sociality by securing religiosity and volunteering (Barr et al. 2005). Civility has constituted sociality by inducing fairness and trust (Vera-Toscano et al. 2013). Communication has weaved sociality regarding social cohesion, participation, and trust (Miyata et al. 2008; Rothstein and Uslaner 2005). Communitarianism constitutes sociality by espousing caring, civility, collective identity, commonweal orientation, community, dutifulness or responsibility, education or socialization, equality, interdependence, loyalty, mentoring, patriotism, reciprocity, relatedness, self-discipline, servicing including volunteering, settlement, social construction, social participation, solidarity, and trust (Delanty 2009; Frazer 1999; Moore 2010; Speth 2012). Compliance or subordination has constituted sociality by raising patriotism and impeding violence and acceptance of deviants and outsiders (Pulkkinen et al. 2009; Schwartz et al. 2014; Van Hootegem et al. 2000; Yeo and Chu 2018). Conventionality has buttressed sociality by enhancing patriotism and faith in religion and discouraging protesting and accepting deviants and outsiders (Costa et al. 2023; Datler et al. 2013; Meuleman et al. 2019; Schwartz et al. 2014). Egalitarianism has underpinned sociality by enhancing empathy, support for welfare, and trust in government and impeding radicalism (Faricy and Ellis 2014; Lauriola et al. 2015; Lucas and Kteily 2018; Roosma et al. 2014). Interrelatedness has buttressed sociality by securing attachment, donation, prosocial behavior, social inclusion, and social interaction (Feeney and Collins 2001; Uskul et al. 2004; Z. Xin et al. 2017). Legal responsiveness has buttressed sociality by dismissing radicalism (Muthuswamy 2022). Prosociality has constituted sociality by civility, consolidating connectedness, cooperation, religiosity, responsibility, and volunteering (Hample 2018; Marsh and Dik 2021; Musick and Wilson 2008; Nelson-Coffey et al. 2023; Shahzalal and Adnan 2022). Moreover, prosociality underlies sociality by enhancing citizenship, loyalty, social cohesion, socializing, and trust and diminishing self-interest (Dovidio et al. 2006; Hawley 2014; Kisliuk and Weißmuller 2023; Music 2014). Solidarity has constituted sociality by enhancing attachment and dampening tolerance for deviance (Stafford et al. 2005; Woosnam et al. 2018). Temperance has buttressed sociality by enhancing generativity and impeding crime, risking, and violence (Y. Cheung et al. 2014; Koegl and Day 2019; Peterson and Klohnen 1995; Welch et al. 2008).

Conversely, norms for crime and against sociality have stemmed from co-offenders, friend or peer delinquency, and school crime (Hoffmann 2023; Nguyen and McGloin 2013; Tanner-Smith et al. 2013). Moreover, norms for crime and against sociality can stem from commodification to popularize aggression, alienation, brutality, competition, conflict, crime, disruption, heterogeneity, immigration, individualism and individualization, inequality, normlessness, opportunism, protesting, struggle, toxicity, unfairness, and working-class (Benson and Simpson 2018; Hallsworth and Young 2010; Karstedt 2010; Lilly et al. 2011; McLaughlin 2010; Reiner 2016; Salisbury 2013; Sidanius and Pratto 1999; J. Wo et al. 2016).

Justification or tolerance for misdeeds engages association, communication, conviction, entitlement or claiming rights, evaluation, neutralization, and willingness regarding misdeeds (Denver and Pickett 2022; Forsyth and Ward 2022; Hadlington and Knight 2022; Matthews and Channon 2016; Mededovic and Kovacevic 2021; Schumpe et al. 2020). Neutralization comprises dehumanizing victims and separating responsibility (Matthews and Channon 2016). Conversely, such justification dismisses disapproval of misdeeds and support for control over misdeeds (Barkan and Cohn 2005; Mededovic and Kovacevic 2021). An example of such justification is the rape myth (Joseph and Black 2012). This justification jeopardizes sociality by withdrawing power, utility, ideals, and norms for sociality and securing power, utility, ideals, and norms against sociality, as predicated on the voluntaristic mechanisms of analytical functionalism. Notably, this justification has dampened sociality by triggering violence (van Hiel et al. 2007). Violence has undermined sociality by breeding antisociality, crime and recidivism, blaming, conflict, hostility, rejecting others, and impairing agreeableness, morality, and responsibility (Asendorpf et al. 2008; Del Bove et al. 2008; Morrison 2006; Scholte et al. 2009; Vitaro et al. 2007).

Justification for misdeeds also obstructs sociality by reflecting or conveying power, utility, ideals, and norms against sociality. Alternatively, this justification reflects inadequate power, utility, ideals, and norms for sociality. Such reflection exercises the voluntaristic mechanisms of power realization, utility optimization, ideal calibration, and norm conformity in analytical functionalism. The power realization mechanism engages conflict, questing, and the force field where forces clash (Schumpe et al. 2020; Spini et al. 2008). This mechanism generates and uses power to attain the fulfillment function. The utility optimization mechanism realizes rational choice (Spini et al. 2008). This mechanism applies cost-benefit analysis or calculation to maintain the adaptation function. The ideal calibration mechanism stands on affirmation, cognitive association, and identification (Montgomery et al. 2004). This mechanism highlights attitudes, beliefs, and values to achieve the latency function. The norm conformity mechanism builds on information processing, learning, and norming or normalizing (Forsyth and Ward 2022; Song et al. 2017; Waterman et al. 2022). This mechanism emphasizes internalizing norms to achieve the integration function. Norms against justification for misdeeds have flowed from conventional media (Forsyth and Ward 2022).

Power reflected by justification for misdeeds to undermine sociality has stemmed from anger, contempt, Machiavellianism, masculinity, narcissism, psychopathy, sadism, and sensation-seeking (Joseph and Black 2012; Mededovic and Kovacevic 2021; Tausch et al. 2011). Anger has jeopardized sociality by eroding social integration and fomenting protesting and violence and its tolerance (Krahe 2013; Molm 2008; Passini 2019; Tausch et al. 2011). Moreover, anger can dampen sociality by breeding crime and radicalism (Brant 2019; Larson et al. 2020). Contempt has impeded sociality by diminishing policy agreement (Tausch et al. 2011). Moreover, contempt can cause radicalism to hinder sociality (Koomen and van der Pligt 2016). Machiavellianism has impaired sociality by eroding commitment and satisfaction in relationships and breeding abuse and misbehavior (Brewer and Abell 2017; Jones and Paulhus 2009). Masculinity has hindered sociality by weakening regard (Bond et al. 2000). Besides, masculinity espouses aggression and dominance to constrain sociality (Courtenay 2000; Hoyck and Gutmann 2006). Narcissism has impeded sociality by breeding aggression and misbehavior (Tracy et al. 2009). Besides, narcissism dismisses discipline, empathy, friendship, humor, morality, and responsibility and embraces exploitation, lying, rage, rivalry, and violence to undermine sociality (Cichocka et al. 2024; Kilminster 2008; Twenge and Campbell 2009). Psychopathy has undermined sociality by withdrawing prosocial behavior and breeding radicalism, victimization, and violence (Ehrensuft et al. 2003; Krahe 2013; Soliman et al. 2016; Thielmann et al. 2020). Besides, psychopathy embraces antisociality, manipulation, and radicalism to inhibit sociality (Johnston and Bose 2020; Krupp et al. 2012; Welsh and Lenzenweger 2021). Sadism has impaired sociality by boosting deviance and obstructing prosocial behavior (Emer and Poepsel 2021; Masui 2023). Moreover, sadism can brew radicalism, suicide, and violence to undermine sociality (Kral 2019; Larson et al. 2020; J. Turner 2007). As such, sadism fuels terrorism to eradicate sociality (Sternberg and Sternberg 2008). Sensation-seeking has impaired sociality by reducing civic engagement and fomenting doping (Foschi and Lauriola 2014).

Conversely, justification for misdeeds has reflected inadequate self-efficacy and social skills to achieve sociality (Ozer and Bertelsen 2019; Tausch et al. 2011). Self-efficacy has sustained sociality by raising civic engagement, donation, government and social trust, leadership, political participation, prosocial behavior, and social activity (Bednall et al. 2013; Frye 2007; Gnambs and Batinic 2012; Huber et al. 2022; Mangum 2012; Rahn 2008; Pei and Pan 2018; Yao and Enright 2019). Social skills have facilitated sociality by raising civility, civic engagement, political participation, prosocial behavior, social cohesion, and social trust (Foschi and Lauriola 2014; Halvorsen 2007; Letki 2008).

Disutility reflected by justification for misdeeds to discourage sociality has rested on abuse or victimization experienced, crime or violence experienced, frustration, hardship, injustice appraised, meaninglessness, and stress experienced (Hovermann and Messner 2019; Ray and Kort-Butler 2020; Song et al. 2017; Schumpe et al. 2020; Song et al. 2017; Tausch et al. 2011). Victimization experienced has impaired sociality by eroding social trust (Olivera 2015). Conversely, crime, victimization, or violence experienced has hurt sociality by activating conflict and migration (Bar-Tal and Halperin 2013; Ramesh et al. 2019). Frustration has hindered sociality by reducing communication (Vanhee et al. 2018). Hardship has impaired sociality by dampening trust and fomenting social exclusion experienced, suicide, and victimization experienced (Economou et al. 2016; Reeskens and Vandecasteele 2017; Ross and Mirowsky 2009). Injustice experienced has worsened sociality regarding civility, cooperation, community identification, political participation, and social trust as opposed to protesting (A. Hu 2013; Lawrence and Daniels 1997; Sunshine and Tyler 2003; Tyler and Degoey 1995; van Prooijen et al. 2008; Wenzel 2000). Meaninglessness has hampered sociality by lowering civic practice, responsibility, and volunteering and raising rejection experience (Duffy and Raque-Bogdan 2010; Summers and Falco 2020; Twenge et al. 2003). Stress experienced has undermined sociality by eroding civility, forgiveness, generativity, relationship quality and satisfaction, social integration, social support received, and trust and heightening conflict, maltreatment, substance abuse, suicide, and violence (Atkinson et al. 2005; Dutton et al. 2016; Gelles 2007; Grzywacz and Almeida 2008; Jackson et al. 2006; Sobeck et al. 2020; Toussaint et al. 2016).

Ideals for dominance and fighting have underlain justification for misdeeds to hamper sociality (Crowson 2009; Spini et al. 2008). The ideal for domination has inhibited sociality by reducing altruism, attachment security, and coalition building and breeding lying (Hample 2018; Sinn and Hayes 2018). Fighting has undermined sociality by breeding antisociality, crime and recidivism, blaming, conflict, hostility, rejecting others, and impairing agreeableness, morality, and responsibility (Asendorpf et al. 2008; Del Bove et al. 2008; Morrison 2006; Scholte et al. 2009; Vitaro et al. 2007).

Conversely, justification for misdeeds has reflected ideals against conservatism, conventional media use, punishment, and social desirability to erode sociality (Douglas 2006; Forsyth and Ward 2022; Garland et al. 2017; Hovermann and Messner 2019; Ray and Kort-Butler 2020). Conservatism sustains sociality by nurturing empathy, loyalty, prosocial behavior, religiousness, and sacrifice (Dutton and Rayner-Hilles 2022). Moreover, conservatism underpins sociality by maintaining allegiance or loyalty, attachment, civility, community, conformity, cooperation, discipline, ethnocentrism, honesty, humility, intimacy, legality, morality, nationalism, obedience, order, partnership, patriotism, peace, responsibility, sharing, trust, and xenophobia (Dutton and Rayner-Hilles 2022; Heilman and Kusev 2020; Hickson 2013; Lakoff 2009; Rhodes-Purdy et al. 2023; Scruton 2014; Yoos 2007; Zuk and Zuk 2020). Conversely, conservatism upholds sociality by condemning dehumanizing, evilness, revolution, sexuality, terrorism, and transgression (Dutton and Rayner-Hilles 2022; Malka and Soto 2011; Scruton 2014; Suhay 2015). Conventionality has buttressed sociality by enhancing patriotism and faith in religion and discouraging protesting and accepting deviants and outsiders (Costa et al. 2023; Datler et al. 2013; Meuleman et al. 2019; Schwartz et al. 2014). Punishment or punishing characterizes sociality (Fowers 2015). Besides, punishment endorses prosociality to maintain sociality (Gausel et al. 2012). Social desirability has upheld sociality by advancing altruism, empathy, perspective-taking, and the ideal for benevolence and diminishing suicide and violence (Krumrei-Mancuso 2017; Pulkkinen et al. 2009).

Norms against violence have diminished justification for misdeeds to attain sociality (Waterman et al. 2022). Conversely, the norms of deprivation, grievance, inequality, poverty, and retaliation have underlain justification for misdeeds to obstruct sociality (Simon et al. 2001; Tadjoeddin 2013; You and Khagram 2005). Deprivation experienced erodes sociality by breeding conflict (J. Turner 2013b). Grievance has undermined sociality by fomenting resistance and impeding social capital and trust (Pulkkinen et al. 2009; Webber and Huxley 2007). The norm of inequality has impeded sociality by eroding social capital, support for redistribution and welfare, sympathy, trust, and volunteering (Busemeyer 2013; Hitlin and Harkness 2018; Lipford and Yandle 2009; Oishi et al. 2011; Portes and Vickstrom 2011). Conversely, the norm of inequality has impaired sociality by provoking crime and violence (Ousey and Lee 2013; van Wilsem 2007).

Acceptance of Deviants

Deviants or unconventional people cover addicts, alcoholics, homosexuals, psychopaths, and psychiatric patients. For instance, deviants exhibit aggression, depression, extremism, doping, fandom, rule-breaking, or rule-violation (S. Burt et al. 2019; Eggert and Green et al. 2009; North et al. 2005). Deviance has impeded sociality by impairing morality and triggering doping, recidivism, rejection received, and violence (Abbey et al. 2012; Bowen and Wretman 2014; Tsakpinoglou and Poulin 2017). Such impedance works through power, utility, ideals, and norms reduced for or increased against sociality offered or reflected by deviance with the voluntaristic mechanisms of analytical functionalism. These mechanisms activate power realization, utility optimization, ideal calibration, and norm conformity to achieve the requisite functions. The power realization mechanism hinges on attachment and conflict (S. Henry 2009; Kaplan et al. 2013). Attachment enhances power based on security. The utility optimization mechanism applies contracting and deterrence involving reward and punishment (Kaplan et al. 2013; Y. Yau 2014). Herein, contracting specifies expected reward and cost. The ideal calibration mechanism balances control, constraint, and self-categorization (Kaplan et al. 2013; Seddig 2020). Herein, internal control reduces deviance, whereas external control breeds deviance. The norm conformity mechanism engages association, bonding, labeling, learning, social construction, social interaction, and social reaction (Herman-Kinney 2003; Kaplan et al. 2013; J. Williams 2011). Herein, others' social reaction is the basis for others' social labeling, such that a deviant label provokes deviance.

Power for driving sociality suffering in deviance has stemmed from close friendship, dominance, and family resources (Boman and Mowen 2019; Dishion and Kavanagh 2000; E. Green et al. 2009). Friendship has constituted sociality by enhancing community attachment, compliance, donation, gratitude, political participation, social cohesion, social desirability, social integration, and social trust (Corcoran 2013; Fahmy 2006; Gundert and Hohendanner 2015; Keillor et al. 2001; Kende et al. 2022; Opp 2001; Rotkirch 2014). Dominance has enabled sociality by facilitating nationalism and patriotism (MuBotter 2024). Family resources have facilitated sociality by increasing civic engagement, civility, community involvement, compliance, donation, social interaction, and trust (Alnsour and Meaton 2009; Apinunmahakul and Devlin 2008; Doff and Kleinhans 2011; Norris and Inglehart 2009; Oliver 2003; Shin 2012; Traunmuller 2011). Conversely, family resources have furnished sociality by preventing cheating and crime (Cerin and Leslie 2008; Ozbay 2008).

Utility for attracting sociality suffering in deviance has rested on intimacy and satisfaction (K. Chou 2000; G. Wu et al. 2007). Intimacy has constituted sociality by boosting relationship satisfaction and social support received and dampening rejection expected (Arseth et al. 2009; Hand et al. 2013). Satisfaction has advanced sociality by strengthening political participation, social cohesion, social and government trust, and volunteering (E. Chan 2014; Flavin and Keane 2011; Rochelle 2015).

Conversely, deviance has reflected disutility in abuse, conflict, resentment, and threats experienced to discourage sociality (Boman and Mowen 2019; Chen and Liu 2019; Yeh 2011; Yeh et al. 2010). Abuse experienced has impaired sociality by eroding social trust (Olivera 2015). Conversely, abuse experienced has hurt sociality by activating conflict and migration (Bar-Tal and Halperin 2013; Ramesh et al. 2019). Conflict has impeded sociality regarding donation and trust as opposed to violence (Farmer and Fedor 2001; Farrington 2018; Kunovich and Hodson 1999). Resentment experienced has disturbed sociality by eroding closeness and prosocial behavior (Bockler et al. 2021; K. Lin et al. 2013). Threats received have inhibited sociality by reducing cohesion and triggering conflict and resistance (Lubbers et al. 2006; B. Rick et al. 2006).

Ideals for rationalizing sociality deficient in deviance have favored careers, legality, and prosociality (L. Chen 2019; Costello and Hope 2016; Huiras et al. 2000). The ideal for a career has built sociality by increasing dependence and pleasing others (Willner et al. 2020). Legality has buttressed sociality by dismissing radicalism (Muthuswamy 2022). Prosociality has constituted sociality by civility, consolidating connectedness, cooperation, religiosity, responsibility, and volunteering (Hample 2018; Marsh and Dik 2021; Musick and Wilson 2008; Nelson-Coffey et al. 2023; Shahzalal and Adnan 2022). Moreover, prosociality underlies sociality by enhancing citizenship, loyalty, social cohesion, socializing, and trust and diminishing self-interest (Dovidio et al. 2006; Hawley 2014; Kisliuk and WeiBmuller 2023; Music 2014). Conversely, deviance has reflected the ideal against family attachment to weaken sociality (Silbereisen et al. 2002). Family attachment has constituted sociality by boosting social cohesion and social support receipt (Espvall and Dellgren 2008).

Norms against sociality underlying deviance have popularized deviance and rule-breaking or violation (Boman and Mowen 2019; S. Burt et al. 2019). Rule-breaking or violation has undermined sociality by diminishing patriotism and triggering violence and acceptance of deviants and outsiders (Pulkkinen et al. 2009; Schwartz et al. 2014; Van Hootegem et al. 2000; Yeo and Chu 2018).

Conversely, deviance has reflected norms against fairness, serving, and supportiveness to distract sociality (Koumenta 2015). The norm of fairness has upheld sociality by elevating morality and prosocial behavior (Barber 2004; McCaffoee 2016). Service orientation has established sociality by enhancing friendship and love (Fehr and Broughton 2001). Supportiveness has advanced sociality by raising affection, civic engagement, fairness, friendship quality, kindness, likability, moral behavior, popularity, relatedness, religiosity, social well-being, and volunteering (Barry et al. 2012; Gest et al. 2005; Layous et al. 2012; Markiewicz et al. 2001; Martela and Ryan 2016; Marzana et al. 2012; Masterson 2001; Shillington et al. 2021; L. Taylor et al. 2018; Wright and Li 2011). Conversely, supportiveness has built sociality by reducing delinquency and violence (Mesch 2009).

Doping or drug abuse, as addictive deviance, functions for recreation, relaxation, and stress relief (Engle and Kasser 2005; Hathaway 2003). Meanwhile, doping features drug dependence and withdrawal symptoms (Sussman and Ames 2001). Doping has hampered sociality by withdrawing power, utility, ideals, and norms for sociality and creating power, utility, ideals, and norms against sociality. Such hampering rests on the voluntaristic mechanisms of analytical functionalism. These mechanisms engage cognitive processing, communication, learning, and social construction (Arce and Winkelman 2021). Hence, doping can jeopardize sociality, featuring altruism, empathy, and healing (Arce and Winkelman 2021).

Power for driving sociality reduced by doping can rest on fitness and rationality (Arce and Winkelman 2021; Sussman and Ames 2001). Fitness has uplifted sociality by boosting community sense, morality, popularity, social activity, social cohesion, social integration, social trust, social well-being, and volunteering (Huxhold et al. 2014; Jorgensen et al. 2010; Son and Wilson 2012; Tolsma et al. 2009; Yu and Chiu 2016). Conversely, fitness has sustained sociality by preventing loneliness (Koromeckyj-Cox et al. 2007). Rationality has championed sociality by dampening aggression and antisociality (DiGiuseppe et al. 2017). Conversely, doping has evolved from depression to weaken power to drive sociality. Depression has eroded sociality by breeding conflict, hate, hostility perceived, loneliness, revenge, risking, suicide, and violence (Cacioppo and Hawkley 2009; Economou et al. 2016; Haner et al. 2020; Morokoff et al. 2009; Mullet et al. 2005; Proulx et al. 2004; H. Smith et al. 2016; E. Wright et al. 2015). Conversely, depression has attenuated sociality by impeding benevolence, closeness experienced, fairness, forgiveness, gratitude, honesty, leadership, love, social integration, teamwork, and volunteering (Blanchard et al. 2021; Cornwall 2009; Holzel et al. 2011; Mancini et al. 2011; Mullet et al. 2005; Thoits and Hewitt 2001).

Disutility created by doping to impede sociality has evolved from victimization experienced (Kendler et al. 2006; Krahe 2013). Victimization experienced has impaired sociality by eroding social trust (Olivera 2015). Conversely, victimization experienced has hurt sociality by activating conflict and migration (Bar-Tal and Halperin 2013; Ramesh et al. 2019).

The ideal against sociality generated by doping has favored violence (Stogner et al. 2014). Violence has undermined sociality by breeding antisociality, crime and recidivism, blaming, conflict, hostility, rejecting others, and impairing agreeableness, morality, and responsibility (Asendorpf et al. 2008; Del Bove et al. 2008; Morrison 2006; Scholte et al. 2009; Vitaro et al. 2007).

Doping also reduces sociality by drawing power, utility, ideals, and norms against sociality and withdrawing power, utility, ideals, and norms for sociality. Accordingly, the reduction hinges on the voluntaristic mechanisms of power realization, utility optimization, ideal calibration, and norm conformity in analytical functionalism. These mechanisms engage cognitive control and processing, conditioning based on reward and punishment, learning, modeling, and reinforcement (Bardo et al. 2003; Bunringer et al. 2008; Sussman and Ames 2001).

Power for driving sociality to prevent doping has built on adaptation, health, and self-control (Spohn and Kaplan 2000; Stogner et al. 2014). Adaptation has secured sociality regarding partnership, social adjustment, and satisfaction as opposed to discord (Chow et al. 2014; Mitchell 2005). Self-control has buttressed sociality by enhancing generativity and impeding crime, risking, and violence (Y. Cheung et al. 2014; Koegl and Day 2019; Peterson and Klohnen 1995; Welch et al. 2008). Conversely, doping has arisen from emotional and physical problems and negative affectivity to impair sociality (C. Chen et al. 2009; Manning et al. 2018). Doping can also arise from frustration and isolation experienced to impede sociality (Sussman and Ames 2001). Emotional and physical problems have obstructed sociality by diminishing community attachment, social capital, and social trust (G. Brown et al. 2004; Congdon 2010; Ross and Mirowsky 2009). Negative affectivity has eroded sociality by impeding government trust and morality and provoking violence (Guerin 2003; Huesmann et al. 2006; Sun et al. 2013).

Disutility underlying doping for discouraging sociality has stemmed from anxiety, loneliness, and stress (Siddaway et al. 2018; Hatch 2007; Kelly et al. 2022). Anxiety has disrupted sociality by breeding interpersonal problems, loneliness, risking, suicide, and violence (Dutton et al. 2016; Gillath et al. 2005; Pulkkinen et al. 2009; Trumbo et al. 2008). Conversely, anxiety has undermined sociality by reducing donation, friendship, humor, political participation, prosocial behavior, and social well-being (Best and Krueger 2010; Hewstone et al. 2005; Litman et al. 2017; Kuiper and Nicholl 2004; Zhong 2010). Loneliness has impaired sociality by weakening reciprocity, social capital, and social cohesion and provoking suicide (C. Cheng et al. 2019; Espvall and Dellgren 2008). Stress experienced has undermined sociality by eroding civility, forgiveness, generativity, relationship quality and satisfaction, social integration, social support received, and trust and heightening conflict, maltreatment, substance abuse, suicide, and violence (Atkinson et al. 2005; Dutton et al. 2016; Gelles 2007; Grzywacz and Almeida 2008; Jackson et al. 2006; Sobeck et al. 2020; Toussaint et al. 2016).

Ideals for sociality to prevent doping have valorized conventionality and religiosity (Hatch 2007; Sussman and Ames 2001). Conventionality has buttressed sociality by enhancing patriotism and faith in religion and discouraging protesting and accepting deviants and outsiders (Costa et al. 2023; Datler et al. 2013; Meuleman et al. 2019; Schwartz et al. 2014). Religiosity has sustained sociality by fostering civic engagement, civility, cohesion, compliance, donation, empathy, morality, patriotism, prejudice against deviants and outsiders, prosocial behavior, social trust, and volunteering (Apinunmahakul and Devlin 2008; Corcoran et al. 2011; Ishio 2010; Keyes 2002; Kim and Wilcox 2013; Ravanera et al. 2003; van Tienen et al. 2011; Weisberg 2005; Wuthnow 2004). Conversely, religiosity has secured sociality by reducing crime, deviance, individualism, protesting, and sexuality (Andrews et al. 2015; Coffe and Geys 2007; Guo et al. 2008; Skerkat and Ellison 1999; Spilka et al. 2003). Moreover, religiosity realizes sociality regarding altruism, community, ethicality, groupism, sharing, and solidarity (Franks et al. 2013; Lichterman 2012; Peifer 2010; Spilka et al. 2003; Stavrova and Siegers 2014). Religiosity also upholds sociality by featuring altruism, attachment, caring, community, compassion, harmony, hospitality, love, morality, obedience, other-centeredness, peace, trust, unity, xenophobia (Ager and Ager 2011; Fontana 2003; Harris et al. 2018; Horell 2014; Paterson 2018; Shorey et al. 2018; Simpson et al. 2008; Spilka et al. 2003; Tenorio and Lo 2011; Werbner 2010). Conversely, religiosity maintains sociality by dismissing individualism, oppression, sexuality, and violence (Fontana 2003; Horell 2014; Spilka et al. 2003). Doping also arises from ideals challenging moralism and civilization exemplified by Confucianism and morality (Hathaway 2003; Levesque and Benoit 2020; Truong et al. 2020). Civilization constitutes sociality by establishing civility, loyalty, social contact, and social identification (Collins 2001; Hudson 2023). Besides, civilization embraces legality, relational quality, social capital, social cohesion, and social quality and dismisses violence (Phillips 2006; Rindermann 2018; Szakolczai 2001). Confucianism has championed sociality regarding association, civility, and collectivism as opposed to violence (Y. Lin et al. 2021; Shin 2012; Stotzer 2014). Moralism has sustained sociality by boosting gratitude (Pohling et al. 2010). Moreover, moralism can enhance sociality regarding social trust (Bersot and Arrigo 2015; Steinhardt 2012). Inherently, moralism embraces altruism, consensus, legality, obligation, and virtue to maintain sociality (R. Brown 2018).

Conversely, ideals against sociality underlying doping have favored violence (Stogner et al. 2014). Violence has undermined sociality by breeding antisociality, crime and recidivism, blaming, conflict, hostility, rejecting others, and impairing agreeableness, morality, and responsibility (Asendorpf et al. 2008; Del Bove et al. 2008; Morrison 2006; Scholte et al. 2009; Vitaro et al. 2007). Doping arises from the ideals of individualism and voluntarism, which means self-determinism (Levesque and Benoit 2020). Individualism has weakened sociality by reducing civic engagement, religiousness, social cohesion, and volunteering (Church 2010; Green and Janmaat 2011; J. He et al. 2014; Hener et al. 2016; Leong 2008; Pollack and Pickel 2007; Whitford et al. 2006). Conversely, individualism has impeded sociality by bolstering acceptance of outsiders, competition, crime, extremity, self-enhancement, protesting, and violence (Church 2010; J. He et al. 2014; Karstedt 2010; Leong 2008;

Li and Song 1992; Pollack and Pickel 2007; Whitford et al. 2006). Voluntarism can fuel protesting to disrupt sociality (Tsai 2019).

Norms underlying doping can support doping to weaken sociality (Sussman and Ames 2001). The norm for doping has reflected the norm of social disorganization to hinder sociality (Cattarello 2000).

Homosexuality smacks of aggression, domination, intolerance, mental illness, promiscuity, risking, and victimization (Cameron et al. 2005; Lingiadi and Capozzi 2004; Stanton and Maier 2004). Currently, homosexuality arises from capitalism, which affords flexibility, freedom or liberty, and rights to displace communality (Valocchi 2020). Hence, homosexuality benefits from public support (Smith and Windes 2000). Inherently, homosexuality represents an act or behavior involving attraction or fantasy, desire, and identity or self-identification (Rich et al. 2018; Wolfe 2008). Homosexuality impedes sociality by withdrawing power, utility, ideals, and norms for sociality and generating power, utility, ideals, and norms against sociality with the voluntaristic mechanisms of analytical functionalism. These mechanisms engage coping or stress management, identification, internalization, and understanding involving power, utility, ideals, and norms (Bond 2017; Henderson and Hodges 2007; Rith and Diamond 2013).

Power for driving sociality reduced by homosexuality has stemmed from health (Rosario and Schrinshaw 2013). Health has uplifted sociality by boosting community sense, morality, popularity, social activity, social cohesion, social integration, social trust, social well-being, and volunteering (Huxhold et al. 2014; Jorgensen et al. 2010; Son and Wilson 2012; Tolsma et al. 2009; Yu and Chiu 2016). Conversely, health has sustained sociality by preventing loneliness (Koromeckyj-Cox et al. 2007). Besides, homosexuality has bred disorders, illness, morbidity, and sensation-seeking to weaken power for driving sociality (Rosario and Schrinshaw 2013; Simoni et al. 2013). Disorders have covered anxiety, attention deficit, autism, conduct, eating, hyperactivity, and substance use (A. Cheung et al. 2018; Cochran and Mays 2013; Rosario and Schrinshaw 2013; Vrangalova and Savin-Williams 2014). As such, disorders have obstructed sociality by diminishing community attachment, social capital, and social trust (G. Brown et al. 2004; Congdon 2010; Ross and Mirowsky 2009). Illness or morbidity has eroded sociality by impeding volunteering (Wuthnow 2004). Morality has constituted sociality by boosting volunteering and inhibiting violence (Piquero and Hickman 2002; Whitford et al. 2006). Sensation-seeking has impaired sociality by reducing civic engagement and fomenting doping (Foschi and Lauriola 2014).

Disutility generated by homosexuality to discourage sociality has arisen from anxiety, depression, distress, infection, internalizing problems, loneliness, mental health problems, relationship dissolution, risk, and victimization (Cameron et al. 2005; A. Cheung et al. 2018; Compton 2013; Rosario and Schrinshaw 2013; Stotzer 2014; van Griensven et al. 2004; Vrangalova and Savin-Williams 2014). Anxiety has disrupted sociality by breeding interpersonal problems, loneliness, risking, suicide, and violence (Dutton et al. 2016; Gillath et al. 2005; Pulkkinen et al. 2009; Trumbo et al. 2008). Conversely, anxiety has undermined sociality by reducing donation, friendship, humor, political participation, prosocial behavior, and social well-being

(Best and Krueger 2010; Hewstone et al. 2005; Litman et al. 2017; Kuiper and Nicholl 2004; Zhong 2010). Depression has eroded sociality by breeding conflict, hate, hostility perceived, loneliness, revenge, risking, suicide, and violence (Cacioppo and Hawkley 2009; Economou et al. 2016; Haner et al. 2020; Morokoff et al. 2009; Mullet et al. 2005; Proulx et al. 2004; H. Smith et al. 2016; E. Wright et al. 2015). Conversely, depression has attenuated sociality by impeding benevolence, closeness experienced, fairness, forgiveness, gratitude, honesty, leadership, love, social integration, teamwork, and volunteering (Blanchard et al. 2021; Cornwall 2009; Holzel et al. 2011; Mancini et al. 2011; Mullet et al. 2005; Thoits and Hewitt 2001). Distress has undermined sociality by fomenting resistance and impeding social capital and trust (Pulkkinen et al. 2009; Webber and Huxley 2007). Infection or risk has eroded sociality by weakening social integration and social trust (Hammer et al. 2009; Lindstrom and Rosvall 2015). Conversely, infection or risk has dampened sociality by raising social exclusion (Hammer et al. 2009). Loneliness has impaired sociality by weakening reciprocity, social capital, and social cohesion and provoking suicide (C. Cheng et al. 2019; Espvall and Dellgren 2008). Mental health problems have undermined sociality by withdrawing prosocial behavior and breeding radicalism, victimization, and violence (Ehrensuft et al. 2003; Krahe 2013; Soliman et al. 2016; Thielmann et al. 2020). Relationship dissolution can diminish sociality by shaking attachment security (Demo and Buehler 2013). Victimization experienced has impaired sociality by eroding social trust (Olivera 2015),

Conversely, homosexuality has lowered utility based on intimacy and self-esteem to attract sociality (van Griensven et al. 2004). Intimacy has constituted sociality by boosting relationship satisfaction and social support received and dampening rejection expected (Arseth et al. 2009; Hand et al. 2013). Self-esteem has buttressed sociality by raising attachment security, political participation, and prosociality and preventing suicide (Kitayama and Markus 2000; Tracy et al. 2009).

Ideals reduced by homosexuality for rationalizing sociality have accentuated conformity, religiosity, and social desirability (R. Anderson et al. 2017; Vrangalova and Savin-Williams 2014). Conformity has constituted sociality by raising patriotism and impeding violence and acceptance of deviants and outsiders (Pulkkinen et al. 2009; Schwartz et al. 2014; Van Hootegem et al. 2000; Yeo and Chu 2018). The ideal for conformity has built sociality regarding xenophobia or rejection of outsiders (Costa et al. 2023). Religiosity has sustained sociality by fostering civic engagement, civility, cohesion, compliance, donation, empathy, morality, patriotism, prejudice against deviants and outsiders, prosocial behavior, social trust, and volunteering (Apinunmahakul and Devlin 2008; Corcoran et al. 2011; Ishio 2010; Keyes 2002; Kim and Wilcox 2013; Ravanera et al. 2003; van Tienen et al. 2011; Weisberg 2005; Wuthnow 2004). Conversely, religiosity has secured sociality by reducing crime, deviance, individualism, protesting, and sexuality (Andrews et al. 2015; Coffe and Geys 2007; Guo et al. 2008; Skerkat and Ellison 1999; Spilka et al. 2003). Moreover, religiosity realizes sociality regarding altruism, community, ethicality, groupism, sharing, and solidarity (Franks et al. 2013; Lichterman 2012; Peifer 2010; Spilka et al. 2003; Stavrova and Siegers 2014). Religiosity also upholds sociality by featuring altruism, attachment, caring, community, compassion, harmony, hospitality, love, morality, obedience, other-centeredness, peace, trust, unity, xenophobia (Ager and Ager 2011; Fontana 2003; Harris et al. 2018; Horell 2014; Paterson 2013; Shorey et al. 2018; Simpson et al. 2008; Spilka et al. 2003; Tenorio and Lo 2011; Werbner 2010). Conversely, religiosity maintains sociality by dismissing individualism, oppression, sexuality, and violence (Fontana 2003; Horell 2014; Spilka et al. 2003). Social desirability has buttressed sociality by raising altruism, benevolence value, and empathy and perspective-taking and suppressing violence and its tolerance (Douglas 2006; Fisher and Katz 2000; Krumrei-Mancuso 2017; Pulkkinen et al. 2009).

Conversely, homosexuality has bolstered ideals for crime, dispute, molesting, promiscuity, risking, sexuality, substance abuse, suicide, and violence to jeopardize sociality (Cameron et al. 2005; Hughes 2006; Rosario and Schrinshaw 2013). Crime, including molesting, has impaired sociality by reducing community involvement, prosocial behavior, and social trust and fomenting avoidance, protesting, risking, victimization, and violence (Brayne 2014; McNeeley and Yuan 2017; Broadbent and Papadopoulos 2011; Sun and Wang 2012; Wittebrood and Nieuwbeerta 2000; Zhong 2010). Dispute has impeded sociality regarding donation and trust as opposed to violence (Farmer and Fedor 2001; Farrington 2018; Kunovich and Hodson 1999). Promiscuity can breed crime to hinder sociality (Walsh 2011). The ideal for risking has disrupted sociality by generating crime, hate, and violence (Farrington 2018; Hawdon et al. 2019; Merdian et al. 2017). The ideal for sexuality has disrupted sociality by breeding risking (Moran et al. 2021). Sexuality or its ideal has also hurt sociality by fomenting isolation experienced and aggression (Vrangalova and Bukberg 2015). Substance abuse raised by homosexuality has covered alcohol, cigarettes, and drugs (Cochran and Mays 2013; G. Li et al. 2023; Simoni et al. 2013; Tabaac et al. 2016; Vrangalova and Savin-Williams 2014). As such, substance abuse has impaired sociality by fomenting crime, risking, suicide, victimization, and violence (Krahe 2013; Stogner et al. 2014; Tanner-Smith et al. 2013; Theall et al. 2003). Conversely, substance abuse has eroded sociality by reducing civic engagement (Bruch et al. 2010). The ideal for suicide has impeded sociality by fomenting radicalism (Soliman et al. 2016). Violence has undermined sociality by breeding antisociality, crime and recidivism, blaming, conflict, hostility, rejecting others, and impairing agreeableness, morality, and responsibility (Asendorpf et al. 2008; Del Bove et al. 2008; Morrison 2005; Scholte et al. 2009; Vitaro et al. 2007).

Acceptance of homosexuals obstructs sociality by conveying underlying power, utility, ideals, and norms against sociality or withdrawing underlying power, utility, ideals, and norms for sociality with the voluntaristic mechanisms of analytical functionalism. These mechanisms engage contact, elaboration, and structuring to handle power, utility, ideals, and norms (Horn 2013; Macmillan and Baiocchi 2010; Stewart 2008).

Power for driving sociality to resist acceptance of homosexuals has drained due to deprivation (Meuleman et al. 2019). Deprivation has undermined sociality by reducing civic participation, trust, social connection, and volunteering (Caputo 2010; Stephens et al. 2014; R. Walker et al. 2010). Conversely, deprivation has disrupted sociality by creating isolation, relationship problems, and social exclusion experienced (Dhal et al. 2008; Stephens et al. 2014; R. Walker et al. 2010). Acceptance of homosexuals has risen from inadequate power in cultural capital to drive sociality (Slootmaeckers and Lievens 2014). Cultural capital has sustained sociality by enhancing civic engagement, organizational participation, political interest, religiosity, and social trust (Campagna et al. 2020; Freitag 2003b; Guillen et al. 2011; Prior 2019; Wuthnow 2004).

Ideals underlying acceptance of homosexuals to dismiss sociality have espoused alcoholism, cosmopolitanism, entitlement, homosexuality, liberalism, and sexual permissiveness (Barker and Tinnick 2006; Loftus 2001; Marsh and Brown 2011; Motschenbacher 2013; Patrick et al. 2013; Rowatt et al. 2009). Alcoholism has impaired sociality by raising risking, victimization, and violence (Eakins et al. 2022; Krahe 2013; Zavala and Guadalupe-Diaz 2019). Cosmopolitanism opposes sociality by downplaying attachment, collective identity, communality, localism, nationalism, and patriotism (Baildon and Alviar-Martin 2020; Bray 2013; Caruana 2014; Delanty 2009; Sorge 2008). Conversely, cosmopolitanism contradicts sociality by hailing autonomy, diversity, foreignness, fusion, individualism, and liberalism (Corstange and York 2018; Delanty 2009; Held 2010; Herrmann 2023). As such, cosmopolitanism has eroded sociality by discounting religiosity and raising liberalism and acceptance of deviants and outsiders (Costa et al. 2023; Motschenbacher 2013; Norris and Inglehart 2009). Entitlement has impaired sociality by eroding compliance and relatedness and provoking narcissism and hostility (Moeller et al. 2009; Piff 2014; Zitek and Jordan 2019). Homosexuality has hindered sociality by breeding crime, dispute, loneliness, molesting, relationship dissolution, risking, suicide, victimization, and violence (R. Anderson et al. 2017; Cameron et al. 2005; Compton 2013; Hughes 2006; Rosario and Schrinshaw 2013; Tabaac et al. 2016).

Conversely, homosexuality has obstructed sociality by eroding conformity, intimacy, and social desirability (R. Anderson et al. 2017; van Griensven et al. 2004; Vrangalova and Savin-Williams 2014). Liberalism has impeded sociality regarding morality, normativity, and social order (Feinberg et al. 2019). Sexual permissiveness has disrupted sociality by initiating crime and risking (Donahue et al. 2013; Moran et al. 2021). Conversely, acceptance of homosexuals has built on ideals against conformity, conservatism, nationalism, religiosity, and traditionalism to impede sociality (Gaines and Garand 2010; Meuleman et al. 2019; Motschenbacher 2013; Patrick et al. 2013; Yeo and Chu 2018). Conformity has constituted sociality by raising patriotism and impeding violence and acceptance of deviants and outsiders (Pulkkinen et al. 2009; Schwartz et al. 2014; Van Hootegem et al. 2000; Yeo and Chu 2018). The ideal for conformity has built sociality regarding xenophobia or rejection of outsiders (Costa et al. 2023). Conservatism sustains sociality by nurturing empathy, loyalty, prosocial behavior, religiousness, and sacrifice (Dutton and Rayner-Hilles 2022). Moreover, conservatism underpins sociality by maintaining allegiance or loyalty, attachment, civility, community, conformity, cooperation, discipline, ethnocentrism, honesty, humility, intimacy, legality, morality, nationalism, obedience, order, partnership, patriotism, peace, responsibility, sharing, trust, and xenophobia (Dutton and Rayner-Hilles 2022; Heilman and Kusev 2020; Hickson 2013; Lakoff

2009; Rhodes-Purdy et al. 2023; Scruton 2014; Yoos 2007; Zuk and Zuk 2020). Conversely, conservatism upholds sociality by condemning dehumanizing, evilness, revolution, sexuality, terrorism, and transgression (Dutton and Rayner-Hilles 2022; Malka and Soto 2011; Scruton 2014; Suhay 2015). Nationalism has underpinned sociality by fostering attachment, intolerance against deviance, patriotism, political participation, religiousness, social inclusion, trust in government, and xenophobia, and diminishing protesting (N. Chen 2012; Flanagan and Lee 2000; Huddy et al. 2021; Li and Brewer 2004; Osborne et al. 2017; Pinto et al. 2020; Rippl et al. 2010). Religiosity has sustained sociality by fostering civic engagement, civility, cohesion, compliance, donation, empathy, morality, patriotism, prejudice against deviants and outsiders, prosocial behavior, social trust, and volunteering (Apinunmahakul and Devlin 2008; Corcoran et al. 2011; Ishio 2010; Keyes 2002; Kim and Wilcox 2013; Ravanera et al. 2003; van Tienen et al. 2011; Weisberg 2005; Wuthnow 2004). Conversely, religiosity has secured sociality by reducing crime, deviance, individualism, protesting, and sexuality (Andrews et al. 2015; Coffe and Geys 2007; Guo et al. 2008; Skerkat and Ellison 1999; Spilka et al. 2003). Moreover, religiosity realizes sociality regarding altruism, community, ethicality, groupism, sharing, and solidarity (Franks et al. 2013; Lichterman 2012; Peifer 2010; Spilka et al. 2003; Stavrova and Siegers 2014). Religiosity also upholds sociality by featuring altruism, attachment, caring, community, compassion, harmony, hospitality, love, morality, obedience, other-centeredness, peace, trust, unity, xenophobia (Ager and Ager 2011; Fontana 2003; Harris et al. 2018; Horell 2014; Paterson 2018; Shorey et al. 2018; Simpson et al. 2008; Spilka et al. 2003; Tenorio and Lo 2011; Werbner 2010). Conversely, religiosity maintains sociality by dismissing individualism, oppression, sexuality, and violence (Fontana 2003; Horell 2014; Spilka et al. 2003). Traditionalism has buttressed sociality by enhancing patriotism and faith in religion and discouraging protesting and accepting deviants and outsiders (Costa et al. 2023; Datler et al. 2013; Meuleman et al. 2019; Schwartz et al. 2014). Acceptance of homosexuals also evolves from ideals against altruism such as childrearing, Christianity, Confucianism, feminism, and moralism (Blanc 2005; McVeigh and Diaz 2009; Viefhues-Bailey 2010; Wagner and Hayes 2022). Altruism has constituted sociality by boosting attachment, civic engagement, friendship quality, likability, moral behavior, popularity, relatedness and diminishing loneliness and violence (Bond and Kwan 2000; W. Chen et al. 2022; Layous et al. 2012; Markiewicz et al. 2001; Martela and Ryan 2016; Mesch 2009; Na and Paternoster 2019; L. Taylor et al. 2018; Wright and Li 2011). Christianity dispels acceptance of homosexuals by favoring compassion, desert, healing, health, love, majoritarianism, marriage, patriarchy, patriotism, procreation, and respectability, as opposed to aggression or violence, choice, harm, nihilism, pluralism, selfishness, sin, and tolerance for deviance (Burack 2008; Viefhues-Bailey 2010). Feminism disdains acceptance of homosexuals by demeaning violence (de la Ossa 2016). As such, Christianity has buttressed sociality by securing conformity, donation, and morality and impeding cosmopolitanism (Hollinger 2017; Phillips and Smith 2008). Feminism, as introduced by the community institution to frame sociality, idealizes philanthropy and social interaction (Phillips 2002). Besides, feminism upholds sociality by embracing caring, closeness, cooperation, empathy, equality, justice, and solidarity (Hutchings 2010; Sanderson et al. 2005). Feminism has also buttressed sociality regarding solidarity (van Breen et al. 2017). Moralism has sustained sociality by boosting gratitude (Pohling et al. 2010). Moreover, moralism can enhance sociality regarding social trust (Bersot and Arrigo 2015; Steinhardt 2012). Inherently, moralism embraces altruism, consensus, legality, obligation, and virtue to maintain sociality (R. Brown 2018).

Norms against sociality underlying acceptance of homosexuals can foreground globalization and Westernization (Y. Hu 2016; Roberts 2019). Globalization has impeded sociality by eroding patriotism (Kunovich 2009). Westernization has dampened sociality by provoking protesting and the norm of hostility (Kwan and Law 1994; Zhu and Rosen 1994). Hostility impedes sociality by embodying competition, conflict, protesting, and violence (Canary et al. 2013; Koerner 2018; Renger et al. 2020; Webster and Kirkpatrick 2006).

Psychopathy registers antisociality and dark personality (Fox et al. 2015; March 2019). Furthermore, psychopathy counts as criminality (Fox et al. 2015). Inherently, psychopathy features antisociality, boldness, callousness or unemotionality, coldheartedness, disinhibition, dominance, greed, impulsiveness, manipulativeness, and meanness (Krupp et al. 2012; Mussel and Hewig 2016; Satchell et al. 2018; Welsh and Lenzenweger 2021). As such, psychopathy opposes sociality by draining power, utility, ideals, and norms for sociality and breeding power, utility, ideals, and norms against sociality with the voluntaristic mechanisms of analytical functionalism. Accordingly, power drives or resists sociality through the power realization mechanism. Utility attracts or distracts sociality through the utility optimization mechanism. Ideals rationalize or refute sociality through the ideal calibration mechanism. Norms assimilate or dissimilate sociality through the norm conformity mechanism. The impacts of psychopathy on sociality rest affordance and social interaction provided by psychopathy (Fox et al. 2015; Thielmann et al. 2020).

Power reflected by psychopathy to resist sociality resides in dark personality and dependence (March 2019; Thielmann et al. 2020). Dark personality impedes sociality by dampening justice and morality (Douglass et al. 2023). Dependence has impaired sociality by hindering social capital, social cohesion, social trust, and equality value, and engendering protesting and suicide (Cornwall 2009; Granzin and Haggard 2000; Konarska 2005; Van Vugt et al. 2003; Zanin et al. 2013). Moreover, psychopathy embraces antisociality, callousness, greed, and impulsiveness as power to resist sociality (Krupp et al. 2012; Mussel and Hewig 2016; Satchell et al. 2018; Welsh and Lenzenweger 2021). Antisociality has impeded sociality by impairing morality and triggering doping, recidivism, rejection received, and violence (Abbey et al. 2012; Bowen and Wretman 2014; Tsakpinoglou and Poulin 2017). Callousness has impaired sociality by breeding aggression, antisocial behavior, deviance, and violence and impeding empathy (Camara et al. 2025; Stulhofer 2021; M. Wang et al. 2015). Greed has hindered sociality by dampening prosocial behavior (Thielmann et al. 2020). Impulsiveness has impeded sociality by diminishing prosocial behavior and engendering protesting, radicalism, and violence (Breakwell 2007; Koehler and Fiebig 2019; Thielmann et al. 2020; Wright and DeLisi 2016). Furthermore, psychopathy can incubate recklessness to reduce power for sociality (Fox et al.

2015). Recklessness has disrupted sociality by generating crime, hate, and violence (Farrington 2018; Hawdon et al. 2019; Merdian et al. 2017). Ideals justifying crime to impede sociality espouse entitlement, individualism, and liberalism (Waiton 2008; Wright and DeLisi 2016). Conversely, psychopathy can reduce community attachment, guardianship received, self-control, and social skills as power to drive sociality (Fox et al. 2015). Community attachment has facilitated sociality regarding cooperation, networking, and trust (Groves et al. 2000; Molitor et al. 2011; Rochelle 2015). Guardianship received has sustained sociality. Guardianship received has bolstered sociality by enhancing affiliative humor and attenuating aggressive humor (Erickson and Feldstein 2007). Self-control has buttressed sociality by enhancing generativity and impeding crime, risking, and violence (Y. Cheung et al. 2014; Koegl and Day 2019; Peterson and Klohnen 1995; Welch et al. 2008). Social skills have facilitated sociality by raising civility, civic engagement, political participation, prosocial behavior, social cohesion, and social trust (Foschi and Lauriola 2014; Halvorsen 2007; Letki 2008). Furthermore, psychopathy can reflect inadequate social bonding to drive sociality (Fox et al. 2015). Social bonding has constituted sociality regarding connectedness, friendship, giving, and social interaction (Eberl 2020; Liebler and Sandefur 2002; Nelson-Coffey et al. 2023; Phan et al. 2009).

Utility reduced by psychopathy to distract sociality has rested on success experienced (Welsh and Lenzenweger 2021). Success or achievement has induced sociality by enhancing love and trust (Nezlek et al. 2008; Rieger and Wang 2021). Moreover, psychopathy can diminish achievement and gain as utility to attract sociality (Fox et al. 2015; Short 2018). Gain received has buttressed sociality by boosting compliance, institutional trust, political participation, prosocial behavior, and recourse (Davis-Lipman et al. 2007; Grimes 2006; Kirchler and Maciejovsky 2001; Pattie et al. 2004; Premo et al. 2018). Conversely, psychopathy has heightened disutility in risk, thus distracting sociality (Satchell et al. 2018). Risk has eroded sociality by weakening social integration and social trust (Hammer et al. 2009; Lindstrom and Rosvall 2015). Conversely, risk has dampened sociality by raising social exclusion (Hammer et al. 2009). Moreover, psychopathy can breed conflict as disutility to distract sociality (Fox et al. 2015). Conflict has impeded sociality regarding donation and trust as opposed to violence (Farmer and Fedor 2001; Farrington 2018; Kunovich and Hodson 1999).

Ideals against sociality raised by psychopathy have emphasized polygyny or promiscuity and violence (Z. Han et al. 2017; Mededovic and Kovacevic 2021). Polygyny or promiscuity can breed crime to hinder sociality (Walsh 2011). Violence has undermined sociality by fomenting crime and tolerance for violence (Markowitz 2001; Tanner-Smith et al. 2013). Moreover, psychopathy can induce ideals for bullying, doping, and radicalism to refute sociality (Fox et al. 2015; Johnston and Bose 2020). Bullying has dampened sociality by raising aggressiveness, antisociality, blaming, conflict, crime and recidivism, hostility, and social rejection (Asendorpf et al. 2008; Morrison 2006; Del Bove et al. 2008; Vitaro et al. 2007). Conversely, bullying has impeded sociality by inhibiting agreeableness and morality (Del Bove et al. 2008; Scholte et al. 2009). Doping has impaired sociality by dampening civic engagement (Bruch et al. 2010). Conversely, doping has disrupted sociality by engendering crime, risking, suicide, victimization, and violence (Krahe 2013; Stogner et al. 2014; Tanner-Smith et al. 2013; Theall et al. 2003). Radicalism has undermined sociality by raising violence and diminishing collective practice and confidence in government (Achilov 2016; Levi and Strker 2000). Conversely, psychopathy has diminished ideals for feminism and prosociality to hinder sociality (Douglass et al. 2023; Thielmann et al. 2020). Feminism has also buttressed sociality regarding solidarity (van Breen et al. 2017). Prosociality has constituted sociality by civility, consolidating connectedness, cooperation, religiosity, responsibility, and volunteering (Hample 2018; Marsh and Dik 2021; Musick and Wilson 2008; Nelson-Coffey et al. 2023; Shahzalal and Adnan 2022). Moreover, prosociality underlies sociality by enhancing citizenship, loyalty, social cohesion, socializing, and trust and diminishing self-interest (Dovidio et al. 2006; Hawley 2014; Kisliuk and WeiBmuller 2023; Music 2014). Moreover, psychopathy has dampened the ideal for morality, thus impeding sociality (Johnston and Bose 2020). Morality has championed sociality by boosting volunteering and inhibiting violence (Piquero and Hickman 2002; Whitford et al. 2006).

Norms reduced by psychopathy can reside in parental supervision (Fox et al. 2015). Parental supervision received has sustained sociality by preventing violence (Farrington 2007). More generally, supervision received can prevent crime, thus upholding sociality (Brezina and Agnew 2013). Conversely, psychopathy can foster peer delinquency as a norm to dissimilate sociality (Fox et al. 2015). Peer delinquency has brewed aggression, antisociality, delinquency, recidivism, social rejection experienced, victimization, and violence and inhibited conformity and prosocial behavior, thus undermining sociality (Bhochhibhoya et al. 2021; Carlo et al. 2014; Carson 2013; Deptula and Cohen 2004; Grant et al. 2019; Holloway et al. 2022; H. Ma et al. 2007; Nivette et al. 2021). Psychopathy can also reflect deviant bonding as a norm to resist sociality (Fox et al. 2015). The deviant norm has weakened sociality by increasing relocation (Snyder et al. 2015).

Acceptance of or tolerance for deviance impedes sociality by draining power, utility, ideals, and norms for sociality and engendering power, utility, ideals, and norms against sociality to operate the voluntaristic mechanisms of analytical functionalism. These mechanisms apply power for driving or resisting sociality, utility to attract or distract sociality, ideals to rationalize or refute sociality, and norms to assimilate or dissimilate sociality.

Power underlying tolerance for deviance has stemmed from aggressiveness to impair sociality (Stanley et al. 2014). Aggressiveness has undermined sociality by fomenting crime and tolerance for violence (Markowitz 2001; Tanner-Smith et al. 2013).

Utility weakening tolerance for deviance has involved justice to buttress sociality (Rade et al. 2018). Justice experienced has warranted sociality regarding civility, cooperation, community identification, political participation, and social trust as opposed to protesting (A. Hu 2013; Lawrence and Daniels 1997; Sunshine and Tyler 2003; Tyler and Degoey 1995; van Prooijen et al. 2008; Wenzel 2000).

Ideals reduced by tolerance for deviance have accentuated government and institutional trust to maintain sociality (R. Chan 2012; Morris and Klesner 2010). Government trust has constituted sociality by sustaining compliance, conformity, nationalism, political participation, and preventing protesting (Rhodes-Purdy et al. 2023; Ulbig 2002; van der Meer and van Ingen 2009; V. Vu 2021). Institutional trust has constituted sociality by enhancing civic engagement, civility, compliance, legalism, political participation, prosocial behavior, responsibility, and social trust (Coffe and van der Lippe 2010; Grimes 2006; Jakobsen 2010; Seifert 2018; Stagnaro et al. 2017; Stolle and Micheletti 2013). Conversely, institutional trust has maintained sociality by preventing risking (Ehrke et al. 2023). Tolerance for deviance has declined with ideals for conservatism, government or statism, legality, morality, order, and religiosity (Gibson 2013; Gustavsson 2012; Lehmann et al. 2021; Markus 2001; Verkuyten 2023). Conservatism sustains sociality by nurturing empathy, loyalty, prosocial behavior, religiousness, and sacrifice (Dutton and Rayner-Hilles 2022). Moreover, conservatism underpins sociality by maintaining allegiance or loyalty, attachment, civility, community, conformity, cooperation, discipline, ethnocentrism, honesty, humility, intimacy, legality, morality, nationalism, obedience, order, partnership, patriotism, peace, responsibility, sharing, trust, and xenophobia (Dutton and Rayner-Hilles 2022; Heilman and Kusev 2020; Hickson 2013; Lakoff 2009; Rhodes-Purdy et al. 2023; Scruton 2014; Yoos 2007; Zuk and Zuk 2020). Conversely, conservatism upholds sociality by condemning dehumanizing, evilness, revolution, sexuality, terrorism, and transgression (Dutton and Rayner-Hilles 2022; Malka and Soto 2011; Scruton 2014; Suhay 2015). The ideal for government or statism has sustained sociality by dampening protesting (Schofer and Fourcade-Gourinchas 2001). Legality has buttressed sociality by dismissing radicalism (Muthuswamy 2022). Morality has constituted sociality by boosting volunteering and inhibiting violence (Piquero and Hickman 2002; Whitford et al. 2006). The ideal for order has bred sociality based on confidence in the business institution (Costa et al. 2023). The ideal for religion or religiosity has sustained sociality by fostering civic engagement, civility, cohesion, compliance, donation, empathy, morality, patriotism, prejudice against deviants and outsiders, prosocial behavior, social trust, and volunteering (Apinunmahakul and Devlin 2008; Corcoran et al. 2011; Ishio 2010; Keyes 2002; Kim and Wilcox 2013; Ravanera et al. 2003; van Tienen et al. 2011; Weisberg 2005; Wuthnow 2004). Conversely, religiosity has secured sociality by reducing crime, deviance, individualism, protesting, and sexuality (Andrews et al. 2015; Coffe and Geys 2007; Guo et al. 2008; Sherkat and Ellison 1999; Spilka et al. 2003). Moreover, religiosity realizes sociality regarding altruism, community, ethicality, groupism, sharing, and solidarity (Franks et al. 2013; Lichterman 2012; Peifer 2010; Spilka et al. 2003; Stavrova and Siegers 2014). Religiosity also upholds sociality by featuring altruism, attachment, caring, community, compassion, harmony, hospitality, love, morality, obedience, other-centeredness, peace, trust, unity, xenophobia (Ager and Ager 2011; Fontana 2003; Harris et al. 2018; Horell 2014; Paterson 2018; Shorey et al. 2018; Simpson et al. 2008; Spilka et al. 2003; Tenorio and Lo 2011; Werbner 2010). Conversely, religiosity maintains sociality by dismissing individualism, oppression, sexuality, and violence (Fontana 2003; Horell 2014; Spilka et al. 2003). Tolerance for deviance dismisses the ideal for conformity, thus hindering sociality (Coffe and Geys 2007). The ideal for conformity has built sociality regarding xenophobia or rejection of outsiders (Costa et al. 2023). Tolerance for deviance declines with ideals for culture or culturalism, paternalism, repentance, and responsibility, thus shaking sociality (A. Cohen 2014; Garland et al. 2017; Verkuyten and Yogeeswaran 2017). Culturalism constitutes sociality by maintaining xenophobia and dismissing tolerance for diversity (Verkuyten and Yogeeswaran 2017; Wessendorf 2008). Paternalism prioritizes caring in an overriding way (Arneson 2005). As such, paternalism upholds sociality by valorizing morality and protection and denouncing suicide (Arneson 2005; Kullgen 1995). Repentance has elevated sociality by enhancing donation (Bednall et al. 2013). Moreover, repentance upholds sociality by espousing compassion (K. Lee et al. 2017). Responsibility has fostered sociality regarding compliance, morality, and xenophobia as opposed to violence (Bussey 2020; Granzin and Olsen 1998; Kaurin 2020; Milner and Myers 2007).

Conversely, tolerance for deviance has bred the ideal for protesting to undermine sociality (Lodewijkx et al. 2008). Protesting has impaired sociality by escalating distancing and radicalism and dampening moral motivation (Kutlaca et al. 2020; Vestergren et al. 2017). Besides, protesting impedes sociality by embracing antisociality, conflict, extremism, hostility, incivility, illegality, rioting, social exclusion, terrorism, and violence (Renger et al. 2020; Kaplan and Liu 2000; S. Lo 2021; McCright and Dunlap 2008; Morselli and Passini 2018; Smidt 2020; Stewart et al. 2012; Swart et al. 2020; Tan and Snow 2015). Moreover, tolerance for deviance has arisen from ideals for individualism, liberalism or freedom, and political disagreement to weaken sociality (Gibson 2013; Markus 2001; Mutz and Mondak 2006). Individualism has weakened sociality by reducing civic engagement, religiousness, social cohesion, and volunteering (Church 2010; Green and Janmaat 2011; J. He et al. 2014; Hener et al. 2016; Leong 2008; Pollack and Pickel 2007; Whitford et al. 2006). Conversely, individualism has impeded sociality by bolstering acceptance of outsiders, competition, crime, extremity, self-enhancement, protesting, and violence (Church 2010; J. He et al. 2014; Karstedt 2010; Leong 2008; Li and Song 1992; Pollack and Pickel 2007; Whitford et al. 2006). Liberalism has impeded sociality regarding morality, normativity, and social order (Feinberg et al. 2019). Violence has undermined sociality by breeding antisociality, crime and recidivism, blaming, conflict, hostility, rejecting others, and impairing agreeableness, morality, and responsibility (Asendorpf et al. 2008; Del Bove et al. 2008; Morrison 2006; Scholte et al. 2009; Vitaro et al. 2007).

Norms dispelling tolerance for deviance have popularized morality and parenthood to uphold sociality (Eibach et al. 2009; Verkuyten 2023). The norm for morality has maintained sociality by developing morality and dampening self-interest (A. Liu et al. 2025; J. Wright et al. 2017). Morality has championed sociality by boosting volunteering and inhibiting violence (Piquero and Hickman 2002; Whitford et al. 2006). Parenthood has buttressed sociality by raising civic engagement, generativity, and invitation received and eroding crime and removal (Kim and Wilcox 2013; Richmond 2003; Savolainen 2009; Schwadel 2012).

Justification for Unconventional Sexuality

Unconventional sexuality or its permissiveness involves abortion, adultery, divorce, eroticism, extramarital sex, homosexuality, infidelity, masturbation, pornography consumption, premarital sex, promiscuity, prostitution, sexual perversity, and sexting (Alparone et al. 2024; Y. Hu 2016; Kraaykamp and van Eijck 2005; Primoratz 1999; Schafer 2011; van Oosten and Vandenbosch 2020; Vauclair and Fischer 2011). Sexual perversity covers exhibitionism, fetishism, homosexuality, masochism, necrophilia, pedophilia, sadism, transvestism, voyeurism, and zoophilia (Primoratz 1999). Sexuality, particularly unconventional sexuality, is shameful, frightening, and threatening and counts as a taboo (Brown and Weigel 2018; Mollon 2005). As such, unconventional sexuality inhibits sociality by draining power, utility, ideals, and norms for sociality and engendering power, utility, ideals, and norms against sociality with the voluntaristic mechanisms of analytical functionalism. These mechanisms engage power realization, utility optimization, ideal calibration, and norm conformity.

Power for sociality weakened by unconventional sexuality has rested on attachment security (Dunkel et al. 2016). Attachment security has driven sociality by boosting appreciation received, communication, love, and responsiveness and diminishing distancing, ignoring, interpersonal problems, and intrusiveness (Alonso-Arbiol et al. 2007; Gillath et al. 2005; Lavy et al. 2010; Lemay et al. 2007; McCarthy and Maughan 2010). Furthermore, attachment security can secure sociality and its components of caring, companionship, compassion, donation, intimacy, marriage, prosocial behavior, recourse, relatedness, self-help group attendance, social support received, and social trust (Brown and Brown 2006; Carter 2016; Collins et al. 2011; Fowers 2015; Juhl et al. 2019; Meng and Chen 2014; Preves and Mortimer 2013; Tomlinson et al. 2018). Conversely, attachment security can sustain sociality by preventing conflict, deviance, fighting, flight, hate, loneliness, threatening, victimization, and violence (Caughlin et al. 2013; S. Henry 2009; Manassis 2017; Milner and Myers 2007; Ponti and Tani 2019; Rempel and Burris 2005; Rokach 2019; Spitzberg and Cupach 2014). Unconventional sexuality has arisen from deficient conscientiousness, emotional stability, relatedness or relational quality, self-efficacy, social support received, and warmth as power to drive sociality (Browning et al. 2005; Cohen and Fromme 2002; de Jong et al. 2012; Kraaykamp and van Eijck 2005; Markey and Markey 2007; Pearson et al. 2006). Conscientiousness has elevated sociality by consolidating attachment, compliance, order value, responsibility, social desirability, and volunteering reducing deviance, violence, and justification for unconventional sexuality (Bekkers 2005; de Jong et al. 2012; Fraley et al. 2011; Gotzsche-Astrup 2020; Mondak and Hurwitz 2012; Mullet et al. 2005; Saucier and Skrzypinska 2006; Twardawski et al. 2021; Wright and DeLisi 2016). Emotional stability has maintained sociality by fostering attachment security, civic engagement, coordination, forgiveness, nationalism, relatedness, and socializing and preventing crime and hostility (Bekkers 2005; Fraley et al. 2011; Hounkpatin et al. 2015; Kalish 2008; Marks 1996; Mullet et al. 2005; Pulkkinen et al. 2009; Schbley and McCauley 2005; Ward and Forney 2020). Relatedness has consolidated sociality by consolidating sharing, social interaction, and relationship satisfaction (Downie et al. 2008; Frazer 1999; Wickham and Knee 2012). Social integration has constituted sociality by strengthening cooperation and preventing suicide (Duberstein et al. 2004; Lepkowski and Couper 2002). Self-efficacy has sustained sociality by raising civic engagement, donation, government and social trust, leadership, political participation, prosocial behavior, and social activity (Bednall et al. 2013; Frye 2007; Gnambs and Batinic 2012; Huber et al. 2022; Mangum 2012; Rahn 2008; Pei and Pan 2018; Yao and Enright 2019). Social support received has strengthened sociality by enhancing attachment, gratitude, political participation, prosocial behavior, recourse, respect, responsibility, social integration, and social well-being (Boezeman and Ellemers 2008; Fahmy 2006; Phipps 2003; Williams and Galliher 2006; R. Wright et al. 2009; Zeldin et al. 2016; Zeng et al. 2024). Conversely, social support received has boosted sociality by preventing aggression, conflict, delinquency, doping, externalizing, hyperactivity, loneliness, runaway, sexuality, suicide, and violence (Bernardon et al. 2011; Browning et al. 2005; Hayslip et al. 2000; Nieuwenhuis et al. 2017; Pearson and Wilkinson 2013; Terzi-Unsal and Karei 2005; Wight et al. 2006; R. Wright et al. 2009). Warmth has fostered sociality by enhancing attachment (Fraley et al. 2011; J. Sun et al. 2018). Xenophobia has constituted sociality by boosting patriotism and social cohesion (Granzin and Olsen 1998; Wang and Chen 2004).

Conversely, unconventional sexuality reduces power for sociality by contracting disease (Bompani and Brown 2015). Disease has eroded sociality by impeding volunteering (Wuthnow 2004). Morality has constituted sociality by boosting volunteering and inhibiting violence (Piquero and Hickman 2002; Whitford et al. 2006). Alternatively, unconventional sexuality has arisen from disorders and mental illness to weaken power for sociality (Harris et al. 2002; C. Paul et al. 2000). Disorders have obstructed sociality by diminishing community attachment, social capital, and social trust (G. Brown et al. 2004; Congdon 2010; Ross and Mirowsky 2009). Mental illness has undermined sociality by withdrawing prosocial behavior and breeding radicalism, victimization, and violence (Ehrensuft et al. 2003; Krahe 2013; Soliman et al. 2016; Thielmann et al. 2020).

Disutility reduced by unconventional sexuality to inhibit sociality has rested on control experienced, depression, disrespect experienced, isolation experienced, and stress experienced (Donahue et al. 2013; Ein-Dor and Hirschberger 2012; Kettrey 2016; Upchurch et al. 1999; Vrangalova and Bukberg 2015). Control experienced has worsened sociality by breeding violence (Felson and Outlaw 2007). Depression has eroded sociality by breeding conflict, hate, hostility perceived, loneliness, revenge, risking, suicide, and violence (Cacioppo and Hawkley 2009; Economou et al. 2016; Haner et al. 2020; Morokoff et al. 2009; Mullet et al. 2005; Proulx et al. 2004; H. Smith et al. 2016; E. Wright et al. 2015). Conversely, depression has attenuated sociality by impeding benevolence, closeness experienced, fairness, forgiveness, gratitude, honesty, leadership, love, social integration, teamwork, and volunteering (Blanchard et al. 2021; Cornwall 2009; Holzel et al. 2011; Mancini et al. 2011; Mullet et al. 2005; Thoits and Hewitt 2001). Disrespect contradicts sociality regarding caring and equality (Renger and Reese 2017). Unconventional sexuality has also arisen from distress and stress experienced as disutility against sociality (Ein-Dor and Hirschberger 2012; South et al. 2005). Distress has undermined sociality by fomenting resistance and impeding social capital and trust (Pulkkinen et al. 2009; Webber and Huxley 2007). Stress experienced has undermined sociality by eroding civility, forgiveness, generativity, relationship quality and satisfaction, social integration, social support received, and trust and heightening conflict, maltreatment, substance abuse, suicide, and violence (Atkinson et al. 2005; Dutton et al. 2015; Gelles 2007; Grzywacz and Almeida 2008; Jackson et al. 2006; Sobeck et al. 2020; Toussaint et al. 2016). Unconventional sexuality can arise from loss and trauma as disutility against sociality (Alparone et al. 2024; Jackson and Scott 2010). Loss experienced has hindered sociality by eroding compliance and government trust and fomenting suicide (Kirchler and Maciejovsky 2001; Nicholls and Picou 2012). Trauma has worsened sociality by eroding social cohesion, social support received and breeding delinquency, independence, and suicide (Darling et al. 2007; J. Hong et al. 2012; Liu and Tein 2005; Nakashima et al. 2013; Rojas et al. 2017).

Conversely, unconventional sexuality can reduce happiness as utility for attracting sociality (Soble 2008). Happiness has uplifted sociality by consolidating altruism, conformism, cooperation, donation, liking for people, prosociality, sociability, and trust and social trust (Fetvadjiev and He 2019; A. Hu 2013; Lyubomirsky et al. 2006; Y. Pan et al. 2023; Wang and Graddy 2008). Unconventional sexuality has arisen from inadequate empathy experienced, relational satisfaction, and self-esteem as utility to attract sociality (Bearman and Bruckner 2001; Erin and Friel 2001; Evans et al. 2004). Empathy embodies social support (X. Li 2023). Social support received has buttressed sociality by enhancing attachment, political participation, prosocial behavior, recourse, relational expectancy, respect received, social integration, social responsibility, and social well-being (Boezeman and Ellemers 2008; Fahmy 2006; Garst et al. 2021; Hitlin 2006; Williams and Galliher 2006; R. Wright et al. 2009; Zeldin et al. 2016). Conversely, social support has sustained sociality by preventing aggression, conflict, delinquency, externalizing behavior, loneliness, runaway, suicide, and violence (Bernardon et al. 2011; Hayslip et al. 2000; Nieuwenhuis et al. 2017; Pearson and Wilkinson 2013; Phipps 2003; Terzi-Unsal and Karei 2005; Wight et al. 2006; R. Wright et al. 2009). Relations satisfaction constitutes sociality by registering social integration (Y. Wong et al. 2011). Self-esteem has buttressed sociality by raising attachment security, political participation, and prosociality and preventing suicide (Kitayama and Markus 2000; Tracy et al. 2009). Unconventional sexuality can arise from inadequate resolution and satisfaction to attract sociality (Alparone et al. 2024; Jackson and Scott 2010). Resolution experienced has maintained sociality by raising civility, government and social trust, and political participation and dampening deviance (Backman and Nilsson 2011; Fahmy 2006; Marschall and Stolle 2004; Nicholls and Picou 2012). Satisfaction has advanced sociality by strengthening political participation, social cohesion, social and government trust, and volunteering (E. Chan 2014; Flavin and Keane 2011; Rochelle 2015).

Ideals against sociality generated by unconventional sexuality have hailed aggression, alcoholism, and doping or substance abuse generated by unconventional sexuality (Donahue et al. 2013; Vrangalova and Bukberg 2015). Aggression has undermined sociality by breeding antisociality, crime and recidivism, blaming, conflict, hostility, rejecting others, and impairing agreeableness, morality, and responsibility (Asendorpf et al. 2008; Del Bove et al. 2008; Morrison 2006; Scholte et al. 2009; Vitaro et al. 2007). Alcoholism has impaired sociality by raising risking, victimization, and violence (Eakins et al. 2022; Krahe 2013; Zavala and Guadalupe-Diaz 2019). Doping has impaired sociality by dampening civic engagement (Bruch et al. 2010). Conversely, doping has disrupted sociality by engendering crime, risking, suicide, victimization, and violence (Krahe 2013; Stogner et al. 2014; Tanner-Smith et al. 2013; Theall et al. 2003). Unconventional sexuality engendered the ideal for risking to impair sociality (Carpentier 2017). The ideal for risking has disrupted sociality by generating crime, hate, and violence (Farrington 2018; Hawdon et al. 2019; Merdian et al. 2017). Unconventional sexuality has arisen from ideals for bullying, delinquency, independence, risking to inhibit sociality (Evans et al. 2004; South et al. 2005; Treger and Schmitt 2019; Volk et al. 2015). Bullying has undermined sociality by fomenting crime and tolerance for violence (Markowitz 2001; Tanner-Smith et al. 2013). Delinquency has undermined sociality by worsening attachment, empathy, helpfulness, morality, relational quality, sociability, and social capital (Cheung and Cheung 2006; Hoffmann et al. 2013; Keijsers et al. 2011). Conversely, delinquency has disrupted sociality by enhancing antisocial behavior, conflict, suicide, and victimization (Carson 2013; Cutler et al. 2001; P. Lau et al. 2005). Unconventional sexuality can evolve from ideals for individualism to hinder sociality (Alparone et al. 2024). Individualism has weakened sociality by reducing civic engagement, religiousness, social cohesion, and volunteering (Church 2010; Green and Janmaat 2011; J. He et al. 2014; Hener et al. 2016; Leong 2008; Pollack and Pickel 2007; Whitford et al. 2006). Conversely, individualism has impeded sociality by bolstering acceptance of outsiders, competition, crime, extremity, self-enhancement, protesting, and violence (Church 2010; J. He et al. 2014; Karstedt 2010; Leong 2008; Li and Song 1992; Pollack and Pickel 2007; Whitford et al. 2006). Unconventional sexuality rests on ideals for hedonism, liberalism, libertarianism, and queer theory to dampen sociality (Jackson and Scott 2010; Nixon 2008; Primoratz 1999). Hedonism, liberalism, and libertarianism prioritize pleasure (Jackson and Scott 2010; Soble 2008; Primoratz 1999). Hedonism has impeded sociality by dampening communitarianism, legalism, and patriotism (Bore et al. 2005; Schwartz et al. 2014). Liberalism has obstructed sociality regarding morality, normativity, and social order (Feinberg et al. 2019). Libertarianism has dampened sociality by weakening cooperation and patriotism and championing cynicism, protesting, and tolerance for deviance (Eggert and Giugni 2015; Flanagan and Lee 2003; Kertzer et al. 2014). The ideal of queer theory denounces community, identity or role, and tradition and accentuates antisociality, individuality, performativity, and self-expression (Kirsch 2000). Notably, the queer ideal undermines sociality by vindicating anarchy, antisociality, and conflict and dismissing morality and normativity (Nicholas 2014; Smith and Windes 2000; Wiegman 2017; Zanghellini 2020).

Conversely, unconventional sexuality has arisen from ideals against belongingness, conformity, conservatism, interdependence, morality, religiosity, and traditionalism to impede sociality (Cohen and Fromme 2002; de Jong et al. 2012; Donner et al. 2024; Goff and Goddard 1999; Jung 2016; Treger and Schmitt 2019). Ideals for Christianity, particularly Catholicism, can reduce unconventional sexuality, thus sustaining sociality (Berard 1999; Soble 2008). Christianity refutes abortion and prioritizes celibacy, faithfulness, forgiveness, heterosexuality, monogamy, and procreation (Pruss 2013). Catholicism upholds love and denounces contraception (Soble 2008). Unconventional sexuality contradicts ideals for adulthood, natural law, naturalism, socialism, utilitarianism, and universalism to undermine sociality (Gresle-Favier 2010; Primoratz 1999; Soble 2008). The ideal for adulthood treasures responsibility (Gresle-Favier 2010). The ideal for natural law favors celibacy, love, naturalness, procreation, and salvation and denounces idolizing, lechery, lust, and objectification (Soble 2008). Naturalism refutes fetishism, homosexuality, and libertinism (Primoratz 1999). Socialism rejects alienation, commodification, prostitution, and subjection and cherishes equality and monogamy (Primoratz 1999; Soble 2008). Utilitarianism condemns sadomasochism as a basis for unconventional sexuality (Soble 2008). Universalism opposes adultery, commodification, homosexuality, objectification, prostitution, and selfishness and treasures devotion, dignity, heterosexuality, love, marital commitment, and respect (Primoratz 1999; Soble 2008).

Norms underlying unconventional sexuality against sociality have popularized autonomy, liberaty, sexuality and its unconventional forms, and Westernization (Barry 2007; Guo et al. 2008; Y. Hu 2016; Lyons et al. 2011; Vauclair and Fischer 2011). Conversely, unconventional sexuality has arisen from norms against government and traditionalism to hinder sociality (Barry 2007; Jung 2016). Unconventional sexuality can change with norms disseminated or learned through normalization, social construction, social bonding, social interaction, social labeling, and socialization (Hannah and Kitzinger 2001; Jackson and Scott 2010; Jung 2016; Olmstead et al. 2019; P. Wright 2022).

Promiscuity, including polygyny, as unconventional sexuality, worsens sociality by engaging power, utility, ideals, and norms against sociality or draining power, utility, ideals, and norms for sociality through the voluntaristic mechanisms of analytical functionalism. These mechanisms wield power to drive or resist sociality, utility to attract or distract sociality, ideals to rationalize or refute sociality, and norms to assimilate or dissimilate sociality.

Power reduced by promiscuity to disrupt sociality stems from disease (Kampf 2008). Disease has eroded sociality by impeding volunteering (Wuthnow 2004). Promiscuity has arisen from powerlessness to sustain sociality due to psychopathy (Z. Han et al. 2017). Psychopathy has undermined sociality by withdrawing prosocial behavior and breeding radicalism, victimization, and violence (Ehrensuft et al. 2003; Krahe 2013; Soliman et al. 2016; Thielmann et al. 2020).

Disutility underlying promiscuity for distracting sociality has originated from victimization, including abuse, rape, and violence experienced (Dunkle et al., 2004). Victimization experienced has impaired sociality by eroding social trust (Olivera

2015). Conversely, victimization experienced has hurt sociality by activating conflict and migration (Bar-Tal and Halperin 2013; Ramesh et al. 2019). Moreover, promiscuity reflects inadequate intimacy as disutility to distract sociality (Noller 2006). Intimacy has constituted sociality by boosting relationship satisfaction and social support received and dampening rejection expected (Arseth et al. 2009; Hand et al. 2013).

Ideals developed by promiscuity to distract sociality can valorize antisociality and crime (Farrington 2010; Walsh 2011). Antisociality has impeded sociality by impairing morality and triggering doping, recidivism, rejection received, and violence (Abbey et al. 2012; Bowen and Wretman 2014; Tsakpinoglou and Poulin 2017). Crime has impaired sociality by reducing community involvement, prosocial behavior, and social trust and fomenting avoidance, protesting, risking, victimization, and violence (Brayne 2014; McNeeley and Yuan 2017; Broadbent and Papadopoulos 2011; Sun and Wang 2012; Wittebrood and Nieuwbeerta 2000; Zhong 2010). Promiscuity has arisen from ideals for alcoholism and doping to impair sociality (Dunkle et al. 2004). Alcoholism has impaired sociality by raising risking, victimization, and violence (Eakins et al. 2022; Krahe 2013; Zavala and Guadalupe-Diaz 2019). Doping has impaired sociality by dampening civic engagement (Bruch et al. 2010). Moreover, promiscuity stands on the ideal for queer theory to weaken sociality (Jeffreys 2012). The queer ideal undermines sociality by vindicating anarchy, antisociality, and conflict and dismissing morality and normativity (Nicholas 2014; Smith and Windes 2000; Wiegman 2017; Zanghellini 2020). Conversely, promiscuity has developed from ideals against binding morality to impair sociality (Donner et al. 2024). Morality has championed sociality by boosting volunteering and inhibiting violence (Piquero and Hickman 2002; Whitford et al. 2006).

Norms sustaining promiscuity have popularized economic dependence and inadequate income to disrupt sociality (Price et al. 2014). Such norms have impaired sociality by eroding political participation, volunteering, and government, institutional, and social trust (Inglehart 2003; Marien 2011; Traunmuller 2011; van Oorschot and Arts 2005).

Acceptance of Outsiders

Outsiders, including foreigners, immigrants, and refugees, feature dependency, panicking, segregation, stressfulness, and unemployment (Boeri et al. 2002; Hombrados-Mendieta et al. 2013; KhosraviNik 2010; Painter-Davis et al. 2010; Roemer 2006). Conversely, outsiders lack income, nationalism, skillfulness, and solidarity (Millar 2013; Roemer 2006). With these features, outsiders are deficient in sociality by generating or drawing power, utility, ideals, and norms against sociality and reducing or draining power, utility, ideals, and norms for sociality, hinging on the voluntaristic mechanisms of analytical functionalism. These mechanisms engage power realization, utility optimization, ideal calibration, and norm conformity to shape sociality. Specifically, these mechanisms involve assimilation concerning norms and production concerning power use (Kivisto and Faist 2010; Boert et al. 2012).

Power for sociality reduced by outsider status has evolved from employment, health, marriage, and social capital (Fanning et al. 2011; Islam et al. 2006; Ravanera et al. 2003; Thornton et al. 2007). Employment has facilitated sociality by elevating civic engagement, community involvement, donation, philanthropy value, political discussion, political participation, social capital, social functioning, social cohesion experienced, social interaction, and social trust (Anciaes et al. 2017; Fridberg and Kangas 2008b; Kerrissey and Schofer 2013; H. Lu et al. 2002; Ross and Mirowsky 2009; Tsai 2006). Conversely, employment has safeguarded sociality by lessening crime, relocation, and social exclusion experienced (Groot et al. 2007; Kleinhans 2009; Savolainen 2009). Health has uplifted sociality by boosting community sense, morality, popularity, social activity, social cohesion, social integration, social trust, social well-being, and volunteering (Huxhold et al. 2014; Jorgensen et al. 2010; Son and Wilson 2012; Tolsma et al. 2009; Yu and Chiu 2016). Conversely, health has sustained sociality by preventing loneliness (Koromeckyj-Cox et al. 2007). Intelligence has raised sociality by facilitating donation and social capital and reducing criminality and protesting (Cornwall 2009; Feinstein and Bynner 2006; Paterson 2008; Piferi et al. 2006). Social capital has consolidated sociality by raising civic engagement, community involvement, donation, political involvement, social trust, and volunteering (Bekkers et al. 2008; Broadbent and Papadopoulos 2011; Brown and Ferris 2007; Chua et al. 2021; Narayan and Cassidy 2001). Conversely, social capital has strengthened sociality by erasing violence (Pulkkinen et al. 2009). Moreover, outsider status may lower power based on income and solidarity, thus hindering sociality (Roemer 2006). Income has upheld sociality by boosting civic engagement, community attachment and involvement, civic dutifulness, civility, conformity value, neighboring, political interest and participation, political and social trust, prosocial behavior, social capital, social integration, social interaction, social support received, social well-being, and volunteering (Bjornberg and Latta 2007; Chang 2009; Djupe and Lewis 2015; Frei et al. 2009; Kerrissey and Schofer 2013; Letki 2006; McCabe 2014; Patulny and Morris 2012; Son and Wilson 2012; Sun and Wang 2012; Swaroop and Morenoff 2006; Ulbig 2002). Conversely, income has maintained sociality by dampening alienation, discrimination experienced, migration, protesting, relocation, social deprivation experienced, social exclusion experienced, victimization, and violence (Broom et al. 2013; Brown and Connell 2004; Buck 2001; Rijken and Groenewegen 2008; V. Taylor et al. 2009; Weakliem and Borch 2006). Solidarity has constituted sociality by enhancing attachment and dampening tolerance for deviance (Stafford et al. 2005; Woosnam et al. 2018).

Conversely, outsider status has bred dysfunction, poverty, social exclusion experienced, and unemployment to weaken power for driving sociality (Bask 2005; Herd et al. 2008; Posthumus et al. 2013). Dysfunction has weakened sociality by eroding social capital, social cohesion, social trust, and volunteering (Cornwall 2009; Granzin and Haggard 2000; Tang 2006; Zanin et al. 2013). Conversely, dysfunction has impeded sociality by instigating protesting and suicide (Van Vugt et al. 2003). Moreover, outsider status may breed dependency, symptoms, and unemployment to weaken power for driving sociality (Boeri et al. 2002; Borjas 1999; Roemer 2006). Dependency has impaired sociality by hindering social capital, social cohesion, social trust, and equality value, and engendering protesting and suicide (Cornwall 2009; Granzin and Haggard 2000; Konarska 2005; Van Vugt et al. 2003; Zanin et al. 2013). Symptoms have eroded sociality by impeding volunteering (Wuthnow 2004). Unemployment has impeded sociality by dissolving social capital, social cohesion, and trust (Espvall and Dellgren 2008; Manturuk et al. 2010; Reeskens and Vandecasteele 2017). Conversely, unemployment has hurt sociality by breeding conflict experienced, moving, protesting, threats experienced, and victimization (Bramley and Morgan 2003; Kaukinen 2004; Lewin-Epstein et al. 2003; Schneider 2007; Su and Feng 2013). .

Disutility generated by outsider status to inhibit sociality has rested on depression and fear (Kitchen and Williams 2010; Lofors and Sundquist 2007). Depression has eroded sociality by breeding conflict, hate, hostility perceived, loneliness, revenge, risking, suicide, and violence (Cacioppo and Hawkley 2009; Economou et al. 2016; Haner et al. 2020; Morokoff et al. 2009; Mullet et al. 2005; Proulx et al. 2004; H. Smith et al. 2016; E. Wright et al. 2015). Conversely, depression has attenuated sociality by impeding benevolence, closeness experienced, fairness, forgiveness, gratitude, honesty, leadership, love, social integration, teamwork, and volunteering (Blanchard et al. 2021; Cornwall 2009; Holzel et al. 2011; Mancini et al. 2011; Mullet et al. 2005; Thoits and Hewitt 2001). Fear has disrupted sociality by breeding interpersonal problems, loneliness, risking, suicide, and violence (Dutton et al. 2016; Gillath et al. 2005; Pulkkinen et al. 2009; Trumbo et al. 2008). Conversely, fear has undermined sociality by reducing donation, friendship, humor, political participation, prosocial behavior, and social well-being (Best and Krueger 2010; Hewstone et al. 2005; Litman et al. 2017; Kuiper and Nicholl 2004; Zhong 2010). Moreover, outsider status involves stress as disutility to distract sociality (Hombrados-Mendieta et al. 2013). Stress has undermined sociality by eroding civility, forgiveness, generativity, relationship quality and satisfaction, social integration, social support received, and trust and heightening conflict, maltreatment, substance abuse, suicide, and violence (Atkinson et al. 2005; Dutton et al. 2016; Gelles 2007; Grzywacz and Almeida 2008; Jackson et al. 2006; Sobeck et al. 2020; Toussaint et al. 2016). Conversely, outsider status has diminished life satisfaction as utility to attract sociality (Ambrey and Fleming 2014). Life satisfaction has incubated sociality regarding political participation, social cohesion, social trust, and volunteering (E. Chan 2014; Flavin and Keane 2011; Rochelle 2015).

Ideals for sociality hindered by outsider status have emphasized birth, civic engagement, community attachment, egalitarianism, political participation, social cohesion, social trust, and volunteering (Anton and Lawrence 2014; K. Brown et al. 2014; R. King 2005; Ravanera et al. 2003; Saunders and Wong 2012; Sonderskov 2011; Stromblad and Myrberg 2013). Birth has raised sociality by enhancing civic engagement, community involvement, conformism, donation, social capital, social cohesion, social integration, social interaction, social support received, and volunteering (Apinunmahakul and Devlin 2008; Bjornberg and Ekbrand 2008; Frei et al. 2009; Ghimire 2021a; Kleinhans et al. 2007; Magdol and Bessel 2003; Taniguichi and Thomas 2011; Wilkinson 2008; Xiao 2000; Xu and Lai 2002). Conversely, birth has advanced sociality by reducing social distance and violence (Broom et al. 2013; Tsai 2006). Meanwhile, outsider status has raised ideals for migration, sleep, and suicide to oppose sociality (Gurak and Kritz 2000; Hamermesh 2019). Migration has impeded sociality by diminishing social integration (Kearns and Whitley 2015). The ideal for sleeping or sleepiness has bred crime to disrupt sociality (Raine and Venables 2017). The ideal for suicide has impeded sociality by fomenting radicalism (Soliman et al. 2016). Moreover, outsider status may breed the ideal for segregation to diminish sociality (Painter-Davis et al. 2010). Segregation characterizes social exclusion (Smets and Salman 2008). Social exclusion has impeded sociality by fueling crime, doping, and violence (Barry and Hullett 1998).

The norm for sociality hindered by outsider status has popularized social control (Lilly et al. 2011). The norm for social control has enhanced sociality by raising civic engagement, government trust, political participation, and recourse (Su and Feng 2013; Z. Han et al. 2017; F. Lee 2012; Palmer et al. 2011). Conversely, the norm for social control has safeguarded sociality by dampening victimization and violence (Hansen-Nord et al. 2014; E. Wright et al. 2015). Outsider status has grown with the norm against unionization to impede sociality (Boert et al. 2012). The norm for unionization has bolstered unemployment and the norm for conflict to disrupt sociality (Van Dyke et al. 2007; White and Smith 1994). Unemployment has impeded sociality by dissolving social capital, social cohesion, and trust (Espvall and Dellgren 2008; Manturuk et al. 2010; Reeskens and Vandecasteele 2017). Conversely, unemployment has hurt sociality by breeding conflict experienced, moving, protesting, threats experienced, and victimization (Bramley and Morgan 2003; Kaukinen 2004; Lewin-Epstein et al. 2003; Schneider 2007; Su and Feng 2013). The norm for conflict has impaired sociality by fomenting protesting and resistance (Schatzman 2005; Sorens 2011).

Acceptance of outsiders or xenophilia impedes sociality by generating or drawing power, utility, ideals, and norms against sociality and dampening or draining power, utility, ideals, and norms for sociality through the voluntaristic mechanisms of analytical functionalism. Specifically, these mechanisms employ power, utility, ideals, and norms to trigger acculturation, categorization, construction, deprivation, and differentiation (Mols and Jetten 2017; Stawarz and Muller 2020; Valenty and Sylvia 2004).

Power for sociality weakening xenophilia or foreigner support has resided in friendliness (Kraaykamp and van Eijck 2005). Friendliness has enabled sociality regarding prosocial behavior (Foschi and Lauriola 2014).

Ideals for rationalizing sociality weakening xenophilia have accentuated assimilation, Christianity, conformity, conservatism, culturalism, nationalism, nativism, patriotism, political interest, religiosity, solidarity, and tradition (Al-Kire et al. 2022; Bello 2016; Carter and Perez 2016; Erhart 2016; Huddy et al. 2021; Ishii 2009; Leong 2008; Lancee and Pardos-Prado 2013; Schwartz et al. 2014; Van Hootegem et al. 2000). Assimilation reflects social integration as opposed to discrimination experienced to buttress sociality (Walters et al. 2007; Zick et al. 2001). Christianity has buttressed sociality by securing conformity, donation, and morality, and impeding cosmopolitanism (Hollinger 2017; Phillips and Smith 2008). The ideal for conformity has built sociality regarding xenophobia or rejection of outsiders (Costa et al. 2023). Conservatism sustains sociality by nurturing empathy, loyalty, prosocial behavior, religiousness, and sacrifice (Dutton and Rayner-Hilles 2022). Moreover, conservatism underpins sociality by maintaining allegiance or loyalty, attachment, civility, community, conformity, cooperation, discipline, ethnocentrism, honesty, humility, intimacy, legality, morality, nationalism, obedience, order, partnership, patriotism, peace, responsibility, sharing, trust, and xenophobia (Dutton and Rayner-Hilles 2022; Heilman and Kusev 2020; Hickson 2013; Lakoff 2009; Rhodes-Purdy et al. 2023; Scruton 2014; Yoos 2007; Zuk and Zuk 2020). Conversely, conservatism upholds sociality by condemning dehumanizing, evilness, revolution, sexuality, terrorism, and transgression (Dutton and Rayner-Hilles 2022; Malka and Soto 2011; Scruton 2014; Suhay 2015). Culturalism constitutes sociality by maintaining xenophobia and dismissing tolerance for diversity (Verkuyten and Yogeeswaran 2017; Wessendorf 2008). Nationalism has underpinned sociality by fostering attachment, intolerance against deviance, patriotism, political participation, religiousness, social inclusion, trust in government, and xenophobia, and diminishing protesting (N. Chen 2012; Flanagan and Lee 2000; Huddy et al. 2021; Li and Brewer 2004; Osborne et al. 2017; Pinto et al. 2020; Rippl et al. 2010). Nativism constitutes sociality by espousing communitarianism and community, cooperation, familiarity, harmony, nationalism, patriotism, reciprocity, social participation, and xenophobia (Gregg 2003; Macedo 2021; Ng and Kennedy 2019; Zhang and Gu 2022). Patriotism has constituted sociality by raising government trust, nationalism, prosocial behavior or prosociality, social cohesion, volunteering, and xenophobia (Beyerlein and Sikkink 2008; Gross et al. 2004; Ishii 2009; Straume and Odeen 2010). Political interest has elevated sociality by raising civic engagement, civic and social motivation, civility, and discussion as opposed to protesting (Gil de Zuniga et al. 2017; Lee and Chan 2011; Pattie et al. 2004). Religiosity has sustained sociality by fostering civic engagement, civility, cohesion, compliance, donation, empathy, morality, patriotism, prejudice against deviants and outsiders, prosocial behavior, social trust, and volunteering (Apinunmahakul and Devlin 2008; Corcoran et al. 2011; Ishio 2010; Keyes 2002; Kim and Wilcox 2013; Ravanera et al. 2003; van Tienen et al. 2011; Weisberg 2005; Wuthnow 2004). Conversely, religiosity has secured sociality by reducing crime, deviance, individualism, protesting, and sexuality (Andrews et al. 2015; Coffe and Geys 2007; Guo et al. 2008; Skerkat and Ellison 1999; Spilka et al. 2003). Moreover, religiosity realizes sociality regarding altruism, community, ethicality, groupism, sharing, and solidarity (Franks et al. 2013; Lichterman 2012; Peifer 2010; Spilka et al. 2003; Stavrova and Siegers 2014). Religiosity also upholds sociality by featuring altruism, attachment, caring, community, compassion, harmony, hospitality, love, morality, obedience, other-centeredness, peace, trust, unity, xenophobia (Ager and Ager 2011; Fontana 2003; Harris et al. 2018; Horell 2014; Paterson 2018; Shorey et al. 2018; Simpson et al. 2008; Spilka et al. 2003; Tenorio and Lo 2011; Werbner 2010). Solidarity has constituted sociality by enhancing attachment and dampening tolerance for deviance (Stafford et al. 2005; Woosnam et al. 2018). The ideal for tradition has buttressed sociality by enhancing patriotism and faith in religion and discouraging protesting and accepting deviants (Costa et al. 2023; Datler et al. 2013; Meuleman et al. 2019; Schwartz et al. 2014). Moreover, xenophilia can arise from ideals against ingroup cooperation and status to undermine sociality (D'Ancona and Angeles 2018; Francois and Magni-Berton 2013). Xenophilia also stands on the ideal against responsibility to erode sociality (Van Hootegem et al. 2000). Cooperation has constituted sociality regarding attachment and trustworthiness as opposed to argument (Gerbasi and Cook 2008; Hample 2018; Tak 2017). Ingroup status has constituted sociality regarding connectedness, friendship, giving, and social interaction (Eberl 2020; Liebler and Sandefur 2002; Nelson-Coffey et al. 2023; Phan et al. 2009).

Conversely, xenophilia has arisen from ideals for internationalism, liberalism, relocation, and multiculturalism to impede sociality (Bessudnov 2016; Esses et al. 2005; Igarashi 2021; Mangum 2019). Similarly, xenophilia stands on ideals for cosmopolitanism and neoliberalism to challenge sociality (Andreouli and Figgou 2019; Herrmann 2023). Internationalism opposes sociality by downplaying attachment, collective identity, communality, localism, nationalism, and patriotism (Baildon and Alviar-Martin 2020; Bray 2013; Caruana 2014; Delanty 2009; Sorge 2008). Conversely, internationalism contradicts sociality by hailing autonomy, diversity, foreignness, fusion, individualism, and liberalism (Corstange and York 2018; Delanty 2009; Held 2010; Herrmann 2023). As such, internationalism has eroded sociality by discounting religiosity and raising liberalism and acceptance of deviants and outsiders (Costa et al. 2023; Motschenbacher 2013; Norris and Inglehart 2009). Liberalism has impeded sociality regarding morality, normativity, and social order (Feinberg et al. 2019). Relocation has impeded sociality by diminishing social integration (Kearns and Whitley 2015). Multiculturalism obstructs sociality by denouncing assimilation, embracing unrest, and standing on independence (Pehrson et al. 2011; Verkuyten 2005).

Norms against sociality underlying xenophilia have popularized individualism, multiculturalism, protesting, and unemployment (Branton et al. 2015; Leong 2008; Mahfud et al. 2018; Van Hootegem et al. 2000). Individualism has weakened sociality by reducing civic engagement, religiousness, social cohesion, and volunteering (Church 2010; Green and Janmaat 2011; J. He et al. 2014; Hener et al. 2016; Leong 2008; Pollack and Pickel 2007; Whitford et al. 2006). Conversely, individualism has impeded sociality by bolstering acceptance of outsiders, competition, crime, extremity, self-enhancement, protesting, and violence (Church 2010; J. He et al. 2014; Karstedt 2010; Leong 2008; Li and Song 1992; Pollack and Pickel 2007; Whitford et al. 2006). Protesting has impaired sociality by escalating distancing and radicalism and dampening moral motivation (Kutlaca et al. 2020; Vestergren et al. 2017). Besides, protesting impedes sociality by embracing antisociality, conflict, extremism, hostility, incivility, illegality, rioting, social exclusion, terrorism, and violence (Renger et al. 2020; Kaplan and Liu 2000; S. Lo 2021; McCright and Dunlap 2008; Morselli and Passini 2018; Smidt 2020; Stewart et al. 2012; Swart et al. 2020; Tan and Snow 2015). Unemployment has impeded sociality by dissolving social capital, social cohesion, and trust (Espvall and Dellgren 2008; Manturuk et al. 2010; Reeskens and Vandecasteele 2017). Conversely, unemployment has hurt sociality by breeding conflict experienced, moving, protesting, threats experienced, and victimization (Bramley and Morgan 2003; Kaukinen 2004; Lewin-Epstein et al. 2003; Schneider 2007; Su and Feng 2013). Meanwhile, xenophilia has arisen from norms against conservatism and republicanism to weaken sociality (Boeri et al. 2002; Valenty and Sylvia 2004). Republicanism upholds sociality regarding citizenship, the commonweal, interdependence, morality, nationalism, publicity, responsibility, social adaptation, and solidarity (Delanty 2009; Honohan 2002).

Xenophobia features nationalism, paternalism, protectionism, and traditionalism (Biggs and Knauss 2012; Huddy et al. 2021; Jayaratne et al. 2006). As such, xenophobia builds sociality by offering or drawing power, utility, ideals, and norms for sociality and removing and draining power, utility, ideals, and norms against sociality based on the voluntaristic mechanisms of analytical functionalism. These mechanisms engage appraisal, competition, and conflict concerning power, utility, ideals, and norms (Banks and Valentino 2012; M. Cooper et al. 2021; Pardos-Prado 2011).

Power for sociality buttressing xenophobia has rested on income (T. Wilson 2001). Income has upheld sociality by boosting civic engagement, community attachment and involvement, civic dutifulness, civility, conformity value, neighboring, political interest and participation, political and social trust, prosocial behavior, social capital, social integration, social interaction, social support received, social well-being, and volunteering (Bjornberg and Latta 2007; Chang 2009; Djupe and Lewis 2015; Frei et al. 2009; Kerrissey and Schofer 2013; Letki 2006; McCabe 2014; Patulny and Morris 2012; Son and Wilson 2012; Sun and Wang 2012; Swaroop and Morenoff 2006; Ulbig 2002). Conversely, income has maintained sociality by dampening alienation, discrimination experienced, migration, protesting, relocation, social deprivation experienced, social exclusion experienced, victimization, and violence (Broom et al. 2013; Brown and Connell 2004; Buck 2001; Rijken and Groenewegen 2008; V. Taylor et al. 2009; Weakliem and Borch 2006).

Utility attracting sociality underlying xenophobia has stemmed from gratification (Dambrun et al. 2006). Gratification has advanced sociality by strengthening political participation, social cohesion, social and government trust, and volunteering (E. Chan 2014; Flavin and Keane 2011; Rochelle 2015).

Ideals for sociality consolidated by xenophobia have extolled assimilation, nativism, patriotism, and social cohesion (Granzin and Olsen 1998; Kunst et al. 2016; Wolsko et al. 2006). Assimilation reflects social integration as opposed to discrimination experienced to buttress sociality (Walters et al. 2007; Zick et al. 2001). Nativism constitutes sociality by espousing communitarianism and community, cooperation, familiarity, harmony, nationalism, patriotism, reciprocity, social participation, and xenophobia (Gregg 2003; Macedo 2021; Ng and Kennedy 2019; Zhang and Gu 2022). Patriotism has constituted sociality by raising government trust, nationalism, prosocial behavior or prosociality, social cohesion, volunteering, and xenophobia (Beyerlein and Sikkink 2008; Gross et al. 2004; Ishii 2009; Straume and Odeen 2010). Social cohesion has constituted sociality by enhancing attachment and dampening tolerance for deviance (Stafford et al. 2005; Woosnam et al. 2018). Moreover, xenophobia features the ideals of nationalism, paternalism, protectionism, and traditionalism to build sociality (Biggs and Knauss 2012; Huddy et al.

2021; Jayaratne et al. 2006). Nationalism has underpinned sociality by fostering attachment, intolerance against deviance, patriotism, political participation, religiousness, social inclusion, trust in government, and xenophobia, and diminishing protesting (N. Chen 2012; Flanagan and Lee 2000; Huddy et al. 2021; Li and Brewer 2004; Osborne et al. 2017; Pinto et al. 2020; Rippl et al. 2010). Paternalism prioritizes caring in an overriding way (Arneson 2005). As such, paternalism upholds sociality by valorizing morality and protection and denouncing suicide (Arneson 2005; Kullgen 1995). Protectionism upholds collectivism and communitarianism to sustain sociality (Hindman 2009). Besides, protection has bolstered sociality by enhancing affiliative humor and attenuating aggressive humor (Erickson and Feldstein 2007). Traditionalism has buttressed sociality by enhancing patriotism and faith in religion and discouraging protesting and accepting deviants and outsiders (Costa et al. 2023; Datler et al. 2013; Meuleman et al. 2019; Schwartz et al. 2014). Xenophobia rests on the ideals of collectivism or groupism, communitarianism, conservatism, culturalism, evolutionism, functionalism or organicism, Judeo-Christianity, and republicanism to enrich sociality (Elias and Feagin 2016; Feinberg et al. 2012; Marotta 2017; Zienkowski 2017). Collectivism has constituted sociality by securing civility, cooperation, prosocial behavior, and religiousness and preventing extremism (Hample 2018; Harzing 2006; Oyserman et al. 1998; Saucier and Skrzypinska 2006; Thielmann et al. 2020). For xenophobia, communitarianism treasures community, ties, and unity (Amin 2012). Communitarianism constitutes sociality by espousing caring, civility, collective identity, commonweal orientation, community, dutifulness or responsibility, education or socialization, equality, interdependence, loyalty, mentoring, patriotism, reciprocity, relatedness, self-discipline, servicing including volunteering, settlement, social construction, social participation, solidarity, and trust (Delanty 2009; Frazer 1999; Moore 2010; Speth 2012). Conservatism sustains sociality by nurturing empathy, loyalty, prosocial behavior, religiousness, and sacrifice (Dutton and Rayner-Hilles 2022). Moreover, conservatism underpins sociality by maintaining allegiance or loyalty, attachment, civility, community, conformity, cooperation, discipline, ethnocentrism, honesty, humility, intimacy, legality, morality, nationalism, obedience, order, partnership, patriotism, peace, responsibility, sharing, trust, and xenophobia (Dutton and Rayner-Hilles 2022; Heilman and Kusev 2020; Hickson 2013; Lakoff 2009; Rhodes-Purdy et al. 2023; Scruton 2014; Yoos 2007; Zuk and Zuk 2020). Conversely, conservatism upholds sociality by condemning dehumanizing, evilness, revolution, sexuality, terrorism, and transgression (Dutton and Rayner-Hilles 2022; Malka and Soto 2011; Scruton 2014; Suhay 2015). Culturalism constitutes sociality by maintaining xenophobia and dismissing tolerance for diversity (Verkuyten and Yogeeswaran 2017; Wessendorf 2008). For xenophobia, evolutionism highlights civilization (Elias and Feagin 2016). Moreover, evolutionism treasures adaptation to facilitate sociality (J. Turner et al. 2020). Adaptation has secured sociality regarding partnership and social adjustment and satisfaction as opposed to discord (Chow et al. 2014; Mitchell 2005). Civilization constitutes sociality by establishing civility, loyalty, social contact, and social identification (Collins 2001; Hudson 2023). Besides, civilization embraces legality, relational quality, social capital, social cohesion, and social quality and dismisses violence (Phillips 2006; Rindermann 2018; Szakolczai 2001). Xenophobia has built on ideals for politics, religiosity, and social responsibility (Fredman et al. 2017; Jayaratne et al. 2006; Nijs et al. 2022). The ideal for politics has elevated sociality by raising civic engagement, civic and social motivation, civility, and discussion as opposed to protesting (Gil de Zuniga et al. 2017; Lee and Chan 2011; Pattie et al. 2004). Religiosity has sustained sociality by fostering civic engagement, civility, cohesion, compliance, donation, empathy, morality, patriotism, prejudice against deviants and outsiders, prosocial behavior, social trust, and volunteering (Apinunmahakul and Devlin 2008; Corcoran et al. 2011; Ishio 2010; Keyes 2002; Kim and Wilcox 2013; Ravanera et al. 2003; van Tienen et al. 2011; Weisberg 2005; Wuthnow 2004). Conversely, religiosity has secured sociality by reducing crime, deviance, individualism, protesting, and sexuality (Andrews et al. 2015; Coffe and Geys 2007; Guo et al. 2008; Skerkat and Ellison 1999; Spilka et al. 2003). Moreover, religiosity realizes sociality regarding altruism, community, ethicality, groupism, sharing, and solidarity (Franks et al. 2013; Lichterman 2012; Peifer 2010; Spilka et al. 2003; Stavrova and Siegers 2014). Religiosity also upholds sociality by featuring altruism, attachment, caring, community, compassion, harmony, hospitality, love, morality, obedience, other-centeredness, peace, trust, unity, xenophobia (Ager and Ager 2011; Fontana 2003; Harris et al. 2018; Horell 2014; Paterson 2018; Shorey et al. 2018; Simpson et al. 2008; Spilka et al. 2003; Tenorio and Lo 2011; Werbner 2010). Conversely, religiosity maintains sociality by dismissing individualism, oppression, sexuality, and violence (Fontana 2003; Horell 2014; Spilka et al. 2003). Social responsibility has constituted sociality by inducing fairness and trust (Vera-Toscano et al. 2013).

Conversely, xenophobia discounts the ideal of multiculturalism to uphold sociality (Leong and Ward 2006). Multiculturalism obstructs sociality by denouncing assimilation, embracing unrest, and standing on independence (Pehrson et al. 2011; Verkuyten 2005). Xenophobia stands on ideals against cosmopolitanism, liberalism, and neoliberalism to boost sociality (S. Kim 2012; Marotta 2017; Hobfoll 2018). Cosmopolitanism opposes sociality by downplaying attachment, collective identity, communality, localism, nationalism, and patriotism (Baildon and Alviar-Martin 2020; Bray 2013; Caruana 2014; Delanty 2009; Sorge 2008). Conversely, cosmopolitanism contradicts sociality by hailing autonomy, diversity, foreignness, fusion, individualism, and liberalism (Corstange and York 2018; Delanty 2009; Held 2010; Herrmann 2023). As such, cosmopolitanism has eroded sociality by discounting religiosity and raising liberalism and acceptance of deviants and outsiders (Costa et al. 2023; Motschenbacher 2013; Norris and Inglehart 2009). Liberalism has impeded sociality regarding morality, normativity, and social order (Feinberg et al. 2019). Neoliberalism espouses atomization and silos and disregards ethics and social services to undermine sociality (Lobao et al. 2014; Lakoff 2009; Rhodes-Purdy et al. 2023; Smart 2003).

The norm for sociality disseminated by xenophobia has popularized similarity or commonality (Granzin and Olsen 1998). Similarity has upheld sociality by enhancing social cohesion, social interaction, and trust and social trust (Stokman et al. 2013; Xiang et al. 2016). Xenophobia has arisen from norms for Catholicism, collectivism, and republicanism to foster sociality (Leong and Ward 2006; McVeigh et al. 2004; Valenty and Sylvia 2004). Catholicism has enhanced sociality by raising conformism and volunteering and dampening the value of independence and radicalism (Bekkers 2010; Devos et al. 2002; Fjellvang 2011). Catholicism has also safeguarded sociality by inculcating cooperation and interdependence (Bellah et al. 1991). The norm for collectivism has strengthened sociality by raising intimacy and institutional trust (Georgas et al. 1997; McAllister 1999). Republicanism upholds sociality regarding citizenship, the commonweal, interdependence, morality, nationalism, publicity, responsibility, social adaptation, and solidarity (Delanty 2009; Honohan 2002). Conversely, xenophobia has arisen from the norm against injustice to enable sociality (Dixon et al. 2010). The norm against injustice has upheld sociality by elevating morality and prosocial behavior (Barber 2004; McCaffoee 2016).

Trust in Others

Trust in others or social trust is an expectation of goodwill (Mingo and Faggiano 2020). Social trust characterizes social capital, cohesion, and resources (B. Six 2014; Sundquist and Yang 2007). Inherently, social trust features cooperativeness, investment, and kindness (Bellemare and Kroger 2007; Habibis et al. 2016; Rahn 2008). As such, social trust constitutes sociality by generating and drawing power, utility, ideals, and norms for sociality and diminishing and draining power, utility, ideals, and norms against sociality with the voluntaristic mechanisms of analytical functionalism. Specifically, these mechanisms engage attachment, exchange, investment, learning, sharing, socialization, and verifying concerning power, utility, ideals, and norms (Adongo et al. 2019; Burke and Stets 2009; Buskens and Raub 2013; Carter 2016; McKnight and Chervany 2006; Stolle and Harell 2013).

Power strengthened by social trust to drive sociality has resided in health, social support received, and survival (Barefoot et al. 1998; Mata and Pendakur 2014). Health has uplifted sociality by boosting community sense, morality, popularity, social activity, social cohesion, social integration, social trust, social well-being, and volunteering (Huxhold et al. 2014; Jorgensen et al. 2010; Son and Wilson 2012; Tolsma et al. 2009; Yu and Chiu 2016). Conversely, health has sustained sociality by preventing loneliness (Koromeckyj-Cox et al. 2007). Social support received has strengthened sociality by enhancing attachment, gratitude, political participation, prosocial behavior, recourse, respect, responsibility, social integration, and social well-being (Boezeman and Ellemers 2008; Fahmy 2006; Phipps 2003; Williams and Galliher 2006; R. Wright et al. 2009; Zeldin et al. 2016; Zeng et al. 2024). Conversely, social support received has boosted sociality by preventing aggression, conflict, delinquency, doping, externalizing, hyperactivity, loneliness, runaway, sexuality, suicide, and violence (Bernardon et al. 2011; Browning et al. 2005; Hayslip et al. 2000; Nieuwenhuis et al. 2017; Pearson and Wilkinson 2013; Terzi-Unsal and Karei 2005; Wight et al. 2006; R. Wright et al. 2009). Survival can sustain morality and social commitment to uplift sociality (Narvaez 2014; Ogolsky and Monk 2018). Social trust has benefitted from agreeableness, familiarity, friendship, knowledge, language proficiency, moderateness, self-efficacy, and sociability to provide power to drive sociality (Freitag and Bauer 2016; Halvorsen 2007; Kende et al. 2022; Lancee and Dronkers 2011; McCabe 2012; Pattie et al. 2004; Rahn 2008). Agreeableness has fostered sociality by enhancing attachment (Fraley et al. 2011). Familiarity or knowledge has raised sociality by enhancing cooperation, prosocial behavior, social cohesion, social trust, and volunteering (de Groot and Steg 2009; Lepkowski and Couper 2002; Pattie et al. 2004; Simon-Bemd and Steffens 2000; Volker et al. 2007;). Friendship has constituted sociality by enhancing community attachment, compliance, donation, gratitude, political participation, social cohesion, social desirability, social integration, and social trust (Corcoran 2013; Fahmy 2006; Gundert and Hohendanner 2015; Keillor et al. 2001; Kende et al. 2022; Opp 2001; Rotkirch 2014). Language proficiency has enabled sociality by elevating nationalism and social trust (Cai et al. 2022; Lancee and Dronkers 2011). Moderateness can boost sociality by enhancing marriage, marital and relational quality, and social cohesion (Hornsey and Jetten 2004; Forte 2001; SunWolf 2008). Self-efficacy has sustained sociality by raising civic engagement, donation, government and social trust, leadership, political participation, prosocial behavior, and social activity (Bednall et al. 2013; Frye 2007; Gnambs and Batinic 2012; Huber et al. 2022; Mangum 2012; Rahn 2008; Pei and Pan 2018; Yao and Enright 2019). Sociability has enhanced sociality by raising civic engagement, civility, political participation, prosocial behavior, and social cohesion (Foschi and Lauriola 2014; Letki 2008). Conversely, dysfunction and uncontrollability have weakened social trust to impede power to drive sociality (B. B. Williams et al. 1999; Zanin et al. 2013). Dysfunction has weakened sociality by eroding social capital, social cohesion, social trust, and volunteering (Cornwall 2009; Granzin and Haggard 2000; Tang 2006; Zanin et al. 2013). Uncontrollability has dampened sociality regarding social trust (Burke and Stets 1999). Social trust has prevented illness, thus maintaining power to drive sociality (Ahnquist et al. 2012). Illness has eroded sociality by impeding volunteering (Wuthnow 2004).

Utility or benefit can arise from social trust to attract sociality (Adongo et al. 2019). As such, social trust generates profit and revenue to secure sociality (Jarvinen and Branders 2020). Social trust has created well-being or wellness as utility to attract sociality (Almakaeva et al. 2018). Such well-being has included happiness, intimacy, life control, living standards, pride, and satisfaction (Abascal 2015; A. Hu 2013; Newton 1999; Rothstein and Uslaner 2005; Steinhardt 2012). Such satisfaction has covered democracy, economy, finance, life, public affairs, and volunteering (Almakaeva et al. 2018; Cais et al. 2021; Jung and Kwon 2011; Shao et al. 2021; Sun and Wang 2012). Satisfaction has eroded sociality by strengthening political participation, social cohesion, social and government trust, and volunteering (E. Chan 2014; Flavin and Keane 2011; Rochelle 2015). More generally, well-being has uplifted sociality by consolidating altruism, conformism, cooperation, donation, liking for people, prosociality, sociability, and trust and social trust (Fetvadjiev and He 2019; A. Hu 2013; Lyubomirsky et al. 2006; Y. Pan et al. 2023; Wang and Graddy 2008). Additionally, well-being sustains sociality by enabling civilization, fairness, forgiveness, intimacy, kindness, love, loyalty, modesty, morality, open-mindedness, social intelligence, and societal functioning (Cummins 2016; D'raven and Pasha-Zaidi 2016; Meadows 2014). Social trust furthermore has arisen from equality, reciprocity, security, windfalls, and expectations for living standards and reciprocity as utility to attract sociality (Barrera 2007; Glaeser et al. 2000; Molm et al. 2007; Uslaner 2002; Yamagishi et al. 1998). Equality experienced can sustain sociality by preventing crime and illegality (Kyriacou 2020). Reciprocity has constituted sociality by fostering prosocial behavior (Thielmann et al. 2020). Reciprocity experienced has elevated sociality by triggering affiliating, civic engagement, prosocial behavior, and social interaction and opposed to discriminating against others (Dovidio et al. 2006; Gui et al. 2020; Tusicisny 2017; Stadtfeld and Pentland 2015). Security has buttressed sociality regarding civility, social capital, and trust (Curley 2010; Watson et al. 2021; Williamson 2002). Windfalls received have buttressed sociality by boosting compliance, institutional trust, political participation, prosocial behavior, and recourse (Davis-Lipman et al. 2007; Grimes 2006; Kirchler and Maciejovsky 2001; Pattie et al. 2004; Premo et al. 2018). Living standards have enhanced sociality by elevating satisfaction with the nation, social capital, social interaction, and social trust (Booth and Richard 1998; S. Chan et al. 2022; Cummins et al. 2003; Moyano-Diaz and Palomo-Velez 2018).

Conversely, disutility against sociality distracting social trust has rested on conflict, discrimination experienced, distress, fear, hardship, inequality experienced, ostracism experienced, risk, stress, unemployment, and victimization (Alesina and La Ferrara 2002; Burke and Stets 1999; Cais et al. 2021; Lindstrom and Rosvall 2015; Mewes et al. 2021; Olivera 2015; Rodrigo-Gonzalez et al. 2019; Shao et al. 2021; Uslaner 2002). Social trust has reduced loneliness as disutility against sociality (Edara 2021). Conflict has impeded sociality regarding donation and trust as opposed to violence (Farmer and Fedor 2001; Farrington 2018; Kunovich and Hodson 1999). Discrimination experienced can foment violence to undermine sociality (White et al. 2015). Distress has undermined sociality by fomenting resistance and impeding social capital and trust (Pulkkinen et al. 2009; Webber and Huxley 2007). Fear has disrupted sociality by breeding interpersonal problems, loneliness, risking, suicide, and violence (Dutton et al. 2016; Gillath et al. 2005; Pulkkinen et al. 2009; Trumbo et al. 2008). Conversely, fear has undermined sociality by reducing donation, friendship, humor, political participation, prosocial behavior, and social well-being (Best and Krueger 2010; Hewstone et al. 2005; Litman et al. 2017; Kuiper and Nicholl 2004; Zhong 2010). Hardship has impaired sociality by dampening trust and fomenting social exclusion experienced, suicide, and victimization experienced (Economou et al. 2016; Reeskens and Vandecasteele 2017; Ross and Mirowsky 2009). Inequality experienced can engender crime and illegal behavior to obstruct sociality (Kyriacou 2020). Ostracism experienced has disrupted sociality by reducing prosocial behavior and engendering illegal association (Bockler et al. 2021; Zamperini et al. 2020). Risk has eroded sociality by weakening social integration and social trust (Hammer et al. 2009; Lindstrom and Rosvall 2015). Conversely, risk has dampened sociality by raising social exclusion (Hammer et al. 2009). Stress has undermined sociality by eroding civility, forgiveness, generativity, relationship quality and satisfaction, social integration, social support received, and trust and heightening conflict, maltreatment, substance abuse, suicide, and violence (Atkinson et al. 2005; Dutton et al. 2016; Gelles 2007; Grzywacz and Almeida 2008; Jackson et al. 2006; Sobeck et al. 2020; Toussaint et al. 2016). Unemployment has impeded sociality by dissolving social capital, social cohesion, and trust (Espvall and Dellgren 2008; Manturuk et al. 2010; Reeskens and Vandecasteele 2017). Conversely, unemployment has hurt sociality by breeding conflict experienced, moving, protesting, threats experienced, and victimization (Bramley and Morgan 2003; Kaukinen 2004; Lewin-Epstein et al. 2003; Schneider 2007; Su and Feng 2013). Victimization experienced has impaired sociality by eroding social trust (Olivera 2015). Conversely, victimization experienced has hurt sociality by activating conflict and migration (Bar-Tal and Halperin 2013; Ramesh et al. 2019).

Ideals raised by social trust to rationalize sociality have valorized attachment, civic conformity and engagement, civility, donation or charitable contribution, group involvement, government trust, institutional confidence, political participation, social inclusion, trustworthiness, and volunteering (Burke and Stets 1999; Cisterna et al. 2022; Coffe and van der Lippe 2010; Stolle and Micheletti 2013; Uslaner 2000; Delhey et al. 2011; Sonderskov 2011; Yamagishi et al. 1999). Attachment has constituted sociality by boosting relationship satisfaction and social support received and dampening rejection expected (Arseth et al. 2009; Hand et al. 2013). Civic engagement has propped sociality by strengthening attachment, civility, collective behavior, discussion, donation, neighboring, patriotism, prosociality, social capital, socialism, trust, and volunteering and impeding cheating and individualism (Coffe and Geys 2007; Gilberbloom and Markham 1995; Kerrissey and Schofer 2013; Mata and Pendakur 2014; Ozbay 2008; Pattie et al. 2004; Pena-Lopez and Sanchez-Santos 2016; Rahn 2008; Richey 2011; Tak 2017; M. Tang 2011; Taniguchi 2013; Yip et al. 2007). Civility has constituted sociality by inducing fairness and trust (Vera-Toscano et al. 2013). Additionally, civility maintains sociality by enhancing the commonweal, community, equality, friendship, reciprocity, and social capital (Hudson 2023). Donation has constituted sociality by consolidating charity, service value, social capital, social trust, and volunteering (Bekkers 2010; Chang 2009; Foster et al. 2001; Uslaner 2000). Group involvement has fostered sociality regarding cohesion, common identity, and identification (Fischer et al. 2007). Government trust has constituted sociality by sustaining compliance, conformity, nationalism, political participation, and preventing protesting (Rhodes-Purdy et al. 2023; Ulbig 2002; van der Meer and van Ingen 2009; V. Vu 2021). Institutional confidence has constituted sociality by enhancing civic engagement, civility, compliance, legalism, political participation, prosocial behavior, responsibility, and social trust (Coffe and van der Lippe 2010; Grimes 2006; Jakobsen 2010; Seifert 2018; Stagnaro et al. 2017; Stolle and Micheletti 2013). Conversely, institutional confidence has maintained sociality by preventing risking (Ehrke et al. 2023). Tolerance for deviance has declined with ideals for conservatism, government or statism, legality, morality, order, and religiosity (Gibson 2013; Gustavsson 2012; Lehmann et al. 2021; Markus 2001; Verkuyten 2023). Political participation has buttressed sociality regarding civility

(Campbell 2003). Social inclusion experienced has constituted sociality by strengthening cooperation and preventing suicide (Duberstein et al. 2004; Lepkowski and Couper 2002). Trustworthiness has constituted sociality, strengthening justness and likability (Molm et al. 2003; Gerbasi and Cook 2008). Moreover, trustworthiness can maintain sociality by boosting intimacy, cooperation experienced, dependency experienced, and trust experienced (Harvey and Wenzel 2006; O'Keefe 2002; Seifert 2018; Yamagishi et al. 2005). Volunteering has championed social trust and confidence in the political institution and reduced tolerance (Richey 2010; Richey and Ikeda 2009; Woolley 2003). Similarly, social trust elevates ideals for collaboration, cooperation, and sharing to enhance sociality (Jarvinen and Branders 2020). Social trust has arisen from ideals for charity, civic engagement, connection or relatedness, consideration, contact, donation, morality, neighboring, political interest and participation, religion, social integration, social interaction to rationalize sociality (Campbell 2011; Dyck 2012; Goodman 2015; Freitag 2003b; Kende et al. 2022; Lundasen et al. 2013; Rahn 2008; Rodrigo-Gonzalez et al. 2019; Rothstein and Uslaner 2005; Uslaner 2002; Zanin 2017). Collaboration or cooperation has strengthened sociality regarding attachment and trustworthiness as opposed to argument (Gerbasi and Cook 2008; Hample 2018; Tak 2017). Sharing has raised sociality by facilitating donating (Piferi et al. 2006). Moreover, sharing maintains sociality by involving social closeness, commitment, contribution, and gifting (Godoy et al. 2007; Murray and Holmes 2008).

Norms for sociality underlying social trust have popularized bonding, cohesiveness, equality, fairness, justice, and support (A. Hu 2013; Steinhardt 2012; Z. Su et al. 2019; Vera-Toscano et al. 2013). Bonding has constituted sociality regarding connectedness, friendship, giving, and social interaction (Eberl 2020; Liebler and Sandefur 2002; Nelson-Coffey et al. 2023; Phan et al. 2009). The norm for cohesiveness has supported sociality by enhancing civic engagement, community favor, government trust, political participation, and recourse and dampening violence (Z. Han et al. 2017; F. Lee 2012; Palmer et al. 2011; Pulkkinen et al. 2009; Su and Feng 2013; Whitham 2012). The norm for equality has fostered sociality by championing cohesion and its experience, fairness, justice, social capital, sympathy, trust, and volunteering (Eriksson et al. 2015; Green et al. 2003; Hitlin and Harkness 2018; Musick and Wilson 2008; Oishi et al. 2011; Portes and Vickstrom 2011; van Oorschot and Arts 2005). Trust developed by the norm for equality has covered institutions and people (Lundasen et al. 2013; van Oorschot and Arts 2005). Conversely, the norm for equality sustains sociality by preventing corruption, crime, social exclusion experienced, and violence (Reardon and Bischoff 2011; Uslaner 2008; Ousey and Lee 2013; van Wilsem 2007). The norm for fairness or justice has upheld sociality by elevating morality and prosocial behavior (Barber 2004; McCaffree 2016). The norm for support has elevated sociality by enhancing association, civic engagement, political participation, and recourse (Kampen 2010; F. Lee 2012; Palmer et al. 2011; Su and Feng 2013).

Conversely, social trust has developed from norms against corruption, crime, disorder, inequality, risk, and stress to assimilate sociality (Ross and Mirowsky 2009; Snijders and Keren 1999; Uslaner 2002; J. You 2012; Zanin 2017). The norm for corruption has undermined sociality by disrupting institutional trust (Morris and Klesner 2010). The norm of crime has jeopardized sociality by inhibiting community involvement and prosocial behavior and raising victimization (Broadbent and Papadopoulos 2011; Jacobs and Carmichael 2002; Zhong 2010). The norm for the disorder has eroded sociality by weakening community attachment and social capital and fomenting victimization (G. Brown et al. 2004; Congdon 2010; Like 2011). The norm for risk has impaired sociality by provoking protesting (Scafuto and La Barbera 2016). Moreover, the risk norm can hurt sociality by generating opposition to the establishment (P. Brown 2020). Social trust has furthermore diminished perceived norms for corruption and risk to sustain sociality (Ariely and Uslaner 2017; Macias 2015).

Current Findings

Factor analysis of the World Values Survey attitudinal data in the fifth and sixth waves identified seven factors based on maximum likelihood extraction and varimax rotation (see Table 2.1). These factors were confidence in institutions ($\alpha = .920$ with 17 items), justification for misdeeds ($\alpha = .844$ with 9 items), justification for unconventional sexuality ($\alpha = .866$ with 4 items), acceptance of outsiders ($\alpha = .749$ with 4 items), acceptance of deviants ($\alpha = .684$ with 5 items), trust in other people ($\alpha = .736$ with 5 items), and faith in religion ($\alpha = .716$ with 3 items). As such, these factors maintained satisfactory internal consistency reliability by taking simple averages based on their respective items.

Subsequently, factor analysis of the seven attitudinal factors after removing their acquiescence effects revealed their (second-order) common factor of sociality (see Table 2.2). Notably, refutation against misdeeds, refutation against unconventional sexuality, rejection of outsiders, and rejection of deviants were the reverses of justification for misdeeds, justification for unconventional sexuality, acceptance of outsiders, and acceptance of deviants, respectively. While six of the attitudes manifested positive factor loadings on the common factor, faith in religion exhibited a negative loading ($\lambda = -.243$). The latter thus revised the original expectation for sociality so that religious faith was a negative indicator of sociality instead. Besides, the loadings of rejection of deviants, trust in other people, and confidence in institutions on the sociality factor were not striking. The generally low loadings reflected that the attitudes originally represented independent, orthogonal factors based on factor analysis to maintain their independence. Hence, the attitudes were relatively independent and loosely connected to reveal sociality.

The current finding showed that faith in religion negatively represented sociality, such that irreligion registered sociality. Supporting the current finding, existing research findings have indicated that religious faith or religiosity impedes sociality by engendering or drawing power, utility, ideals, and norms against sociality and

Table 2.1 Factor loadings on attitudes

Item	Institutions	Misdeed	Sexuality	Outsider	Religion	Other	Deviant
Q123	.750	–.038	.063	–.074	–.150	–.025	–.001
Q122	.738	–.042	.081	–.085	–.125	–.013	–.009
Q124	.659	–.053	.053	–.083	–.147	.027	.006
Q118	.656	.030	–.104	–.001	.255	.116	.026
Q117	.654	.075	–.202	.036	.464	.105	.040
Q119	.629	–.063	.020	–.063	–.053	.035	.044
Q126	.616	.019	.054	.016	.028	.088	–.009
Q121	.609	–.025	–.172	.032	–.117	.008	.153
Q115	.595	.052	–.141	–.021	.493	.090	.030
Q114	.592	.000	–.055	.082	.298	.152	–.023
Q120	.592	.006	–.013	–.033	–.009	.060	–.006
Q112	.584	.021	–.101	.066	.080	.136	.021
Q110	.577	.022	–.112	.137	.052	.094	.051
Q116	.566	.106	–.191	.008	.536	.128	.018
Q111	.557	.032	–.130	.124	.056	.059	.079
Q113	.505	.006	–.021	.079	.326	.195	–.054
Q109	.495	–.045	–.078	.066	.035	.114	.007
Q202	–.023	.794	.097	.084	–.061	–.002	–.063
Q201	–.045	.787	.118	.015	–.070	–.021	–.071
Q200	–.037	.774	–.002	.006	–.048	.028	–.001
Q199	–.048	.657	.134	–.020	–.069	–.050	–.078
Q208	.009	.651	.184	.131	.034	–.001	–.013
Q210	–.031	.633	.146	–.006	.142	.002	.023
Q207	–.039	.537	.446	.068	.064	.035	–.039
Q198	.043	.485	.013	–.018	.028	–.065	.018
Q209	.085	.424	.071	–.042	.136	–.077	.029
Q205	–.131	.230	.765	–.056	.055	.024	–.094
Q206	–.130	.225	.753	–.138	.203	.002	–.190
Q204	–.099	.369	.670	.019	.090	.070	–.061
Q203	–.092	.304	.637	–.043	–.047	.070	–.200
Q41	.023	.041	–.028	.684	–.057	–.032	–.015
Q37	.008	.058	–.031	.671	–.058	.001	–.064
Q44	.017	.030	–.021	.613	–.102	–.001	–.017
Q39	.035	–.022	–.019	.573	–.092	–.030	.190
Q147	–.026	–.043	–.108	.158	–.524	.131	–.065
Q108	.208	.016	–.217	.183	–.496	.144	–.020
Q149	–.092	–.015	–.085	.121	–.419	.088	–.033

(continued)

Table 2.1 (continued)

Item	Institutions	Misdeed	Sexuality	Outsider	Religion	Other	Deviant
Q106	.136	–.027	.093	–.076	–.191	.735	–.018
Q107	.110	–.012	.153	–.103	–.086	.724	–.032
Q105	.102	.022	.001	.039	.014	.606	–.023
Q104	.166	–.096	–.006	–.008	–.024	.396	.023
Q103	.218	–.067	–.178	.083	.035	.329	.020
Q36	–.004	–.062	.006	–.224	.090	–.007	.626
Q42	.017	–.065	–.017	–.041	–.051	.025	.593
Q40	.032	–.005	–.193	.113	.044	–.004	.572
Q38	.098	.064	–.124	.198	.193	–.089	.537
Q43	.109	–.048	–.208	.326	–.190	.040	.422

Note. % variance explained = 61.9

Fwilful = willfulness, fgreed = greed, fbeat = violence, fnpride = nation, fauthor = authorities, Q130 = democracy, Q99 = noncompetition, Q66 = willingness to fight for the country

	Item
	Confidence in institutions
Q123	Having confidence in women's organizations
Q 117	Having confidence in the parliament
Q122	Having confidence in environmental organizations
Q118	Having confidence in the civil service
Q115	Having confidence in the government
Q114	Having confidence in courts
Q124	Having confidence in charitable organizations
Q116	Having confidence in political parties
Q119	Having confidence in universities
Q126	Having confidence in the country
Q121	Having confidence in banks
Q112	Having confidence in labor unions
Q110	Having confidence in the press
Q120	Having confidence in major companies
Q111	Having confidence in television
Q113	Having confidence in the police
Q109	Having confidence in armed forces
	Justification for misdeeds
Q202	Someone accepting a bribe in the course of duties being justifiable
Q201	Cheating on taxes being justifiable
Q200	Stealing property being justifiable

(continued)

Table 2.1 (continued)

	Item
Q199	Avoiding a fare on public transport being justifiable
Q208	Man's beating his wife being justifiable
Q210	Violence against others being justifiable
Q207	Suicide being justifiable
Q198	Claiming non-entitled government benefits being justifiable
Q209	Parents' beating children being justifiable
	Justification for unconventional sexuality
Q205	Divorce being justifiable
Q206	Sex before marriage being justifiable
Q204	Abortion being justifiable
Q203	Homosexuality being justifiable
	Faith in religion
Q108	Having confidence in churches
Q147	Being a religious person
Q149	Believing in hell
	Trust in other people
Q107	Trusting people of another nationality
Q106	Trusting people of another religion
Q105	Trusting people you meet for the first time
Q104	Trusting people you know personally
Q103	Trusting your neighborhood
	Acceptance of outsiders
Q41	Liking to have people of a different religion as neighbors
Q37	Liking to have people of a different race as neighbors
Q44	Liking to have people who speak a different language as neighbors
Q39	Liking to have immigrants or foreign workers as neighbors
	Acceptance of deviants
Q36	Liking to have drug addicts as neighbors
Q42	Liking to have heavy drinkers as neighbors
Q40	Liking to have homosexuals as neighbors
Q38	Liking to have people who have AIDS as neighbors
Q43	Liking to have unmarried couples living together as neighbors

Table 2.2 Factor loadings on sociality

Attitude	Sociality
Confidence in institutions	.448
Refutation against misdeeds	.761
Refutation against unconventional sexuality	.625
Faith in religion	–.243
Rejection of outsiders	.530
Rejection of deviants	.174
Trust in other people	.446

hindering or draining power, utility, ideals, and norms for sociality through the voluntaristic mechanisms of analytical functionalism. These mechanisms engage attribution, compulsion, conflict, identification, learning, meaning-making, and social inclusion and integration (Forsyth 2003; Pfeifer 2019; Spilka et al. 2003).

Power for sociality weakened by religiosity has rested on employment, family functioning experienced, and health (J. Ma et al. 2009; Ravanera et al. 2003; Yamaoka 2008). Employment has facilitated sociality by elevating civic engagement, community involvement, donation, philanthropy value, political discussion, political participation, social capital, social functioning, social cohesion experienced, social interaction, and social trust (Anciaes et al. 2017; Fridberg and Kangas 2008b; Kerrissey and Schofer 2013; H. Lu et al. 2002; Ross and Mirowsky 2009; Tsai 2006). Conversely, employment has safeguarded sociality by lessening crime, relocation, and social exclusion experienced (Groot et al. 2007; Kleinhans 2009; Savolainen 2009). Family functioning experienced represents interdependency and social capital (Parke 2004; White et al. 2015). Moreover, family functioning features attentiveness, caring, compassion, empathy, mutuality, and socialization (Herr 2012; Parke 2004). As such, family functioning experienced has facilitated sociality by raising social support received and reducing social avoidance (F. Liu et al. 2024). Health has uplifted sociality by boosting community sense, morality, popularity, social activity, social cohesion, social integration, social trust, social well-being, and volunteering (Huxhold et al. 2014; Jorgensen et al. 2010; Son and Wilson 2012; Tolsma et al. 2009; Yu and Chiu 2016). Conversely, health has sustained sociality by preventing loneliness (Koromeckyj-Cox et al. 2007). Power for sociality to dampen religiosity has stemmed from income and social class (Fjellvang 2011; Spilka et al. 2003). Income has upheld sociality by boosting civic engagement, community attachment and involvement, civic dutifulness, civility, conformity value, neighboring, political interest and participation, political and social trust, prosocial behavior, social capital, social integration, social interaction, social support received, social well-being, and volunteering (Bjornberg and Latta 2007; Chang 2009; Djupe and Lewis 2015; Frei et al. 2009; Kerrissey and Schofer 2013; Letki 2006; McCabe 2014; Patulny and Morris 2012; Son and Wilson 2012; Sun and Wang 2012; Swaroop and Morenoff 2006; Ulbig 2002). Conversely, income has maintained sociality by dampening alienation, discrimination experienced, migration, protesting, relocation, social deprivation experienced, social exclusion experienced, victimization, and violence (Broom et al. 2013; Brown and Connell 2004; Buck 2001; Rijken and Groenewegen 2008; V. Taylor et al. 2009; Weakliem and Borch 2006). Social class has sustained sociality by raising adaptation, civic engagement, cohesion, institutional and political trust, organizational involvement and membership, prosocial behavior, social capital, social support received, and volunteering (E. Chan 2014; Elchardus and De Keere 2013; La Grange 2011; Lennartsson 2010; Letki 2008; Mutaner et al. 2002; Wallace and Pichler 2009; Wuthnow 2004; Yeh et al. 2013; Zhong 2010). Conversely, social class has maintained sociality by preventing crime and social exclusion experienced (Agnew and Brezina 2010; Buck 2001). Moreover, power for sociality to impede religiosity can hinge on attachment (Yuchtman-Yaar 2002). Attachment has constituted sociality by boosting relationship satisfaction and social support received and dampening rejection expected (Arseth et al. 2009; Hand et al. 2013).

Conversely, religiosity has engendered illness and social distance to weaken power for driving sociality (Pedahzur and Canetti-Nisim 2004; Yamaoka 2008). Illness has eroded sociality by impeding volunteering (Wuthnow 2004). Social distance has worsened sociality by diminishing donation, political evaluation, and social interaction (Bekkers 2010; Belanger and Aarts 2006). Conversely, social distance has weakened sociality by breeding radicalism and protesting (Borbach and Gessler 2020; Pedahzur and Canetti-Nisim 2004). Religiosity has arisen from hatred to furnish power against sociality (Rip et al. 2012). Hatred has eroded sociality by fueling deviance and tolerance for violence and inhibiting prosocial behavior (Emer and Poepsel 2021; Mededovic and Kovacevic 2021; Masui 2023). Moreover, hatred can dampen sociality by engendering radicalism, suicide, and violence (Kral 2019; Larson et al. 2020; J. Turner 2007). Religiosity can emerge from narcissism to engender power against sociality (Fontana 2003). Narcissism has impeded sociality by breeding aggression and misbehavior (Tracy et al. 2009). Besides, narcissism dismisses discipline, empathy, friendship, humor, morality, and responsibility and embraces exploitation, lying, rage, rivalry, and violence to undermine sociality (Cichocka et al. 2024; Kilminster 2008; Twenge and Campbell 2009). Religiosity can evolve from dependency to weaken power for sociality (Spilka et al. 2003). Dependency has impaired sociality by hindering social capital, social cohesion, social trust, and equality value, and engendering protesting and suicide (Cornwall 2009; Granzin and Haggard 2000; Konarska 2005; Van Vugt et al. 2003; Zanin et al. 2013).

Utility for sociality reduced by religiosity has resided in well-being (Michalos et al. 2005). Such well-being has covered neighborhood satisfaction (Ayalon et al. 1993). Neighborhood satisfaction has fostered sociality by enhancing attachment, community involvement, volunteering, and social capital (Cummins et al. 2003; Long and Perkins 2007; Xu 2007). More generally, well-being has uplifted sociality by consolidating altruism, conformism, cooperation, donation, liking for people, prosociality, sociability, and trust and social trust (Fetvadjiev and He 2019; A. Hu 2013; Lyubomirsky et al. 2006; Y. Pan et al. 2023; Wang and Graddy 2008). Additionally, well-being sustains sociality by enabling civilization, fairness, forgiveness, intimacy, kindness, love, loyalty, modesty, morality, open-mindedness, social intelligence, and societal functioning (Cummins 2016; D'raven and Pasha-Zaidi 2016; Meadows 2014).

Conversely, religiosity has engendered marginalization experienced as disutility against sociality (Wuthnow 2004). Marginalization experienced has disturbed sociality by eroding closeness and prosocial behavior (Bockler et al. 2021; K. Lin et al. 2013). Religiosity has also arisen from conflict, dying, status inconsistency, and war as disutility against sociality (A. Miller 1995; Sasaki 1979; Immerzeel and van Tubergen 2013; Wuthnow 2004). Conflict has impeded sociality regarding donation and trust as opposed to violence (Farmer and Fedor 2001; Farrington 2018; Kunovich and Hodson 1999). Resentment experienced has disturbed sociality by eroding closeness and prosocial behavior (Bockler et al. 2021; K. Lin et al. 2013). Dying can dampen sociality by fomenting aggression (Reeve 2021). Status inconsistency can disrupt sociality by breeding conflict (J. Turner 2013b). War dampens sociality by triggering crime and religiousness (Immerzeel and van Tubergen 2013; Reiner 2016). Religiosity can arise from guilt and helplessness as disutility against sociality (Forsyth 2003). Guilt can erode sociality by diminishing relatedness (Stafford 2015). Helplessness can impede sociality by breeding religiousness (Forsyth 2003). Helplessness can impede sociality by breeding religiousness (Forsyth 2003). Religiosity also evolves from the disutility of stress to distract sociality (Spilka et al. 2003). Stress has undermined sociality by eroding civility, forgiveness, generativity, relationship quality and satisfaction, social integration, social support received, and trust and heightening conflict, maltreatment, substance abuse, suicide, and violence (Atkinson et al. 2005; Dutton et al. 2016; Gelles 2007; Grzywacz and Almeida 2008; Jackson et al. 2006; Sobeck et al. 2020; Toussaint et al. 2016).

Ideals for sociality weakened by religiosity have identified civic engagement, government trust, humanitarianism, institutional trust, localism, moral obligation, nationalism, social interaction, social welfare, and survival (Ayalon et al. 1993; Chappell and Prince 1997; Coffe and Geys 2007; Gill 2004; Kunovich 2009; Pakulshi and Tranter 2000; Shmueli 1999; Suh et al. 2012; Urbatsch 2014). Civic engagement has propped sociality by strengthening attachment, civility, collective behavior, discussion, donation, neighboring, patriotism, prosociality, social capital, socialism, trust, and volunteering and impeding cheating and individualism (Coffe and Geys 2007; Gilberbloom and Markham 1995; Kerrissey and Schofer 2013; Mata and Pendakur 2014; Ozbay 2008; Pattie et al. 2004; Pena-Lopez and Sanchez-Santos 2016; Rahn 2008; Richey 2011; Tak 2017; M. Tang 2011; Taniguchi 2013; Yip et al. 2007). Government trust has constituted sociality by sustaining compliance, conformity, nationalism, political participation, and preventing protesting (Rhodes-Purdy et al. 2023; Ulbig 2002; van der Meer and van Ingen 2009; V. Vu 2021). Humanitarianism has enhanced sociality by activating political participation (Foschi and Lauriola 2014). Besides, humanitarianism upholds sociality by embracing altruism, caring, coalitions, empathy, justice, other orientation, pity, prosociality, responsibility, and solidarity (Angelis and Pensini 2024; Bendixsen 2018; Brigg 2018; Chouliaraki 2013; Hoekstra 2021). Institutional trust has constituted sociality by enhancing civic engagement, civility, compliance, legalism, political participation, prosocial behavior, responsibility, and social trust (Coffe and van der Lippe 2010; Grimes 2006; Jakobsen 2010; Seifert 2018; Stagnaro et al. 2017; Stolle and Micheletti 2013). Conversely, institutional trust has maintained sociality by preventing risking (Ehrke et al. 2023). Localism constitutes sociality by espousing communitarianism and community, cooperation, familiarity, harmony, nationalism, patriotism, reciprocity, social participation, and xenophobia (Gregg 2003; Macedo 2021; Ng and Kennedy 2019; Zhang and Gu 2022). Moral obligation has sustained sociality by boosting gratitude (Pohling et al. 2010). Nationalism has underpinned sociality by fostering attachment, intolerance against deviance, patriotism, political participation, religiousness, social inclusion, trust in government, and xenophobia, and diminishing protesting (N. Chen 2012; Flanagan and Lee 2000; Huddy et al. 2021; Li and Brewer 2004; Osborne et al. 2017; Pinto et al. 2020; Rippl et al. 2010). Social interaction has realized sociality by consolidating altruism, compliance, cooperation, donation, morality, political participation, reciprocity, social trust, and volunteering (Guillen et al. 2011; Dixon and McKeown 2021; Lucas and Livingston 2014; Musick 2000; Rodrigo-Gonzalez et al. 2019; Rubin and Step 2000). The ideal for social welfare has championed sociality by consolidating government trust (U. Kim et al. 2002). Survival can sustain morality and social commitment to uplift sociality (Narvaez 2014; Ogolsky and Monk 2018). Similarly, ideals for conservatism and political engagement to rationalize sociality have weakened religiosity (Corstange and York 2018; Schlenker et al. 2012). Conservatism sustains sociality by nurturing empathy, loyalty, prosocial behavior, religiousness, and sacrifice (Dutton and Rayner-Hilles 2022). Moreover, conservatism underpins sociality by maintaining allegiance or loyalty, attachment, civility, community, conformity, cooperation, discipline, ethnocentrism, honesty, humility, intimacy, legality, morality, nationalism, obedience, order, partnership, patriotism, peace, responsibility, sharing, trust, and xenophobia (Dutton and Rayner-Hilles 2022; Heilman and Kusev 2020; Hickson 2013; Lakoff 2009; Rhodes-Purdy et al. 2023; Scruton 2014; Yoos 2007; Zuk and Zuk 2020). Conversely, conservatism upholds sociality by condemning dehumanizing, evilness, revolution, sexuality, terrorism, and transgression (Dutton and Rayner-Hilles 2022; Malka and Soto 2011; Scruton 2014; Suhay 2015). Political engagement has buttressed sociality regarding civility (Campbell 2003). An additional ideal repelling religiosity to rationalize sociality is socialism (Browning and Cooper 2004). Socialism maintained in the community institution to frame sociality anticipates association, cooperation, equality, harmony, and mutuality as opposed to conflict (Powell 2007). Besides, socialism has enhanced sociality regarding cooperation and discussion as opposed to crime (Collier 2001; Lilly et al. 2011; Sanderson 2001).

Conversely, religiosity has raised ideals for freedom, hawkishness, hedonism, pornographic consumption, protesting, radicalism, self-enhancement, substance abuse, and tolerance for deviance to challenge sociality (Booth and Martin 1998; Datler et al. 2013; Gibson 2013; MacInnis and Hodson 2016; Norris 2002; Pedahzur and Canetti-Nisim 2004). The ideal for freedom has impeded sociality regarding morality, normativity, and social order (Feinberg et al. 2019). Hawkishness has impaired sociality by provoking violence (Krahe 2013). Furthermore, hawkishness can obstruct sociality by diminishing protection and social competence (Dinic and

Bodroza 2021; Ting-Toomey 2004). Hedonism has impeded sociality by dampening communitarianism, legalism, and patriotism (Bore et al. 2005; Schwartz et al. 2014). The ideal for pornography has disrupted sociality by engendering the ideal for violence (Hald and Malamuth 2015). Moreover, the ideal for pornography can impede sociality by raising delinquency (Stevens et al. 2011). Protesting has impaired sociality by escalating distancing and radicalism and dampening moral motivation (Kutlaca et al. 2020; Vestergren et al. 2017). Besides, protesting impedes sociality by embracing antisociality, conflict, extremism, hostility, incivility, illegality, rioting, social exclusion, terrorism, and violence (Renger et al. 2020; Kaplan and Liu 2000; S. Lo 2021; McCright and Dunlap 2008; Morselli and Passini 2018; Smidt 2020; Stewart et al. 2012; Swart et al. 2020; Tan and Snow 2015). Radicalism has undermined sociality by raising violence and diminishing collective practice and confidence in government (Achilov 2016; Levi and Strker 2000). Self-enhancement maintains sociality by espousing attachment (Raeff 2010). Substance abuse has impaired sociality by fomenting crime, risking, suicide, victimization, and violence (Krahe 2013; Stogner et al. 2014; Tanner-Smith et al. 2013; Theall et al. 2003)). Conversely, substance abuse has eroded sociality by reducing civic engagement (Bruch et al. 2010). Deviance has ruined sociality by provoking social exclusion experienced (Backman and Nilsson 2011). Furthermore, religiosity espouses ideals against sociality as for the afterlife and heaven, extremism, and supernaturalness (Fontana 2003; Rip et al. 2012). Religiosity has arisen from hierarchicalism as an ideal against sociality (Saucier and Skrzypinska 2006). Religiosity may also breed the ideal for violence to undermine sociality (Muluk et al. 2013). The ideal for the afterlife would sustain sociality by impeding risking (Kasser 2016). Extremism has impeded sociality by provoking protesting (Moreira et al. 2018). The ideal for supernaturalness can hamper sociality by fomenting risking (Parker and Stanworth 2005).

Norms for sociality impeded by religiosity have popularized security (Coffe and Geys 2007). The norm for security has enhanced sociality by maintaining neighboring, social cohesion, and trust and reducing aggression and opposition (Barbarin and Richter 2001; Grannis 2009; Rochelle 2015). The norm for government has embraced communitarianism, coordination, institutionalism, and republicanism to uphold sociality (Chahboun 2024; Jessop 2016; Prokhovnik 2008). Institutionalism maintains sociality by emphasizing communication, relatedness, and social order (Jessop 2016). Religiosity has also arisen from norms against government to disrupt sociality (Corstange and York 2018). The norm for government has embraced communitarianism, coordination, institutionalism, and republicanism to uphold sociality (Chahboun 2024; Jessop 2016; Prokhovnik 2008). Institutionalism maintains sociality by emphasizing communication, relatedness, and social order (Jessop 2016). Conversely, religiosity can evolve from norms for individualization and inequality to impede sociality (Jasso 2002; Lane 1991). The norm for individualization inhibits sociality by featuring competition, deintegration, disembeddedness, disengagement, independence, inequality, risk, and self-indulgence (Bauman 2001; Beck and Beck-Gernsheim 2002; Burgess 2018; Dannreuther and Perren 2013; Krys et al. 2019; Stankov et al. 2014). The norm for inequality has impeded sociality by eroding social capital, support for redistribution and welfare, sympathy, trust, and volunteering (Busemeyer 2013; Hitlin and Harkness 2018; Lipford and Yandle 2009; Oishi et al. 2011; Portes and Vickstrom 2011). Conversely, the norm for inequality has impaired sociality by provoking crime and violence (Ousey and Lee 2013; van Wilsem 2007).

Hence, current and existing findings indicate faith in religion as a negative indicator of sociality. Religious faith thus opposes the positive indicators of sociality, including confidence in institutions, refutation against misdeeds, refutation against unconventional sexuality, rejection of outsiders, rejection of deviants, and trust in other people.

Chapter 3
Functioning of Personal Characteristics for Social Attitudes

Personal characteristics provide and register power, utility, ideals, and norms to fulfill functions required for social attitudes. These characteristics include gender, age, education, irreligion, marital status, living arrangements, parental immigration status, employment, work conditions, family income, and survey interest. Marital status includes being married, cohabited, divorced, separated, widowed, and unmarried. Living arrangements cover children and parents. Parental immigration covers the father and mother. Employment covers the status and sector. Employment status includes full-time employment, part-time employment, self-employment, retirement, homemaking, studying, and unemployment. Employment sectors cover public, private business, and nonprofit organization employment. Work conditions cover intellectual, creative, independent, and supervisory work. Meanwhile, social attitudes comprise confidence in institutions, refutation against misdeeds, refutation against unconventional sexuality, unfaith in religion, rejection of outsiders, rejection of deviants, and trust in other people to reflect sociality.

According to analytical functionalism, sociality regarding the seven social attitudes builds on power, utility, ideals, and norms regarding sociality. Such building hinges on the voluntaristic mechanisms of power realization to drive, utility optimization to attract, ideal calibration to rationalize, and norm conformity to assimilate sociality. The power, utility, ideals, and norms evolve from personal characteristics, as existing knowledge and current findings indicate.

Existing Knowledge

Personal characteristics generate and register power, utility, ideals, and norms to influence sociality and its attitudinal components. The influence is positive when the power, utility, ideals, and norms support or spring from sociality or social involvement. Conversely, the impact is negative when the power, utility, ideals, and norms

C.-k. Cheung, *Social Attitudes in the Early 21st Century*,
https://doi.org/10.1007/978-981-96-9705-2_3

obstruct or deviate from sociality or social involvement. Power rests on agency, arousal, assets, authority, capital, coercion, control, discipline, disposition, domination, functioning, income, information, knowledge, material, motivation, needs, prestige, prominence, resources, rules, skill, social class, social status, structure, and wealth (Dolinski 2016; Grealish et al. 2017; Haugaard 2020; C. Leung et al. 2014; Piven and Cloward 2005). Power bases comprise care received, health, knowledge, membership, material, and transcendence (Liu and Pratto 2018). Specifically, power for sociality has unfolded as attachment, attention, empathy, and punishment (Campos-Castillo and Hitlin 2013; Molm 1997). Utility inheres in achievement, belongingness, blessing received, company, comfort, enjoyment, fun, praise received, pride, savoring, satisfaction, security, and well-being (Ambrey and Fleming 2014; Haller and Hadler 2006; Isham et al. 2006; Jau and Hodgson 2018; Kubayashi and Kerbo 2012; Pavani and Colombo 2024). Ideals embody attitudes, beliefs, desires, evaluations, favors, goals, ideologies, identities, interests, intentions, opinions, preferences, prejudices, sentiments, values, willingness, and worldviews (Burton et al. 2021; Fabrigar et al. 2014; Ottati et al. 2014; Read and Simon 2012; Greenberg and Arndt 2012; Zunick et al. 2017). Norms are collective power, utility, and ideals. Hence, norms represent collective capital and identity (Huddy 2013; Kleinhans 2009). Specifically, norms characterize cultures, definitions, exposures, frames, institutions, media, persuasions, propaganda, roles, social constructions, and socialization (Chaney 2014; Jensen 2007; Klandermans and van Stekelenburg 2013; Kral 2019; Lahey and Waldman 2007; Markowitz 2001; Proctor and Niemeyer 2019; Wahlstrom 2011). Meanwhile, power driving sociality can stem from adaptability, agency, attrachment, care received, certainty, categorization, homophily, manipulation received, mentalizing, motivation, punishment, signaling ability as power realization, social intelligence, and stress (Boer and Fischer 2013; Fowers 2015; Phithakkitnukoon and Smoreda 2016; Tomasello 2014; Tuomela 2007). Utility attracting sociality can arise from exchange, collaboration, games, interdependence, reciprocity, and reward (Fowers 2015; Tuomela 2007). Ideals rationalizing sociality can favor collective identity, communality, and collective goals (Fowers 2015; Tomasello 2014; Tuomela 2007). Norms assimilating sociality can derive from culture, institutions, learning, and social interaction (Cottrell et al. 2007; Fowers 2015; Tuomela 2007).

Gender

Female gender (vs. male gender) is likely to maintain sociality regarding confidence in institutions, refutation against misdeeds, refutation against unconventional sexuality, unfaith in religion, rejection of outsiders, rejection of deviants, and trust in other people. Such maintenance engages the voluntaristic mechanisms of analytical functionalism to apply power, utility, ideals, and norms generated by female gender. These mechanisms exercise power realization, utility optimization, ideal calibration, and norm conformity. Power realization underlying gender impacts engages biological and biosocial functioning, dominance, evolution or constitution due to natural selection, overload, resources, status, supplies, and subordination (Feingold 1994; Fyall and Gazley 2015; Hopcroft 2016; Rundman and Glick 2008). Utility optimization underlying gender impacts engages exchange, expectancy, and social demand (Renfrow and Howard 2013; Valiente 2018). Ideal calibration underlying gender impacts engages (personal) construction and schemata (Franklin 2012). Norm conformity underlying gender impacts engages culture, learning, objectification, role, social construction, and social expectation (Carli 2013; Franklin 2012; Grijalva et al. 2015; Guimond et al. 2013; Kurz and Donaghue 2013).

Power for sociality arising from female gender has stemmed from agreeableness, cognitive complexity, extraversion, friendship, friends' provision, mastery, and political efficacy (Carbery and Buhrmester 1998; Caprara and Vecchione 2017; de Vries and Megathlin 2009; Dyck and Lascher 2009; Feingold 1994; S. Fer 2012; Hansen et al. 2012). Agreeableness has fostered sociality by enhancing attachment (Fraley et al. 2011). Moreover, agreeableness constitutes sociality by featuring communicn, compliance, cooperation, empathy, helping, intimacy, morality, politeness, prosociality, respect, solidarity, sympathy, understanding, warmth, and unity (Dinic and Bodroza 2021; Graziano and Tobin 2009; J. Sun et al. 2018). Cognitive complexity embraces resilience to enable sociality (R. Berger 2015). Resilience has attracted sociality by raising bonding and inhibiting crime and violence (Fields and McNamara 2003; Hoffman 2003; Solomon and Roloff 2018). Furthermore, resilience sustains sociality by embodying or fostering adaptation and legality (Hoffman 2003; Ungar 2012). Resilience also underlies sociality by demonstrating altruism, attractiveness, communication or conversation, community, compassion, empathy or perspective-taking, negotiation, peacefulness, relationality, relatedness, social capital or resourcefulness, social cohesion, and social competence (Elfers et al. 2024; Hjemdal et al. 2015; Jones and d'Errico 2019; Kelley et al. 2019; Kent and Davis 2010; Ungar 2010; Zautra 2014). Extraversion has buttressed sociality by fostering attachment, civic engagement, civility, donation, humor, nationalism, political participation, social capital, socializing, volunteering, and favor for civic and political participation (Bekkers 2010; C. Cheng et al. 2019; Fraley et al. 2011; Gotzsche-Astrup 2020; Hample 2018; Omoto et al. 2010; Schbley and McCauley 2005; Vernon et al. 2008; Ward and Forney 2020). Friendship has constituted sociality by enhancing community attachment, compliance, donation, gratitude, political participation, social cohesion, social desirability, social integration, and social trust (Corcoran 2013; Fahmy 2006; Gundert and Hohendanner 2015; Keillor et al. 2001; Kende et al. 2022; Opp 2001; Rotkirch 2014). Mastery has enhanced sociality by uplifting social trust (Burke and Stets 1999). Political efficacy facilitates sociality by raising donation, leadership, political discussion, and trust and lessening violence (X. Fu 2018; Huber et al. 2022; Sandovici and Davis 2010; Tausch et al. 2011; Weeks et al. 2017).

Utility for sociality arising from female gender has resided in interaction quality, life satisfaction, membership quality, purposefulness, relatedness, and relationship satisfaction (Hepper et al. 2020; Molana and Adams 2019; Prins et al. 1993; Tiliouine et al. 2006). Interaction quality, relatedness, or relationship satisfaction has consolidated sociality by consolidating sharing, social interaction, and relationship satisfaction (Downie et al. 2008; Frazer 1999; Wickham and Knee 2012). Life satisfaction has incubated sociality regarding political participation, social cohesion, social trust, and volunteering (E. Chan 2014; Flavin and Keane 2011; Rochelle 2015). Membership quality constitutes social capital (Child and Nikolova 2020). Social capital has consolidated sociality by raising civic engagement, community involvement, donation, political involvement, social trust, and volunteering (Bekkers et al. 2008; Broadbent and Papadopoulos 2011; Brown and Ferris 2007; Chua et al. 2021; Narayan and Cassidy 2001). Conversely, social capital has strengthened sociality by erasing violence (Pulkkinen et al. 2009). Purposefulness has underlain sociality by boosting civic practice, responsibility, and volunteering and reducing rejection experience (Duffy and Raque-Bogdan 2010; Summers and Falco 2020; Twenge et al. 2003). Conversely, disutility against sociality reduced by female gender has involved anger, political alienation, rejection experienced, and victimization (Charles and Carstensen 2008; de Coster 2005; Kaplan and Liu 2000; Weakliem and Borch 2006). Anger has jeopardized sociality by eroding social integration and fomenting protesting and violence and its tolerance (Krahe 2013; Molm 2008; Passini 2019; Tausch et al. 2011). Moreover, anger can dampen sociality by breeding crime and radicalism (Brant 2019; Larson et al. 2020). Rejection experienced has disturbed sociality by eroding closeness and prosocial behavior (Bockler et al. 2021; K. Lin et al. 2013). Political alienation erodes sociality regarding government trust (Kabashima et al. 2000). Victimization experienced has impaired sociality by eroding social trust (Olivera 2015). Conversely, victimization experienced has hurt sociality by activating conflict and migration (Bar-Tal and Halperin 2013; Ramesh et al. 2019).

Ideals for sociality maintained by female gender have valorized altruism, benevolence, caring, civic engagement, civility, conformity, cooperation, egalitarianism, friendship, government, government trust, patriotism, political agreement, political approval, recourse, tax paying, traditionalism, and transcendence (Caprara and Vecchione 2017; E. Daniel et al. 2022; Dietz et al. 2002; Eagly et al. 2004; S. Fer 2012; Hample 2018; Hooghe et al. 2015; Kunovich 2009; Lippa 2005; Maule and Goidel 2003; Morris and Klesner 2010; Norris 2011; Rentziou et al. 2011; Saunders and Wong 2012; Tamres et al. 2002; Treiman and Gartner 2006; Wallace and Pichler 2009; Wuthnow 2004). Altruism has constituted sociality by boosting attachment, civic engagement, friendship quality, likability, moral behavior, popularity, relatedness and diminishing loneliness and violence (Bond and Kwan 2000; W. Chen et al. 2022; Layous et al. 2012; Markiewicz et al. 2001; Martela and Ryan 2016; Mesch 2009; Na and Paternoster 2019; L. Taylor et al. 2018; Wright and Li 2011). Benevolence has upheld sociality by enhancing government trust and likability (Patricio et al. 2022). Caring has constituted sociality by securing religiosity and volunteering (Barr et al. 2005). Civic engagement has propped sociality by strengthening attachment, civility, collective behavior, discussion, donation, neighboring, patriotism, prosociality, social capital, socialism, trust, and volunteering and impeding cheating and individualism (Coffe and Geys 2007; Gilberbloom and Markham 1995; Kerrissey and Schofer 2013; Mata and Pendakur 2014; Ozbay 2008; Pattie et al. 2004; Pena-Lopez and Sanchez-Santos 2016; Rahn 2008; Richey 2011;

Tak 2017; M. Tang 2011; Taniguchi 2013; Yip et al. 2007). Civility has constituted sociality by inducing fairness and trust (Vera-Toscano et al. 2013). Additionally, civility maintains sociality by enhancing the commonweal, community, equality, friendship, reciprocity, and social capital (Hudson 2023). The ideal for conformity has built sociality regarding xenophobia or rejection of outsiders (Costa et al. 2023). Cooperation has strengthened sociality regarding attachment and trustworthiness as opposed to argument (Gerbasi and Cook 2008; Hample 2018; Tak 2017). Egalitarianism has underpinned sociality by enhancing empathy, support for welfare, and trust in government and impeding radicalism (Faricy and Ellis 2014; Lauriola et al. 2015; Lucas and Kteily 2018; Roosma et al. 2014). The ideal for friendship has fostered sociality by embracing help, honesty, respect, similarity, and trust (Galupo and Gonzalez 2013; Wuthnow 2004). The ideal for government has sustained sociality by dampening protesting (Schofer and Fourcade-Gourinchas 2001). Political agreement and approval reflect government trust (McGraw et al. 2002). Government trust has constituted sociality by sustaining compliance, conformity, nationalism, political participation, and preventing protesting (Rhodes-Purdy et al. 2023; Ulbig 2002; van der Meer and van Ingen 2009; V. Vu 2021). Patriotism has consolidated sociality by uplifting prosociality, social cohesion, volunteering, and xenophobia (Granzin and Olsen 1998; Ishii 2009; Straume and Odeen 2010; Vida and Reardon 2008; Y. Yang et al. 2010). Recourse reflects sociality regarding affiliation and social support received (Ledbetter et al. 2013; Sullivan 2001). Tax-paying buttressed sociality by representing compliance (Kirchler et al. 2006). Traditionalism has buttressed sociality by enhancing patriotism and faith in religion and discouraging protesting and accepting deviants and outsiders (Costa et al. 2023; Datler et al. 2013; Meuleman et al. 2019; Schwartz et al. 2014). Transcending has advanced sociality by raising prosocial behavior and social inclusion (Guan et al. 2009; Heilman and Kusev 2020). Female gender also enhances sociality by embracing communality (Diekman and Schneider 2010). Communality developed from female gender comprises caring, helping, and nurturing (Fyall and Gazley 2015). Communality has constituted sociality by securing civility, cooperation, prosocial behavior, and religiousness and preventing extremism (Hample 2018; Harzing 2006; Oyserman et al. 1998; Saucier and Skrzypinska 2006; Thielmann et al. 2020). Conversely, ideals against sociality diminished by female gender have emphasized aggression, cosmopolitanism, cynicism, independence, individualism, individualist attribution, neoliberalism, privatization, protesting, and sexual desire (Cornell and Grimes 2015; Hample 2018; Jakobsen 2010; Kirk and Papachristos 2011; Larsen 2006; Lippa 2005; Norris and Inglehart 2009; Pichler 2009; Prins et al. 1993; Welzel 2013). Aggression has undermined sociality by breeding antisociality, crime and recidivism, blaming, conflict, hostility, rejecting others, and impairing agreeableness, morality, and responsibility (Asendorpf et al. 2008; Del Bove et al. 2008; Morrison 2006; Scholte et al. 2009; Vitaro et al. 2007). Cosmopolitanism has eroded sociality by discounting religiosity and raising liberalism and acceptance of deviants and outsiders (Costa et al. 2023; Motschenbacher 2013; Norris and Inglehart 2009). Cynicism has undermined sociality by eroding government and social trust, patriotism, and political participation and raising competition (Flanagan and

Lee 2003; Guan et al. 2010; Uslaner 2002; van der Meer and van Ingen 2009). Independence has impeded sociality by reducing justification for the system and the norm for legitimacy (Blanchar and Eidelman 2013). Individualism has weakened sociality by reducing civic engagement, religiousness, social cohesion, and volunteering (Church 2010; Green and Janmaat 2011; J. He et al. 2014; Hener et al. 2016; Leong 2008; Pollack and Pickel 2007; Whitford et al. 2006). Conversely, individualism has impeded sociality by bolstering acceptance of outsiders, competition, crime, extremity, self-enhancement, protesting, and violence (Church 2010; J. He et al. 2014; Karstedt 2010; Leong 2008; Li and Song 1992; Pollack and Pickel 2007; Whitford et al. 2006). Voluntarism can fuel protesting to disrupt sociality (Tsai 2019). Neoliberalism espouses atomization and silos and disregards ethics and social services to undermine sociality (Lobao et al. 2014; Lakoff 2009; Rhodes-Purdy et al. 2023; Smart 2003). Featuring denationalization, privatization hinders sociality by raising foreign ownership (Denisova et al. 2009; Tang 1998). Protesting has impaired sociality by escalating distancing and radicalism and dampening moral motivation (Kutlaca et al. 2020; Vestergren et al. 2017). Besides, protesting impedes sociality by embracing antisociality, conflict, extremism, hostility, incivility, illegality, rioting, social exclusion, terrorism, and violence (Renger et al. 2020; Kaplan and Liu 2000; S. Lo 2021; McCright and Dunlap 2008; Morselli and Passini 2018; Smidt 2020; Stewart et al. 2012; Swart et al. 2020; Tan and Snow 2015). Sexual desire has disrupted sociality by breeding risking (Moran et al. 2021).

Norms against sociality reduced by female gender have populatized problems, risks, and violence (Niemi et al. 1999; Scharrer 2008; Trumbo et al. 2008). The norm for problems has impaired sociality by jeopardizing civility, government and social trust, and political participation and breeding deviance (Backman and Nilsson 2011; Fahmy 2006; Marschall and Stolle 2004; Nicholls and Picou 2012). The norm for risk has impaired sociality by provoking protesting (Scafuto and La Barbera 2016). Moreover, the risk norm can hurt sociality by generating opposition to the establishment (P. Brown 2020). The norm for violence has weakened sociality by boosting antisocial behavior and victimization (Ehrensuft et al. 2003; Krahe 2013).

Age

Age is likely to generate power, utility, ideals, and norms to elevate sociality through the voluntaristic mechanisms of power realization, utility optimization, ideal calibration, and norm conformity to achieve the functions of sociality. Power realization can engage activity, adaptation, balance, capital, maturity, and resiliency (Charles and Carstensen 2009; Marcum 2013; Michaeli et al. 2022; Von Krogh and Wallin 2011). Maturity comprises agreeableness, conscientiousness, emotional stability, positivity, and reflectivity (Michaeli et al. 2022). Ideal calibration can accentuate closeness, friendship, generativity, kinship, presentness, and time-limitedness as opposed to self-centeredness (Crafter et al. 2019; Morgan and Robinson 2013; Ramsey and Gentzler 2015; Wagner and Lang 2011). Notably, sociality covers confidence in institutions, refutation against misdeeds, refutation against unconventional sexuality, unfaith in religion, rejection of outsiders, rejection of deviants, and trust in other people.

Power for sociality increased by age has stemmed from affordability, agreeableness, empathy, extraversion, family functioning, knowledge, maturity, organizational membership, self-efficacy, social network homogeneity and proximity, and stability (Bleidorn et al. 2013; Brundidge and Rice 2009; Carreras 2018; Fuller-Iglesias and Antonucci 2016; Fung and Ng 2006; Hallerod 2006; Juhl et al. 2019; Molana and Adams 2019; Price et al. 2006; Roberts and DelVecchio 2000; Smith and Hamon 2012). Affordability has advanced sociality by elevating recourse and responsibility (A. He 2019; J. Chen 2012). Agreeableness has fostered sociality by enhancing attachment (Fraley et al. 2011). Moreover, agreeableness constitutes sociality by featuring communion, compliance, cooperation, empathy, helping, intimacy, morality, politeness, prosociality, respect, solidarity, sympathy, understanding, warmth, and unity (Dinic and Bodroza 2021; Graziano and Tobin 2009; J. Sun et al. 2018). Empathy has elevated sociality by facilitating prosocial behavior (Fraser et al. 2012). Extraversion has buttressed sociality by fostering attachment, civic engagement, civility, donation, humor, nationalism, political participation, social capital, socializing, volunteering, and favor for civic and political participation (Bekkers 2010; C. Cheng et al. 2019; Fraley et al. 2011; Gotzsche-Astrup 2020; Hample 2018; Omoto et al. 2010; Schbley and McCauley 2005; Vernon et al. 2008; Ward and Forney 2020). Family functioning experienced represents interdependency and social capital (Parke 2004; White et al. 2015). Moreover, family functioning features attentiveness, caring, compassion, empathy, mutuality, and socialization (Herr 2012; Parke 2004). As such, family functioning experienced has facilitated sociality by raising social support received and reducing social avoidance (F. Liu et al. 2024). Generally, knowledge has raised sociality by enhancing cooperation, prosocial behavior, social cohesion, social trust, and volunteering (de Groot and Steg 2009; Lepkowski and Couper 2002; Pattie et al. 2004; Simon-Bemd and Steffens 2000; Volker et al. 2007;). Maturity has upheld sociality by encouraging conformity and prosocial behavior (Fetvadjiev and He 2019). Moreover, maturity sustains sociality by featuring conformity, generativity, harmony, intimacy, morality, social interest, understanding as opposed to rebellion (Browning and Cooper 2004; Hale 1999; Hendry and Kloep 2012; Hwang and Chang 2009). Organizational membership has constituted sociality by strengthening institutional commitment and conformity (Vartanian and Hopkinson 2010). Social network homogeneity and proximity constitute social capital (Caulkins 2009; Rivera 2018). Social capital has consolidated sociality by raising civic engagement, community involvement, donation, political involvement, social trust, and volunteering (Bekkers et al. 2008; Broadbent and Papadopoulos 2011; Brown and Ferris 2007; Chua et al. 2021; Narayan and Cassidy 2001). Conversely, social capital has strengthened sociality by erasing violence (Pulkkinen et al. 2009). Stability has secured sociality, including civic engagement, cohesion, neighboring, and relational quality, as opposed to violence (Pulkkinen et al. 2009; C. Ross et al. 2000; Swaroop and Morenoff 2006; Villarreal and Silva 2006).

Conversely, power or dispositions against sociality reduced by age have involved hostility, impulsivity, and neuroticism (Meuleman et al. 2019; Tirmizi et al. 2009). Hostility impedes sociality by embodying competition, conflict, protesting, and violence (Canary et al. 2013; Koerner 2018; Renger et al. 2020; Webster and Kirkpatrick 2006). Impulsivity has impeded sociality by diminishing prosocial behavior and engendering protesting, radicalism, and violence (Breakwell 2007; Koehler and Fiebig 2019; Thielmann et al. 2020; Wright and DeLisi 2016). Neuroticism has impaired sociality by reducing attachment security, civic engagement, coordination, forgiveness, nationalism, relatedness, and socializing and generating crime and hostility (Bekkers 2005; Fraley et al. 2011; Hounkpatin et al. 2015; Kalish 2008; Marks 1996; Mullet et al. 2005; Pulkkinen et al. 2009; Schbley and McCauley 2005; Ward and Forney 2020).

Utility for sociality elevated by age has lain in the community sense, gratitude, identity achievement, meaningfulness, resilience, satisfaction, self-confidence, self-esteem, and positive affect or emotion generally (Chen and Davey 2009; Cherry et al. 2023; Ferssizidis et al. 2010; Howe 2010; Sneed et al. 2006; Krumrei-Mancuso 2017; A. Lau et al. 2008; Steger et al. 2009; Tomas et al. 2013). Gratitude constitutes sociality through expressing or raising morality, social awareness, liking, and understanding and reducing avoidance (Eibach et al. 2015; Tudge et al. 2022; Kloos et al. 2022). Identity achievement facilitates sociality by raising belongingness (Reese et al. 2019). Meaningfulness has underlain sociality by boosting civic practice, responsibility, and volunteering and reducing rejection experience (Duffy and Raque-Bogdan 2010; Summers and Falco 2020; Twenge et al. 2003). Resilience has attracted sociality by raising bonding and inhibiting crime and violence (Fields and McNamara 2003; Hoffman 2003; Solomon and Roloff 2018). Furthermore, resilience sustains sociality by embodying or fostering adaptation and legality (Hoffman 2003; Ungar 2012). Resilience also underlies sociality by demonstrating altruism, attractiveness, communication or conversation, community, compassion, empathy or perspective-taking, negotiation, peacefulness, relationality, relatedness, social capital or resourcefulness, social cohesion, and social competence (Elfers et al. 2024; Hjemdal et al. 2015; Jones and d'Errico 2019; Kelley et al. 2019; Kent and Davis 2010; Ungar 2010; Zautra 2014). Satisfaction has covered life, the nation, and relationships (Chen and Davey 2009; Ferssizidis et al. 2010; Russell et al. 2008). The sense of community constitutes sociality (Fowers 2015). Satisfaction has advanced sociality by strengthening political participation, social cohesion, social and government trust, and volunteering (E. Chan 2014; Flavin and Keane 2011; Rochelle 2015). Well-being has uplifted sociality by consolidating altruism, conformism, cooperation, donation, liking for people, prosociality, sociability, and trust and social trust (Fetvadjiev and He 2019; A. Hu 2013; Lyubomirsky et al. 2006; Y. Pan et al. 2023; Wang and Graddy 2008). Self-confidence or self-esteem has buttressed sociality by raising attachment security, political participation, and prosociality and preventing suicide (Kitayama and Markus 2000; Tracy et al. 2009). Positive affect has maintained sociality by raising government trust and patriotism (Hunt et al. 2019; Turner and Stets 2005).

Disutility against sociality diminished by age has lain in anger, depression, financial stress and strain, jealousy, neighborhood disorder, and negative affect generally (Bauer et al. 2008; Caplan and Schooler 2007; Charles and Carstensen 2008; Ferssizidis et al. 2010; Stanley et al. 2014; Villarreal and Silva 2006). Anger has jeopardized sociality by eroding social integration and fomenting protesting and violence and its tolerance (Krahe 2013; Molm 2008; Passini 2019; Tausch et al. 2011). Moreover, anger can dampen sociality by breeding crime and radicalism (Brant 2019; Larson et al. 2020). Financial stress or strain has impaired economic satisfaction, health, and even self-transcendence, which connects the self to nature and/or other people (Reeskens and Vandecasteele 2017). Jealousy has hampered sociality by fomenting aggression and violence (Felson and Outlaw 2007). Neighborhood disorder has eroded sociality by weakening community attachment and social capital and fomenting victimization (G. Brown et al. 2004; Congdon 2010; Like 2011). Negative affect has undermined sociality by fomenting resistance and impeding social capital and trust (Pulkkinen et al. 2009; Webber and Huxley 2007).

Ideals for sociality fostered by age have highlighted accommodating, altruism, birth, community attachment, conservatism, generativity, influencing others, interpersonal interaction, interdependence, marriage, moralism, morality, organizational involvement, political discussion, political identification, sharing, traditionalism, trust, transcendence, and volunteering (Boulianne et al. 2022; E. Daniel et al. 2022; Clark 2004a; Cornelis et al. 2009; Lu and Kao 2002; Gubernskaya 2010; Howe 2010; Inglehart 2003; Isaacowitz et al. 2003; Kaufmann et al. 2012; Krumrei-Mancuso 2017; Moticjunaite and Kravchenko 2008; Norris and Inglehart 2009; Nussio 2019; Penningroth and Scott 2012; Sneed et al. 2006; Y. Zhang et al. 2005). Accommodation can sustain sociality by raising loving (Aron et al. 2006). Moreover, accommodation experienced has constituted sociality by strengthening cooperation and preventing suicide (Duberstein et al. 2004; Lepkowski and Couper 2002). Altruism has constituted sociality by boosting attachment, civic engagement, friendship quality, likability, moral behavior, popularity, relatedness and diminishing loneliness and violence (Bond and Kwan 2000; W. Chen et al. 2022; Layous et al. 2012; Markiewicz et al. 2001; Martela and Ryan 2016; Mesch 2009; Na and Paternoster 2019; L. Taylor et al. 2018; Wright and Li 2011). Birth has raised sociality by enhancing civic engagement, community involvement, conformism, donation, social capital, social cohesion, social integration, social interaction, social support received, and volunteering (Apinunmahakul and Devlin 2008; Bjornberg and Ekbrand 2008; Frei et al. 2009; Ghimire 2021a; Kleinhans et al. 2007; Magdol and Bessel 2003; Taniguichi and Thomas 2011; Wilkinson 2008; Xiao 2000; Xu and Lai 2002). Conversely, birth has advanced sociality by reducing social distance and violence (Broom et al. 2013; Tsai 2006). Community attachment has facilitated sociality regarding cooperation, networking, and trust (Groves et al. 2000; Molitor et al. 2011; Rochelle 2015). Conservatism sustains sociality by nurturing empathy, loyalty, prosocial behavior, religiousness, and sacrifice (Dutton and Rayner-Hilles 2022). Moreover, conservatism underpins sociality by maintaining allegiance or loyalty, attachment, civility, community, conformity, cooperation, discipline, ethnocentrism, honesty, humility, intimacy, legality, morality, nationalism, obedience, order, partnership, patriotism, peace, responsibility, sharing, trust, and xenophobia (Dutton and Rayner-Hilles 2022; Heilman and Kusev 2020; Hickson 2013; Lakoff 2009; Rhodes-Purdy et al. 2023; Scruton 2014; Yoos 2007; Zuk and Zuk 2020). Conversely, conservatism upholds sociality by condemning dehumanizing, evilness, revolution, sexuality, terrorism, and transgression. Generativity means caring and concern for others (Cote 2000; Peterson and Klohnen 1995). As such, generativity has enhanced sociality by raising helping value and political participation (Peterson and Klohnen 1995). Social influence has enhanced sociality by boosting attachment, empathy, giving, punishment, and xenophobia (Campos-Castillo and Hitlin 2013; Molm 1997; Schwartz et al. 2014). Social interaction has realized sociality by consolidating altruism, compliance, cooperation, donation, morality, political participation, reciprocity, social trust, and volunteering (Guillen et al. 2011; Dixon and McKeown 2021; Lucas and Livingston 2014; Musick 2000; Rodrigo-Gonzalez et al. 2019; Rubin and Step 2000). Interdependence has buttressed sociality by securing attachment, donation, prosocial behavior, social inclusion, and social interaction (Feeney and Collins 2001; Uskul et al. 2004; Z. Xin et al. 2017). Marriage has consolidated sociality by enhancing community attachment, community evaluation, community involvement, civic engagement, closeness experienced, donation, friendship satisfaction, neighboring, political participation, prosocial behavior, reciprocity, relationship quality, social capital, social cohesion, social integration, social interaction, social support received, and trust (W. Chang 2009; Cornwall 2009; Degenne et al. 2004; Flavin and Keane 2011; Frye 2007; Kerrissey and Schofer 2013; Lizardo 2006; Louis and Zhao 2002; Mata and Pendakur 2014; McCabe 2014; Prezza et al. 2001; Ross and Mirowsky 2009; Sampson and Raudenbush 2004; Swaroop and Morenoff 2006; Tolsma et al. 2009). Conversely, marriage has upheld sociality by reducing crime, discrimination experienced, loneliness, social exclusion experienced, tolerance for deviance, and violence (Carr and Friedman 2005; Coffe and Geys 2007; Koromeckyj-Cox et al. 2007; Savolainen 2009; E. Wojcieszak and Mutz 2009; E. Wright et al. 2015). Moralism has sustained sociality by boosting gratitude (Pohling et al. 2010). Moreover, moralism can enhance sociality regarding social trust (Bersot and Arrigo 2015; Steinhardt 2012). Inherently, moralism embraces altruism, consensus, legality, obligation, and virtue to maintain sociality (R. Brown 2018). Morality has constituted sociality by boosting volunteering and inhibiting violence (Piquero and Hickman 2002; Whitford et al. 2006). Organizational involvement has fostered sociality by enhancing attachment, civility, political participation, social integration, socialism (favor), and trust (Geys 2012; Guillen et al. 2011; Pattie et al. 2004; Tak 2017). Political participation has buttressed sociality regarding civility (Campbell 2003). Sharing has constituted sociality by strengthening leadership and neighboring (Dubois et al. 2020; Grannis 2009). Moreover, sharing constitutes sociality regarding friendship (Launay and Dunbar 2015). Sharing can also underlie sociality by boosting morality, punishment, and social cohesion (N. Duncan 2017; Delton and Krasnow 2017). Traditionalism has buttressed sociality by enhancing patriotism and faith in religion and discouraging protesting and acceptance of deviants and outsiders (Costa et al. 2023; Datler et al. 2013; Meuleman et al. 2019; Schwartz et al. 2014). Trust has constituted sociality through donation, involvement, and volunteering (Uslaner 2000). Transcending has advanced sociality by raising prosocial behavior and social inclusion (Guan et al. 2009; Heilman and Kusev 2020).

Volunteering has constituted sociality by raising altruism, charity orientation, civic motivation, donation, helping, moral responsibility, political participation, social integration, and social and government trust (Foster et al. 2001; Isham et al. 2006; Richey 2010; Richey and Ikeda 2009; Wiepking and Maas 2009). Conversely, volunteering has safeguarded sociality by preventing deviance and its tolerance, delinquency, and loneliness (Gillath et al. 2005; J. Wilson 2000; Woolley 2003). Conversely, ideals against sociality diminished by age have hailed addiction, capitalism, deviance and its tolerance, globalization, hedonism, privatization, protesting, risking, and self-focus (Charles and Carstensen 2008; Cheung and Lai 2020; Defoe et al. 2015; Edwards 2006; Hraba et al. 2001; Howe 2010; Tao and Thogersen 2019; Tilley 2002; Vauclair and Fischer 2011; Wilska 2002). Addiction has hampered sociality by withdrawing power, utility, ideals, and norms for sociality and creating power, utility, ideals, and norms against sociality. The ideal for capitalism impedes sociality by boosting narcissism and disrupting mutuality (De Vos 2010; Young and Reynolds 2017). Moreover, the ideal for capitalism undermines sociality by embracing competition, conflict, and egoism (Bernstein 2012; S. Hall 2014; LaMothe 2012). Conversely, the ideal for capitalism weakens sociality by dispelling collectivism, reciprocity, socialism, and statism (Beardsworth 2011; Bernstein 2012).

A norm for sociality raised by age has popularized equality (Barker and Tinnick 2006). The norm for equality has fostered sociality by championing cohesion and its experience, fairness, justice, social capital, sympathy, trust, and volunteering (Eriksson et al. 2015; Green et al. 2003; Hitlin and Harkness 2018; Musick and Wilson 2008; Oishi et al. 2011; Portes and Vickstrom 2011; van Oorschot and Arts 2005).

Mid-age, or the reverse of age squared, is likely to dampen sociality by restraining power, utility, ideals, and norms for sociality. Notably, age squared means old or young in the presence of age in linear regression analysis.

Power for sociality weakened by mid-age has rested on affordability, family incomes, friendship, organizational membership, and savings (Anderson and Nevitte 2006; Apinunmahakul and Devlin 2008; Hallerod 2006; Prouteau and Wolff 2008; van Praag and Ferrer-I-Carbonell 2004). Affordability has advanced sociality by elevating recourse and responsibility (A. He 2019; J. Chen 2012). Family income has buttressed sociality by raising civility, civic engagement, community involvement, compliance, donation, friendliness, nationalism, political participation, social capital, social integration, social interaction, social support received, social trust (Alnsour and Meaton 2009; Crowder et al. 2006; Doff and Kleinhans 2011; Kleinhans et al. 2007; La Grange and Yip 2001; Lennartsson 2010; Norris and Inglehart 2009; Oliver 2003; Shin 2012; Wiepking and Maas 2009; Q. Xu et al. 2010). Conversely, family income has sustained sociality by preventing crime, discrimination experienced, sleeping, and social exclusion experienced (Cerin and Leslie 2008; Hamermesh 2019; Moore and Aweiss 2003; Stanley et al. 2011).

Utility for sociality reduced by mid-age has involved well-being, including democracy, environment, financial, housing, job, leisure, and marital satisfaction (Graham and Pettinato 2002b; van Praag and Ferrer-I-Carbonell 2004; van Praag et al. 2003; Zagorski 2011). Satisfaction has advanced sociality by strengthening political participation, social cohesion, social and government trust, and volunteering (E. Chan 2014; Flavin and Keane 2011; Rochelle 2015). Well-being has uplifted sociality by consolidating altruism, conformism, cooperation, donation, liking for people, prosociality, sociability, and trust and social trust (Fetvadjiev and He 2019; A. Hu 2013; Lyubomirsky et al. 2006; Y. Pan et al. 2023; Wang and Graddy 2008). Conversely, disutility for sociality enhanced by mid-age has arisen from political alienation (Coffe and Geys 2007). Political alienation erodes sociality regarding government trust (Kabashima et al. 2000).

Ideals for sociality dampened by mid-age have treasured charity, civic engagement, community participation, political participation, political and social trust, social cohesion, social interaction, and volunteering (Brown and Ferris 2007; Fridberg and Kangas 2008b; Glaeser and Gottlieb 2006; Ikeda and Richey 2005; Marien 2011; Richey 2007; Traunmuller 2011; van Tienen et al. 2011; Wilkinson 2008). The ideal for charity upholds sociality by embracing altruism, compassion, mercy, and volunteering (Apinunmahakul and Devlin 2008; Eggemeier and Fritz 2020; Musick and Wilson 2008; Pommier et al. 2020). Civic engagement has propped sociality by strengthening attachment, civility, collective behavior, discussion, donation, neighboring, patriotism, prosociality, social capital, socialism, trust, and volunteering and impeding cheating and individualism (Coffe and Geys 2007; Gilberbloom and Markham 1995; Kerrissey and Schofer 2013; Mata and Pendakur 2014; Ozbay 2008; Pattie et al. 2004; Pena-Lopez and Sanchez-Santos 2016; Rahn 2008; Richey 2011; Tak 2017; M. Tang 2011; Taniguchi 2013; Yip et al. 2007). Community participation has facilitated sociality regarding cooperation, networking, and trust (Groves et al. 2000; Molitor et al. 2011; Rochelle 2015). Political trust has constituted sociality by sustaining compliance, conformity, nationalism, political participation, and preventing protesting (Rhodes-Purdy et al. 2023; Ulbig 2002; van der Meer and van Ingen 2009; V. Vu 2021). Social trust has constituted sociality through donation, involvement, and volunteering (Uslaner 2000). Social cohesion has constituted sociality by enhancing attachment and dampening tolerance for deviance (Stafford et al. 2005; Woosnam et al. 2018). Social interaction has realized sociality by consolidating altruism, compliance, cooperation, donation, morality, political participation, reciprocity, social trust, and volunteering (Guillen et al. 2011; Dixon and McKeown 2021; Lucas and Livingston 2014; Musick 2000; Rodrigo-Gonzalez et al. 2019; Rubin and Step 2000). Volunteering has constituted sociality by raising altruism, charity orientation, civic motivation, donation, helping, moral responsibility, political participation, social integration, and social and government trust (Foster et al. 2001; Isham et al. 2006; Richey 2010; Richey and Ikeda 2009; Wiepking and Maas 2009).

Conversely, an ideal against sociality raised by mid-age has emphasized religiosity (Apinunmahakul and Devlin 2008). Religiosity has hindered sociality by reducing nationalism and social interaction and engendering protesting, marginalization experienced, radicalism, and social distance (Ayalon et al. 1993; Kunovich 2009; Norris 2002; Pedahzur and Canetti-Nisim 2004; Wuthnow 2004).

The norm for sociality diminished by mid-age has popularized government responsiveness (T. Shi 2000). The norm for government responsiveness has upgraded sociality by advancing justice perceived, social harmony perceived, and institutional, political, and social trust and preventing suicide (Grimes 2006; Heatherington and Globetti 2002; Helliwell 2006; R. Taylor et al. 2015; Wong and Shik 2011; C. Wong et al. 2005).

Education

Education, also indicated by graduation age, represents human capital, learning, social position, and study interest (Dolton et al. 2004; Horowitz 2018; Nordin 2011; Papastephanon 2015). As such, education is likely to sustain sociality by generating power, utility, ideals, and norms to achieve functions required for sociality. Such generation applies the voluntaristic mechanisms of power realization, utility optimization, ideal calibration, and norm conformity. Specifically, these mechanisms engage credentials, enlightenment, human capital, ideological refinement, instruction, social identity, and social interest (Horowitz 2018; Kuppens et al. 2018; Wodtke 2012; Yair 2003). Instruction poses challenge, competition, excitation, and surprise to build creativity and self-discovery (Yair 2003).

Power for sociality enhanced by education has rested on civic skill, conscientiousness, earnings or income, empathy, employment, friendship, health and mental health, intelligence, knowledge, mastery, memory, organizational membership, physical functioning, self-efficacy, social class, social competence, social networking, social support received, verbal ability, and youthfulness (Bullock 2021; Cerin and Leslie 2008; Corcoran et al. 2011; Keightley et al. 2006; Keyes 2002; Miyata et al. 2008; Pettigrew 2002; Prouteau and Wolff 2008; Rossi 2001; Schnittker and Behrman 2012; Shin 2012; Straughn and Andriot 2011; Stavrova and Ehlebracht 2018; Stevens et al. 2001; van Praag and Frijters 1999; Verba et al. 1995). Civic, social competence, or social skills have facilitated sociality by raising civility, civic engagement, political participation, prosocial behavior, social cohesion, and social trust (Foschi and Lauriola 2014; Halvorsen 2007; Letki 2008). Conscientiousness has elevated sociality by consolidating attachment, compliance, order value, responsibility, social desirability, and volunteering reducing deviance, violence, and justification for unconventional sexuality (Bekkers 2005; de Jong et al. 2012; Fraley et al. 2011; Gotzsche-Astrup 2020; Mondak and Hurwitz 2012; Mullet et al. 2005; Saucier and Skrzypinska 2006; Twardawski et al. 2021; Wright and DeLisi 2016). Income has upheld sociality by boosting civic engagement, community attachment and involvement, civic dutifulness, civility, conformity value, neighboring, political interest and participation, political and social trust, prosocial behavior, social capital, social integration, social interaction, social support received, social well-being, and volunteering (Bjornberg and Latta 2007; Chang 2009; Djupe and Lewis 2015; Frei et al. 2009; Kerrissey and Schofer 2013; Letki 2006; McCabe 2014; Patulny and Morris 2012; Son and Wilson 2012; Sun and Wang 2012; Swaroop and Morenoff 2006; Ulbig 2002). Conversely, income has maintained sociality by dampening alienation, discrimination experienced, migration, protesting, relocation, social deprivation experienced, social exclusion experienced, victimization, and violence (Broom et al. 2013; Brown and Connell 2004; Buck 2001; Rijken and Groenewegen 2008; V. Taylor et al. 2009; Weakliem and Borch 2006). Empathy has elevated sociality by facilitating prosocial behavior (Fraser et al. 2012). Employment has facilitated sociality by elevating civic engagement, community involvement, donation, philanthropy value, political discussion, political participation, social capital, social functioning, social cohesion experienced, social interaction, and social trust (Anciaes et al. 2017; Fridberg and Kangas 2008b; Kerrissey and Schofer 2013; H. Lu et al. 2002; Ross and Mirowsky 2009; Tsai 2006). Conversely, employment has safeguarded sociality by lessening crime, relocation, and social exclusion experienced (Groot et al. 2007; Kleinhans 2009; Savolainen 2009). Friendship has constituted sociality by enhancing community attachment, compliance, donation, gratitude, political participation, social cohesion, social desirability, social integration, and social trust (Corcoran 2013; Fahmy 2006; Gundert and Hohendanner 2015; Keillor et al. 2001; Kende et al. 2022; Opp 2001; Rotkirch 2014). Health has uplifted sociality by boosting community sense, morality, popularity, social activity, social cohesion, social integration, social trust, social well-being, and volunteering (Huxhold et al. 2014; Jorgensen et al. 2010; Son and Wilson 2012; Tolsma et al. 2009; Yu and Chiu 2016). Intelligence has raised sociality by facilitating donation and social capital and reducing criminality and protesting (Cornwall 2009; Feinstein and Bynner 2006; Paterson 2008; Piferi et al. 2006). Generally, knowledge has raised sociality by enhancing cooperation, prosocial behavior, social cohesion, social trust, and volunteering (de Groot and Steg 2009; Lepkowski and Couper 2002; Pattie et al. 2004; Simon-Bemd and Steffens 2000; Volker et al. 2007). Mastery has enhanced sociality by uplifting social trust (Burke and Stets 1999). Memory has facilitated sociality by strengthening role-taking (Henry et al. 2009). Moreover, memory can maintain sociality by preventing suicide (Van Orden et al. 2010). Organizational membership has constituted sociality by strengthening institutional commitment and conformity (Vartanian and Hopkinson 2010). Physical functioning has sustained sociality by enriching social capital (Cornwall 2009). Self-efficacy has sustained sociality by raising civic engagement, donation, government and social trust, leadership, political participation, prosocial behavior, and social activity (Bednall et al. 2013; Frye 2007; Gnambs and Batinic 2012; Huber et al. 2022; Mangum 2012; Rahn 2008; Pei and Pan 2018; Yao and Enright 2019). Social class has sustained sociality by raising adaptation, civic engagement, cohesion, institutional and political trust, organizational involvement and membership, prosocial behavior, social capital, social support received, and volunteering (E. Chan 2014; Elchardus and De Keere 2013; La Grange 2011; Lennartsson 2010; Letki 2008; Mutaner et al. 2002; Wallace and Pichler 2009; Wuthnow 2004; Yeh et al. 2013; Zhong 2010).

Conversely, social class has maintained sociality by preventing crime and social exclusion experienced (Agnew and Brezina 2010; Buck 2001). Social networking or social capital has consolidated sociality by raising civic engagement, community involvement, donation, political involvement, social trust, and volunteering (Bekkers et al. 2008; Broadbent and Papadopoulos 2011; Brown and Ferris 2007; Chua et al. 2021; Narayan and Cassidy 2001). Conversely, social capital has strengthened sociality by erasing violence (Pulkkinen et al. 2009). Social support received has strengthened sociality by enhancing attachment, gratitude, political participation, prosocial behavior, recourse, respect, responsibility, social integration, and social well-being (Boezeman and Ellemers 2008; Fahmy 2006; Phipps 2003; Williams and Galliher 2006; R. Wright et al. 2009; Zeldin et al. 2016; Zeng et al. 2024). Conversely, social support received has boosted sociality by preventing aggression, conflict, delinquency, doping, externalizing, hyperactivity, loneliness, runaway, sexuality, suicide, and violence (Bernardon et al. 2011; Browning et al. 2005; Hayslip et al. 2000; Nieuwenhuis et al. 2017; Pearson and Wilkinson 2013; Terzi-Unsal and Karei 2005; Wight et al. 2006; R. Wright et al. 2009). Verbal ability has maintained sociality by fostering leadership and dampening delinquency (Brugman et al. 2003; D. Chan 2007). Youthfulness has sustained sociality regarding volunteering (Reed and Selbee 2000).

Conversely, education has reduced poverty and vulnerability to maintain power to drive sociality (Langenderfer and Shimp 2001; K. Wang et al. 2013). Poverty has undermined sociality by reducing civic participation, trust, social connection, and volunteering (Caputo 2010; Stephens et al. 2014; R. Walker et al. 2010). Conversely, poverty has disrupted sociality by creating isolation, relationship problems, and social exclusion experienced (Dhal et al. 2008; Stephens et al. 2014; R. Walker et al. 2010). Vulnerability has worsened sociality by evoking ostracism experienced, radicalism, threat experienced, threatening, and violence (Ferguson and McAuley 2020; Lohman 2006; Pauwels and De Waele 2014; Poon et al. 2020; Thomsen and Birkmose 2015). Moreover, vulnerability can impair sociality by breeding divorce, nimbyism, stigmatizing, and victimization experienced and diminishing xenophobia (Badurdeen et al. 2022; Dum et al. 2017; Dijker and Koomen 2007; Lancee and Pardos-Prado 2013; Zavala and Guadalupe-Diaz 2019).

Utility for sociality raised by education has sprung from benefit, opportunity, security, and well-being, including living standard quality, self-esteem and satisfaction with living standards, safety, and security (Cerin and Leslie 2008; Emler and Frazer 1999; Hraba et al. 2001; James and Amato 2013; Mau 2005a; Yienprugsawan et al. 2010; Whyte and Gao 2009). Benefit or opportunity received has sustained sociality by enhancing civic engagement, compliance, institutional trust, political participation, prosocial behavior, and recourse (Davis-Lipman et al. 2007; Grimes 2006; Islam et al. 2006; Kirchler and Maciejovsky 2001; Pattie et al. 2004; Premo et al. 2018). Security has buttressed sociality regarding civility, social capital, and trust (Curley 2010; Watson et al. 2021; Williamson 2002). Well-being has uplifted sociality by consolidating altruism, conformism, cooperation, donation, liking for people, prosociality, sociability, and trust and social trust (Fetvadjiev and He 2019; A. Hu 2013; Lyubomirsky et al. 2006; Y. Pan et al. 2023; Wang and Graddy

2008). Conversely, disutility against sociality dampened by education has arisen from constraint, control, crime, discrimination, political alienation, social exclusion, threat, and victimization experienced (Backman and Nilsson 2011; Jones and Ferguson 2009; Kaukinen 2004; Raijman et al. 2003; Stavrova and Ehlebracht 2018; Weakliem and Borch 2006). Constraint or control experienced has worsened sociality by breeding violence (Felson and Outlaw 2007). Crime or victimization experienced has impaired sociality by eroding social trust (Olivera 2015). Conversely, crime or victimization experienced has hurt sociality by activating conflict and migration (Bar-Tal and Halperin 2013; Ramesh et al. 2019). Discrimination experienced can foment violence to undermine sociality (White et al. 2015). Social exclusion experienced has disturbed sociality by eroding closeness and prosocial behavior (Bockler et al. 2021; K. Lin et al. 2013). Political alienation erodes sociality regarding government trust (Kabashima et al. 2000). Threat experienced has inhibited sociality by reducing cohesion and triggering conflict and resistance (Lubbers et al. 2006; B. Rick et al. 2006).

Ideals for sociality fostered by education have highlighted charity, citizen identity or citizenship, civic duty, civic engagement, civility, communitarianism, community attachment, community involvement, conformism, conservatism, cooperation, coordination, donation, equality or egalitarianism, moralism, morality, neighbor networking, patriotism, political discussion, political interest, political participation, recourse, redistribution, social cohesion, socialism, traditionalism, trust, volunteering, xenophobia or hostility against foreignness (Billiet et al. 2003; Briggs et al. 1999; Brown and Ferris 2007; Bullock 2021; E. Chan 2014; Chen and Ren 2016; Clark 2004a; Cornwall 2009; Djupe and Lewis 2015; Gilberbloom and Markham 1995; Holbrook et al. 2003; Kerrissey and Schofer 2013; Kung 2003; Miyata et al. 2008; Norris 2011; Norris and Inglehart 2009; Pakulshi and Tranter 2000; Pichler 2009; Ulbig 2002; Volker et al. 2007; Zhu and Ke 2001; Zumbrunnen and Gangl 2008). Charity embodies sociality regarding compassion, giving, mercy, and volunteering (Apinunmahakul and Devlin 2008; Eggemeier and Fritz 2020; Pommier et al. 2020). Citizenship or civic dutifulness has constituted sociality by inducing fairness and trust (Vera-Toscano et al. 2013). Civic engagement has propped sociality by strengthening attachment, civility, collective behavior, discussion, donation, neighboring, patriotism, prosociality, social capital, socialism, trust, and volunteering and impeding cheating and individualism (Coffe and Geys 2007; Gilberbloom and Markham 1995; Kerrissey and Schofer 2013; Mata and Pendakur 2014; Ozbay 2008; Pattie et al. 2004; Pena-Lopez and Sanchez-Santos 2016; Rahn 2008; Richey 2011; Tak 2017; M. Tang 2011; Taniguchi 2013; Yip et al. 2007). Civility has constituted sociality by inducing fairness and trust (Vera-Toscano et al. 2013). Communitarianism constitutes sociality by espousing caring, civility, collective identity, commonweal orientation, community, dutifulness or responsibility, education or socialization, equality, interdependence, loyalty, mentoring, patriotism, reciprocity, relatedness, self-discipline, servicing including volunteering, settlement, social construction, social participation, solidarity, and trust (Delanty 2009; Frazer 1999; Moore 2010; Speth 2012). Community attachment or involvement has facilitated sociality regarding cooperation, networking, and trust (Groves et al. 2000; Molitor et al.

2011; Rochelle 2015). Conformism has constituted sociality by raising patriotism and impeding violence and acceptance of deviants and outsiders (Pulkkinen et al. 2009; Schwartz et al. 2014; Van Hootegem et al. 2000; Yeo and Chu 2018). Conservatism sustains sociality by nurturing empathy, loyalty, prosocial behavior, religiousness, and sacrifice (Dutton and Rayner-Hilles 2022). Moreover, conservatism underpins sociality by maintaining allegiance or loyalty, attachment, civility, community, conformity, cooperation, discipline, ethnocentrism, honesty, humility, intimacy, legality, morality, nationalism, obedience, order, partnership, patriotism, peace, responsibility, sharing, trust, and xenophobia (Dutton and Rayner-Hilles 2022; Heilman and Kusev 2020; Hickson 2013; Lakoff 2009; Rhodes-Purdy et al. 2023; Scruton 2014; Yoos 2007; Zuk and Zuk 2020). Conversely, conservatism upholds sociality by condemning dehumanizing, evilness, revolution, sexuality, terrorism, and transgression (Dutton and Rayner-Hilles 2022; Malka and Soto 2011; Scruton 2014; Suhay 2015). Political participation has buttressed sociality regarding civility (Campbell 2003). Cooperation has constituted sociality regarding attachment and trustworthiness as opposed to argument (Gerbasi and Cook 2008; Hample 2018; Tak 2017). Coordination has constituted sociality by strengthening agreeableness, empathy, morality, and social capital (Halevy et al. 2019). Donation has constituted sociality by consolidating charity, service value, social capital, social trust, and volunteering (Bekkers 2010; Chang 2009; Foster et al. 2001; Uslaner 2000). The ideal for equality or egalitarianism has underpinned sociality by enhancing empathy, support for welfare, and trust in government and impeding radicalism (Faricy and Ellis 2014; Lauriola et al. 2015; Lucas and Kteily 2018; Roosma et al. 2014). Moralism has sustained sociality by boosting gratitude (Pohling et al. 2010). Moreover, moralism can enhance sociality regarding social trust (Bersot and Arrigo 2015; Steinhardt 2012). Inherently, moralism embraces altruism, consensus, legality, obligation, and virtue to maintain sociality (R. Brown 2018). Morality has constituted sociality by boosting volunteering and inhibiting violence (Piquero and Hickman 2002; Whitford et al. 2006). Neighbor networking has elevated sociality by raising consulting and influencing (Hays and Kogl 2007). Patriotism has constituted sociality by raising government trust, nationalism, prosocial behavior or prosociality, social cohesion, volunteering, and xenophobia (Beyerlein and Sikkink 2008; Gross et al. 2004; Ishii 2009; Straume and Odeen 2010). Political discussion or participation has buttressed sociality regarding civility (Campbell 2003). Political interest has elevated sociality by raising civic engagement, civic and social motivation, civility, and discussion as opposed to protesting (Gil de Zuniga et al. 2017; Lee and Chan 2011; Pattie et al. 2004). Recourse reflects sociality regarding affiliation and social support received (Ledbetter et al. 2013; Sullivan 2001). The ideal for redistribution has reflected sociality regarding social trust (Nagayoshi and Sato 2014). Social cohesion has constituted sociality by enhancing attachment and dampening tolerance for deviance (Stafford et al. 2005; Woosnam et al. 2018). Socialism maintained in the community institution to frame sociality anticipates association, cooperation, equality, harmony, and mutuality as opposed to conflict (Powell 2007). Besides, socialism has enhanced sociality regarding cooperation and discussion as opposed to crime (Collier 2001; Lilly et al. 2011; Sanderson 2001). Traditionalism in community involvement upholds dependency, dutifulness, groupness, loyalty, obedience, order, and religiosity to foster sociality (Heckscher 2015). Additionally, traditionalism has buttressed sociality by enhancing patriotism and faith in religion and discouraging protesting and acceptance of deviants and outsiders (Costa et al. 2023; Datler et al. 2013; Meuleman et al. 2019; Schwartz et al. 2014). Trust has constituted sociality through donation, involvement, and volunteering (Uslaner 2000). Volunteering has constituted sociality by raising altruism, charity orientation, civic motivation, donation, helping, moral responsibility, political participation, social integration, and social and government trust (Foster et al. 2001; Isham et al. 2006; Richey 2010; Richey and Ikeda 2009; Wiepking and Maas 2009). Xenophobia has constituted sociality by boosting patriotism and social cohesion (Granzin and Olsen 1998; Wang and Chen 2004). Conversely, ideals against sociality dampened by education have cherished crime, deviance, discrimination, individualist attribution, protesting, religiosity, resistance, and violence and its tolerance (Atkinson et al. 2005; Backman and Nilsson 2011; Behr et al. 2014; Immerzeel and van Tubergen 2013; Larsen 2006; B. Lee et al. 2004; Lubbers et al. 2006; T. Simon et al. 2001; Wilson and Dunham 2001). Tolerance for crime or violence has provoked violence (van Hiel et al. 2007). Violence has undermined sociality by breeding antisociality, crime and recidivism, blaming, conflict, hostility, rejecting others, and impairing agreeableness, morality, and responsibility (Asendorpf et al. 2008; Del Bove et al. 2008; Morrison 2006; Scholte et al. 2009; Vitaro et al. 2007). Deviance has ruined sociality by provoking social exclusion experienced (Backman and Nilsson 2011). Discrimination has weakened sociality by hindering friendship (A. Thomas et al. 2016). Individualism has weakened sociality by reducing civic engagement, religiousness, social cohesion, and volunteering (Church 2010; Green and Janmaat 2011; J. He et al. 2014; Hener et al. 2016; Leong 2008; Pollack and Pickel 2007; Whitford et al. 2006). Conversely, individualism has impeded sociality by bolstering acceptance of outsiders, competition, crime, extremity, self-enhancement, protesting, and violence (Church 2010; J. He et al. 2014; Karstedt 2010; Leong 2008; Li and Song 1992; Pollack and Pickel 2007; Whitford et al. 2006). Protesting has impaired sociality by escalating distancing and radicalism and dampening moral motivation (Kutlaca et al. 2020; Vestergren et al. 2017). Besides, protesting impedes sociality by embracing antisociality, conflict, extremism, hostility, incivility, illegality, rioting, social exclusion, terrorism, and violence (Renger et al. 2020; Kaplan and Liu 2000; S. Lo 2021; McCright and Dunlap 2008; Morselli and Passini 2018; Smidt 2020; Stewart et al. 2012; Swart et al. 2020; Tan and Snow 2015). Religiosity has hindered sociality by reducing nationalism, social interaction and engendering protesting, marginalization experienced, radicalism, and social distance (Ayalon et al. 1993; Kunovich 2009; Norris 2002; Pedahzur and Canetti-Nisim 2004; Wuthnow 2004). Resistance has impaired sociality by eroding solidarity and fomenting deviance (Foy et al. 2014; J. Williams 2011).

Norms for sociality promoted by education have stressed equality and justice (Barker and Tinnick 2006; Bullock 2021). The norm for equality has fostered sociality by championing cohesion and its experience, fairness, justice, social capital, sympathy, trust, and volunteering (Eriksson et al. 2015; Green et al. 2003; Hitlin and

Harkness 2018; Musick and Wilson 2008; Oishi et al. 2011; Portes and Vickstrom 2011; van Oorschot and Arts 2005). The norm for justice has upheld sociality by elevating morality and prosocial behavior (Barber 2004; McCaffoee 2016).

Conversely, norms against sociality reduced by education have featured corruption, crime, problems, prostitution, and risk (Morris and Klesner 2010; Nabi and Sullivan 2001; Sjoberg 2003; Swader and Vorobeva 2015). The norm for corruption has undermined sociality by disrupting institutional trust (Morris and Klesner 2010). The norm of crime has jeopardized sociality by inhibiting community involvement and prosocial behavior and raising victimization (Broadbent and Papadopoulos 2011; Jacobs and Carmichael 2002; Zhong 2010). The norm for problems has impaired sociality by jeopardizing civility, government and social trust, and political participation and breeding deviance (Backman and Nilsson 2011; Fahmy 2006; Marschall and Stolle 2004; Nicholls and Picou 2012). Prostitution has impaired sociality by generating antisocial behavior, escape, relationship loss, and sexual abuse experienced (Dalla 2006; Swedin and Priebe 2007). The norm for risk has impaired sociality by provoking protesting (Scafuto and La Barbera 2016). Moreover, the risk norm can hurt sociality by generating opposition to the establishment (P. Brown 2020).

Irreligion

Irreligion is likely to uphold sociality by fostering power, utility, ideals, and norms for sociality and diminishing power, disutility, ideals, and norms against sociality. Such upholding exercises the voluntaristic mechanisms of power realization, utility optimization, ideal calibration, and norm conformity. These mechanisms engage encouraging, learning, social control, and social networking (French et al. 2008; Sallquist et al. 2010; C. Smith 2003).

Power against sociality prevented by irreligion lies in wrathfulness (Lehmann and Gorsuch 2017). Wrathfulness has jeopardized sociality by eroding social integration and fomenting protesting and violence and its tolerance (Krahe 2013; Molm 2008; Passini 2019; Tausch et al. 2011). Moreover, wrathfulness can dampen sociality by breeding crime and radicalism (Brant 2019; Larson et al. 2020). Irreligion has also lessened power fueling narcissism and psychopathy to maintain sociality (Y. Lee et al. 2023). Narcissism has impeded sociality by breeding aggression and misbehavior (Tracy et al. 2009). Besides, narcissism dismisses discipline, empathy, friendship, humor, morality, and responsibility and embraces exploitation, lying, rage, rivalry, and violence to undermine sociality (Cichocka et al. 2024; Kilminster 2008; Twenge and Campbell 2009). Psychopathy has undermined sociality by withdrawing prosocial behavior and breeding radicalism, victimization, and violence (Ehrensuft et al. 2003; Krahe 2013; Soliman et al. 2016; Thielmann et al. 2020). Besides, psychopathy embraces antisociality, manipulation, and radicalism to inhibit sociality (Johnston and Bose 2020; Krupp et al. 2012; Welsh and Lenzenweger 2021).

Ideals for sociality fostered by irreligion have espoused citizenship and community participation (Kim and Wilcox 2013; Kuperus and Asante 2021). Citizenship has constituted sociality by inducing fairness and trust (Vera-Toscano et al. 2013). Community participation has facilitated sociality regarding cooperation, networking, and trust (Groves et al. 2000; Molitor et al. 2011; Rochelle 2015). Moreover, irreligion has fostered ideals against cosmopolitanism and discrimination to establish sociality (Chui and Leung 2014; Forman 2001). Cosmopolitanism opposes sociality by downplaying attachment, collective identity, communality, localism, nationalism, and patriotism (Baildon and Alviar-Martin 2020; Bray 2013; Caruana 2014; Delanty 2009; Sorge 2008). Conversely, cosmopolitanism contradicts sociality by hailing autonomy, diversity, foreignness, fusion, individualism, and liberalism (Corstange and York 2018; Delanty 2009; Held 2010; Herrmann 2023). As such, cosmopolitanism has eroded sociality by discounting religiosity and raising liberalism and acceptance of deviants and outsiders (Costa et al. 2023; Motschenbacher 2013; Norris and Inglehart 2009). Discrimination has weakened sociality by hindering friendship (A. Thomas et al. 2016).

Marital Status

Marital status, including marriage, cohabitation, divorce, separation, widowhood, and unmarried status, is likely to influence sociality by affecting power, utility, ideals, and norms for or against sociality. The influence builds on the voluntaristic mechanisms of power realization, utility optimization, ideal calibration, and norm conformity in analytical functionalism.

Marriage has enhanced power based on social capital, social integration, and social support received to drive sociality (W. Chang 2009; Lizardo 2006; Mata and Pendakur 2014). Social capital has consolidated sociality by raising civic engagement, community involvement, donation, political involvement, social trust, and volunteering (Bekkers et al. 2008; Broadbent and Papadopoulos 2011; Brown and Ferris 2007; Chua et al. 2021; Narayan and Cassidy 2001). Conversely, social capital has strengthened sociality by erasing violence (Pulkkinen et al. 2009). Social integration has constituted sociality by enhancing cooperation and preventing suicide (Duberstein et al. 2004; Lepkowski and Couper 2002). Social support received has strengthened sociality by enhancing attachment, gratitude, political participation, prosocial behavior, recourse, respect, responsibility, social integration, and social well-being (Boezeman and Ellemers 2008; Fahmy 2006; Phipps 2003; Williams and Galliher 2006; R. Wright et al. 2009; Zeldin et al. 2016; Zeng et al. 2024). Conversely, social support received has boosted sociality by preventing aggression, conflict, delinquency, doping, externalizing, hyperactivity, loneliness, runaway, sexuality, suicide, and violence (Bernardon et al. 2011; Browning et al. 2005; Hayslip et al. 2000; Nieuwenhuis et al. 2017; Pearson and Wilkinson 2013; Terzi-Unsal and Karei 2005; Wight et al. 2006; R. Wright et al. 2009). Moreover, marriage has maintained power to drive sociality by prevention dysfunction (Li and Chung 2008). Dysfunction has weakened sociality by eroding social capital, social cohesion, social trust, and volunteering (Cornwall 2009; Granzin and Haggard 2000; Tang 2006; Zanin et al. 2013).

Conversely, dysfunction has impeded sociality by instigating protesting and suicide (Van Vugt et al. 2003). Moreover, outsider status may breed dependency, symptoms, and unemployment to weaken power for driving sociality (Boeri et al. 2002; Borjas 1999; Roemer 2006).

Marriage has generated utility for sociality based on well-being, including community evaluation, interaction and relationship quality, satisfaction, and self-esteem (Carrieri 2012; McMullin and Cairney 2004; Molana and Adams 2019; Sampson and Raudenbush 2004). Community evaluation has elevated sociality by building social capital, order, and cohesion (Rupp et al. 2020; Sampson and Raudenbush 2004). Relationship quality features attachment, closeness, friendship, security, and sharing (Hample 2018; Koerner 2018; Mikulincer and Shaver 2018; Van Lear et al. 2006). Satisfaction raised by marriage has covered achievement, family, finance, friendship, health, life, and living standards (Distante 2013; Koromeckyj-Cox et al. 2007; Mitrut and Wolff 2011; Prezza et al. 2001; Yienprugsawan et al. 2010). Satisfaction has advanced sociality by strengthening political participation, social cohesion, social and government trust, and volunteering (E. Chan 2014; Flavin and Keane 2011; Rochelle 2015). Self-esteem has buttressed sociality by raising attachment security, political participation, and prosociality and preventing suicide (Kitayama and Markus 2000; Tracy et al. 2009). Generally, well-being has uplifted sociality by consolidating altruism, conformism, cooperation, donation, liking for people, prosociality, sociability, and trust and social trust (Fetvadjiev and He 2019; A. Hu 2013; Lyubomirsky et al. 2006; Y. Pan et al. 2023; Wang and Graddy 2008).

Conversely, marriage has reduced disutility against sociality by eroding discrimination, social exclusion, and victimization experienced (Carr and Friedman 2005; Ross and Mirowsky 2009; Wojcieszak and Mutz 2009). Discrimination experienced can foment violence to undermine sociality (White et al. 2015). Social exclusion experienced has disturbed sociality by eroding closeness and prosocial behavior (Bockler et al. 2021; K. Lin et al. 2013). Victimization experienced has impaired sociality by eroding social trust (Olivera 2015). Conversely, victimization experienced has hurt sociality by activating conflict and migration (Bar-Tal and Halperin 2013; Ramesh et al. 2019).

Marriage has buttressed ideals for charity, civic engagement, community attachment and involvement, donation, family functioning, government responsibility, neighboring, political participation, prosocial behavior, protection or relief, reciprocity, social cohesion, social interaction, and trust to rationalize sociality (Bednall et al. 2013; Brown and Ferris 2007; Degenne et al. 2004; Flavin and Keane 2011; Magee 2008; Mata and Pendakur 2014; McCabe 2014; Okun et al. 1998; Prezza et al. 2001; Ross and Mirowsky 2009; Smith and Hamon 2012; Swaroop and Morenoff 2006; Tolsma et al. 2009; Tsai 2006; K. Wang et al. 2013). The ideal for charity upholds sociality by embracing altruism, compassion, mercy, and volunteering (Apinunmahakul and Devlin 2008; Eggemeier and Fritz 2020; Musick and Wilson 2008; Pommier et al. 2020). Civic engagement has propped sociality by strengthening attachment, civility, collective behavior, discussion, donation, neighboring, patriotism, prosociality, social capital, socialism, trust, and volunteering and impeding cheating and individualism (Coffe and Geys 2007; Gilberbloom and Markham 1995;

Kerrissey and Schofer 2013; Mata and Pendakur 2014; Ozbay 2008; Pattie et al. 2004; Pena-Lopez and Sanchez-Santos 2016; Rahn 2008; Richey 2011; Tak 2017; M. Tang 2011; Taniguchi 2013; Yip et al. 2007). Community attachment or involvement has facilitated sociality regarding cooperation, networking, and trust (Groves et al. 2000; Molitor et al. 2011; Rochelle 2015). Donation has constituted sociality by consolidating charity, service value, social capital, social trust, and volunteering (Bekkers 2010; Chang 2009; Foster et al. 2001; Uslaner 2000). Family functioning has constituted sociality by enhancing cohesion and social support receipt (Espvall and Dellgren 2008; Rook and Ituarte 1999). The ideal for government has sustained sociality by dampening protesting (Schofer and Fourcade-Gourinchas 2001). Neighboring has elevated sociality by raising consulting and influencing (Hays and Kogl 2007). Political participation has buttressed sociality regarding civility (Campbell 2003). Prosocial behavior has constituted sociality by civility, consolidating connectedness, cooperation, religiosity, responsibility, and volunteering (Hample 2018; Marsh and Dik 2021; Musick and Wilson 2008; Nelson-Coffey et al. 2023; Shahzalal and Adnan 2022). Moreover, prosocial behavior underlies sociality by enhancing citizenship, loyalty, social cohesion, socializing, and trust and diminishing self-interest (Dovidio et al. 2006; Hawley 2014; Kisliuk and WeiBmuller 2023; Music 2014). Protection has bolstered sociality by enhancing affiliative humor and attenuating aggressive humor (Erickson and Feldstein 2007). Reciprocity has constituted sociality by fostering prosocial behavior (Thielmann et al. 2020). Social cohesion has constituted sociality by enhancing attachment and dampening tolerance for deviance (Stafford et al. 2005; Woosnam et al. 2018). Social interaction has realized sociality by consolidating altruism, compliance, cooperation, donation, morality, political participation, reciprocity, social trust, and volunteering (Guillen et al. 2011; Dixon and McKeown 2021; Lucas and Livingston 2014; Musick 2000; Rodrigo-Gonzalez et al. 2019; Rubin and Step 2000). Trust has constituted sociality through donation, involvement, and volunteering (Uslaner 2000). Moreover, marriage has supported ideals against crime, deviance or its tolerance, and violence to rationalize sociality (Savolainen 2009; Coffe and Geys 2007; E. Wright et al. 2015). Crime has impaired sociality by reducing community involvement, prosocial behavior, and social trust and fomenting avoidance, protesting, risking, victimization, and violence (Brayne 2014; McNeeley and Yuan 2017; Broadbent and Papadopoulos 2011; Sun and Wang 2012; Wittebrood and Nieuwbeerta 2000; Zhong 2010). Deviance has ruined sociality by provoking social exclusion experienced (Backman and Nilsson 2011). Violence has undermined sociality by fomenting crime and tolerance for violence (Markowitz 2001; Tanner-Smith et al. 2013).

Marriage has engaged norms for closeness to assimilate sociality (Cornwall 2009). Closeness has constituted sociality by boosting relationship satisfaction and social support received and dampening rejection expected (Arseth et al. 2009; Hand et al. 2013).

Cohabitation has reduced disutility against sociality stemming from depression (Silverstein and Ruiz 2006). Depression has eroded sociality by breeding conflict, hate, hostility perceived, loneliness, revenge, risking, suicide, and violence (Cacioppo and Hawkley 2009; Economou et al. 2016; Haner et al. 2020; Morokoff et al. 2009;

Mullet et al. 2005; Proulx et al. 2004; H. Smith et al. 2016; E. Wright et al. 2015). Conversely, depression has attenuated sociality by impeding benevolence, closeness experienced, fairness, forgiveness, gratitude, honesty, leadership, love, social integration, teamwork, and volunteering (Blanchard et al. 2021; Cornwall 2009; Holzel et al. 2011; Mancini et al. 2011; Mullet et al. 2005; Thoits and Hewitt 2001).

Cohabitation has strengthened power for sociality based on employment. Employment has facilitated sociality by elevating civic engagement, community involvement, donation, philanthropy value, political discussion, political participation, social capital, social functioning, social cohesion experienced, social interaction, and social trust (Anciaes et al. 2017; Fridberg and Kangas 2008b; Kerrissey and Schofer 2013; H. Lu et al. 2002; Ross and Mirowsky 2009; Tsai 2006). Conversely, employment has safeguarded sociality by lessening crime, relocation, and social exclusion experienced (Groot et al. 2007; Kleinhans 2009; Savolainen 2009).

Cohabitation has diminished the ideal against sociality that prefers suicide (Abrutyn and Mueller 2014). The ideal for suicide has impeded sociality by fomenting radicalism (Soliman et al. 2016). Meanwhile, cohabitation has secured the ideal for sociality favoring traditionalism (Brynin et al. 2009). Traditionalism has buttressed sociality by enhancing patriotism and faith in religion and discouraging protesting and accepting deviants and outsiders (Costa et al. 2023; Datler et al. 2013; Meuleman et al. 2019; Schwartz et al. 2014).

Divorce has eroded power for sociality based on dependability (Allemand et al. 2015). Dependability can sustain sociality by boosting or maintaining cooperation, intimacy, and social capital (X. Chen et al. 2015; Harvey and Wenzel 2006; Yamagishi et al. 2005).

Divorce can generate disutility against sociality due to dissatisfaction (Demo and Buehler 2013). Dissatisfaction has obstructed sociality by reducing political participation, social cohesion, social and government trust, and volunteering (E. Chan 2014; Flavin and Keane 2011; Rochelle 2015).

Widowhood has disrupted utility for sociality stemming from life satisfaction (Tiliouine et al. 2006). Life satisfaction has incubated sociality regarding political participation, social cohesion, social trust, and volunteering (E. Chan 2014; Flavin and Keane 2011; Rochelle 2015).

Unmarriage has sustained sociality by raising social support received (Degenne et al. 2004). Social support received has strengthened sociality by enhancing attachment, gratitude, political participation, prosocial behavior, recourse, respect, responsibility, social integration, and social well-being (Boezeman and Ellemers 2008; Fahmy 2006; Phipps 2003; Williams and Galliher 2006; R. Wright et al. 2009; Zeldin et al. 2016; Zeng et al. 2024). Conversely, social support received has boosted sociality by preventing aggression, conflict, delinquency, doping, externalizing, hyperactivity, loneliness, runaway, sexuality, suicide, and violence (Bernardon et al. 2011; Browning et al. 2005; Hayslip et al. 2000; Nieuwenhuis et al. 2017; Pearson and Wilkinson 2013; Terzi-Unsal and Karei 2005; Wight et al. 2006; R. Wright et al. 2009).

Living Arrangement

Living arrangement covers living with parents and children or the number of children. Such arrangement is likely to secure sociality by developing power, utility, ideals, and norms to achieve functions required for sociality. The development hinges on the voluntaristic mechanisms of power realization, utility optimization, ideal calibration, and norm conformity based on analytical functionalism. Specifically, these mechanisms engage resource gathering and distribution (Segrin and Flora 2019).

Living with parents has cultivated ideals for prosociality and voting to uplift sociality (Janmaat and Mons 2023). Prosociality has constituted sociality by civility, consolidating connectedness, cooperation, religiosity, responsibility, and volunteering (Hample 2018; Marsh and Dik 2021; Musick and Wilson 2008; Nelson-Coffey et al. 2023; Shahzalal and Adnan 2022). Moreover, prosociality underlies sociality by enhancing citizenship, loyalty, social cohesion, socializing, and trust and diminishing self-interest (Dovidio et al. 2006; Hawley 2014; Kisliuk and WeiBmuller 2023; Music 2014). Voting has engendered sociality by boosting civic and community participation and neighboring (Djupe and Lewis 2015; Dorff 2017; Hays and Kogl 2007). Conversely, living with parents has enhanced the ideal against violence to rationalize sociality (Kaufman-Parks et al. 2017). Violence has undermined sociality by breeding antisociality, crime and recidivism, blaming, conflict, hostility, rejecting others, and impairing agreeableness, morality, and responsibility (Asendorpf et al. 2008; Del Bove et al. 2008; Morrison 2006; Scholte et al. 2009; Vitaro et al. 2007). Living with parents has dampened the disutility of failure and victimization to maintain sociality (Gil and Molina 2007; Oksanen et al. 2014). Failure has impeded sociality by activating risking and suicide (Piquero et al. 2010; Simon and Masters 2024). Victimization experienced has impaired sociality by eroding social trust (Olivera 2015). Conversely, victimization experienced has hurt sociality by activating conflict and migration (Bar-Tal and Halperin 2013; Ramesh et al. 2019).

The number of children enhances power for sociality based on health, family functioning experienced, knowledge, mastery, organizational membership, social capital, social integration, and social support received (Apinunmahakul and Devlin 2008; Bjornberg and Ekbrand 2008; Frei et al. 2009; Kleinhans et al. 2007; Lelli 2008; Menahem 2001; Smith and Hamon 2012; Thoits and Hewitt 2001). Health has uplifted sociality by boosting community sense, morality, popularity, social activity, social cohesion, social integration, social trust, social well-being, and volunteering (Huxhold et al. 2014; Jorgensen et al. 2010; Son and Wilson 2012; Tolsma et al. 2009; Yu and Chiu 2016). Conversely, health has sustained sociality by preventing loneliness (Koromeckyj-Cox et al. 2007). Moreover, family functioning features attentiveness, caring, compassion, empathy, mutuality, and socialization (Herr 2012; Parke 2004). As such, family functioning experienced has facilitated sociality by raising social support received and reducing social avoidance (F. Liu et al. 2024). Generally, knowledge has raised sociality by enhancing cooperation, prosocial behavior, social cohesion, social trust, and volunteering (de Groot and

Steg 2009; Lepkowski and Couper 2002; Pattie et al. 2004; Simon-Bemd and Steffens 2000; Volker et al. 2007). Mastery has enhanced sociality by uplifting social trust (Burke and Stets 1999). Organizational membership has constituted sociality by strengthening institutional commitment and conformity (Vartanian and Hopkinson 2010). Social capital has consolidated sociality by raising civic engagement, community involvement, donation, political involvement, social trust, and volunteering (Bekkers et al. 2008; Broadbent and Papadopoulos 2011; Brown and Ferris 2007; Chua et al. 2021; Narayan and Cassidy 2001). Conversely, social capital has strengthened sociality by erasing violence (Pulkkinen et al. 2009). Social integration has constituted sociality by enhancing cooperation and preventing suicide (Duberstein et al. 2004; Lepkowski and Couper 2002). Social support received has strengthened sociality by enhancing attachment, gratitude, political participation, prosocial behavior, recourse, respect, responsibility, social integration, and social well-being (Boezeman and Ellemers 2008; Fahmy 2006; Phipps 2003; Williams and Galliher 2006; R. Wright et al. 2009; Zeldin et al. 2016; Zeng et al. 2024). Conversely, social support received has boosted sociality by preventing aggression, conflict, delinquency, doping, externalizing, hyperactivity, loneliness, runaway, sexuality, suicide, and violence (Bernardon et al. 2011; Browning et al. 2005; Hayslip et al. 2000; Nieuwenhuis et al. 2017; Pearson and Wilkinson 2013; Terzi-Unsal and Karei 2005; Wight et al. 2006; R. Wright et al. 2009). Moreover, the number of children has lessened economic hardship to maintain power to drive sociality (Muhlau 2014). Economic hardship has impaired sociality by dampening trust and fomenting social exclusion experienced, suicide, and victimization experienced (Economou et al. 2016; Reeskens and Vandecasteele 2017; Ross and Mirowsky 2009).

The number of children fosters utility for sociality based on well-being, including self-esteem, social quality, satisfaction with family, health, life, marriage, and the neighborhood (Savolainen et al. 2001; Guo and Huang 2005; Parkes et al. 2002; Sarracino 2010; Thoits and Hewitt 2001; van Praag and Ferrer-I-Carbonell 2004). Self-esteem has buttressed sociality by raising attachment security, political participation, and prosociality and preventing suicide (Kitayama and Markus 2000; Tracy et al. 2009). Social quality constitutes sociality by embracing social actualization, acceptance, adjustment, coherence, cohesion, contribution, empowerment, evaluation, inclusion, integration, life satisfaction, relatedness, resourcefulness, and security (Keyes and Shapiro 2004; Phillips 2006; Shapiro and Keyes 2008; Xie et al. 2022; van Praag and Ferrer-I-Carbonell 2004). Satisfaction has advanced sociality by strengthening political participation, social cohesion, social and government trust, and volunteering (E. Chan 2014; Flavin and Keane 2011; Rochelle 2015). Generally, well-being has uplifted sociality by consolidating altruism, conformism, cooperation, donation, liking for people, prosociality, sociability, and trust and social trust (Fetvadjiev and He 2019; A. Hu 2013; Lyubomirsky et al. 2006; Y. Pan et al. 2023; Wang and Graddy 2008). Moreover, the number of children has maintained security experienced to secure utility to attract sociality (Coffe and Geys 2007). Security experienced has buttressed sociality regarding civility, social capital, and trust (Curley 2010; Watson et al. 2021; Williamson 2002). Conversely, the number of children has reduced disutility against sociality arising from social distance experienced (Tsai 2006). Social distance has worsened sociality by diminishing donation, political evaluation, and social interaction (Bekkers 2010; Belanger and Aarts 2006). Conversely, social distance has weakened sociality by breeding radicalism and protesting (Borbath and Gessler 2020; Pedahzur and Canetti-Nisim 2004).

The number of children cultivates ideals for sociality prizing charity, civic engagement, conformism, donation, law enforcement, recourse, social cohesion, social interaction, social welfare, traditionalism, trust, and volunteering (Apinunmahakul and Devlin 2008; Brown and Ferris 2007; Eger 2010; Fridberg and Kangas 2008b; Kulik 2002; Magdol and Bessel 2003; Marschall and Stolle 2004; Palmer et al. 2011; Taniguichi and Thomas 2011; Timberlake et al. 2003; Wilkinson 2008; Xiao 2000). The ideal for charity upholds sociality by embracing altruism, compassion, mercy, and volunteering (Apinunmahakul and Devlin 2008; Eggemeier and Fritz 2020; Musick and Wilson 2008; Pommier et al. 2020). Civic engagement has propped sociality by strengthening attachment, civility, collective behavior, discussion, donation, neighboring, patriotism, prosociality, social capital, socialism, trust, and volunteering and impeding cheating and individualism (Coffe and Geys 2007; Gilberbloom and Markham 1995; Kerrissey and Schofer 2013; Mata and Pendakur 2014; Ozbay 2008; Pattie et al. 2004; Pena-Lopez and Sanchez-Santos 2016; Rahn 2008; Richey 2011; Tak 2017; M. Tang 2011; Taniguchi 2013; Yip et al. 2007). Conformism has constituted sociality by raising patriotism and impeding violence and acceptance of deviants and outsiders (Pulkkinen et al. 2009; Schwartz et al. 2014; Van Hootegem et al. 2000; Yeo and Chu 2018). Donation has constituted sociality by consolidating charity, service value, social capital, social trust, and volunteering (Bekkers 2010; Chang 2009; Foster et al. 2001; Uslaner 2000). Legalism has maintained sociality by preventing radicalism (Muthuswamy 2022). Recourse reflects sociality regarding affiliation and social support received (Ledbetter et al. 2013; Sullivan 2001). Social cohesion has constituted sociality by enhancing attachment and dampening tolerance for deviance (Stafford et al. 2005; Woosnam et al. 2018). Social interaction has realized sociality by consolidating altruism, compliance, cooperation, donation, morality, political participation, reciprocity, social trust, and volunteering (Guillen et al. 2011; Dixon and McKeown 2021; Lucas and Livingston 2014; Musick 2000; Rodrigo-Gonzalez et al. 2019; Rubin and Step 2000). The ideal for social welfare has championed sociality by consolidating government trust (U. Kim et al. 2002). Traditionalism has buttressed sociality by enhancing patriotism and faith in religion and discouraging protesting and acceptance of deviants and outsiders (Costa et al. 2023; Datler et al. 2013; Meuleman et al. 2019; Schwartz et al. 2014). Trust has constituted sociality through donation, involvement, and volunteering (Uslaner 2000). Volunteering has constituted sociality by raising altruism, charity orientation, civic motivation, donation, helping, moral responsibility, political participation, social integration, and social and government trust (Foster et al. 2001; Isham et al. 2006; Richey 2010; Richey and Ikeda 2009; Wiepking and Maas 2009). Moreover, the number of children incubates ideals against crime, migration, relocation, suicide, and violence to rationalize sociality (Akers and Kaukinen 2009; Broom et al. 2013; Duberstein et al. 2004; Kleinhans 2009; Richmond 2003). Crime has impaired sociality by reducing community involvement, prosocial behavior, and social trust and fomenting avoidance, protesting, risking, victimization, and violence (Brayne 2014; McNeeley and Yuan 2017; Broadbent and Papadopoulos 2011; Sun and Wang 2012; Wittebrood and Nieuwbeerta 2000; Zhong 2010). Promiscuity has arisen from ideals for alcoholism and doping to impair sociality (Dunkle et al. 2004). Migration has impeded sociality by diminishing social integration (Kearns and Whitley 2015). Relocation has impeded sociality by diminishing social integration (Kearns and Whitley 2015). The ideal for suicide has impeded sociality by fomenting radicalism (Soliman et al. 2016). Violence has undermined sociality by breeding antisociality, crime and recidivism, blaming, conflict, hostility, rejecting others, and impairing agreeableness, morality, and responsibility (Asendorpf et al. 2008; Del Bove et al. 2008; Morrison 2006; Scholte et al. 2009; Vitaro et al. 2007).

Parental Immigrant Status

Parental immigrant status is likely to impede sociality by weakening power, utility, ideals, and norms for sociality. This weakening engages the voluntaristic mechanisms of power realization, utility optimization, ideal calibration, and norm conformity posited in analytical functionalism. Specifically, the mechanisms involve assimilation and production (Boert et al. 2012; Kivisto and Faist 2010).

Power for sociality reduced by immigrant status has stemmed from employment, health, marriage, and social capital (Fanning et al. 2011; Islam et al. 2006; Ravanera et al. 2003; Thornton et al. 2007). involvement, donation, philanthropy value, political discussion, political participation, social capital, social functioning, social cohesion experienced, social interaction, and social trust (Anciaes et al. 2017; Fridberg and Kangas 2008b; Kerrissey and Schofer 2013; H. Lu et al. 2002; Ross and Mirowsky 2009; Tsai 2006). Conversely, employment has safeguarded sociality by lessening crime, relocation, and social exclusion experienced (Groot et al. 2007; Kleinhans 2009; Savolainen 2009). Health has uplifted sociality by boosting community sense, morality, popularity, social activity, social cohesion, social integration, social trust, social well-being, and volunteering (Huxhold et al. 2014; Jorgensen et al. 2010; Son and Wilson 2012; Tolsma et al. 2009; Yu and Chiu 2016). Conversely, health has sustained sociality by preventing loneliness (Koromeckyj-Cox et al. 2007). Marriage has consolidated sociality by enhancing community attachment, community evaluation, community involvement, civic engagement, closeness experienced, donation, friendship satisfaction, neighboring, political participation, prosocial behavior, reciprocity, relationship quality, social capital, social cohesion, social integration, social interaction, social support received, and trust (W. Chang 2009; Cornwall 2009; Degenne et al. 2004; Flavin and Keane 2011; Frye 2007; Kerrissey and Schofer 2013; Lizardo 2006; Louis and Zhao 2002; Mata and Pendakur 2014; McCabe 2014; Prezza et al. 2001; Ross and Mirowsky 2009; Sampson and Raudenbush 2004; Swaroop and Morenoff 2006; Tolsma et al. 2009). Conversely, marriage has upheld sociality by reducing crime, discrimination experienced, loneliness, social exclusion experienced, tolerance for deviance, and violence (Carr and Friedman 2005; Coffe and Geys 2007; Koromeckyj-Cox et al. 2007; Savolainen 2009; E. Wojcieszak and Mutz 2009; E. Wright et al. 2015). Social capital has consolidated sociality by raising civic engagement, community involvement, donation, political involvement, social trust, and volunteering (Bekkers et al. 2008; Broadbent and Papadopoulos 2011; Brown and Ferris 2007; Chua et al. 2021; Narayan and Cassidy 2001). Conversely, social capital has strengthened sociality by erasing violence (Pulkkinen et al. 2009). Moreover, immigrant status has engendered dysfunction, poverty, and unemployment to weaken power driving sociality (Herd et al. 2008; Kurz et al. 2005; Posthumus et al. 2013). Dysfunction has weakened sociality by eroding social capital, social cohesion, social trust, and volunteering (Cornwall 2009; Granzin and Haggard 2000; Tang 2006; Zanin et al. 2013). Conversely, dysfunction has impeded sociality by instigating protesting and suicide (Van Vugt et al. 2003). Poverty has undermined sociality by reducing civic participation, trust, social connection, and volunteering (Caputo 2010; Stephens et al. 2014; R. Walker et al. 2010). Conversely, poverty has disrupted sociality by creating isolation, relationship problems, and social exclusion experienced (Dhal et al. 2008; Stephens et al. 2014; R. Walker et al. 2010). Unemployment has impeded sociality by dissolving social capital, social cohesion, and trust (Espvall and Dellgren 2008; Manturuk et al. 2010; Reeskens and Vandecasteele 2017). Conversely, unemployment has hurt sociality by breeding conflict experienced, moving, protesting, threats experienced, and victimization (Bramley and Morgan 2003; Kaukinen 2004; Lewin-Epstein et al. 2003; Schneider 2007; Su and Feng 2013).

Utility for sociality impaired by immigrant status has rested on well-being, including life satisfaction and relationship quality (Ambrey and Fleming 2014; Fridberg and Kangas 2008a). Life satisfaction has incubated sociality regarding political participation, social cohesion, social trust, and volunteering (E. Chan 2014; Flavin and Keane 2011; Rochelle 2015). Relationship quality has constituted sociality by increasing xenophobia (Yun and Kim 2008). Generally, well-being has uplifted sociality by consolidating altruism, conformism, cooperation, donation, liking for people, prosociality, sociability, and trust and social trust (Fetvadjiev and He 2019; A. Hu 2013; Lyubomirsky et al. 2006; Y. Pan et al. 2023; Wang and Graddy 2008). Disutility against sociality created by immigrant status has arisen from depression, economic hardship, fear, and social exclusion experienced (Bask 2005; Fridberg and Kangas 2008; Kitchen and Williams 2010; Lofors and Sundquist 2007). Depression has eroded sociality by breeding conflict, hate, hostility perceived, loneliness, revenge, risking, suicide, and violence (Cacioppo and Hawkley 2009; Economou et al. 2016; Haner et al. 2020; Morokoff et al. 2009; Mullet et al. 2005; Proulx et al. 2004; H. Smith et al. 2016; E. Wright et al. 2015). Conversely, depression has attenuated sociality by impeding benevolence, closeness experienced, fairness, forgiveness, gratitude, honesty, leadership, love, social integration, teamwork, and volunteering (Blanchard et al. 2021; Cornwall 2009; Holzel et al. 2011; Mancini et al. 2011; Mullet et al. 2005; Thoits and Hewitt 2001). Economic hardship has impaired sociality by dampening trust and fomenting social exclusion experienced, suicide, and victimization experienced (Economou et al. 2016; Reeskens and Vandecasteele 2017; Ross and Mirowsky 2009). Fear has disrupted sociality by breeding interpersonal problems, loneliness, risking, suicide, and violence (Dutton et al. 2016; Gillath et al. 2005; Pulkkinen et al. 2009; Trumbo et al. 2008). Conversely, fear has undermined sociality by reducing donation, friendship, humor, political participation, prosocial behavior, and social well-being (Best and Krueger 2010; Hewstone et al. 2005; Litman et al. 2017; Kuiper and Nicholl 2004; Zhong 2010). Social exclusion experienced has disturbed sociality by eroding closeness and prosocial behavior (Bockler et al. 2021; K. Lin et al. 2013).

Ideals for sociality downplayed by immigrant status have espoused birth, civic engagement, community attachment, egalitarianism, political participation, social cohesion, social trust, and volunteering (Anton and Lawrence 2014; K. Brown et al. 2014; R. King 2005; Ravanera et al. 2003; Saunders and Wong 2012; Sonderskov 2011; Stromblad and Myrberg 2013). Birth has raised sociality by enhancing civic engagement, community involvement, conformism, donation, social capital, social cohesion, social integration, social interaction, social support received, and volunteering (Apinunmahakul and Devlin 2008; Bjornberg and Ekbrand 2008; Frei et al. 2009; Ghimire 2021a; Kleinhans et al. 2007; Magdol and Bessel 2003; Taniguchi and Thomas 2011; Wilkinson 2008; Xiao 2000; Xu and Lai 2002). Conversely, birth has advanced sociality by reducing social distance and violence (Broom et al. 2013; Tsai 2006). Civic engagement has propped sociality by strengthening attachment, civility, collective behavior, discussion, donation, neighboring, patriotism, prosociality, social capital, socialism, trust, and volunteering and impeding cheating and individualism (Coffe and Geys 2007; Gilberbloom and Markham 1995; Kerrissey and Schofer 2013; Mata and Pendakur 2014; Ozbay 2008; Pattie et al. 2004; Pena-Lopez and Sanchez-Santos 2016; Rahn 2008; Richey 2011; Tak 2017; M. Tang 2011; Taniguchi 2013; Yip et al. 2007). Community attachment has facilitated sociality regarding cooperation, networking, and trust (Groves et al. 2000; Molitor et al. 2011; Rochelle 2015). Egalitarianism has underpinned sociality by enhancing empathy, support for welfare, and trust in government and impeding radicalism (Faricy and Ellis 2014; Lauriola et al. 2015; Lucas and Kteily 2018; Roosma et al. 2014). Political participation has buttressed sociality regarding civility (Campbell 2003). Social cohesion has constituted sociality by enhancing attachment and dampening tolerance for deviance (Stafford et al. 2005; Woosnam et al. 2018). Social trust has constituted sociality through donation, involvement, and volunteering (Uslaner 2000). Volunteering has constituted sociality by raising altruism, charity orientation, civic motivation, donation, helping, moral responsibility, political participation, social integration, and social and government trust (Foster et al. 2001; Isham et al. 2006; Richey 2010; Richey and Ikeda 2009; Wiepking and Maas 2009). Moreover, immigrant status has fostered ideals for migration, sleeping, and suicide to disturb sociality (Gurak and Kritz 2000; Hamermesh 2019; Hassan 1995). Migration has impeded sociality by diminishing social integration (Kearns and Whitley 2015). The ideal for sleeping or sleepiness has bred crime to disrupt sociality (Raine and Venables 2017). The ideal for suicide has impeded sociality by fomenting radicalism (Soliman et al. 2016).

Norms against impeded by immigrant status have popularized social control (Lilly et al. 2011). The norm for social control has enhanced sociality by raising civic engagement, government trust, political participation, and recourse (Su and Feng 2013; Z. Han et al. 2017; F. Lee 2012; Palmer et al. 2011). Conversely, the norm for social control has safeguarded sociality by dampening victimization and violence (Hansen-Nord et al. 2014; E. Wright et al. 2015).

Employment Status

Employment status covers full-time employment, part-time employment, self-employment, retirement, homemaking, studying, and unemployment. This status is likely to affect sociality by affecting power, utility, ideals, and norms based on the voluntaristic mechanisms of power realization, utility optimization, ideal calibration, and norm conformity. Generally, employment is likely to sustain sociality.

Employment has sustained power for sociality stemming from health, mastery, and self-efficacy (Distante 2013; Hansen et al. 2012; Corcoran et al. 2011). Health has uplifted sociality by boosting community sense, morality, popularity, social activity, social cohesion, social integration, social trust, social well-being, and volunteering (Huxhold et al. 2014; Jorgensen et al. 2010; Son and Wilson 2012; Tolsma et al. 2009; Yu and Chiu 2016). Conversely, health has sustained sociality by preventing loneliness (Koromeckyj-Cox et al. 2007). Mastery has enhanced sociality by uplifting social trust (Burke and Stets 1999). Self-efficacy has sustained sociality by raising civic engagement, donation, government and social trust, leadership, political participation, prosocial behavior, and social activity (Bednall et al. 2013; Frye 2007; Gnambs and Batinic 2012; Huber et al. 2022; Mangum 2012; Rahn 2008; Pei and Pan 2018; Yao and Enright 2019). Conversely, employment has reduced dysfunction, powerlessness, and psychosis to maintain power for driving sociality (Lofors and Sundquist 2007; Ross and Mirowsky 2009). Dysfunction has weakened sociality by eroding social capital, social cohesion, social trust, and volunteering (Cornwall 2009; Granzin and Haggard 2000; Tang 2006; Zanin et al. 2013). Conversely, dysfunction has impeded sociality by instigating protesting and suicide (Van Vugt et al. 2003). Powerlessness has eroded sociality by dampening attachment and giving (Campos-Castillo and Hitlin 2013; Molm 1997). Psychosis has obstructed sociality by diminishing community attachment, social capital, and social trust (G. Brown et al. 2004; Congdon 2010; Ross and Mirowsky 2009).

Employment has secured utility for sociality resting on well-being, including growth, life satisfaction, purposiveness, relatedness, and self-acceptance (Carrieri 2012; Ryff et al. 2004). Growth has upheld sociality by encouraging conformity and prosocial behavior (Fetvadjiev and He 2019). Moreover, growth sustains sociality by featuring conformity, generativity, harmony, intimacy, morality, social interest, and understanding as opposed to rebellion (Browning and Cooper 2004; Hale 1999; Hendry and Kloep 2012; Hwang and Chang 2009). Life satisfaction has incubated sociality regarding political participation, social cohesion, social trust, and volunteering (E. Chan 2014; Flavin and Keane 2011; Rochelle 2015). Purposiveness has underlain sociality by boosting civic practice, responsibility, and volunteering and reducing rejection experience (Duffy and Raque-Bogdan 2010; Summers and Falco 2020; Twenge et al. 2003). Relatedness has consolidated sociality by raising sharing, social interaction, and relationship satisfaction (Downie et al. 2008; Frazer 1999; Wickham and Knee 2012). Self-acceptance has buttressed sociality by raising attachment security, political participation, and prosociality and preventing suicide (Kitayama and Markus 2000; Tracy et al. 2009).

Conversely, employment has reduced depression, distress, and loneliness as disutility distracting sociality. Depression has eroded sociality by breeding conflict, hate, hostility perceived, loneliness, revenge, risking, suicide, and violence (Cacioppo and Hawkley 2009; Economou et al. 2016; Haner et al. 2020; Morokoff et al. 2009; Mullet et al. 2005; Proulx et al. 2004; H. Smith et al. 2016; E. Wright et al. 2015). Conversely, depression has attenuated sociality by impeding benevolence, closeness experienced, fairness, forgiveness, gratitude, honesty, leadership, love, social integration, teamwork, and volunteering (Blanchard et al. 2021; Cornwall 2009; Holzel et al. 2011; Mancini et al. 2011; Mullet et al. 2005; Thoits and Hewitt 2001). Distress has undermined sociality by fomenting resistance and impeding social capital and trust (Pulkkinen et al. 2009; Webber and Huxley 2007). Loneliness has impaired sociality by weakening reciprocity, social capital, and social cohesion and provoking suicide (C. Cheng et al. 2019; Espvall and Dellgren 2008).

Self-employment has afforded power for sociality based on financial adequacy, health, self-efficacy, and social integration (Gundert and Hohendanner 2015; Markowski 2006; Raymo 2015; van Praag and Ferrer-I-Carbonell 2004). Financial adequacy has enabled sociality by raising government trust (Li and Mayraz 2017). Health has uplifted sociality by boosting community sense, morality, popularity, social activity, social cohesion, social integration, social trust, social well-being, and volunteering (Huxhold et al. 2014; Jorgensen et al. 2010; Son and Wilson 2012; Tolsma et al. 2009; Yu and Chiu 2016). Conversely, health has sustained sociality by preventing loneliness (Koromeckyj-Cox et al. 2007). Self-efficacy has sustained sociality by raising civic engagement, donation, government and social trust, leadership, political participation, prosocial behavior, and social activity (Bednall et al. 2013; Frye 2007; Gnambs and Batinic 2012; Huber et al. 2022; Mangum 2012; Rahn 2008; Pei and Pan 2018; Yao and Enright 2019). Social integration has constituted sociality by strengthening cooperation and preventing suicide (Duberstein et al. 2004; Lepkowski and Couper 2002).

Self-employment has furnished utility for sociality springing from life satisfaction and self-esteem (Kluegel et al. 1995; Lane 1991). Life satisfaction has incubated sociality regarding political participation, social cohesion, social trust, and volunteering (E. Chan 2014; Flavin and Keane 2011; Rochelle 2015). Self-esteem has buttressed sociality by raising attachment security, political participation, and prosociality and preventing suicide (Kitayama and Markus 2000; Tracy et al. 2009). Conversely, self-employment has diminished disutility against sociality arising from depression (Lelli 2008). Depression has eroded sociality by breeding conflict, hate, hostility perceived, loneliness, revenge, risking, suicide, and violence (Cacioppo and Hawkley 2009; Economou et al. 2016; Haner et al. 2020; Morokoff et al. 2009; Mullet et al. 2005; Proulx et al. 2004; H. Smith et al. 2016; E. Wright et al. 2015).

Self-employment has fostered the ideal for volunteering to rationalize sociality (Musick and Wilson 2008). Volunteering has constituted sociality by raising altruism, charity orientation, civic motivation, donation, helping, moral responsibility, political participation, social integration, and social and government trust (Foster et al. 2001; Isham et al. 2006; Richey 2010; Richey and Ikeda 2009; Wiepking and Maas 2009).

Retirement has eroded power for sociality based on health, homeownership, mastery, physical functioning, social capital, and social integration (Cornwall 2009; Frei et al. 2009; Lelli 2008; Manturuk et al. 2010; Schieman 2001; E. Smith et al. 2006). Health has uplifted sociality by boosting community sense, morality, popularity, social activity, social cohesion, social integration, social trust, social well-being, and volunteering (Huxhold et al. 2014; Jorgensen et al. 2010; Son and Wilson 2012; Tolsma et al. 2009; Yu and Chiu 2016). Conversely, health has sustained sociality by preventing loneliness (Koromeckyj-Cox et al. 2007). Homeownership has sustained sociality by securing civic engagement, community involvement, donation, friendship, political participation, social capital, social cohesion, social interaction, social trust, and volunteering (Degenne et al. 2004; Ghimire 2021a; Glaeser et al. 2002; Kilburn and Maume 2000; Kang and Kwak 2003; Manturuk et al. 2010; Putnam 2007; Tsai 2006; Wiepking and Maas 2009). Conversely, homeownership has maintained sociality by preventing relocation and victimization (Dawkins 2006; Michalski 2005). Mastery has enhanced sociality by uplifting social trust (Burke and Stets 1999). Physical functioning has sustained sociality by enriching social capital (Cornwall 2009). Social capital has consolidated sociality by raising civic engagement, community involvement, donation, political involvement, social trust, and volunteering (Bekkers et al. 2008; Broadbent and Papadopoulos 2011; Brown and Ferris 2007; Chua et al. 2021; Narayan and Cassidy 2001). Conversely, social capital has strengthened sociality by erasing violence (Pulkkinen et al. 2009). Social integration has constituted sociality by enhancing cooperation and preventing suicide (Duberstein et al. 2004; Lepkowski and Couper 2002). Moreover, due to poverty, retirement has diminished power for sociality (Muffels and Fouarge 2004). Poverty has undermined sociality by reducing civic participation, trust, social connection, and volunteering (Caputo 2010; Stephens et al. 2014; R. Walker et al. 2010). Conversely, poverty has disrupted sociality by creating isolation, relationship problems, and social exclusion experienced (Dhal et al. 2008; Stephens et al. 2014; R. Walker et al. 2010).

Retirement has diminished life satisfaction as utility attracting sociality (Rozer and Kraaykamp 2013). Life satisfaction has incubated sociality regarding political participation, social cohesion, social trust, and volunteering (E. Chan 2014; Flavin and Keane 2011; Rochelle 2015). Conversely, retirement has heightened disutility against sociality arising from threats experienced (Schneider 2007). Threats received have inhibited sociality by reducing cohesion and triggering conflict and resistance (Lubbers et al. 2006; B. Rick et al. 2006).

Retirement has weakened civility, conservatism, coordination, social cohesion, social interaction, and social trust as ideals rationalizing sociality (Cornwall 2009;

Espvall and Dellgren 2008; Pattie et al. 2004; Zanin 2017). Civility has constituted sociality by inducing fairness and trust (Vera-Toscano et al. 2013). Conservatism sustains sociality by nurturing empathy, loyalty, prosocial behavior, religiousness, and sacrifice (Dutton and Rayner-Hilles 2022). Moreover, conservatism underpins sociality by maintaining allegiance or loyalty, attachment, civility, community, conformity, cooperation, discipline, ethnocentrism, honesty, humility, intimacy, legality, morality, nationalism, obedience, order, partnership, patriotism, peace, responsibility, sharing, trust, and xenophobia (Dutton and Rayner-Hilles 2022; Heilman and Kusev 2020; Hickson 2013; Lakoff 2009; Rhodes-Purdy et al. 2023; Scruton 2014; Yoos 2007; Zuk and Zuk 2020). Conversely, conservatism upholds sociality by condemning dehumanizing, evilness, revolution, sexuality, terrorism, and transgression (Dutton and Rayner-Hilles 2022; Malka and Soto 2011; Scruton 2014; Suhay 2015). Social cohesion has constituted sociality by enhancing attachment and dampening tolerance for deviance (Stafford et al. 2005; Woosnam et al. 2018). Social interaction has realized sociality by consolidating altruism, compliance, cooperation, donation, morality, political participation, reciprocity, social trust, and volunteering (Guillen et al. 2011; Dixon and McKeown 2021; Lucas and Livingston 2014; Musick 2000; Rodrigo-Gonzalez et al. 2019; Rubin and Step 2000). Social trust has constituted sociality through donation, involvement, and volunteering (Uslaner 2000).

Retirement has impeded the norm for economic quality to dissimilate sociality (Nielsen et al. 2005). The norm for economic quality has uplifted sociality by raising government support, nationalism, political participation, relationship quality, trust, volunteering, and xenophobia (Cheng and Smyth 2016; Fridberg and Kangas 2008a; Inglehart 2003; Rhodes-Purdy et al. 2023; Traunmuller 2011; van Oorschot and Arts 2005).

Homemaking or homemaker status has withdrawn power for sociality based on financial adequacy, health, mastery, physical functioning, and social capital (Lelli 2008; Schieman 2001; Ross and Mirowsky 1995). Financial adequacy has enabled sociality by raising government trust (Li and Mayraz 2017). Health has uplifted sociality by boosting community sense, morality, popularity, social activity, social cohesion, social integration, social trust, social well-being, and volunteering (Huxhold et al. 2014; Jorgensen et al. 2010; Son and Wilson 2012; Tolsma et al. 2009; Yu and Chiu 2016). Conversely, health has sustained sociality by preventing loneliness (Koromeckyj-Cox et al. 2007). Mastery has enhanced sociality by uplifting social trust (Burke and Stets 1999). Self-efficacy has sustained sociality by raising civic engagement, donation, government and social trust, leadership, political participation, prosocial behavior, and social activity (Bednall et al. 2013; Frye 2007; Gnambs and Batinic 2012; Huber et al. 2022; Mangum 2012; Rahn 2008; Pei and Pan 2018; Yao and Enright 2019). Physical functioning has sustained sociality by enriching social capital (Cornwall 2009). Social capital has consolidated sociality by raising civic engagement, community involvement, donation, political involvement, social trust, and volunteering (Bekkers et al. 2008; Broadbent and Papadopoulos 2011; Brown and Ferris 2007; Chua et al. 2021; Narayan and Cassidy 2001). Conversely, social capital has strengthened sociality by erasing violence (Pulkkinen et al. 2009). Moreover, homemaking or not working has weakened power driving sociality due to homelessness (Lelli 2008). Homelessness represents loneliness that impairs sociality (Rokach 2019).

Homemaking has evolved disutility against sociality arising from depression and threat (Kessler et al. 2004; Schneider 2007). Depression has eroded sociality by breeding conflict, hate, hostility perceived, loneliness, revenge, risking, suicide, and violence (Cacioppo and Hawkley 2009; Economou et al. 2016; Haner et al. 2020; Morokoff et al. 2009; Mullet et al. 2005; Proulx et al. 2004; H. Smith et al. 2016; E. Wright et al. 2015). Conversely, depression has attenuated sociality by impeding benevolence, closeness experienced, fairness, forgiveness, gratitude, honesty, leadership, love, social integration, teamwork, and volunteering (Blanchard et al. 2021; Cornwall 2009; Holzel et al. 2011; Mancini et al. 2011; Mullet et al. 2005; Thoits and Hewitt 2001). Threats experienced have inhibited sociality by reducing cohesion and triggering conflict and resistance (Lubbers et al. 2006; B. Rick et al. 2006).

Homemaking has diminished the ideal for social interaction to dismiss sociality (Lelli 2008). Social interaction has realized sociality by consolidating altruism, compliance, cooperation, donation, morality, political participation, reciprocity, social trust, and volunteering (Guillen et al. 2011; Dixon and McKeown 2021; Lucas and Livingston 2014; Musick 2000; Rodrigo-Gonzalez et al. 2019; Rubin and Step 2000).

Studying or student status has impeded power for sociality based on social capital (Webber and Huxley 2007). Social capital has consolidated sociality by raising civic engagement, community involvement, donation, political involvement, social trust, and volunteering (Bekkers et al. 2008; Broadbent and Papadopoulos 2011; Brown and Ferris 2007; Chua et al. 2021; Narayan and Cassidy 2001).

Studying or student status has bred disutility for sociality arising from anxiety, depression, stress, and victimization (Arsandaux et al. 2021; Hansen-Nord et al. 2014). Anxiety has disrupted sociality by breeding interpersonal problems, loneliness, risking, suicide, and violence (Dutton et al. 2016; Gillath et al. 2005; Pulkkinen et al. 2009; Trumbo et al. 2008). Conversely, anxiety has undermined sociality by reducing donation, friendship, humor, political participation, prosocial behavior, and social well-being (Best and Krueger 2010; Hewstone et al. 2005; Litman et al. 2017; Kuiper and Nicholl 2004; Zhong 2010). Depression has eroded sociality by breeding conflict, hate, hostility perceived, loneliness, revenge, risking, suicide, and violence (Cacioppo and Hawkley 2009; Economou et al. 2016; Haner et al. 2020; Morokoff et al. 2009; Mullet et al. 2005; Proulx et al. 2004; H. Smith et al. 2016; E. Wright et al. 2015). Conversely, depression has attenuated sociality by impeding benevolence, closeness experienced, fairness, forgiveness, gratitude, honesty, leadership, love, social integration, teamwork, and volunteering (Blanchard et al. 2021; Cornwall 2009; Holzel et al. 2011; Mancini et al. 2011; Mullet et al. 2005; Thoits and Hewitt 2001). Stress experienced has undermined sociality by eroding civility, forgiveness, generativity, relationship quality and satisfaction, social integration, social support received, and trust and heightening conflict, maltreatment, substance abuse, suicide, and violence (Atkinson et al. 2005; Dutton et al. 2016; Gelles 2007; Grzywacz and

Almeida 2008; Jackson et al. 2006; Sobeck et al. 2020; Toussaint et al. 2016). Victimization experienced has impaired sociality by eroding social trust (Olivera 2015). Conversely, victimization experienced has hurt sociality by activating conflict and migration (Bar-Tal and Halperin 2013; Ramesh et al. 2019). Moreover, studying has diminished utility for sociality resting on life satisfaction (Rampichini and D'Andrea 1998). Life satisfaction has incubated sociality regarding political participation, social cohesion, social trust, and volunteering (E. Chan 2014; Flavin and Keane 2011; Rochelle 2015).

Student status has eroded ideals for legality and traditionalism to dismiss sociality (Alm and Torpler 2003; Aygun and Imamoglu 2002). Conversely, student status has fostered ideals for protesting, religiosity, and suicide to refute sociality (Arsandaux et al. 2021; Immerzeel and van Tubergen 2013; Olcese et al. 2014). Legality has buttressed sociality by dismissing radicalism (Muthuswamy 2022). Traditionalism has buttressed sociality by enhancing patriotism and faith in religion and discouraging protesting and accepting deviants and outsiders (Costa et al. 2023; Datler et al. 2013; Meuleman et al. 2019; Schwartz et al. 2014).

Student status has triggered the norm for theft to weaken sociality (Winterdyk and Thompson 2008). Theft has bred social avoidance to weaken sociality (Brayne 2014).

Employment Sector

Employment sectors include public, private business, and nonprofit ones. They are likely to facilitate sociality by providing power, utility, ideals, and norms to meet the functions required for sociality.

Public employment has fostered ideals for politics, respect, and teamwork to rationalize sociality (Robichau and Sandberg 2022). The ideal for politics has elevated sociality by raising civic engagement, civic and social motivation, civility, and discussion as opposed to protesting (Gil de Zuniga et al. 2017; Lee and Chan 2011; Pattie et al. 2004). Respect constitutes sociality regarding caring and equality (Renger and Reese 2017). Teamwork has boosted sociality by raising organizational commitment and social cohesion (Carter et al. 2024; Gould-Williams 2005).

Nonprofit organization employment has secured utility for sociality resting on harmony (Ariza-Montes and Lucia-Casademunt 2016). Harmony experienced has induced sociality characterized by adjustment, attunement, civility, compromise, connectedness, interdependency, order, peace, relatedness, respect, sacrifice, selflessness, solidarity, and sympathy as opposed to competition and conflict (Arat and Kerelian 2019; Cheung and Ma 2011; P. Ip 2014; Kjell et al. 2016; Peck 2002; G. Zhang 2006).

Nonprofit organization employment has uplifted ideals for community and relatedness to rationalize sociality (Robichau and Sandberg 2022). The ideal for community constitutes sociality (Fowers 2015). Religiosity also reflects ideals for altruism, groupism or sharing, and nationalism to rationalize sociality (Franks et al. 2013;

Lichterman 2012; Requena and Stanek 2014). Relatedness has consolidated sociality by consolidating sharing, social interaction, and relationship satisfaction (Downie et al. 2008; Frazer 1999; Wickham and Knee 2012).

Work Condition

Work conditions include intellectual, creative, independent, and supervisory work. Intellectual, creative, and independent work are likely to weaken sociality, and supervisory work is likely to enhance sociality. These working conditions are influential because of their generation or withdrawal of power, utility, ideals, and norms to run the voluntaristic mechanisms of analytical functionalism.

Creative work has weakened power for sociality by engendering nervousness (Gelade 1999). Nervousness reflects cheating to impede sociality (Burgoon et al. 2010). Conversely, creative work has impaired power for sociality arising from conscientiousness (Gelade 1999). Conscientiousness has elevated sociality by consolidating attachment, compliance, order value, responsibility, social desirability, and volunteering and reducing deviance, violence, and justification for unconventional sexuality (Bekkers 2005; de Jong et al. 2012; Fraley et al. 2011; Gotzsche-Astrup 2020; Mondak and Hurwitz 2012; Mullet et al. 2005; Saucier and Skrzypinska 2006; Twardawski et al. 2021; Wright and DeLisi 2016).

Independent work has generated disutility against sociality from alienation experienced (Vallas 1988). Alienation experienced has eroded sociality regarding attachment (Bishop et al. 2002).

Supervisory work has enhanced power for sociality stemming from self-efficacy, social capital, and social status (Corcoran et al. 2011; Whyte and Gao 2009; Wuthnow 2002). Self-efficacy has sustained sociality by raising civic engagement, donation, government and social trust, leadership, political participation, prosocial behavior, and social activity (Bednall et al. 2013; Frye 2007; Gnambs and Batinic 2012; Huber et al. 2022; Mangum 2012; Rahn 2008; Pei and Pan 2018; Yao and Enright 2019). Social capital has consolidated sociality by raising civic engagement, community involvement, donation, political involvement, social trust, and volunteering (Bekkers et al. 2008; Broadbent and Papadopoulos 2011; Brown and Ferris 2007; Chua et al. 2021; Narayan and Cassidy 2001). Conversely, social capital has strengthened sociality by erasing violence (Pulkkinen et al. 2009). Social status has enhanced sociality by raising helping and interaction quality (Molana and Adams 2019). Conversely, supervisory work has prevented unemployment, thus maintaining power for sociality (Francesconi and Golsch 2005). Unemployment has impeded sociality by dissolving social capital, social cohesion, and trust (Espvall and Dellgren 2008; Manturuk et al. 2010; Reeskens and Vandecasteele 2017). Conversely, unemployment has hurt sociality by breeding conflict experienced, moving, protesting, threats experienced, and victimization (Bramley and Morgan 2003; Kaukinen 2004; Lewin-Epstein et al. 2003; Schneider 2007; Su and Feng 2013).

Supervisory work has secured utility for sociality from life satisfaction (Rampichini and D'Andrea 1998). Life satisfaction has incubated sociality regarding political participation, social cohesion, social trust, and volunteering (E. Chan 2014; Flavin and Keane 2011; Rochelle 2015).

Supervisory work has enhanced ideals for community service, community welfare, equality, ethics, political participation, and social welfare to rationalize sociality (Fahmy 2006; Kraft and Singhapakdi 1991; Taylor-Gooby et al. 2003). Conversely, supervisory work has weakened ideals against tolerating deviance and protesting to approve sociality (Geser 1998; Jenkins and Wallace 1996). Community service has constituted sociality by raising altruism, charity orientation, civic motivation, donation, helping, moral responsibility, political participation, social integration, and social and government trust (Foster et al. 2001; Isham et al. 2006; Richey 2010; Richey and Ikeda 2009; Wiepking and Maas 2009). Conversely, community service has safeguarded sociality by preventing deviance and its tolerance, delinquency, and loneliness (Gillath et al. 2005; J. Wilson 2000; Woolley 2003). The ideal for community upholds sociality by espousing caring, civility, collective identity, commonweal orientation, community, dutifulness or responsibility, education or socialization, equality, interdependence, loyalty, mentoring, patriotism, reciprocity, relatedness, self-discipline, servicing including volunteering, settlement, social construction, social participation, solidarity, and trust (Delanty 2009; Frazer 1999; Moore 2010; Speth 2012). Egalitarianism has underpinned sociality by enhancing empathy, support for welfare, and trust in government and impeding radicalism (Faricy and Ellis 2014; Lauriola et al. 2015; Lucas and Kteily 2018; Roosma et al. 2014). The ideal for ethics can enhance sociality regarding social trust (Bersot and Arrigo 2015; Steinhardt 2012). Political participation has buttressed sociality regarding civility (Campbell 2003). The ideal for social welfare has championed sociality by consolidating government trust (U. Kim et al. 2002).

Family Income

Family income is likely to consolidate sociality by affording power, utility, ideals, and norms to achieve the functions of sociality. Such achievement leverages the voluntaristic mechanisms of power realization, utility optimization, ideal calibration, and norm conformity integral to analytical functionalism.

Family income has secured power for sociality based on education, financial adequacy, friendliness, health and mental health, knowledge, mastery, organizational membership, self-efficacy, social capital, social integration, social status, and social support received (Apinunmahakul and Devlin 2008; Belzil and Hansen 2020; Cerin and Leslie 2008; Crowder et al. 2006; Kleinhans et al. 2007; La Grange and Yip 2001; Lennartsson 2010; Oshio and Kobayashi 2010; Powdthavee 2009; Shin 2012; Thoits and Hewitt 2001; Whyte and Gao 2009). Education has fostered sociality by raising civic engagement, civility, conformism, crime disapproval, equality support, morality, political discussion, political interest, political participation, socialism, and trust (Bullock 2021; E. Chan 2014; Djupe and Lewis 2015; Gilberbloom and Markham 1995; Kerrissey and Schofer 2013; Miyata et al. 2008; Norris 2011; Norris and Inglehart 2009; Ulbig 2002; Wilson and Dunham 2001). Conversely, education has sustained sociality by reducing political alienation, deviance, prostitution, resistance, and violence and its tolerance (Backman and Nilsson 2011; Coffe and Geys 2007; Lubbers et al. 2006; Michalski 2005; Simon et al. 2001; Swader and Vorobeva 2015). Financial adequacy has enabled sociality by raising government trust (Li and Mayraz 2017). Friendliness has enabled sociality regarding prosocial behavior (Foschi and Lauriola 2014). Health has uplifted sociality by boosting community sense, morality, popularity, social activity, social cohesion, social integration, social trust, social well-being, and volunteering (Huxhold et al. 2014; Jorgensen et al. 2010; Son and Wilson 2012; Tolsma et al. 2009; Yu and Chiu 2016). Conversely, health has sustained sociality by preventing loneliness (Koromeckyj-Cox et al. 2007). Generally, knowledge has raised sociality by enhancing cooperation, prosocial behavior, social cohesion, social trust, and volunteering (de Groot and Steg 2009; Lepkowski and Couper 2002; Pattie et al. 2004; Simon-Bemd and Steffens 2000; Volker et al. 2007;). Mastery has enhanced sociality by uplifting social trust (Burke and Stets 1999). Organizational membership has constituted sociality by strengthening institutional commitment and conformity (Vartanian and Hopkinson 2010). Self-efficacy has sustained sociality by raising civic engagement, donation, government and social trust, leadership, political participation, prosocial behavior, and social activity (Bednall et al. 2013; Frye 2007; Gnambs and Batinic 2012; Huber et al. 2022; Mangum 2012; Rahn 2008; Pei and Pan 2018; Yao and Enright 2019). Social capital has consolidated sociality by raising civic engagement, community involvement, donation, political involvement, social trust, and volunteering (Bekkers et al. 2008; Broadbent and Papadopoulos 2011; Brown and Ferris 2007; Chua et al. 2021; Narayan and Cassidy 2001). Conversely, social capital has strengthened sociality by erasing violence (Pulkkinen et al. 2009). Social integration has constituted sociality by enhancing cooperation and preventing suicide (Duberstein et al. 2004; Lepkowski and Couper 2002). Social status has enhanced sociality by raising helping and interaction quality (Molana and Adams 2019). Social support received has strengthened sociality by enhancing attachment, gratitude, political participation, prosocial behavior, recourse, respect, responsibility, social integration, and social well-being (Boezeman and Ellemers 2008; Fahmy 2006; Phipps 2003; Williams and Galliher 2006; R. Wright et al. 2009; Zeldin et al. 2016; Zeng et al. 2024). Conversely, social support received has boosted sociality by preventing aggression, conflict, delinquency, doping, externalizing, hyperactivity, loneliness, runaway, sexuality, suicide, and violence (Bernardon et al. 2011; Browning et al. 2005; Hayslip et al. 2000; Nieuwenhuis et al. 2017; Pearson and Wilkinson 2013; Terzi-Unsal and Karei 2005; Wight et al. 2006; R. Wright et al. 2009). Conversely, family income has prevented mortality, thus retaining power for sociality (Phelan et al. 2004). Dying can dampen sociality by fomenting aggression (Reeve 2021).

Family income has created utility for sociality based on living standards, neighborhood quality, satisfaction, and self-esteem (Oliver 2003; Woldoff and Ovadia 2009; Whyte and Gao 2009). Satisfaction covers democracy, finance, friendship, housing, life, marriage, the neighborhood, and work (Ambrey and Fleming 2014; Harris 2001; Kwok et al. 2015; Louis and Zhao 2002; Norris 2011; van Praag et al. 2003). Living standards can elevate sociality regarding morality (Narvaez 2014). Neighborhood quality has elevated sociality by building social capital, order, and cohesion (Rupp et al. 2020; Sampson and Raudenbush 2004). Satisfaction has advanced sociality by strengthening political participation, social cohesion, social and government trust, and volunteering (E. Chan 2014; Flavin and Keane 2011; Rochelle 2015). Self-esteem has buttressed sociality by raising attachment security, political participation, and prosociality and by preventing suicide (Kitayama and Markus 2000; Tracy et al. 2009).

Conversely, family income has reduced disutility against sociality stemming from discrimination, economic hardship, social exclusion, stress, and threat experienced (Myer et al. 2008; Posthumus et al. 2013; Stanley et al. 2011; Moore and Aweiss 2003; Raijman et al. 2003). Discrimination experienced can foment violence to undermine sociality (White et al. 2015). Economic hardship has impaired sociality by dampening trust and fomenting social exclusion experienced, suicide, and victimization experienced (Economou et al. 2016; Reeskens and Vandecasteele 2017; Ross and Mirowsky 2009). Social exclusion experienced has disturbed sociality by eroding closeness and prosocial behavior (Bockler et al. 2021; K. Lin et al. 2013). Stress experienced has undermined sociality by eroding civility, forgiveness, generativity, relationship quality and satisfaction, social integration, social support received, and trust and heightening conflict, maltreatment, substance abuse, suicide, and violence (Atkinson et al. 2005; Dutton et al. 2016; Gelles 2007; Grzywacz and Almeida 2008; Jackson et al. 2006; Sobeck et al. 2020; Toussaint et al. 2016). Threats received have inhibited sociality by reducing cohesion and triggering conflict and resistance (Lubbers et al. 2006; B. Rick et al. 2006).

Family income has enhanced ideals for sociality highlighting association commitment, civic engagement, civility, community involvement, compliance, conservatism, donation, friendship, institutional and social trust, national identity, nationalism, political interest and participation, prosociality, republicanism, social interaction, and xenophobia (Alnsour and Meaton 2009; Doff and Kleinhans 2011; Ishio 2010; Kunovich 2009; Layman 1997; Norris 2011; Norris and Inglehart 2009; Oliver 2003; Shin 2012; Straume and Odeen 2010; Traunmuller 2011; Wiepking and Maas 2009; T. Wilson 2001; Q. Xu et al. 2010). Association commitment has fostered sociality regarding connectedness, friendship, giving, and social interaction (Eberl 2020; Liebler and Sandefur 2002; Nelson-Coffey et al. 2023; Phan et al. 2009). Civic engagement has propped sociality by strengthening attachment, civility, collective behavior, discussion, donation, neighboring, patriotism, prosociality, social capital, socialism, trust, and volunteering and impeding cheating and individualism (Coffe and Geys 2007; Gilberbloom and Markham 1995; Kerrissey and Schofer 2013; Mata and Pendakur 2014; Ozbay 2008; Pattie et al. 2004; Pena-Lopez and Sanchez-Santos 2016; Rahn 2008; Richey 2011; Tak 2017; M. Tang 2011; Taniguchi 2013; Yip et al. 2007). Civility has constituted sociality by inducing fairness and trust (Vera-Toscano et al. 2013). Additionally, civility maintains sociality by enhancing the commonweal, community, equality, friendship, reciprocity, and social capital

(Hudson 2023). Community involvement has underlain sociality regarding cooperation, networking, and trust (Groves et al. 2000; Molitor et al. 2011; Rochelle 2015). Compliance has constituted sociality by raising patriotism and impeding violence and acceptance of deviants and outsiders (Pulkkinen et al. 2009; Schwartz et al. 2014; Van Hootegem et al. 2000; Yeo and Chu 2018). Conservatism sustains sociality by nurturing empathy, loyalty, prosocial behavior, religiousness, and sacrifice (Dutton and Rayner-Hilles 2022). Moreover, conservatism underpins sociality by maintaining allegiance or loyalty, attachment, civility, community, conformity, cooperation, discipline, ethnocentrism, honesty, humility, intimacy, legality, morality, nationalism, obedience, order, partnership, patriotism, peace, responsibility, sharing, trust, and xenophobia (Dutton and Rayner-Hilles 2022; Heilman and Kusev 2020; Hickson 2013; Lakoff 2009; Rhodes-Purdy et al. 2023; Scruton 2014; Yoos 2007; Zuk and Zuk 2020). Conversely, conservatism upholds sociality by condemning dehumanizing, evilness, revolution, sexuality, terrorism, and transgression (Dutton and Rayner-Hilles 2022; Malka and Soto 2011; Scruton 2014; Suhay 2015). Donation has constituted sociality by consolidating charity, service value, social capital, social trust, and volunteering (Bekkers 2010; Chang 2009; Foster et al. 2001; Uslaner 2000). Friendship has constituted sociality by enhancing community attachment, compliance, donation, gratitude, political participation, social cohesion, social desirability, social integration, and social trust (Corcoran 2013; Fahmy 2006; Gundert and Hohendanner 2015; Keillor et al. 2001; Kende et al. 2022; Opp 2001; Rotkirch 2014). Trust has constituted sociality through donation, involvement, and volunteering (Uslaner 2000). Nationalism or national identity has underpinned sociality by fostering attachment, intolerance against deviance, patriotism, political participation, religiousness, social inclusion, trust in government, and xenophobia, and diminishing protesting (N. Chen 2012; Flanagan and Lee 2000; Huddy et al. 2021; Li and Brewer 2004; Osborne et al. 2017; Pinto et al. 2020; Rippl et al. 2010). Political interest has elevated sociality by raising civic engagement, civic and social motivation, civility, and discussion as opposed to protesting (Gil de Zuniga et al. 2017; Lee and Chan 2011; Pattie et al. 2004). Political participation has buttressed sociality regarding civility (Campbell 2003). Prosociality has constituted sociality by civility, consolidating connectedness, cooperation, religiosity, responsibility, and volunteering (Hample 2018; Marsh and Dik 2021; Musick and Wilson 2008; Nelson-Coffey et al. 2023; Shahzalal and Adnan 2022). Republicanism upholds sociality regarding citizenship, the commonweal, interdependence, morality, nationalism, publicity, responsibility, social adaptation, and solidarity (Delanty 2009; Honohan 2002). Social interaction has realized sociality by consolidating altruism, compliance, cooperation, donation, morality, political participation, reciprocity, social trust, and volunteering (Guillen et al. 2011; Dixon and McKeown 2021; Lucas and Livingston 2014; Musick 2000; Rodrigo-Gonzalez et al. 2019; Rubin and Step 2000). Xenophobia has constituted sociality by boosting patriotism and social cohesion (Granzin and Olsen 1998; Wang and Chen 2004).

Conversely, family income has dampened ideals against sociality favoring cheating, crime, religiousness, sleeping, and violence (Cerin and Leslie 2008; Hamermesh 2019; Norris and Inglehart 2009; Ozbay 2008; T. Simon et al. 2001). Cheating has eroded honesty to impede sociality (O'Connor et al. 2022). Crime has impaired sociality by reducing community involvement, prosocial behavior, and social trust and fomenting avoidance, protesting, risking, victimization, and violence (Brayne 2014; McNeeley and Yuan 2017; Broadbent and Papadopoulos 2011; Sun and Wang 2012; Wittebrood and Nieuwbeerta 2000; Zhong 2010). Religiousness has hindered sociality by reducing nationalism, social interaction and engendering protesting, marginalization experienced, radicalism, and social distance (Ayalon et al. 1993; Kunovich 2009; Norris 2002; Pedahzur and Canetti-Nisim 2004; Wuthnow 2004). The ideal for sleeping or sleepiness has bred crime to disrupt sociality (Raine and Venables 2017). Violence has undermined sociality by breeding antisociality, crime and recidivism, blaming, conflict, hostility, rejecting others, and impairing agreeableness, morality, and responsibility (Asendorpf et al. 2008; Del Bove et al. 2008; Morrison 2006; Scholte et al. 2009; Vitaro et al. 2007).

Family income has exposed norms for sociality popularizing civility, cohesion, and fairness (Ferriss 2002; van Oorschot and Arts 2005; Viewiebe and Wegener 2000). The norm for civility has constituted sociality by enhancing political trust (Mutz and Reeves 2005). Social cohesion has constituted sociality by enhancing attachment and dampening tolerance for deviance (Stafford et al. 2005; Woosnam et al. 2018). The norm for fairness has upheld sociality by elevating morality and prosocial behavior (Barber 2004; McCaffoee 2016).

Conversely, family income has lessened norms against inequality and risk to assimilate sociality (Castillo 2011; Oliver 2003). The norm of inequality has impeded sociality by eroding social capital, support for redistribution and welfare, sympathy, trust, and volunteering (Busemeyer 2013; Hitlin and Harkness 2018; Lipford and Yandle 2009; Oishi et al. 2011; Portes and Vickstrom 2011). Conversely, the norm of inequality has impaired sociality by provoking crime and violence (Ousey and Lee 2013; van Wilsem 2007). The norm for risk has impaired sociality by provoking protesting (Scafuto and La Barbera 2016). Moreover, the risk norm can hurt sociality by generating opposition to the establishment (P. Brown 2020).

Survey Interest

Survey interest is likely to advance sociality by affording power, utility, ideals, and norms to achieve the functions of sociality. This achievement hinges on the voluntaristic mechanisms of power realization, utility optimization, ideal calibration, and norm conformity.

Power for sociality enhanced by interest has stemmed from knowledge, leadership, nationalism, self-efficacy, social capital, and social competence (Foschi and Lauriola 2014; Scheufele and Shah 2000; Su, Lee, and Borah 2021; Boulianne et al. 2022; Vargas-Salfate et al. 2020; Weeks et al. 2017). Generally, knowledge has raised sociality by enhancing cooperation, prosocial behavior, social cohesion, social trust, and volunteering (de Groot and Steg 2009; Lepkowski and Couper 2002; Pattie et al.

2004; Simon-Bemd and Steffens 2000; Volker et al. 2007). Leadership has enhanced sociality by raising civic engagement (Shah and Scheufele 2006).

Utility for sociality attained by interest has rested on political evaluation and satisfaction (Brosius et al. 2020; Stecker and Tausendpfund 2016). Political evaluation constitutes sociality by unfolding communitarianism and republicanism, which espouse community and solidarity (Pattie et al. 2004). Satisfaction has advanced sociality by strengthening political participation, social cohesion, social and government trust, and volunteering (E. Chan 2014; Flavin and Keane 2011; Rochelle 2015).

Ideals for sociality raised by interest have accentuated civic engagement, civility, government trust, political participation, redistribution, sharing, social desirability, social welfare, and xenophobia (Ballard-Rosa et al. 2017; Boulianne et al. 2022; Campbell 2003; Corr et al. 2013; Lancee and Pardos-Prado 2013; Ryan et al. 2005; Shah and Scheufele 2006; Soler-i-Marti 2015; Xiang and Hmielowski 2017). Civic engagement has propped sociality by strengthening attachment, civility, collective behavior, discussion, donation, neighboring, patriotism, prosociality, social capital, socialism, trust, and volunteering and impeding cheating and individualism (Coffe and Geys 2007; Gilberbloom and Markham 1995; Kerrissey and Schofer 2013; Mata and Pendakur 2014; Ozbay 2008; Pattie et al. 2004; Pena-Lopez and Sanchez-Santos 2016; Rahn 2008; Richey 2011; Tak 2017; M. Tang 2011; Taniguchi 2013; Yip et al. 2007). Civility has constituted sociality by inducing fairness and trust (Vera-Toscano et al. 2013). Government trust has constituted sociality by sustaining compliance, conformity, nationalism, political participation, and preventing protesting (Rhodes-Purdy et al. 2023; Ulbig 2002; van der Meer and van Ingen 2009; V. Vu 2021). Political participation has buttressed sociality regarding civility (Campbell 2003). The ideal for redistribution has reflected sociality regarding social trust (Nagayoshi and Sato 2014). Sharing has raised sociality by facilitating donating (Piferi et al. 2006). Moreover, sharing maintains sociality by involving social closeness, commitment, contribution, and gifting (Godoy et al. 2007; Murray and Holmes 2008). Social desirability has buttressed sociality by raising altruism, benevolence value, and empathy and perspective-taking and by suppressing violence and its tolerance (Douglas 2006; Fisher and Katz 2000; Krumrei-Mancuso 2017; Pulkkinen et al. 2009). The ideal for social welfare has championed sociality by consolidating government trust (U. Kim et al. 2002). Xenophobia has constituted sociality by boosting patriotism and social cohesion (Granzin and Olsen 1998; Wang and Chen 2004).

Current Findings

Using the World Values Survey data, linear regression analysis screened out statistically significant ($p < .001$) predictors of social attitudes in five steps with the stepwise selection procedure. Step 1 showed the time effect. Step 2 additionally screened out significant predictors from national performance factors. Step 3 additionally screened out significant predictors from personal and response characteristics. Response characteristics comprised survey interest and acquiescence, which meant rating everything highly. Step 4 additionally screened out significant predictors from national and personal experiences and practices. Step 5 additionally screened out significant national and personal well-being factors. Step 6 additionally screened out superpower main and interaction factors, with China and the United States as superpowers. Among these steps, Step 3 began to reveal the significant effects of personal characteristics on social attitudes. These steps corresponded to the putative causal or temporal order. Regression analysis estimated net effects, with the control for predictors included in a step and earlier steps. These actual effects partly dovetailed with the expected effects (see Table 3.1).

Confidence in institutions most strongly responded to age, among the personal characteristics. The age effect was weakly positive ($\beta = .080$, see Table 3.2). The next strongest predictor was irreligion, which also exhibited a weak positive effect on confidence in institutions ($\beta = .071$).

Justification for misdeeds most strongly responded to nonprofit organization employment, among the personal characteristics. This effect was weakly positive ($\beta = .126$, see Table 3.3). The next strongest predictor was independent work, which exhibited a weak negative effect on justification for misdeeds ($\beta = -.104$).

Justification for unconventional sexuality most strongly responded to irreligion, among the personal characteristics. This effect was weakly positive ($\beta = .156$, see Table 3.4). The next strongest predictor was nonprofit organization employment, which exhibited a weak positive effect on justification for unconventional sexuality ($\beta = .139$).

Faith in religion most strongly responded to irreligion, among the personal characteristics. This effect was strongly negative ($\beta = -.414$, see Table 3.5). The next strongest predictor was education, which exhibited a weak negative effect on faith in religion ($\beta = .139$).

Acceptance of outsiders most strongly responded to education, among the personal characteristics. This effect was strongly negative ($\beta = -.094$, see Table 3.6). The next strongest predictor was independent work, which exhibited a weak negative effect on acceptance of outsiders ($\beta = -.068$).

Acceptance of deviants most strongly responded to nonprofit organization employment, among the personal characteristics. This effect was strongly negative ($\beta = -.105$, see Table 3.7). The next strongest predictor was graduation age, which exhibited a weak negative effect on acceptance of deviants ($\beta = -.097$).

Trust in others most strongly responded to family income and nonprofit organization employment, among the personal characteristics. These effects were weakly positive ($\beta = .062$, see Table 3.8). The next strongest predictor was age, which exhibited a weak positive effect on trust in others ($\beta = .058$) (Table 3.8).

Contrary to expectation, confidence in institutions received negative effects from education, graduation age, survey interest, and supervisory work. Nevertheless, confidence in institutions has received a negative effect from education (S. Chi et al. 2021).

Table 3.1 Expected and actual effects of personal characteristics on sociality

Predictor	Expected	Actual						
		Institution	Anti-misdeed	Anti-sex	Anti-faith	Anti-outsider	Anti-deviant	Other
Female	+	+	+		–		–	
Age	+	+	+		+			+
Education	+	–			+	+	–	
Graduation age	+	–		–	+	+	+	
Irreligious	+	+		–	+	+		
Family income	+			–	+	+	+	+
Age squared	+	+						+
Married	+			+		–		
Cohabited	+				+			
Divorced	–	–		–		–		
Separated	–							–
Widowed	–			+	–	–		
Unmarried	+							+
Kid	+		–	+	–			
Mother immigrant	–	–	–	–				
Father immigrant	–					+	+	
Living with parents	+			+	+	–		
Full-time employment	+			+	–		–	
Part-time employment	+			+	–		–	
Self-employment	+							
Retired	–	–		+	–			

(continued)

Table 3.1 (continued)

Predictor	Expected	Actual						
		Institution	Anti-misdeed	Anti-sex	Anti-faith	Anti-outsider	Anti-deviant	Other
Homemaking	–							
Student	–	–	–				+	
Unemployed	–							
Public employment	+		–	–	+		+	
Private business employment	+			–	+			
Nonprofit organization employment	+		–	–	+	–	+	+
Intellectual work	–			–				
Creative work	–	–	–			–	–	
Independent work	+		+	+		+		
Supervision	+	–			+		+	
Earner status	+						–	+
Earner employed	+	+		–		+	+	+
Survey interest	+	–		+		+	+	+

Note Sociality unfolded in social attitudes in terms of confidence in institutions, refutation against misdeeds, refutation against unconventional sexuality, unfaith in religion, rejection of outsiders, rejection of deviants, and trust in others
+ positive effect. –negative effect

Table 3.2 Significant ($p <$ .001) standardized effects of personal characteristics on confidence in institutions

Predictor	(3)	(4)	(5)
Acquiescence	.525	.544	.565
Female	.055	.048	.046
Age	.080	.059	.046
Education	− .049	− .068	− .079
Creative work	− .052	− .055	− .047
Irreligious	.071	.051	.053
Retired	− .042	− .024	− .020
Graduation age	− .024	− .008n	− .004n
Student	− .027	− .025	− .020
Mother immigrant	− .021	− .025	− .017
Survey interest	− .021	− .007n	− .007n
Age squared	.017	.017	.016
Earner employed	.019	.015	.006n
Supervision	− .017	− .017	− .019
Divorce	− .014	− .013	− .010n
Full-time employment	.014n	.023	.027
Separated	− .010n	− .012n	− .009n
Widowed	.012n	.014	.015
Earner status	− .015n	− .015n	− .010n
Homemaking	− .013n	− .004n	− .002n
R^2	.364	.386	.401

n: $p > .001$

Table 3.3 Significant ($p <$ .001) standardized effects of personal characteristics on justification for misdeeds

Predictor	(3)	(4)
Acquiescence	.132	.153
Female	− .026	− .023
Age	− .044	− .046
Nonprofit organization employment	.126	.123
Mother immigrant	.047	.046
Student	.040	.037
Public employment	.048	.047
Independent work	− .104	− .095
Creative work	.073	.067
Kid	.025	.024
Graduation age	.014n	.018
R^2	.062	.069

n: $p > .001$

Table 3.4 Significant ($p < .001$) standardized effects of personal characteristics on justification for unconventional sexuality

Predictor	(3)	(4)	(5)
Acquiescence	.078	.106	.116
Female	.026	.020	.022
Age	− .012n	− .026	− .027
Education	− .004n	− .020	− .017
Nonprofit organization employment	.139	.037	.036
Irreligious	.156	.149	.149
Earner employed	.063	.039	.043
Intellectual work	.098	.090	.083
Graduation age	.044	.038	.036
Independent work	− .078	− .030	− .020n
Public employment	.080	.025	.024
Private business employment	.055	.024	.022
Part-time employment	− .053	− .027	− .028
Full-time employment	− .055	− .035	− .036
Divorce	.025	.023	.022
Retired	− .030	− .008n	− .010n
Survey interest	− .029	− .017	− .015
Kid	− .026	− .014	− .015n
Family income	.022	.029	.040
Mother immigrant	.018	.011n	.007n
Living with parents	− .023	− .018	− .018
Married	− .030	− .039	− .036
Widowed	− .020	− .025	− .025
Self-employed	− .014n	− .021	− .020
Supervision	.012n	− .004n	− .004n
Student	.013n	− .010n	− .012
R^2	.238	.275	.280

n: $p > .001$

The negative effects of education, graduation age, and supervisory work on confidence in institutions reflect the contradiction between the power of control or domination in education, graduate age, and supervisory work and the ideal for compliance or submission in confidence in institutions. Education or graduate age registers the power of control (Papastephanon 2015). Supervisory work means controlling (Nee and Cao 2002). Meanwhile, confidence in institutions features agreement, commitment, constraint, and regulation to represent compliance or submission (Cox 2016; Lowndes and Roberts 2013; W. Scott 2008). The negative effects of the contradiction

Table 3.5 Significant ($p < .001$) standardized effects of personal characteristics on faith in religion

Predictor	(3)	(4)	(5)
Acquiescence	.209	.181	.184
Female	.040	.048	.047
Age	– .014	.009	.005
Education	– .062	– .045	– .042
Irreligious	– .414	– .410	– .409
Nonprofit organization employment	– .053	– .005	– .005
Kid	.034	.026	.025
Supervision	– .024	– .021	– .021
Part-time employment	.042	.009	.009
Retired	.024	.003	.003
Private business employment	– .037	– .015	– .015
Public employment	– .032	– .003	– .003
Graduation age	– .020	– .012	– .011
Cohabited	– .019	– .012	– .012
Full-time employment	.019	– .004	– .004
Family income	– .016	– .024	– .021
Widowed	.012	.012	.012
Living with parents	– .012	– .011	– .012
R^2	.524	.544	.550

n: $p > .001$

thus represent force theory as an overarching mechanism for incorporating analytical functionalism. Force theory posits that contradicting forces from two factors produce a negative effect between the factors (Ambrose 2002; Cheung 2013, 2024). Force covers power, utility, ideals, and norms.

Contrary to expectation, refutation against misdeeds received negative effects from the number of children, public employment, and nonprofit organization employment. These effects reflect the contradiction between refutation against or ideal for misdeeds and the power of the number of children, public employment, and nonprofit organization employment for misdeeds. The number of children has afforded domestic violence and tolerance for deviance and eroded prosociality to bolster misdeeds (Bjornberg and Ekbrand 2008; Coffe and Geys 2007; Fox et al. 2002). Public employment has enhanced help and respect for deviants to justify misdeeds (Freund 2005; Robichau and Sandberg 2022). Nonprofit organization employment has accentuated the value of clients, who are likely deviant and thus socially excluded, to justify misdeeds (Robichau and Sandberg 2022). Therefore, the negative effects of contradiction follow force theory, which posits the negative impact of contradictory forces.

Table 3.6 Significant ($p < .001$) standardized effects of personal characteristics on acceptance of outsiders

Predictor	(3)	(4)	(5)
Acquiescence	.240	.241	.263
Female	.006n	.005n	.007n
Age	.018n	.004n	− .006n
Education	− .094	− .103	− .099
Graduation age	− .052	− .031	− .031
Nonprofit organization employment	.044	.027	.029
Independent work	− .068	− .062	− .056
Earner employed	− .033	− .032	− .030
Married	.046	.026	.029
Creative work	.041	.028	.023
Irreligious	.034	.037	.041
Family income	− .021	− .014n	.001n
Living with parents	.027	.019	.019
Survey interest	− .020	− .015n	− .013n
Kid	.018n	.030	.029
Father immigrant	− .016	− .009n	− .009n
Widowed	.020	.010	.011n
Divorced	.018	.015	.014n
R^2	.166	.182	.188

n: $p > .001$

Contrary to expectation, refutation against unconventional sexuality received negative effects from family income, employment, family earner employment, and irreligion, and positive effects from retirement and widowhood. In other words, irreligion, family income, employment, and family earner employment supported unconventional sexuality, and retirement and widowhood rejected unconventional sexuality. Sexuality has risen with family income and mother employment (Y. Hu 2016; Yeung and Hu 2016). Moreover, sexuality has declined with widowhood (Jung 2016). Employment has sustained normlessness and protesting and eroded support for the traditional gender role to buttress unconventionality (Kerrissey and Schofer 2013; Moen et al. 1997; Ross and Mirowsky 2009). Irreligion has supported unconventional sexuality, including homosexuality queer theory (Cochran et al. 2004; Gaines and Garand 2010). Retirement has rejected homosexuality and violence to impede unconventionality (Macmillan and Baiocchi 2010; Michalski 2005). Widowhood has obstructed sociality by dampening relatedness, social interaction, social support received, social welfare support, and volunteering and fomented suicide and victimization (Duberstein et al. 2004; J. Ha et al. 2016; Lelli 2008; Like 2011; Patulny and Morris 2012; Taniguchi 2013). Hence, the negative and positive effects follow force

Table 3.7 Significant ($p < .001$) standardized effects of personal characteristics on acceptance of deviants

Predictor	(3)	(4)
Acquiescence	.272	.297
Female	.030	.032
Age	.048	.034
Education	.025	.029
Nonprofit organization employment	− .105	− .106
Graduation age	− .097	− .090
Public employment	− .075	− .073
Earner employed	− .065	− .063
Student	− .033	− .036
Supervision	− .051	− .048
Full-time employment	.042	.043
Part-time employment	.032	.032
Survey interest	− .027	− .023
Father immigrant	− .023	− .022
Earner status	.023	.021
Family income	− .024	− .006n
Creative work	.023	.019
Life satisfaction		− .078
Health		− .046
Security		.029
R^2	.182	.192

n: $p > .001$

Table 3.8 Significant ($p < .001$) standardized effects of personal characteristics on trust in others

Predictor	(3)	(4)	(5)
Female	− .007n	− .008n	− .008n
Age	.058	.060	.059
Family income	.062	.060	.059
Nonprofit organization employment	.062	.075	.074
Survey interest	.042	.042	.043
Earner employed	.026	.029	.029
Separated	− .031	− .030	− .030
Unmarried	.029	.029	.029
Earner status	.029	.027	.026
Age squared	.023	.023	.023
R^2	.039	.040	.042

n: $p > .001$

theory, which posits compatibility and contradiction as positive and negative causes, respectively.

Contrary to expectation, faith in religion rose with female gender, the number of children, and employment. Religious faith has risen with female gender and the number of children (Ghimire 2021a; Ishii and Watanable 2023). Employment has supported donation and philanthropy (Foster et al. 2001; Fridberg and Kangas 2008b). This support characterizes religious faith (Ager and Ager 2011). The positive effects female gender, the number of children, and employment on religious faith thus embody force theory, which emphasizes the compatibility of forces among factors.

Contrary to expectation, refutation against outsiders or xenophobia declined with marriage, parent coresidence, and nonprofit organization employment and increased with father immigration. Marriage has favored immigration to impede xenophobia (Reichman and Kenney 1997). Parent coresidence has fostered prosociality and weakened delinquency, prejudice, victimization experienced, and violence to maintain sociality (Andersson et al. 2010; Dennison and Swisher 2019; Kaufman-Parks et al. 2017; Oksanen et al. 2014). Nonprofit organization employment has dampened racism to inhibit xenophobia (Brolis et al. 2018). Immigration has eroded egalitarianism and volunteering to sustain xenophobia (Ravanera et al. 2003; Saunders and Wong 2012). Egalitarianism has obstructed racism to weaken xenophobia (Hartmann et al. 2017). Volunteering has advanced social network heterogeneity to diminish xenophobia (Patulny and Morris 2012). Hence, marriage, parent coresidence, and nonprofit organization employment generate forces against xenophobia, whereas immigration transmits force for xenophobia. Force theory incorporates power, utility, ideals, and norms in analytical functionalism.

Contrary to expectation, rejection of deviants reduced with female gender, education, employment, and family earner status and increased with father immigration. Female gender has dampened civility, conformism, conservatism, and political participation to diminish rejection of deviants (Kim and Wilcox 2013; Norris and Inglehart 2009; Stromblad and Myrberg 2013; Ulbig 2002). Civility dismisses antisociality, bullying, crime, resistance, and violence and upholds compliance, legality, normativity, obedience, and unity to resist deviance (Abizadeh 2010; Bannister and O'Sullivan 2013; Edyvane 2017; Hudson 2023; Jukes et al. 2018; D. Lin 2017; Williamson 2002). Conservativism has fostered abidance and conformism to reject deviance (Feinberg et al. 2019; Lane and Sulikowski 2017). Moreover, conservatism embraces conformity, legality, and loyalty and dismisses dissent, homosexuality, terrorism, and transgression to reject deviance (Dutton and Rayner-Hilles 2022; Heilman and Kusev 2020; Malka and Soto 2011; Scruton 2014; Sidanius and Pratto 1999; Yoos 2007). Political participation has buttressed civility to reject deviance (J. Berry et al. 1993). Conversely, female gender has engendered egalitarianism, multiculturalism, and radicalism to withdraw deviant rejection (Hagan et al. 1999; Pehrson et al. 2011; Saunders and Wong 2012). Egalitarianism has supported empathy and homosexuality to accept deviance (Brewer 2003; Lucas and Kteily 2018). Empathy has reduced problem avoidance to accept deviance (Momonoki and Ishii 2023). Multiculturalism espouses radicalism and unrest to accept deviance (Delanty 2009;

Pehrson et al. 2011). Radicalism has bred protesting and violence to accept deviance (Li and Song 1992; Pauwels and De Waele 2014). Essentially, radicalism registers deviance (Kruglanski et al. 2017). Education has supported crime, equality, homosexuality, minorities, and protesting and rejected law and its enforcement and restrictiveness to tolerance for deviance (Bullock 2021; Barkan and Cohn 2005; Datler et al. 2013; Olson et al. 2006; Tang 2009; Timberlake et al. 2003; Wodtke 2012; Woodrum 1992). Employment has fostered diversity, normlessness, and protesting and eroded traditionalism to accept deviance (Kerrissey and Schofer 2013; Moen et al. 1997; Ross and Mirowsky 2009; Stalker 2008). Immigration has bred fear of crime and dampened contact with crime to reject deviance (Brayne 2014; Kitchen and Williams 2010). Meanwhile, deviance features illegality and subculture (Vauclair and Fischer 2011; J. Williams 2011). As such, rejecting deviants stands on the force of immigration and declines with the forces of female gender, education, and employment in the lens of force theory.

Chapter 4
Functioning of Personal Experiences for Social Attitudes

Personal experiences cluster into seven factors in the World Values Survey. Experience factors are economic hardship, neighborhood nuisance, victimization, security, family saving, health, and life satisfaction. These experiences are likely to influence social attitudes from the perspective of sociality underlying the attitudes. Attitudes reflecting sociality are confidence in institutions, refutation against misdeeds, refutation against unconventional sexuality, unfaith in religion, rejection of outsiders, rejection of deviants, and trust in other people. According to analytical functionalism, experiences generate power, utility, ideals, and norms to activate voluntaristic mechanisms to influence sociality. Voluntaristic mechanisms engage power realization, utility optimization, ideal calibration, and norm conformity with personal experiences.

Existing Knowledge

Sociality encompasses altruism, attachment, bonding, caring, collective identity, communication, community, conformity, conscientiousness, conservation, cooperation, dependence, emotional stability, extraversion, fairness or justice, friendship, gifting, gregariousness, grouping, helping, honesty, honoring, institutionalization, leadership, learning, membership, morality, networking, normativity, openmindedness, organization, participation, punishment, rapport, reciprocity, relating, role-taking, sharing, social interaction, socializing, supporting, sympathy, teaching, trust, trustworthiness, and xenophobia (Boer and Fischer 2013; Capraro 2024; Cottrell et al 2007; Fenwick 2008; Fowers 2015; Koster 2013; M. Ma 2021; Marres 2017; Phithakkitnukoon and Smoreda 2016; Ratner et al. 2023; Rogers et al. 2014; Tomasello 2020). Conversely, sociality rejects aggression, autonomy, individualism,

C.-k. Cheung, *Social Attitudes in the Early 21st Century*,
https //doi.org/10.1007/978-981-96-9705-2_4

misanthropy, raging, risking, and stealing (Bissell 2010; Fowers 2015; Hughes et al. 2017). Individualism comprises independence, individuation, and self-interest (Fowers 2015).

Economic Hardship

Economic hardship is likely to retard sociality by eroding power, utility, ideals, and norms for sociality. Such erosion engages the voluntaristic mechanisms of power realization, utility optimization, ideal calibration, and norm conformity to maintain the functions of sociality based on analytical functionalism.

Power for sociality weakened by economic hardship has rested on health (Ahnquist et al. 2012). Health has uplifted sociality by boosting community sense, morality, popularity, social activity, social cohesion, social integration, social trust, social well-being, and volunteering (Huxhold et al. 2014; Jorgensen et al. 2010; Son and Wilson 2012; Tolsma et al. 2009; Yu and Chiu 2016). Conversely, health has sustained sociality by preventing loneliness (Koromeckyj-Cox et al. 2007). Moreover, economic hardship has engendered normlessness, weakening the power to drive sociality (Ross and Mirowsky 2009). Normlessness has impeded sociality by raising radicalism and support for violence (Troian et al. 2019). Moreover, normlessness inhibits sociality by disregarding consensus and foregrounding isolation (Troian et al. 2019; Zhao and Cao 2010).

Utility for sociality deprived by economic hardship has resided in well-being, including economic satisfaction (Reeskens and Vandecasteele 2017). Economic satisfaction has upheld sociality by dampening hostility (Rhodes-Purdy et al. 2023). More generally, well-being has uplifted sociality by consolidating altruism, conformism, cooperation, donation, liking for people, prosociality, sociability, and trust and social trust (Fetvadjiev and He 2019; A. Hu 2013; Lyubomirsky et al. 2006; Y. Pan et al. 2023; Wang and Graddy 2008). Additionally, well-being sustains sociality by enabling civilization, fairness, forgiveness, intimacy, kindness, love, loyalty, modesty, morality, open-mindedness, social intelligence, and societal functioning (Cummins 2016; D'raven and Pasha-Zaidi 2016; Meadows 2014). Conversely, economic hardship has brewed depression, distress, economic strain, and victimization as disutility to distract sociality (Ahnquist et al. 2012; Akiyama and Antonucci 2002; Aytac and Rankin 2009; Ross and Mirowsky 2009). Depression has eroded sociality by breeding conflict, hate, hostility perceived, loneliness, revenge, risking, suicide, and violence (Cacioppo and Hawkley 2009; Economou et al. 2016; Haner et al. 2020; Morokoff et al. 2009; Mullet et al. 2005; Proulx et al. 2004; H. Smith et al. 2016; E. Wright et al. 2015). Conversely, depression has attenuated sociality by impeding benevolence, closeness experienced, fairness, forgiveness, gratitude, honesty, leadership, love, social integration, teamwork, and volunteering (Blanchard et al. 2021; Cornwall 2009; Holzel et al. 2011; Mancini et al. 2011; Mullet et al. 2005; Thoits and Hewitt 2001). Distress has undermined sociality by fomenting resistance and impeding social capital and trust (Pulkkinen et al. 2009; Webber and

Huxley 2007). Generally, strain has undermined sociality by fomenting resistance and impeding social capital and trust (Pulkkinen et al. 2009; Webber and Huxley 2007). Victimization experienced has impaired sociality by eroding social trust (Olivera 2015). Conversely, victimization experienced has hurt sociality by activating conflict and migration (Bar-Tal and Halperin 2013; Ramesh et al. 2019). Economic hardship has reflected loss and social exclusion as disutility to distract sociality (Robila 2006; Robinaugh et al. 2016). The loss experienced has hindered sociality by eroding compliance and government trust and fomenting suicide (Kirchler and Maciejovsky 2001; Nicholls and Picou 2012). Social exclusion has impeded sociality by fueling crime, doping, and violence (Barry and Hullett 1998).

Ideals for sociality dispelled by economic hardship have accentuated social welfare and trust (Blomberg and Kroll 1999; Ross and Mirowsky 2009). The ideal for social welfare has championed sociality by consolidating government trust (U. Kim et al. 2002). Trust diminished by economic hardship has included political and social trust (Reeskens and Vandecasteele 2017). Political trust has constituted sociality by sustaining compliance, conformity, nationalism, political participation, and preventing protesting (Rhodes-Purdy et al. 2023; Ulbig 2002; van der Meer and van Ingen 2009; V. Vu 2021). Social trust has constituted sociality through donation, involvement, and volunteering (Uslaner 2000). Conversely, economic hardship has fomented suicide to erase the ideal for sociality (Economou et al. 2016). The ideal for suicide has impeded sociality by fomenting radicalism (Soliman et al. 2016).

Norms against sociality underlying economic hardship have popularized recession, poverty, and social exclusion (Muhlau 2014; Robila 2006). The norm for recession blocks sociality by breeding discrimination, individualism, inequality and polarization, migration, and protesting and lessening nationalism (A. Kim 2004). The norm for poverty has worsened civic engagement, civility, community involvement, donation, relatedness, social trust, and volunteering and fomented cynicism, suicide, theft, violence, and victimization to impair sociality (Abascal 2015; Broadbent and Papadopoulos 2011; J. Brown 2016; Graddy and Wang 2009; Hagan et al. 2016; Krahe 2013; Nepal et al. 2011; Piatkowska 2020; C. Ross et al. 2000; Stoll 2001; Wuthnow 2004). The norm for social exclusion has obstructed sociality by diminishing political participation and breeding inequality (Dawson 2021; Dorling 2010). Furthermore, the norm for social exclusion can undermine sociality by creating crime and revolution (Castells 2000; Goodwin 2005).

Neighborhood Nuisance

Neighborhood nuisance reflects deprivation, disadvantage, disorder, and problems in the surrounding community (Congdon 2010). Such nuisance covers alcohol consumption, drug selling, police interference, robbery, and racist behavior. Hence, neighborhood nuisance indicates incivility, poverty, and stress (G. Brown et al. 2004; Vartanian 1999; B. Williams et al. 1999). Neighborhood nuisance is likely to hamper sociality by attenuating power, utility, ideals, and norms to maintain the functions of sociality, considering analytical functionalism. This nuisance experienced exerts its influence through the voluntaristic mechanisms of power realization, utility optimization, ideal calibration, and norm conformity.

Power for sociality weakened by neighborhood nuisance has resulted from its creation of normlessness (Ross and Mirowsky 2009). Normlessness has impeded sociality by raising radicalism and support for violence (Troian et al. 2019). Moreover, normlessness inhibits sociality by disregarding consensus and foregrounding isolation (Troian et al. 2019; Zhao and Cao 2010). Furthermore, neighborhood nuisance has reduced earnings and social capital as power to drive sociality (Congdon 2010; Vartanian 1999). Earnings or income has upheld sociality by boosting civic engagement, community attachment and involvement, civic dutifulness, civility, conformity value, neighboring, political interest and participation, political and social trust, prosocial behavior, social capital, social integration, social interaction, social support received, social well-being, and volunteering (Bjornberg and Latta 2007; Chang 2009; Djupe and Lewis 2015; Frei et al. 2009; Kerrissey and Schofer 2013; Letki 2006; McCabe 2014; Patulny and Morris 2012; Son and Wilson 2012; Sun and Wang 2012; Swaroop and Morenoff 2006; Ulbig 2002). Conversely, income has maintained sociality by dampening alienation, discrimination experienced, migration, protesting, relocation, social deprivation experienced, social exclusion experienced, victimization, and violence (Broom et al. 2013; Brown and Connell 2004; Buck 2001; Rijken and Groenewegen 2008; V. Taylor et al. 2009; Weakliem and Borch 2006). Social capital has consolidated sociality by raising civic engagement, community involvement, donation, political involvement, social trust, and volunteering (Bekkers et al. 2008; Broadbent and Papadopoulos 2011; Brown and Ferris 2007; Chua et al. 2021; Narayan and Cassidy 2001). Conversely, social capital has strengthened sociality by erasing violence (Pulkkinen et al. 2009). Power for sociality diminishing neighborhood nuisance experienced has stemmed from resiliency (Ferretti et al. 2024). Resiliency has facilitated sociality by raising bonding and inhibiting crime and violence (Fields and McNamara 2003; Hoffman 2003; Solomon and Roloff 2018). Furthermore, resiliency sustains sociality by embodying or fostering adaptation and legality (Hoffman 2003; Ungar 2012). Resiliency also buttresses sociality by demonstrating altruism, attractiveness, communication or conversation, community, compassion, empathy or perspective-taking, negotiation, peacefulness, relationality, relatedness, social capital or resourcefulness, social cohesion, and social competence (Elfers et al. 2024; Hjemdal et al. 2015; Jones and d'Errico 2019; Kelley et al. 2019; Kent and Davis 2010; Ungar 2010; Zautra 2014).

Utility for sociality reduced by neighborhood nuisance has rested on well-being, including happiness and positive emotion (Hackman et al. 2019; van Praag and Frijters 1999). Well-being has uplifted sociality by consolidating altruism, conformism, cooperation, donation, liking for people, prosociality, sociability, and trust and social trust (Fetvadjiev and He 2019; A. Hu 2013; Lyubomirsky et al. 2006; Y. Pan et al. 2023; Wang and Graddy 2008). Conversely, neighborhood nuisance has created disutility against sociality lying in depression, economic hardship, and negative emotion (Hackman et al. 2019; Pei and Kim 2017; Whelan and Maitre 2013). Depression has eroded sociality by breeding conflict, hate, hostility perceived, loneliness, revenge, risking, suicide, and violence (Cacioppo and Hawkley 2009; Economou et al. 2016; Haner et al. 2020; Morokoff et al. 2009; Mullet et al. 2005; Proulx et al. 2004; H. Smith et al. 2016; E. Wright et al. 2015). Conversely, depression has attenuated sociality by impeding benevolence, closeness experienced, fairness, forgiveness, gratitude, honesty, leadership, love, social integration, teamwork, and volunteering (Blanchard et al. 2021; Cornwall 2009; Holzel et al. 2011; Mancini et al. 2011; Mullet et al. 2005; Thoits and Hewitt 2001). Economic hardship has impaired sociality by dampening trust and fomenting social exclusion experienced, suicide, and victimization experienced (Economou et al. 2016; Reeskens and Vandecasteele 2017; Ross and Mirowsky 2009). Negative emotion has undermined sociality by fomenting resistance and impeding social capital and trust (Pulkkinen et al. 2009; Webber and Huxley 2007). Neighborhood nursance experienced has also risen with anxiety and stress as disutility distracting sociality (Ferretti et al. 2024). Anxiety has disrupted sociality by breeding interpersonal problems, loneliness, risking, suicide, and violence (Dutton et al. 2016; Gillath et al. 2005; Pulkkinen et al. 2009; Trumbo et al. 2008). Conversely, anxiety has undermined sociality by reducing donation, friendship, humor, political participation, prosocial behavior, and social well-being (Best and Krueger 2010; Hewstone et al. 2005; Litman et al. 2017; Kuiper and Nicholl 2004; Zhong 2010). Stress has undermined sociality by eroding civility, forgiveness, generativity, relationship quality and satisfaction, social integration, social support received, and trust and heightening conflict, maltreatment, substance abuse, suicide, and violence (Atkinson et al. 2005; Dutton et al. 2016; Gelles 2007; Grzywacz and Almeida 2008; Jackson et al. 2006; Sobeck et al. 2020; Toussaint et al. 2016).

Ideals for sociality dropped by neighborhood nuisance have cherished community attachment and social trust (G. Brown et al. 2004; Ross and Mirowsky 2009). Community attachment has facilitated sociality regarding cooperation, networking, and trust (Groves et al. 2000; Molitor et al. 2011; Rochelle 2015). Social trust has constituted sociality through donation, involvement, and volunteering (Uslaner 2000).

The norm for sociality diminished by neighborhood nuisance has popularized safety (Kanan and Pruitt 2002). The norm for safety has elevated sociality by raising cohesion, neighboring, networking experienced, and trust and dampening aggression and opposition (Barbarin and Richter 2001; Grannis 2009; Rochelle 2015). Conversely, neighborhood nuisance foregrounds norms for deprivation, incivility, poverty, and stress to disrupt sociality (G. Brown et al. 2004; Congdon 2010; Vartanian 1999; B. Williams et al. 1999). Deprivation experienced erodes sociality by breeding conflict (J. Turner 2013b). Favoritism constitutes corruption (Inglehart and Welzel 2005). Incivility has harmed sociality by reducing fairness and trust (Vera-Toscano et al. 2013). Poverty has undermined sociality by reducing civic participation, trust, social connection, and volunteering (Caputo 2010; Stephens et al. 2014; R. Walker et al. 2010). Conversely, poverty has disrupted sociality by creating isolation, relationship problems, and social exclusion experienced (Dhal et al. 2008; Stephens et al. 2014; R. Walker et al. 2010). The norm for stress can impair sociality by breeding conflict and violence (Piatkowska 2020; Van Dyke and Soule 2002).

Victimization

Victimization essentially involves or necessitates arousal, negative reinforcement, readjustment, and scarring (Russo and Roccato 2010; Shippee 2012). Inherently, victimization covers abuse, assault, battering, bullying, fraud, burglary, disaster, harassment, hate, offense, pain, rape, threat, and violence experienced (Waterman et al. 2022; Wittebrood and Nieuwbeerta 2000). Victimization is likely to erode sociality by draining power, utility, ideals, and norms for sociality as required in analytical functionalism. Such draining results from the voluntaristic mechanisms of power realization, utility optimization, ideal calibration, and norm conformity.

Power for sociality weakened by victimization has evolved from neuroticism, normlessness, and powerlessness (Lincoln et al. 2003; Ross and Mirowsky 2009). Neuroticism has impaired sociality by reducing attachment security, civic engagement, coordination, forgiveness, nationalism, relatedness, and socializing and generating crime and hostility (Bekkers 2005; Fraley et al. 2011; Hounkpatin et al. 2015; Kalish 2008; Marks 1996; Mullet et al. 2005; Pulkkinen et al. 2009; Schbley and McCauley 2005; Ward and Forney 2020). Normlessness has impeded sociality by raising radicalism and support for violence (Troian et al. 2019). Moreover, normlessness inhibits sociality by disregarding consensus and foregrounding isolation (Troian et al. 2019; Zhao and Cao 2010). Powerlessness has eroded sociality by dampening attachment and giving (Campos-Castillo and Hitlin 2013; Molm 1997). Victimization experienced has arisen from inadequate power in employment, guardianship received, mental health, partnership, self-control, social competence, training, and wealth for driving sociality (Hollander 2018; Krahe 2013; Jones and Ferguson 2009; Reese et al. 2021; Rodriguez-Menes and Safranoff 2021; Walton-Moss et al. 2005; Wilcox 2002; Zavala and Guadalupe-Diaz 2019). Employment has facilitated sociality by elevating civic engagement, community involvement, donation, philanthropy value, political discussion, political participation, social capital, social functioning, social cohesion experienced, social interaction, and social trust (Anciaes et al. 2017; Fridberg and Kangas 2008b; Kerrissey and Schofer 2013; H. Lu et al. 2002; Ross and Mirowsky 2009; Tsai 2006). Conversely, employment has safeguarded sociality by lessening crime, relocation, and social exclusion experienced (Groot et al. 2007; Kleinhans 2009; Savolainen 2009). Guardianship received reflects attachment to constitute sociality (Gillath et al. 2016). Self-control has buttressed sociality by enhancing generativity and impeding crime, risking, and violence (Y. Cheung et al. 2014; Koegl and Day 2019; Peterson and Klohnen 1995; Welch et al. 2008). Mental health has sustained sociality by upholding prosocial behavior and erasing radicalism, victimization, and violence (Ehrensuft et al. 2003; Krahe 2013; Soliman et al. 2016; Thielmann et al. 2020). Partnership has constituted sociality by preventing victimization (Jones and Ferguson 2009). Moreover, partnership establishes sociality by maintaining equality and responsibility (Harvie and Manzis 2011; Waiton 2008). Social competence has facilitated sociality by raising civility, civic engagement, political participation, prosocial behavior, social cohesion, and social trust (Foschi and Lauriola 2014; Halvorsen 2007; Letki 2008).

Training has facilitated sociality by strengthening civility, collectivism, and donation (Bond and Lun 2014; Klucarova and He 2021; Y. Lin et al. 2021). Moreover, training sustains sociality by highlighting bridging, caring, gratitude, political participation, and responsibility (Kaczmarek et al. 2014; Phillips 2006; Praszkier 2018; Tracy 2002; Wildemeersch 2014). Wealth has safeguarded sociality by enhancing reciprocity experienced, social capital, social integration, and social trust and preventing migration and victimization (Angelusz and Tardos 2001; K. Chan et al. 2014; Crowder et al. 2006; Hackel and Zaki 2018; Reese et al. 2021; Uslaner 2008). Furthermore, victimization experienced has emerged from disability, disorders, illness, jealousy, and poverty to weaken power driving sociality (Barnawi 2017; Ehrensuft et al. 2003; Kaukinen 2004; Zavala and Guadalupe-Diaz 2019). Disability has weakened sociality by eroding social capital, social cohesion, social trust, and volunteering (Cornwall 2009; Granzin and Haggard 2000; Tang 2006; Zanin et al. 2013). Conversely, disability has impeded sociality by instigating protesting and suicide (Van Vugt et al. 2003). Disorders have obstructed sociality by diminishing community attachment, social capital, and social trust (G. Brown et al. 2004; Congdon 2010; Ross and Mirowsky 2009). Illness has eroded sociality by impeding volunteering (Wuthnow 2004). Jealousy has hampered sociality by fomenting aggression and violence (Felson and Outlaw 2007). Poverty has undermined sociality by reducing civic participation, trust, social connection, and volunteering (Caputo 2010; Stephens et al. 2014; R. Walker et al. 2010). Conversely, poverty has disrupted sociality by creating isolation, relationship problems, and social exclusion experienced (Dhal et al. 2008; Stephens et al. 2014; R. Walker et al. 2010). Victimization can arise from dependency, underclass status, and vulnerability to weaken power to drive sociality (Bornstein 2006; Hicks and Brown 2013; Jacobs and Carmichael 2002). Dependency has impaired sociality by hindering social capital, social cohesion, social trust, and equality value, and engendering protesting and suicide (Cornwall 2009; Granzin and Haggard 2000; Konarska 2005; Van Vugt et al. 2003; Zanin et al. 2013). Underclass status embraces antisocial features to disrupt sociality (Wacquant 2008). Vulnerability has worsened sociality by evoking ostracism experienced, radicalism, threat experienced, threatening, and violence (Ferguson and McAuley 2020; Lohman 2006; Pauwels and De Waele 2014; Poon et al. 2020; Thomsen and Birkmose 2015). Moreover, vulnerability can impair sociality by breeding divorce, nimbyism, stigmatizing, and victimization experienced and diminishing xenophobia (Badurdeen et al. 2022; Dum et al. 2017; Dijker and Koomen 2007; Lancee and Pardos-Prado 2013; Zavala and Guadalupe-Diaz 2019). Victimization can arise from gun ownership to afford power against sociality (Wilcox 2002). Gun ownership has impeded sociality by instigating violence (Krahe 2013).

Utility for sociality eroded by victimization has rested on safety and well-being, including intimacy, satisfaction, and self-respect or self-worth (Fernandes 2018; Hanson et al. 2010; Krahe 2013; Singer et al. 2019). Safety has buttressed sociality regarding civility, social capital, and trust (Curley 2010; Watson et al. 2021; Williamson 2002). Intimacy has constituted sociality by boosting relationship satisfaction and social support received and dampening rejection expected (Arseth et al.

2009; Hand et al. 2013). Satisfaction has advanced sociality by strengthening political participation, social cohesion, social and government trust, and volunteering (E. Chan 2014; Flavin and Keane 2011; Rochelle 2015). Self-respect has buttressed sociality by raising attachment security, political participation, and prosociality and preventing suicide (Kitayama and Markus 2000; Tracy et al. 2009). More generally, well-being has uplifted sociality by consolidating altruism, conformism, cooperation, donation, liking for people, prosociality, sociability, and trust and social trust (Fetvadjiev and He 2019; A. Hu 2013; Lyubomirsky et al. 2006; Y. Pan et al. 2023; Wang and Graddy 2008). Additionally, well-being sustains sociality by enabling civilization, fairness, forgiveness, intimacy, kindness, love, loyalty, modesty, morality, open-mindedness, social intelligence, and societal functioning (Cummins 2016; D'raven and Pasha-Zaidi 2016; Meadows 2014).

Conversely, victimization has engendered disutility against sociality based on anxiety, conflict, depression, fear, guilt, helplessness, problems, and shame (Bar-Tal and Halperin 2013' Gray et al. 2019; Krahe 2013; Krulichova 2019). Anxiety or fear has disrupted sociality by breeding interpersonal problems, loneliness, risking, suicide, and violence (Dutton et al. 2016; Gillath et al. 2005; Pulkkinen et al. 2009; Trumbo et al. 2008). Conversely, anxiety has undermined sociality by reducing donation, friendship, humor, political participation, prosocial behavior, and social well-being (Best and Krueger 2010; Hewstone et al. 2005; Litman et al. 2017; Kuiper and Nicholl 2004; Zhong 2010). Conflict has impeded sociality regarding donation and trust as opposed to violence (Farmer and Fedor 2001; Farrington 2018; Kunovich and Hodson 1999). Depression has eroded sociality by breeding conflict, hate, hostility perceived, loneliness, revenge, risking, suicide, and violence (Cacioppo and Hawkley 2009; Economou et al. 2016; Haner et al. 2020; Morokoff et al. 2009; Mullet et al. 2005; Proulx et al. 2004; H. Smith et al. 2016; E. Wright et al. 2015). Conversely, depression has attenuated sociality by impeding benevolence, closeness experienced, fairness, forgiveness, gratitude, honesty, leadership, love, social integration, teamwork, and volunteering (Blanchard et al. 2021; Cornwall 2009; Holzel et al. 2011; Mancini et al. 2011; Mullet et al. 2005; Thoits and Hewitt 2001). Guilt can erode sociality by diminishing relatedness (Stafford 2015). Helplessness can impede sociality by breeding religiousness (Forsyth 2003). Problems have undermined sociality by eroding civility, forgiveness, generativity, relationship quality and satisfaction, social integration, social support received, and trust and heightening conflict, maltreatment, substance abuse, suicide, and violence (Atkinson et al. 2005; Dutton et al. 2016; Gelles 2007; Grzywacz and Almeida 2008; Jackson et al. 2006; Sobeck et al. 2020; Toussaint et al. 2016). Shame can erode sociality by breeding suicide and violence (Kral 2019; J. Turner 2007). Victimization has arisen from disutility against sociality resting on control received, danger exposed, economic hardship, and incivility (Emery and Wu 2020; Ross and Mirowsky 2009; Wilcox 2002). Control received has worsened sociality by breeding violence (Felson and Outlaw 2007). Danger has eroded sociality by weakening social integration and social trust (Hammer et al. 2009; Lindstrom and Rosvall 2015). Conversely, danger has dampened sociality by raising social exclusion (Hammer et al. 2009). Economic hardship has impaired sociality by dampening trust and fomenting social exclusion experienced, suicide, and victimization experienced (Economou et al. 2016; Reeskens and Vandecasteele 2017; Ross and Mirowsky 2009). Incivility has harmed sociality by reducing fairness and trust (Vera-Toscano et al. 2013). Victimization can arise from burdens received, grievance, and helplessness as disutility against sociality (Doerner and Lab 2012; Jacobs and Carmichael 2002). Grievance has undermined sociality by fomenting resistance and impeding social capital and trust (Pulkkinen et al. 2009; Webber and Huxley 2007).

Ideals for sociality dismissed by victimization have favored helping and social trust (Olivera 2015; Staub and Vollhardt 2008). Helping has constituted sociality by installing civility, connectedness, cooperation, religiosity, responsibility, and volunteering (Hample 2018; Marsh and Dik 2021; Musick and Wilson 2008; Nelson-Coffey et al. 2023; Shahzalal and Adnan 2022). Moreover, helping underlies sociality by enhancing citizenship, loyalty, social cohesion, socializing, and trust and diminishing self-interest (Dovidio et al. 2006; Hawley 2014; Kisliuk and WeiBmuller 2023; Music 2014). Social trust has constituted sociality through donation, involvement, and volunteering (Uslaner 2000). Victimization experienced has arisen from ideals against attachment and closeness to discourage sociality (Ehrensuft et al. 2003; Ponti and Tani 2019). Attachment has constituted sociality by boosting relationship satisfaction and social support received and dampening rejection expected (Arseth et al. 2009; Hand et al. 2013). Closeness has constituted sociality by boosting relationship satisfaction and social support received and dampening rejection expected (Arseth et al. 2009; Hand et al. 2013). Conversely, sociality has raised ideals against sociality prizing doping, crime, cynicism, and violence (Kirk and Papachristos 2011; Lineres 2004; Nabi and Horner 2001; L. Zhang et al. 2007a). Doping has hampered sociality by withdrawing power, utility, ideals, and norms for sociality and creating power, utility, ideals, and norms against sociality. Such hampering rests on the voluntaristic mechanisms of analytical functionalism. These mechanisms engage cognitive processing, communication, learning, and social construction (Arce and Winkelman 2021). Hence, doping can jeopardize sociality, featuring altruism, empathy, and healing (Arce and Winkelman 2021). Crime has impaired sociality by reducing community involvement, prosocial behavior, and social trust and fomenting avoidance, protesting, risking, victimization, and violence (Brayne 2014; McNeeley and Yuan 2017; Broadbent and Papadopoulos 2011; Sun and Wang 2012; Wittebrood and Nieuwbeerta 2000; Zhong 2010). Cynicism has undermined sociality by eroding government and social trust, patriotism, and political participation and raising competition (Flanagan and Lee 2003; Guan et al. 2010; Uslaner 2002; van der Meer and van Ingen 2009). Violence has undermined sociality by breeding antisociality, crime and recidivism, blaming, conflict, hostility, rejecting others, and impairing agreeableness, morality, and responsibility (Asendorpf et al. 2008; Del Bove et al. 2008; Morrison 2006; Scholte et al. 2009; Vitaro et al. 2007). Victimization experienced has arisen from ideals for sexuality and weapon carrying to impair sociality (Krahe 2013; Wilcox 2002). Weapon carrying has impeded sociality by instigating violence (Krahe 2013). Sexuality has eroded sociality by eroding attachment security and evoking aggression (Dunkel et al. 2016; Vrangalova and Bukberg 2015).

Norms against sociality exposed by victimization have popularized abuse, extremity, and risk (Corneille et al. 2001; McNeeley and Yuan 2017; Nabi and Horner 2001). The norm for abuse has weakened sociality by boosting antisocial behavior and victimization (Ehrensuft et al. 2003; Krahe 2013). Extremism includes disrespect and intolerance (Kirkpatrick 2020). Immorality covers aggressiveness, antisociality, callousness, cunning, deceitfulness, egocentrism, glibness, grandiosity, hostility, impulsivity, manipulativeness, irresponsibility, irritability, lying, nervousness, normlessness, parasitism, recklessness, remorselessness, sexuality, shamelessness, unreliability, unresponsiveness, and untruthfulness (D. Jones 2016). The norm for risk has impaired sociality by provoking protesting (Scafuto and La Barbera 2016). Moreover, the risk norm can hurt sociality by generating opposition to the establishment (P. Brown 2020). Victimization experienced has reflected norms for crime, disadvantage, disorder, divorce, homelessness, inequality, poverty, rebellion, torture, victimization, and violence to worsen sociality (Jacobs and Carmichael 2002; Nepal et al. 2011; Like 2011; Patel et al. 2012; Schutte 2015; Sullivan 2014; Waterman et al. 2022). The norm for crime has eroded sociality by weakening community involvement, prosocial behavior, and social trust (Broadbent and Papadopoulos 2011; Zanin 2017; Zhong 2010). The norm for disorder has jeopardized sociality by erasing community attachment, neighborhood safety, social capital, and social trust (G. Brown et al. 2004; Congdon 2010; Kanan and Pruitt 2002; Ross and Mirowsky 2009). The norm for disadvantage or poverty has worsened civic engagement, civility, community involvement, donation, relatedness, social trust, and volunteering and fomented cynicism, suicide, theft, violence, and victimization to impair sociality (Abascal 2015; Broadbent and Papadopoulos 2011; J. Brown 2016; Graddy and Wang 2009; Hagan et al. 2016; Krahe 2013; Nepal et al. 2011; Piatkowska 2020; C. Ross et al. 2000; Stoll 2001; Wuthnow 2004). Divorce can represent attachment security to weaken sociality (Demo and Buehler 2013). Homelessness has weakened sociality by incurring victimization and eroding community involvement and social interaction (Like 2011; Saegert and Winkel 2004; Sumerlin and Norman 1992). The norm for inequality has impeded sociality by eroding social capital, support for redistribution and welfare, sympathy, trust, and volunteering (Busemeyer 2013; Hitlin and Harkness 2018; Lipford and Yandle 2009; Oishi et al. 2011; Portes and Vickstrom 2011). Conversely, the norm for inequality has impaired sociality by provoking crime and violence (Ousey and Lee 2013; van Wilsem 2007). Rebellion has impaired sociality by raising deviance and eroding solidarity (Foy et al. 2014; J. Williams 2011). The norm for torture or violence has undermined sociality by engendering protesting and tolerance for violence (Douglas 2006; Smidt 2020).

Conversely, victimization has obstructed the norm for safety to dissimiate sociality (Kanan and Pruitt 2002). The norm for safety has elevated sociality by raising cohesion, neighboring, networking experienced, and trust and dampening aggression and opposition (Barbarin and Richter 2001; Grannis 2009; Rochelle 2015). Victimization experienced has arisen from norms against collective efficacy, education, employment, and residential stability (Nepal et al. 2011; L. Zhang et al. 2007). Furthermore, the norm for victimization disrupts sociality by triggering revolution (Seoighe 2016). The norm for collective efficacy has supported sociality by enhancing civic engagement, community favor, government trust, political participation, and recourse and dampening violence (Z. Han et al. 2017; F. Lee 2012; Palmer et al. 2011; Pulkkinen et al. 2009; Su and Feng 2013; Whitham 2012). The norm for education has fostered sociality by boosting civic participation, government and social trust, social capital, volunteering, and xenophobia and dampening violence (Cohen and Bolt 2005; Lipford and Yandle 2009; Portes and Vickstrom 2011; Poveda 2011; Rupasingha et al. 2006; Uslaner and Brown 2005). The norm for employment has elevated sociality by reducing migration, victimization, and violence and raising prosocial behavior (DiMaggio and Garip 2011; Hampton 2016; Nepal et al. 2011; Poveda 2011). Residential stability has maintained sociality by fostering social integration (Kearns and Whitley 2015).

Security

Security features happiness and safety (Bina et al. 2020; Rader et al. 2012). Conversely, security dismisses anxiety, conflict, danger, guilt, hostility, pessimism, rejection experienced, and tension (Bina et al. 2020). Security is likely to buttress sociality by affording power, utility, ideals, and norms to complete the functions of sociality required in analytical functionalism. These functions comprise fulfillment based on power realization, adaptation based on utility optimization, latency based on ideal calibration, and integration based on norm conformity.

Power for sociality enhanced by security has stemmed from heatlh, marriage, and social capital (D. Chen et al. 2008; Curley 2010). Health has uplifted sociality by boosting community sense, morality, popularity, social activity, social cohesion, social integration, social trust, social well-being, and volunteering (Huxhold et al. 2014; Jorgensen et al. 2010; Son and Wilson 2012; Tolsma et al. 2009; Yu and Chiu 2016). Conversely, health has sustained sociality by preventing loneliness (Koromeckyj-Cox et al. 2007). Marriage has consolidated sociality by enhancing community attachment, community evaluation, community involvement, civic engagement, closeness experienced, donation, friendship satisfaction, neighboring, political participation, prosocial behavior, reciprocity, relationship quality, social capital, social cohesion, social integration, social interaction, social support received, and trust (W. Chang 2009; Cornwall 2009; Degenne et al. 2004; Flavin and Keane 2011; Frye 2007; Kerrissey and Schofer 2013; Lizardo 2006; Louis and Zhao 2002; Mata and Pendakur 2014; McCabe 2014; Prezza et al. 2001; Ross and Mirowsky 2009; Sampson and Raudenbush 2004; Swaroop and Morenoff 2006; Tolsma et al. 2009). Social capital has consolidated sociality by raising civic engagement, community involvement, donation, political involvement, social trust, and volunteering (Bekkers et al. 2008; Broadbent and Papadopoulos 2011; Brown and Ferris 2007; Chua et al. 2021; Narayan and Cassidy 2001). Conversely, social capital has strengthened sociality by erasing violence (Pulkkinen et al. 2009). Security can advance power for sociality based on civility (Williamson 2002). Civility has constituted sociality by inducing fairness and trust (Vera-Toscano et al. 2013).

Security has arisen from agreeableness, competence, conscientiousness, employment, extraversion, income, and organizational membership to shape power to drive sociality (Becker et al. 1997; Coffe and Geys 2007; Rehm 2016; Sacks and Levi 2010; Valera and Guardia 2014). Agreeableness has fostered sociality by enhancing attachment (Fraley et al. 2011). Moreover, agreeableness constitutes sociality by featuring communion, compliance, cooperation, empathy, helping, intimacy, morality, politeness, prosociality, respect, solidarity, sympathy, understanding, warmth, and unity (Dinic and Bodroza 2021; Graziano and Tobin 2009; J. Sun et al. 2018). Competence has buttressed sociality regarding civic engagement, discussion, donation, leadership, prosocial behavior, social interaction, social trust, and intolerance for violence (Bednall et al. 2013; Frye 2007; Gnambs and Batinic 2012; Mazziotta et al. 2011; Pei and Pan 2018; Rahn 2008; Tausch et al. 2011; Yao and Enright 2019). Conscientiousness has elevated sociality by consolidating attachment, compliance, order value, responsibility, social desirability, and volunteering reducing deviance, violence, and justification for unconventional sexuality (Bekkers 2005; de Jong et al. 2012; Fraley et al. 2011; Gotzsche-Astrup 2020; Mondak and Hurwitz 2012; Mullet et al. 2005; Saucier and Skrzypinska 2006; Twardawski et al. 2021; Wright and DeLisi 2016). Employment has facilitated sociality by elevating civic engagement, community involvement, donation, philanthropy value, political discussion, political participation, social capital, social functioning, social cohesion experienced, social interaction, and social trust (Anciaes et al. 2017; Fridberg and Kangas 2008b; Kerrissey and Schofer 2013; H. Lu et al. 2002; Ross and Mirowsky 2009; Tsai 2006). Conversely, employment has safeguarded sociality by lessening crime, relocation, and social exclusion experienced (Groot et al. 2007; Kleinhans 2009; Savolainen 2009). Extraversion has buttressed sociality by fostering attachment, civic engagement, civility, donation, humor, nationalism, political participation, social capital, socializing, volunteering, and favor for civic and political participation (Bekkers 2010; C. Cheng et al. 2019; Fraley et al. 2011; Gotzsche-Astrup 2020; Hample 2018; Omoto et al. 2010; Schbley and McCauley 2005; Vernon et al. 2008; Ward and Forney 2020). Income has upheld sociality by boosting civic engagement, community attachment and involvement, civic dutifulness, civility, conformity value, neighboring, political interest and participation, political and social trust, prosocial behavior, social capital, social integration, social interaction, social support received, social well-being, and volunteering (Bjornberg and Latta 2007; Chang 2009; Djupe and Lewis 2015; Frei et al. 2009; Kerrissey and Schofer 2013; Letki 2006; McCabe 2014; Patulny and Morris 2012; Son and Wilson 2012; Sun and Wang 2012; Swaroop and Morenoff 2006; Ulbig 2002). Organizational membership has constituted sociality by strengthening institutional commitment and conformity (Vartanian and Hopkinson 2010). Security can benefit from social class to afford power to drive sociality (Taylor-Gooby 2001). Social class has sustained sociality by raising adaptation, civic engagement, cohesion, institutional and political trust, organizational involvement and membership, prosocial behavior, social capital, social support received, and volunteering (E. Chan 2014; Elchardus and De Keere 2013; La Grange 2011; Lennartsson 2010; Letki 2008; Mutaner et al. 2002; Wallace and Pichler 2009; Wuthnow 2004; Yeh et al. 2013; Zhong 2010). Conversely, social class has maintained sociality by preventing crime and social exclusion experienced (Agnew and Brezina 2010; Buck 2001). Security experienced benefits from attachment to build power to drive sociality (La Guardia et al. 2000). Attachment has constituted sociality by boosting relationship satisfaction and social support received and dampening rejection expected (Arseth et al. 2009; Hand et al. 2013).

Conversely, security has reduced poverty to retain power to drive sociality (Muffels and Fouarge 2004). Poverty has undermined sociality by reducing civic participation, trust, social connection, and volunteering (Caputo 2010; Stephens et al. 2014; R. Walker et al. 2010). Conversely, poverty has disrupted sociality by creating isolation, relationship problems, and social exclusion experienced (Dhal et al. 2008; Stephens et al. 2014; R. Walker et al. 2010). Security experienced can benefit from low vulnerability to retain power to drive sociality (Rader et al. 2012). Vulnerability has worsened sociality by evoking ostracism experienced, radicalism, threat experienced, threatening, and violence (Ferguson and McAuley 2020; Lohman 2006; Pauwels and De Waele 2014; Poon et al. 2020; Thomsen and Birkmose 2015). Moreover, vulnerability can impair sociality be breeding divorce, nimbyism, stigmatizing, and victimization experienced and diminishing xenophobia (Badurdeen et al. 2022; Dum et al. 2017; Dijker and Koomen 2007; Lancee and Pardos-Prado 2013; Zavala and Guadalupe-Diaz 2019).

Utility for sociality afforded by security has resided in well-being, including neighborhood quality and satisfaction with the country, life, and neighborhood (Cummins et al. 2003; Frey et al. 2007; Gaitan-Rossi and Shen 2018; R. Jones et al. 2014; Olson et al. 2016; Parkes et al. 2002). Neighborhood quality has elevated sociality by building social capital, order, and cohesion (Rupp et al. 2020; Sampson and Raudenbush 2004). Satisfaction has advanced sociality by strengthening political participation, social cohesion, social and government trust, and volunteering (E. Chan 2014; Flavin and Keane 2011; Rochelle 2015).

Security enhances resilience to maintain utility, attracting sociality (Wouters-Soomers et al. 2022). Resilience has attracted sociality by raising bonding and inhibiting crime and violence (Fields and McNamara 2003; Hoffman 2003; Solomon and Roloff 2018). Furthermore, resilience sustains sociality by embodying or fostering adaptation and legality (Hoffman 2003; Ungar 2012). Resilience also underlies sociality by demonstrating altruism, attractiveness, communication or conversation, community, compassion, empathy or perspective-taking, negotiation, peacefulness, relationality, relatedness, social capital or resourcefulness, social cohesion, and social competence (Elfers et al. 2024; Hjemdal et al. 2015; Jones and d'Errico 2019; Kelley et al. 2019; Kent and Davis 2010; Ungar 2010; Zautra 2014). Security has arisen from ease, equality, government fairness, police effectiveness and legitimacy, and protection experienced as utility to buttress sociality (Carter and Wolfe 2021; Sacks and Levi 2010). Ease experienced has sustained sociality by enhancing political agreement (Shockley and Fairdosi 2015). Equality experienced can bolster sociality by preventing crime and illegality (Kyriacou 2020). Police evaluation embraces compliance, cooperation, obedience, respect, and trust to enhance sociality (Hough 2012; Lowrey-Kinberg et al. 2020; Wahyurudhanto

2022). Protection received reflects attachment to constitute sociality (Gillath et al. 2016).

Conversely, security has reduced aggression experienced, control received, deprivation experienced, fear, and victimization as disutility distracting sociality (Chiricos et al. 2000; Fernandes 2018; Peruzzi 2014; Valera and Guardia 2014). Aggression or victimization experienced experienced has impaired sociality by eroding social trust (Olivera 2015). Conversely, victimization experienced has hurt sociality by activating conflict and migration (Bar-Tal and Halperin 2013; Ramesh et al. 2019). Control received has worsened sociality by breeding violence (Felson and Outlaw 2007). Deprivation has undermined sociality by reducing civic participation, trust, social connection, and volunteering (Caputo 2010; Stephens et al. 2014; R. Walker et al. 2010). Fear has disrupted sociality by breeding interpersonal problems, loneliness, risking, suicide, and violence (Dutton et al. 2016; Gillath et al. 2005; Pulkkinen et al. 2009; Trumbo et al. 2008). Conversely, fear has undermined sociality by reducing donation, friendship, humor, political participation, prosocial behavior, and social well-being (Best and Krueger 2010; Hewstone et al. 2005; Litman et al. 2017; Kuiper and Nicholl 2004; Zhong 2010).

Ideals for sociality sustained by security have valorized support and trust (Pena-Lopez and Sanchez-Santos 2016; Watson et al. 2021). Supporting has constituted sociality by civility, consolidating connectedness, cooperation, religiosity, responsibility, and volunteering (Hample 2018; Marsh and Dik 2021; Musick and Wilson 2008; Nelson-Coffey et al. 2023; Shahzalal and Adnan 2022). Moreover, supporting underlies sociality by enhancing citizenship, loyalty, social cohesion, socializing, and trust and diminishing self-interest (Dovidio et al. 2006; Hawley 2014; Kisliuk and WeiBmuller 2023; Music 2014). Trust has constituted sociality through donation, involvement, and volunteering (Uslaner 2000). Security has arisen from the ideal for confidence in police (Nofziger and Williams 2005).

Norms against sociality diminished by security have popularized disorder and incivility (Kanan and Pruitt 2002). The norm for disorder has jeopardized sociality by erasing community attachment, neighborhood safety, social capital, and social trust (G. Brown et al. 2004; Congdon 2010; Kanan and Pruitt 2002; Ross and Mirowsky 2009). Incivility has harmed sociality by reducing fairness and trust (Vera-Toscano et al. 2013).

Security has arisen from norms against homicide and poverty to maintain sociality (Gaitan-Rossi and Shen 2018). Homicide represents crime (L. Cao et al. 2016). The norm for crime has eroded sociality by weakening community involvement, prosocial behavior, and social trust (Broadbent and Papadopoulos 2011; Zanin 2017; Zhong 2010). Conversely, sociality has benefitted from the norm for income to secure sociality (Kanan and Pruitt 2002). The norm for income has uplifted sociality by raising government support, nationalism, political participation, relationship quality, trust, volunteering, and xenophobia (Cheng and Smyth 2016; Fridberg and Kangas 2008; Inglehart 2003; Rhodes-Purdy et al. 2023; Traunmuller 2011; van Oorschot and Arts 2005).

Family Saving

Family saving constitutes or reflects family income or wealth (Yeung et al. 2002). Family wealth is likely to consolidate sociality by affording power, utility, ideals, and norms underpinning the functions of sociality as required in analytical functionalism. These functions comprise fulfillment based on power realization, adaptation based on utility optimization, latency based on ideal calibration, and integration based on norm conformity. As such, family income has buttressed sociality by raising civility, civic engagement, community involvement, compliance, donation, friendliness, nationalism, political participation, social capital, social integration, social interaction, social support received, social trust (Alnsour and Meaton 2009; Crowder et al. 2006; Doff and Kleinhans 2011; Kleinhans et al. 2007; La Grange and Yip 2001; Lennartsson 2010; Norris and Inglehart 2009; Oliver 2003; Shin 2012; Wiepking and Maas 2009; Q. Xu et al. 2010). Conversely, family income has sustained sociality by preventing crime, discrimination experienced, sleeping, and social exclusion experienced (Cerin and Leslie 2008; Hamermesh 2019; Moore and Aweiss 2003; Stanley et al. 2011).

Health

Health features fitness, functioning, safety as opposed to complaint, illness, impairment, mortality, sleepiness, somatization, symptoms, and underweight (Baker et al. 2009; Cutler and Lleras-Muney 2008; Di Domenico and Fournier 2014; Hagquist and Andrich 2004; Hadden et al. 2003; Hendriksen et al. 2021; Taylor and Distelberg 2016; Uchino et al. 2001). Functionally, health is likely to buttress sociality by engendering power, utility, ideals, and norms based on the voluntaristic mechanisms of analytical functionalism. These mechanisms employ power for power realization, utility for utility optimization, ideals for ideal calibration, and norms for norm conformity.

Power for sociality strengthened by health has resided in financial adequacy, friendship, mastery, memory, resiliency, savings, social integration, social networking, socioeconomic status, social support received, and wisdom (Barrett 1999; Boyle and Joss-Reid 2004; Chakrabarty et al. 2008; Friborg et al. 2002; Groot et al. 2007; Huxhold et al. 2014; Mulatu and Schooler 2002; Pena-Lopez and Sanchez-Santos 2016; Schieman 2001; Son and Wilson 2012; Stevens et al. 2001; Stogner et al. 2014; Webster 2003). Financial adequacy has enabled sociality by raising government trust (Li and Mayraz 2017). Friendship has constituted sociality by enhancing community attachment, compliance, donation, gratitude, political participation, social cohesion, social desirability, social integration, and social trust (Corcoran 2013; Fahmy 2006; Gundert and Hohendanner 2015; Keillor et al. 2001; Kende et al. 2022; Opp 2001; Rotkirch 2014). Mastery has enhanced sociality by uplifting social trust (Burke and Stets 1999). Memory has facilitated sociality by strengthening role-taking (Henry et al. 2009). Moreover, memory can maintain sociality by preventing suicide (Van Orden et al. 2010). Resiliency has facilitated sociality by raising bonding and inhibiting crime and violence (Fields and McNamara 2003; Hoffman 2003; Solomon and Roloff 2018). Furthermore, resilience sustains sociality by embodying or fostering adaptation and legality (Hoffman 2003; Ungar 2012). Resiliency also buttresses sociality by demonstrating altruism, attractiveness, communication or conversation, community, compassion, empathy or perspective-taking, negotiation, peacefulness, relationality, relatedness, social capital or resourcefulness, social cohesion, and social competence (Elfers et al. 2024; Hjemdal et al. 2015; Jones and d'Errico 2019; Kelley et al. 2019; Kent and Davis 2010; Ungar 2010; Zautra 2014). Savings have maintained sociality by elevating social trust and dampening social exclusion experienced (K. Lin et al. 2013; Uslaner 2002). Social integration has constituted sociality by strengthening cooperation and preventing suicide (Duberstein et al. 2004; Lepkowski and Couper 2002). Social networking or social capital has consolidated sociality by raising civic engagement, community involvement, donation, political involvement, social trust, and volunteering (Bekkers et al. 2008; Broadbent and Papadopoulos 2011; Brown and Ferris 2007; Chua et al. 2021; Narayan and Cassidy 2001). Conversely, social capital has strengthened sociality by erasing violence (Pulkkinen et al. 2009). Socioeconomic status has enhanced sociality by raising interaction quality and helping (Molana and Adams 2019). Social support received has strengthened sociality by enhancing attachment, gratitude, political participation, prosocial behavior, recourse, respect, responsibility, social integration, and social well-being (Boezeman and Ellemers 2008; Fahmy 2006; Phipps 2003; Williams and Galliher 2006; R. Wright et al. 2009; Zeldin et al. 2016; Zeng et al. 2024). Conversely, social support received has boosted sociality by preventing aggression, conflict, delinquency, doping, externalizing, hyperactivity, loneliness, runaway, sexuality, suicide, and violence (Bernardon et al. 2011; Browning et al. 2005; Hayslip et al. 2000; Nieuwenhuis et al. 2017; Pearson and Wilkinson 2013; Terzi-Unsal and Karei 2005; Wight et al. 2006; R. Wright et al. 2009). Wisdom has enhanced sociality by establishing attachment security, generativity, and the ideal for social engagement (Webster 2003, 2010). Health has built on adaptation, conscientious, humor, organizational membership, self-control, self-efficacy, and social capital to maintain power to drive sociality (Borgonovi 2008; Maltby et al. 2019; Oshio and Kobayashi 2010; Spohn and Kaplan 2000; Vincens et al. 2018). Adaptation has secured sociality regarding partnership and social adjustment and satisfaction as opposed to discord (Chow et al. 2014; Mitchell 2005). Conscientiousness has elevated sociality by consolidating attachment, compliance, order value, responsibility, social desirability, and volunteering and reducing deviance, violence, and justification for unconventional sexuality (Bekkers 2005; de Jong et al. 2012; Fraley et al. 2011; Gotzsche-Astrup 2020; Mondak and Hurwitz 2012; Mullet et al. 2005; Saucier and Skrzypinska 2006; Twardawski et al. 2021; Wright and DeLisi 2016). Humor has uplifted sociality by raising social interaction and reducing hostility (R. Martin 2007; Nezlek and Derks 2001). Organizational membership has constituted sociality by strengthening institutional commitment and conformity (Vartanian and Hopkinson 2010). Self-control has buttressed sociality by enhancing generativity and impeding crime, risking, and violence (Y. Cheung et al. 2014; Koegl and Day 2019; Peterson and Klohnen 1995; Welch et al. 2008). Self-efficacy has sustained sociality by raising civic engagement, donation, government and social trust, leadership, political participation, prosocial behavior, and social activity (Bednall et al. 2013; Frye 2007; Gnambs and Batinic 2012; Huber et al. 2022; Mangum 2012; Rahn 2008; Pei and Pan 2018; Yao and Enright 2019). Health can benefit from resources as power driving sociality (Vincens et al. 2018). Resources can facilitate sociality by raising social integration and obstructing crime, risking, social exclusion received, and violence (Agnew 2007; Figueredo et al. 2018; Gallie 2004; Lilly et al. 2011; Tsai 2006).

Conversely, health has prevented death, illness, and poverty to maintain power and drive sociality (Bekkers 2008; Dekkers 2008; Yu and Chiu 2016). Dying can dampen sociality by fomenting aggression (Reeve 2021). Status inconsistency can disrupt sociality by breeding conflict (J. Turner 2013b). Illness has eroded sociality by impeding volunteering (Wuthnow 2004). Poverty has undermined sociality by reducing civic participation, trust, social connection, and volunteering (Caputo 2010; Stephens et al. 2014; R. Walker et al. 2010). Conversely, poverty has disrupted sociality by creating isolation, relationship problems, and social exclusion experienced (Dhal et al. 2008; Stephens et al. 2014; R. Walker et al. 2010). Health has arisen from low alcoholism, disability, hostility, neuroticism, and obesity to dampen power against sociality (Carpenter 2019; Carrieri 2012; Finggerman et al. 2008; Gorman et al. 2010; Hendriksen et al. 2021). Alcoholism has impaired sociality by raising risking, victimization, and violence (Eakins et al. 2022; Krahe 2013; Zavala and Guadalupe-Diaz 2019). Disability has weakened sociality by eroding social capital, social cohesion, social trust, and volunteering (Cornwall 2009; Granzin and Haggard 2000; Tang 2006; Zanin et al. 2013). Conversely, disability has impeded sociality by instigating protesting and suicide (Van Vugt et al. 2003). Hostility impedes sociality by embodying competition, conflict, protesting, and violence (Canary et al. 2013; Koerner 2018; Renger et al. 2020; Webster and Kirkpatrick 2006). Neuroticism has impaired sociality by reducing attachment security, civic engagement, coordination, forgiveness, nationalism, relatedness, and socializing and generating crime and hostility (Bekkers 2005; Fraley et al. 2011; Hounkpatin et al. 2015; Kalish 2008; Marks 1996; Mullet et al. 2005; Pulkkinen et al. 2009; Schbley and McCauley 2005; Ward and Forney 2020). Obesity has disrupted sociality by raising discrimination received (Carr and Friedman 2005).

Utility for sociality afforded by health has rested on well-being, including the community sense, positive affect, popularity, self-esteem, social evaluation, social well-being, and satisfaction with the family, finance, life, and marriage (Jorgensen et al. 2010; Koromeckyj-Cox et al. 2007; Mroczek 2004; Plagnol 2011; Rochelle 2015; Son and Wilson 2012; Washburn-Busk et al. 2020; Webster et al. 2014; Zotti et al. 2016). The community sense has constituted sociality by enhancing attachment and dampening tolerance for deviance (Stafford et al. 2005; Woosnam et al. 2018). Positive affect has maintained sociality by raising government trust and patriotism (Hunt et al. 2019; Turner and Stets 2005). Popularity has facilitated sociality by raising belongingness (Reich et al. 2018). Self-esteem has buttressed sociality by raising attachment security, political participation, and prosociality and by preventing suicide (Kitayama and Markus 2000; Tracy et al. 2009). Social evaluation or well-being constitutes sociality by embracing social acceptance, actualization, adjustment, cohesion, contribution, empowerment, inclusion, integration, resources, satisfaction, and security (Keyes and Shapiro 2004; Phillips 2006; Shapiro and Keyes 2008; van Praag and Ferrer-I-Carbonell 2004). Satisfaction has advanced sociality by strengthening political participation, social cohesion, social and government trust, and volunteering (E. Chan 2014; Flavin and Keane 2011; Rochelle 2015). Generally, well-being has uplifted sociality by consolidating altruism, conformism, cooperation, donation, liking for people, prosociality, sociability, and trust and social trust (Fetvadjiev and He 2019; A. Hu 2013; Lyubomirsky et al. 2006; Y. Pan et al. 2023; Wang and Graddy 2008). Besides, health has raised controllability perceived as utility attracting sociality (Tomich and Helgeson 2002). Controllability has enhanced sociality by uplifting social trust (Burke and Stets 1999). Health has stood on meaningfulness, justice perceived, neighborliness experienced, positive emotion, and security as utility attracting sociality (Beaudoin 2009; Lucas et al. 2013; Myers 2008; Svebak et al. 2004). Meaningfulness has underlain sociality by boosting civic practice, responsibility, and volunteering and reducing rejection experience (Duffy and Raque-Bogdan 2010; Summers and Falco 2020; Twenge et al. 2003). Self-creation maintains sociality by espousing attachment (Raeff 2010). Justice experienced has warranted sociality regarding civility, cooperation, community identification, political participation, and social trust as opposed to protesting (A. Hu 2013; Lawrence and Daniels 1997; Sunshine and Tyler 2003; Tyler and Degoey 1995; van Prooijen et al. 2008; Wenzel 2000). Neighborliness is part of neighboring (McDonell et al. 2021). Neighboring received has brewed sociality by enhancing government trust and political participation and preventing violence (Caprara and Vecchione 2017; Stolle and Micheletti 2013; E. Wright et al. 2015). Security upholds sociality by avoiding conflict, hostility, and rejection experience (Bina et al. 2020). As such, security has buttressed sociality regarding civility, social capital, and trust (Curley 2010; Watson et al. 2021; Williamson 2002).

Conversely, health has dampened loneliness and social exclusion experienced as disutility distracting sociality (Backman and Nilsson 2011; Koromeckyj-Cox et al. 2007). Loneliness has impaired sociality by weakening reciprocity, social capital, and social cohesion and provoking suicide (C. Cheng et al. 2019; Espvall and Dellgren 2008). Social exclusion experienced has disturbed sociality by eroding closeness and prosocial behavior (Bockler et al. 2021; K. Lin et al. 2013). Health has benefitted from low anxiety, depression, deprivation experienced, distress, economic hardship and strain, fear, and risk perceived as utility distracting sociality (Aytac et al. 2008; Baker et al. 2009; Hendriksen et al. 2021; Kondo et al. 2008; Mathis et al. 2016; Reynolds and Ross 1998; Rodrigues et al. 2022). Anxiety or fear has disrupted sociality by breeding interpersonal problems, loneliness, risking, suicide, and violence (Dutton et al. 2016; Gillath et al. 2005; Pulkkinen et al. 2009; Trumbo et al. 2008). Conversely, anxiety or fear has undermined sociality by reducing donation, friendship, humor, political participation, prosocial behavior, and social well-being (Best and Krueger 2010; Hewstone et al. 2005; Litman et al. 2017; Kuiper and Nicholl 2004; Zhong

2010). Depression has eroded sociality by breeding conflict, hate, hostility perceived, loneliness, revenge, risking, suicide, and violence (Cacioppo and Hawkley 2009; Economou et al. 2016; Haner et al. 2020; Morokoff et al. 2009; Mullet et al. 2005; Proulx et al. 2004; H. Smith et al. 2016; E. Wright et al. 2015). Conversely, depression has attenuated sociality by impeding benevolence, closeness experienced, fairness, forgiveness, gratitude, honesty, leadership, love, social integration, teamwork, and volunteering (Blanchard et al. 2021; Cornwall 2009; Holzel et al. 2011; Mancini et al. 2011; Mullet et al. 2005; Thoits and Hewitt 2001). Deprivation experienced erodes sociality by breeding conflict (J. Turner 2013b). Favoritism constitutes corruption (Inglehart and Welzel 2005). Distress has undermined sociality by fomenting resistance and impeding social capital and trust (Pulkkinen et al. 2009; Webber and Huxley 2007). Economic hardship has impaired sociality by dampening trust and fomenting social exclusion experienced, suicide, and victimization experienced (Economou et al. 2016; Reeskens and Vandecasteele 2017; Ross and Mirowsky 2009). Risk perceived has impaired sociality by provoking protesting (Scafuto and La Barbera 2016). Moreover, risk perceived can hurt sociality by generating opposition to the establishment (P. Brown 2020). Health can benefit from low exploitation and loss experienced as disutility against sociality (Hobfoll and Schumm 2002; Muntaner and Lynch 2002). Exploitation experienced erodes sociality by breeding conflict (J. Turner 2013b). Loss experienced has hindered sociality by eroding compliance and government trust and fomenting suicide (Kirchler and Maciejovsky 2001; Nicholls and Picou 2012).

Ideals for sociality fostered by health have accentuated morality, social activity, social cohesion, social trust, and volunteering (Michel 2007; Pratt et al. 1996; Tolsma et al. 2009; Yu and Chiu 2016). Morality has championed sociality by boosting volunteering and inhibiting violence (Piquero and Hickman 2002; Whitford et al. 2006). Social activity has realized sociality by consolidating altruism, compliance, cooperation, donation, morality, political participation, reciprocity, social trust, and volunteering (Guillen et al. 2011; Dixon and McKeown 2021; Lucas and Livingston 2014; Musick 2000; Rodrigo-Gonzalez et al. 2019; Rubin and Step 2000). Social cohesion has constituted sociality by enhancing attachment and dampening tolerance for deviance (Stafford et al. 2005; Woosnam et al. 2018). Social trust has constituted sociality through donation, involvement, and volunteering (Uslaner 2000). Volunteering has constituted sociality by raising altruism, charity orientation, civic motivation, donation, helping, moral responsibility, political participation, social integration, and social and government trust (Foster et al. 2001; Isham et al. 2006; Richey 2010; Richey and Ikeda 2009; Wiepking and Maas 2009). Health has benefitted from ideals for civic engagement, conservatism, coping, friendship, grouping, hygiene, organizational attendance, political participation, and social inclusion to rationalize sociality (Akaeda 2021; Borgonovi 2008; Gorman et al. 2010; Hendriksen et al. 2021; Myers 2008; Pearce et al. 2016; Poortinga 2012; Raymo 2015; Thoits and Hewitt 2001). Civic engagement has propped sociality by strengthening attachment, civility, collective behavior, discussion, donation, neighboring, patriotism, prosociality, social capital, socialism, trust, and volunteering and impeding cheating and individualism (Coffe and Geys 2007; Gilberbloom and Markham 1995; Kerrissey and Schofer 2013; Mata and Pendakur 2014; Ozbay 2008; Pattie et al. 2004; Pena-Lopez and Sanchez-Santos 2016; Rahn 2008; Richey 2011; Tak 2017; M. Tang 2011; Taniguchi 2013; Yip et al. 2007). Conservatism sustains sociality by nurturing empathy, loyalty, prosocial behavior, religiousness, and sacrifice (Dutton and Rayner-Hilles 2022). Moreover, conservatism underpins sociality by maintaining allegiance or loyalty, attachment, civility, community, conformity, cooperation, discipline, ethnocentrism, honesty, humility, intimacy, legality, morality, nationalism, obedience, order, partnership, patriotism, peace, responsibility, sharing, trust, and xenophobia (Dutton and Rayner-Hilles 2022; Heilman and Kusev 2020; Hickson 2013; Lakoff 2009; Rhodes-Purdy et al. 2023; Scruton 2014; Yoos 2007; Zuk and Zuk 2020). Conversely, conservatism upholds sociality by condemning dehumanizing, evilness, revolution, sexuality, terrorism, and transgression (Dutton and Rayner-Hilles 2022; Malka and Soto 2011; Scruton 2014; Suhay 2015). Coping is a reaction to a stimulus conditional on attitude. As such, the attitude steers the way of coping with the stimulus. The ideal for friendship has fostered sociality by embracing help, honesty, respect, similarity, and trust (Galupo and Gonzalez 2013; Wuthnow 2004). Grouping has fostered sociality regarding cohesion, common identity, and identification (Fischer et al. 2007). Hygiene upholds sociality by featuring prosociality (Motta and Goren 2021). Organizational attendance has fostered sociality by enhancing attachment, civility, political participation, social integration, socialism (favor), and trust (Geys 2012; Guillen et al. 2011; Pattie et al. 2004; Tak 2017). Political participation has buttressed sociality regarding civility (Campbell 2003). Social inclusion can constitute sociality regarding loving (Aron et al. 2006).

Conversely, health has diminished ideals against sociality prizing doping, religiousness, resistance, risking, and self-destruction (Bergeman and Deboeck 2014; Karekla and Panayiotou 2011; Stogner et al. 2014; Immerzeel and van Tubergen 2013; Wickrama et al. 1995). Doping has hampered sociality by withdrawing power, utility, ideals, and norms for sociality and creating power, utility, ideals, and norms against sociality. Such hampering rests on the voluntaristic mechanisms of analytical functionalism. Religiosity has sustained sociality by fostering civic engagement, civility, cohesion, compliance, donation, empathy, morality, patriotism, prejudice against deviants and outsiders, prosocial behavior, social trust, and volunteering (Apinunmahakul and Devlin 2008; Corcoran et al. 2011; Ishio 2010; Keyes 2002; Kim and Wilcox 2013; Ravanera et al. 2003; van Tienen et al. 2011; Weisberg 2005; Wuthnow 2004). Conversely, religiosity has secured sociality by reducing crime, deviance, individualism, protesting, and sexuality (Andrews et al. 2015; Coffe and Geys 2007; Guo et al. 2008; Skerkat and Ellison 1999; Spilka et al. 2003). Moreover, religiosity realizes sociality regarding altruism, community, ethicality, groupism, sharing, and solidarity (Franks et al. 2013; Lichterman 2012; Peifer 2010; Spilka et al. 2003; Stavrova and Siegers 2014). Religiosity also upholds sociality by featuring altruism, attachment, caring, community, compassion, harmony, hospitality, love, morality, obedience, other-centeredness, peace, trust, unity, xenophobia (Ager and Ager 2011; Fontana 2003; Harris et al. 2018; Horell 2014; Paterson 2018; Shorey et al. 2018; Simpson et al. 2008; Spilka et al. 2003; Tenorio and Lo 2011; Werbner 2010). Conversely, religiosity maintains sociality by dismissing individualism, oppression, sexuality, and violence (Fontana 2003; Horell 2014; Spilka et al. 2003). Health has evolved from ideals against deviance to secure sociality (Spohn and Kaplan 2000). Deviance has ruined sociality by provoking social exclusion experienced (Backman and Nilsson 2011).

Norms for sociality underlying health have popularized community development, education, environmental quality, governance quality, human development, income, organizational membership, political participation, prosperity, safety, social capital, social cohesion, and trust (Akaeda 2021; Eikemo et al. 2008; Franzini et al. 2005; Fujisawa et al. 2009; Hadden et al. 2003; Islam et al. 2006; Lavis and Stoddart 2003; Mathis et al. 2016; Stafford et al. 2005; Subramanian et al. 2001; Ziersch et al. 2005). The norm for community development enhances sociality by consolidating citizenship, collaboration, ownership, partnership, reciprocity, and social capital (S. Ha 2007; Schneider 2006). Furthermore, community development espouses assimilation, civic culture, coalitions, cohesion, collective efficacy and involvement, commonality, communitarianism, consensus, coordination, corporatism, dialogue, discussion, equalizing, gathering, integration, interdependence, interlocking, localism, mutuality, negotiation, networking, normativity, organizing, participation, protection, reciprocity, security, sharing, social life, and solidarity to advance sociality (Brint 2001; Castelloe and Gamble 2005; Chaskin 2001; Chaskin and Joseph 2010; Farmer et al. 2016; Gravenkepper 2007; Hendricks and Rudich 2000; Kelly 2006; Labonne and Chase 2011; Lowe 2001; Midgley and Livermore 2005; Morrison 2005; Nelson et al. 2005; Payne 2006; Reisch 2013; M. Taylor 2011; Wakefield and Poland 2005; Weil and Ohmer 2013). Communitarianism upheld in community development establishes egalitarianism, homogeneity, inclusion, justice, morality, order, redistribution, respect, responsibility, and socialism as opposed to oppression to champion sociality (Fraser 2005; M. Taylor 2011). Conversely, community development opposes discrimination, dispute, fragmentation, marginalization, and threatening to maintain sociality (Capraro 2004; Castelloe and Gamble 2005; Duval-Diop et al. 2010; Reisch 2013; J. Turner 2013a). The norm for education has fostered sociality by boosting civic participation, government and social trust, social capital, volunteering, and xenophobia and dampening violence (Cohen and Bolt 2005; Lipford and Yandle 2009; Portes and Vickstrom 2011; Poveda 2011; Rupasingha et al. 2006; Uslaner and Brown 2005). The norm for environmental quality has secured community attachment and social capital and diminished nimbyism and protesting to consolidate sociality (Cummins et al. 2003; Esaisason 2014; Mesch and Manor 1998; Scafuto and La Barbera 2016). Nimbyism represents distrust to impair sociality (Smith and Marquez 2002). Furthermore, nimbyism can germinate protesting to erode sociality (Esaiasson 2014). The norm for governance quality can secure citizenship and social cohesion and prevent conflict, fragmentation, and threats experienced to install sociality (Bukenya and Golooba-Mutebi 2020; Rhodes-Purdy et al. 2021; Tang 1998; Taylor-Gooby 1991). The norm for human development has maintained donation, legalism, and social trust to secure sociality (Fridberg and Kangas 2008b). The norm for income has uplifted sociality by raising government support, nationalism, political participation, relationship quality, trust, volunteering, and xenophobia (Cheng and Smyth 2016; Fridberg and Kangas 2008;

Inglehart 2003; Rhodes-Purdy et al. 2023; Traunmuller 2011; van Oorschot and Arts 2005). Organizational membership has constituted sociality by strengthening institutional commitment and conformity (Vartanian and Hopkinson 2010). Political participation has buttressed sociality regarding civility (Campbell 2003). The norm for prosperity has uplifted sociality by raising government support, nationalism, political participation, relationship quality, trust, volunteering, and xenophobia (Cheng and Smyth 2016; Fridberg and Kangas 2008; Inglehart 2003; Rhodes-Purdy et al. 2023; Traunmuller 2011; van Oorschot and Arts 2005). The norm for safety has elevated sociality by raising cohesion, neighboring, networking experienced, and trust and dampening aggression and opposition (Barbarin and Richter 2001; Grannis 2009; Rochelle 2015). The norm for social capital or social cohesion has buttressed sociality by strengthening civic engagement, community favor, financial help, institutional trust, political participation, and recourse and prevented violence (Z. Han et al. 2017; F. Lee 2012; Mitrut and Wolff 2011; Palmer et al. 2011; Su and Feng 2013; Whitham 2012; E. Wright et al. 2015). The norm for trust has secured sociality by maintaining civic norm adherence, inclusive orientation, and institutional confidence (Delhey et al. 2011). Health can benefit from norms for security to buttress sociality (Dawes 2020). The norm for security has enhanced sociality by maintaining neighboring, social cohesion, and trust and reducing aggression and opposition (Barbarin and Richter 2001; Grannis 2009; Rochelle 2015).

Conversely, health has benefitted from norms against crime, deprivation, disadvantage, disorder, relocation, uncertainty, and unemployment (Carpiano 2008; Franzini et al. 2005; P. Lu et al. 2021; Poortinga 2012; Stafford et al. 2005; Y. Wang and Li 2020). The norm for crime has eroded sociality by weakening community involvement, prosocial behavior, and social trust (Broadbent and Papadopoulos 2011; Zanin 2017; Zhong 2010). Deprivation or disadvantage experienced erodes sociality by breeding conflict (J. Turner 2013b). The norm for disorder has jeopardized sociality by erasing community attachment, neighborhood safety, social capital, and social trust (G. Brown et al. 2004; Congdon 2010; Kanan and Pruitt 2002; Ross and Mirowsky 2009). Relocation has impeded sociality by diminishing social integration (Kearns and Whitley 2015). Uncertainty has impeded sociality by breeding risking (Van Tongeren et al. 2023). Furthermore, uncertainty can impair sociality by reducing communication satisfaction, intimacy, and social interaction and can provoke protesting (Borch 2013; Theiss 2018). The norm for unemployment has jeopardized sociality by eroding legalism, social capital, social trust, and support for the market, and breeding protesting, radicalism, social exclusion experienced, and violence (L. Berger 2005; Buck 2001; Earl and Soule 2001; Gillham et al. 2019; Hayo 2004; Mitts 2019; Savelkoul et al. 2014; Smiley and Yang 2021).

Life Satisfaction

Life satisfaction signifies achievement, attainment, competence, control, mastery, power, stability, and utility (Ambrey and Fleming 2014; Heidemeier and Staudinger

2012; Kjell et al. 2016). Inherently, life satisfaction features delight, quality, and valuation regarding life (Ellis et al. 2019; Lawton et al. 2002; Qouta et al. 2007). Life satisfaction is likely to champion sociality by engendering power, utility, ideals, and norms to achieve the functions required for sociality. Such achievement hinges on the voluntaristic mechanisms of power realization, utility optimization, ideal calibration, and norm conformity posited in analytical functionalism.

Power for sociality enhanced by life satisfaction has stemmed from health, intelligence, marriage, self-efficacy, social networking, and social support received (Celso et al. 2003; Corcoran et al. 2011; Pena-Lopez and Sanchez-Santos 2016; Schaie 2013; Yoo and Jeong 2017). Health has uplifted sociality by boosting community sense, morality, popularity, social activity, social cohesion, social integration, social trust, social well-being, and volunteering (Huxhold et al. 2014; Jorgensen et al. 2010; Son and Wilson 2012; Tolsma et al. 2009; Yu and Chiu 2016). Conversely, health has sustained sociality by preventing loneliness (Koromeckyj-Cox et al. 2007). Intelligence has raised sociality by facilitating donation and social capital and reducing criminality and protesting (Cornwall 2009; Feinstein and Bynner 2006; Paterson 2008; Piferi et al. 2006). Marriage has consolidated sociality by enhancing community attachment, community evaluation, community involvement, civic engagement, closeness experienced, donation, friendship satisfaction, neighboring, political participation, prosocial behavior, reciprocity, relationship quality, social capital, social cohesion, social integration, social interaction, social support received, and trust (W. Chang 2009; Cornwall 2009; Degenne et al. 2004; Flavin and Keane 2011; Frye 2007; Kerrissey and Schofer 2013; Lizardo 2006; Louis and Zhao 2002; Mata and Pendakur 2014; McCabe 2014; Prezza et al. 2001; Ross and Mirowsky 2009; Sampson and Raudenbush 2004; Swaroop and Morenoff 2006; Tolsma et al. 2009). Conversely, marriage has upheld sociality by reducing crime, discrimination experienced, loneliness, social exclusion experienced, tolerance for deviance, and violence (Carr and Friedman 2005; Coffe and Geys 2007; Koromeckyj-Cox et al. 2007; Savolainen 2009; E. Wojcieszak and Mutz 2009; E. Wright et al. 2015). Self-efficacy has sustained sociality by raising civic engagement, donation, government and social trust, leadership, political participation, prosocial behavior, and social activity (Bednall et al. 2013; Frye 2007; Gnambs and Batinic 2012; Huber et al. 2022; Mangum 2012; Rahn 2008; Pei and Pan 2018; Yao and Enright 2019). Social networking has consolidated sociality by raising civic engagement, community involvement, donation, political involvement, social trust, and volunteering (Bekkers et al. 2008; Broadbent and Papadopoulos 2011; Brown and Ferris 2007; Chua et al. 2021; Narayan and Cassidy 2001). Social support received has strengthened sociality by enhancing attachment, gratitude, political participation, prosocial behavior, recourse, respect, responsibility, social integration, and social well-being (Boezeman and Ellemers 2008; Fahmy 2006; Phipps 2003; Williams and Galliher 2006; R. Wright et al. 2009; Zeldin et al. 2016; Zeng et al. 2024). Conversely, social support received has boosted sociality by preventing aggression, conflict, delinquency, doping, externalizing, hyperactivity, loneliness, runaway, sexuality, suicide, and violence (Bernardon et al. 2011; Browning et al. 2005; Hayslip et al. 2000; Nieuwenhuis et al. 2017; Pearson and Wilkinson 2013; Terzi-Unsal and Karei 2005;

Wight et al. 2006; R. Wright et al. 2009). Life satisfaction has arisen from power based on adaptability, agreeableness, attractiveness, conservatism, control or controllability, conscientiousness, extraversion, financial adequacy, friendship, intelligence, mastery, mindfulness, physical functioning, social capital, social desirability, sociability, socioeconomic status, and wisdom to uplift sociality (Abbott et al. 2011; Chang and Kang 2018; d'Astous and Mouakhar-Klouz 2022; C. Hill 2019; T. Hill et al. 2023; Holliman et al. 2021; Klein 2013; Klussman et al. 2020; C. Li et al. 2017; Orlowski and Wicker 2015; Y. Wang and Li 2020; H. Yuan 2016). Adaptability has secured sociality regarding partnership and social adjustment and satisfaction as opposed to discord (Chow et al. 2014; Mitchell 2005). Agreeableness has fostered sociality by enhancing attachment (Fraley et al. 2011). Moreover, agreeableness constitutes sociality by featuring communion, compliance, cooperation, empathy, helping, intimacy, morality, politeness, prosociality, respect, solidarity, sympathy, understanding, warmth, and unity (Dinic and Bodroza 2021; Graziano and Tobin 2009; J. Sun et al. 2018). Attractiveness has facilitated sociality by raising cooperation received, liking received, and political evaluation (Asendorpf et al. 2011; Jackson et al. 1993; Mulford et al. 1998). Conservatism sustains sociality by nurturing empathy, loyalty, prosocial behavior, religiousness, and sacrifice (Dutton and Rayner-Hilles 2022). Controllability has enhanced sociality by uplifting social trust (Burke and Stets 1999). Conscientiousness has elevated sociality by consolidating attachment, compliance, order value, responsibility, social desirability, and volunteering reducing deviance, violence, and justification for unconventional sexuality (Bekkers 2005; de Jong et al. 2012; Fraley et al. 2011; Gotzsche-Astrup 2020; Mondak and Hurwitz 2012; Mullet et al. 2005; Saucier and Skrzypinska 2006; Twardawski et al. 2021; Wright and DeLisi 2016). Extraversion has buttressed sociality by fostering attachment, civic engagement, civility, donation, humor, nationalism, political participation, social capital, socializing, volunteering, and favor for civic and political participation (Bekkers 2010; C. Cheng et al. 2019; Fraley et al. 2011; Gotzsche-Astrup 2020; Hample 2018; Omoto et al. 2010; Schbley and McCauley 2005; Vernon et al. 2008; Ward and Forney 2020). Financial adequacy has enabled sociality by raising government trust (Li and Mayraz 2017). Friendship has constituted sociality by enhancing community attachment, compliance, donation, gratitude, political participation, social cohesion, social desirability, social integration, and social trust (Corcoran 2013; Fahmy 2006; Gundert and Hohendanner 2015; Keillor et al. 2001; Kende et al. 2022; Opp 2001; Rotkirch 2014). Mastery has enhanced sociality by uplifting social trust (Burke and Stets 1999). Mindfulness has facilitated sociality by raising affiliating, intimacy, and prosocial behavior (D. Berry et al. 2020; Flett 2018; Karremans et al. 2017). Physical functioning has sustained sociality by enriching social capital (Cornwall 2009). Social capital has consolidated sociality by raising civic engagement, community involvement, donation, political involvement, social trust, and volunteering (Bekkers et al. 2008; Broadbent and Papadopoulos 2011; Brown and Ferris 2007; Chua et al. 2021; Narayan and Cassidy 2001). Conversely, social capital has strengthened sociality by erasing violence (Pulkkinen et al. 2009). Social desirability has buttressed sociality by raising altruism, benevolence value, and empathy and perspective-taking and suppressing violence and its tolerance (Douglas 2006;

Fisher and Katz 2000; Krumrei-Mancuso 2017; Pulkkinen et al. 2009). The ideal for social welfare has championed sociality by consolidating government trust (U. Kim et al. 2002). Sociability has enhanced sociality by raising civic engagement, civility, political participation, prosocial behavior, and social cohesion (Foschi and Lauriola 2014; Letki 2008). Socioeconomic status has enhanced sociality by raising helping and interaction quality (Molana and Adams 2019). Wisdom has enhanced sociality by establishing attachment security, generativity, and the ideal for social engagement (Webster 2003, 2010). Life satisfaction can benefit from openness and resources as power to drive sociality (Hadjar and Samuel 2015; Headey 2008). Openness has boosted sociality by enhancing civic orientation and participation, civility, forgiveness, loyalty, political participation, relationship quality, social competence, and volunteering and dampening hostility, and violence (Bekkers 2005; Hounkpatin et al. 2015; Keightley et al. 2006; Labrecque 2014; Marks 1996; Mullet et al. 2005; Peterson and Maiden 1993; Rothmund et al. 2014; van Hiel et al. 2007). Resources can facilitate sociality by raising social integration and obstructing crime, risking, social exclusion received, and violence (Agnew 2007; Figueredo et al. 2018; Gallie 2004; Lilly et al. 2011; Tsai 2006).

Conversely, life satisfaction has resulted from the absence of disability, neuroticism, obesity, powerlessness, and unemployment to maintain power to drive sociality (Brockmann et al. 2009; Kahneman et al. 2010; C. Li et al. 2017; Louis and Zhao 2002; Zotti et al. 2016). Disability has weakened sociality by eroding social capital, social cohesion, social trust, and volunteering (Cornwall 2009; Granzin and Haggard 2000; Tang 2006; Zanin et al. 2013). Conversely, disability has impeded sociality by instigating protesting, and suicide (Van Vugt et al. 2003). Neuroticism has impaired sociality by reducing attachment security, civic engagement, coordination, forgiveness, nationalism, relatedness, and socializing and generating crime and hostility (Bekkers 2005; Fraley et al. 2011; Hounkpatin et al. 2015; Kalish 2008; Marks 1996; Mullet et al. 2005; Pulkkinen et al. 2009; Schbley and McCauley 2005; Ward and Forney 2020). Obesity has disrupted sociality by raising discrimination received (Carr and Friedman 2005). Powerlessness has eroded sociality by dampening attachment and giving (Campos-Castillo and Hitlin 2013; Molm 1997). Unemployment has impeded sociality by dissolving social capital, social cohesion, and trust (Esperwall and Dellgren 2008; Manturuk et al. 2010; Reeskens and Vandecasteele 2017).

Utility for sociality raised by life satisfaction has rested on well-being (Rocke and Lachman 2008). Well-being has uplifted sociality by consolidating altruism, conformism, cooperation, donation, liking for people, prosociality, sociability, and trust and social trust (Fetvadjiev and He 2019; A. Hu 2013; Lyubomirsky et al. 2006; Y. Pan et al. 2023; Wang and Graddy 2008).

Life satisfaction has evolved from utility based on community sense, hope, meaningfulness, police confidence, positive affect, safety, security, self-confidence, self-evaluation, and self-esteem to secure sociality (Bronk et al. 2009; Frederick et al. 2016; Frey et al. 2007; T. Hill et al. 2023; Hudders and Pandelaere 2012; Kong et al. 2014; Moller 2005; Russo-Netzer et al. 2021; Shao et al. 2021). Community sense has underlain sociality regarding cooperation, networking, and trust (Groves et al. 2000; Molitor et al. 2011; Rochelle 2015). Hope has buttressed sociality by preventing migration and suicide (Adnanes 2004). Meaningfulness has underlain sociality by boosting civic practice, responsibility, and volunteering and reducing rejection experience (Duffy and Raque-Bogdan 2010; Summers and Falco 2020; Twenge et al. 2003). Police confidence embraces compliance, cooperation, obedience, respect, and trust to enhance sociality (Hough 2012; Lowrey-Kinberg et al. 2020; Wahyurudhanto 2022). Positive affect has maintained sociality by raising government trust and patriotism (Hunt et al. 2019; Turner and Stets 2005). Safety has buttressed sociality regarding civility, social capital, and trust (Curley 2010; Watson et al. 2021; Williamson 2002). Security upholds sociality by avoiding conflict, hostility, and rejection experience (Bina et al. 2020). Self-confidence, self-evaluation, or self-esteem has buttressed sociality by raising attachment security, political participation, and prosociality and preventing suicide (Kitayama and Markus 2000; Tracy et al. 2009).

Conversely, life satisfaction has reduced deprivation, isolation experienced, loneliness, and loss experienced as utility distracting sociality (Luhmann et al. 2013; Neto and Barros 2003; Richards 2016; Schmitt et al. 2010). Deprivation experienced erodes sociality by breeding conflict (J. Turner 2013). Favoritism constitutes corruption (Inglehart and Welzel 2005). Isolation experienced has disturbed sociality by eroding closeness and prosocial behavior (Bockler et al. 2021; K. Lin et al. 2013). Loneliness has impaired sociality by weakening reciprocity, social capital, and social cohesion and provoking suicide (C. Cheng et al. 2019; Espvall and Dellgren 2008). Loss experienced has hindered sociality by eroding compliance and government trust and fomenting suicide (Kirchler and Maciejovsky 2001; Nicholls and Picou 2012). Life satisfaction has resulted from low disutility based on alienation experienced, conflict, depression, deprivation experienced, discrimination experienced, distress, negative affect, stress, social exclusion experienced, and victimization to sustain sociality (Bellani and D'Ambrosio 2011; Brenig and Proeger 2018; Cheung 1998; Delbosc and Currie 2011; Groot and Van Den Brink 2003; Hudders and Pandelaere 2012; Kirmanoglu and Baslevent 2014; Rettig et al. 1999; Yip et al. 2007). Alienation experienced has eroded sociality regarding attachment (Bishop et al. 2002). Conflict has impeded sociality regarding donation and trust as opposed to violence (Farmer and Fedor 2001; Farrington 2018; Kunovich and Hodson 1999). Depression has eroded sociality by breeding conflict, hate, hostility perceived, loneliness, revenge, risking, suicide, and violence (Cacioppo and Hawkley 2009; Economou et al. 2016; Haner et al. 2020; Morokoff et al. 2009; Mullet et al. 2005; Proulx et al. 2004; H. Smith et al. 2016; E. Wright et al. 2015). Conversely, depression has attenuated sociality by impeding benevolence, closeness experienced, fairness, forgiveness, gratitude, honesty, leadership, love, social integration, teamwork, and volunteering (Blanchard et al. 2021; Cornwall 2009; Holzel et al. 2011; Mancini et al. 2011; Mullet et al. 2005; Thoits and Hewitt 2001). Discrimination experienced can foment violence to undermine sociality (White et al. 2015). Distress or negative affect has undermined sociality by fomenting resistance and impeding social capital and trust (Pulkkinen et al. 2009; Webber and Huxley 2007). Stress has undermined sociality by eroding civility, forgiveness, generativity, relationship quality and satisfaction, social integration, social support received, and trust and heightening conflict, maltreatment, substance abuse, suicide, and violence (Atkinson et al. 2005; Dutton et al. 2016; Gelles 2007; Grzywacz and Almeida 2008; Jackson et al. 2006; Sobeck et al. 2020; Toussaint et al. 2016). Social exclusion experienced has disturbed sociality by eroding closeness and prosocial behavior (Bockler et al. 2021; K. Lin et al. 2013). Victimization experienced has impaired sociality by eroding social trust (Olivera 2015). Conversely, victimization experienced has hurt sociality by activating conflict and migration (Bar-Tal and Halperin 2013; Ramesh et al. 2019). Life satisfaction can suffer from competition and uncertainty as disutility against sociality (Rhodes-Purdy et al. 2023; Scons et al. 2009). Competition has impeded sociality by eroding volunteering (Martinez and McMullin 2004). Uncertainty has impeded sociality by breeding risking (Van Tongeren et al. 2023). Furthermore, uncertainty can impair sociality by reducing communication satisfaction, intimacy, and social interaction and provoke protesting (Borch 2013; Theiss 2018).

Ideals bossted by life satisfaction have prized government trust and social trust, political interest, political participation, social cohesion, and volunteering (E. Chan 2014; Flavin and Keane 2011; Rochelle 2015; Schulz et al. 2000). Government trust has constituted sociality by sustaining compliance, conformity, nationalism, political participation, and preventing protesting (Rhodes-Purdy et al. 2023; Ulbig 2002; van der Meer and van Ingen 2009; V. Vu 2021). Social trust has benefitted from agreeableness, familiarity, friendship, knowledge, language proficiency, moderateness, self-efficacy, and sociability to provide power to drive sociality (Freitag and Bauer 2016; Halvorsen 2007; Kende et al. 2022; Lancee and Dronkers 2011; McCabe 2012; Pattie et al. 2004; Rahn 2008). Political interest has elevated sociality by raising civic engagement, civic and social motivation, civility, and discussion as opposed to protesting (Gil de Zuniga et al. 2017; Lee and Chan 2011; Pattie et al. 2004). Political participation has buttressed sociality regarding civility (Campbell 2003). Social cohesion has constituted sociality by enhancing attachment and dampening tolerance for deviance (Stafford et al. 2005; Woosnam et al. 2018). Volunteering has constituted sociality by raising altruism, charity orientation, civic motivation, donation, helping, moral responsibility, political participation, social integration, and social and government trust (Foster et al. 2001; Isham et al. 2006; Richey 2010; Richey and Ikeda 2009; Wiepking and Maas 2009). Life satisfaction has evolved from ideals for altruism, civic participation, community involvement, contact or social interaction, donation, helping, kindness, morality, national attachment, national identification, nationality favor, networking, organizational attendance, political interest, political participation, prosocial behavior, reciprocity, responsibility, social involvement, social participation, socializing, tradition, trust, voluntary association participation, and volunteering to consolidate sociality (Barrett 1999; Becchetti et al. 2012; Buchanan and Bardi 2010; Caprara and Steca 2005; Chang and Kang 2018; Datler et al. 2013; Edara 2021; Gil-Lacruz et al. 2019; Headey 2010; Helliwell et al. 2010; Klein 2013; Krys et al. 2019; Lim and Putnam 2010; Magnani and Zhu 2018; Nam 2019; Oarga et al. 2015; Pavlova and Silbereisen 2012; Rampichini and D'Andrea 1998; Selim 2008; Thoits and Hewitt 2001; Tsai 2021; H. Yuan 2016; Zdrenka et al. 2015). Altruism or helping has constituted sociality by boosting attachment, civic engagement, friendship quality, likability, moral behavior, popularity, relatedness and diminishing loneliness, and violence (Bond and Kwan 2000; W. Chen et al. 2022; Layous et al. 2012; Markiewicz et al. 2001; Martela and Ryan 2016; Mesch 2009; Na and Paternoster 2019; L. Taylor et al. 2018; Wright and Li 2011). Civic participation has propped sociality by strengthening attachment, civility, collective behavior, discussion, donation, neighboring, patriotism, prosociality, social capital, socialism, trust, and volunteering and impeding cheating and individualism (Coffe and Geys 2007; Gilberbloom and Markham 1995; Kerrissey and Schofer 2013; Mata and Pendakur 2014; Ozbay 2008; Pattie et al. 2004; Pena-Lopez and Sanchez-Santos 2016; Rahn 2008; Richey 2011; Tak 2017; M. Tang 2011; Taniguchi 2013; Yip et al. 2007). Community involvement or social participation has underlain sociality regarding cooperation, networking, and trust (Groves et al. 2000; Molitor et al. 2011; Rochelle 2015). Social interaction has realized sociality by consolidating altruism, compliance, cooperation, donation, morality, political participation, reciprocity, social trust, and volunteering (Guillen et al. 2011; Dixon and McKeown 2021; Lucas and Livingston 2014; Musick 2000; Rodrigo-Gonzalez et al. 2019; Rubin and Step 2000). Donation has constituted sociality by consolidating charity, service value, social capital, social trust, and volunteering (Bekkers 2010; Chang 2009; Foster et al. 2001; Uslaner 2000). Kindness has constituted sociality by securing volunteering (Barr et al. 2005). Morality has championed sociality by boosting volunteering and inhibiting violence (Piquero and Hickman 2002; Whitford et al. 2006). National attachment, identification, or favor has underpinned sociality by fostering attachment, intolerance against deviance, patriotism, political participation, religiousness, social inclusion, trust in government, and xenophobia, and diminishing protesting (N. Chen 2012; Flanagan and Lee 2000; Huddy et al. 2021; Li and Brewer 2004; Osborne et al. 2017; Pinto et al. 2020; Rippl et al. 2010). Networking or social involvement has fostered sociality regarding connectedness, friendship, giving, and social interaction (Eberl 2020; Liebler and Sandefur 2002; Nelson-Coffey et al. 2023; Phan et al. 2009). Organizational attendance or voluntary association participation has fostered sociality by enhancing attachment, civility, political participation, social integration, socialism (favor), and trust (Geys 2012; Guillen et al. 2011; Pattie et al. 2004; Tak 2017). Political interest has elevated sociality by raising civic engagement, civic and social motivation, civility, and discussion as opposed to protesting (Gil de Zuniga et al. 2017; Lee and Chan 2011; Pattie et al. 2004). Political participation has buttressed sociality regarding civility (Campbell 2003). Prosocial behavior has constituted sociality by civility, consolidating connectedness, cooperation, religiosity, responsibility, and volunteering (Hample 2018; Marsh and Dik 2021; Musick and Wilson 2008; Nelson-Coffey et al. 2023; Shahzalal and Adnan 2022). Moreover, prosocial behavior underlies sociality by enhancing citizenship, loyalty, social cohesion, socializing, and trust and diminishing self-interest (Dovidio et al. 2006; Hawley 2014; Kisliuk and WeiBmuller 2023; Music 2014). Reciprocity has constituted sociality by fostering prosocial behavior (Thielmann et al. 2020). Responsibility has eroded the acceptance of outsiders (Granzin and Olsen 1998). Socializing has fostered sociality regarding connectedness, friendship, giving, and social interaction (Eberl 2020; Liebler and Sandefur 2002; Nelson-Coffey et al. 2023; Phan et al. 2009). The ideal for tradition has buttressed sociality by enhancing patriotism and faith in religion and discouraging protesting and acceptance of deviants and outsiders (Costa et al. 2023; Datler et al. 2013; Meuleman et al. 2019; Schwartz et al. 2014). Trust has constituted sociality through donation, involvement, and volunteering (Uslaner 2000). Volunteering has constituted sociality by raising altruism, charity orientation, civic motivation, donation, helping, moral responsibility, political participation, social integration, and social and government trust (Foster et al. 2001; Isham et al. 2006; Richey 2010; Richey and Ikeda 2009; Wiepking and Maas 2009). Conversely, life satisfaction has stood on the ideal against homosexuality to rationalize sociality (Zotti et al. 2016). The ideal for homosexuality has obstructed sociality by countering conformity, conservatism, and nationalism (Gaines and Garand 2010; Motschenbacher 2013; Yeo and Chu 2018).

Norms exposed by life satisfaction have popularized justice (Jia et al. 2020). The norm for justice has raised accommodation, civility, cooperation, government and social trust, political participation, and social support received and reduced protesting to elevate sociality (Davis-Lipman et al. 2007; A. Hu 2013; Lawrence and Daniels 1997; Lipkus and Bissonette 1998; Tyler and Degoey 1995; van Prooijen et al. 2008; Wenzel 2000). Life satisfaction has evolved from norms for Christianity, civic participation, civility, employment, government effectiveness, helpfulness, morality, prosperity, social cohesion, social interaction, social service adequacy, social welfare, socialism, socioeconomic status, trust, voluntary organization membership, and volunteering to elevate sociality (Bohnke 2008; Bond and Lun 2014; Castles 2000; Chang and Kang 2018; Conzo et al. 2017; Helliwell 2006; Michalos and Zumbo 2001; Okulicz-Kozaryn et al. 2014; Orlowski and Wicker 2015; Ovaska and Takashima 2006; Radcliff 2001; Wallace and Pichler 2009; Whiteley et al. 2010; C. Wong et al. 2006; Yip et al. 2007; Yuan 2016; Zeng and Zhang 2022). Christianity has buttressed sociality by securing conformity, donation, and morality, and impeding cosmopolitanism (Hollinger 2017; Phillips and Smith 2008). The norm for civil participation can maintain sociality by consolidating social capital and preventing conflict (Edwards 2004; Langman 2005). Besides, the norm for civil participation constitutes sociality by championing association, civility, communitarianism, community, conservatism, donation, humanism, justice, networking, participation, philanthropy, responsibility, shaming, social democracy, social orientation, socialism, and solidarity (Adloff 2018; Choi 2004; DeLue and Dale 2009; Edwards 2004; O'Mahony 2013; Powell 2007). The norm for civility has enhanced political trust to champion sociality (Mutz and Reeves 2005). The norm for governance effectiveness can secure citizenship and social cohesion and prevent conflict, fragmentation, and threats experienced to install sociality (Bukenya and Golooba-Mutebi 2020; Rhodes-Purdy et al. 2021; Tang 1998; Taylor-Gooby 1991). The norm for helpfulness has raised responsibility, thus enhancing sociality (Shahzalal and Adnan 2022). Morality has championed sociality by boosting volunteering and inhibiting violence (Piquero and Hickman 2002; Whitford et al. 2006). The norm for prosperity or socioeconomic status has uplifted sociality by raising government support, nationalism, political participation, relationship quality, trust, volunteering, and xenophobia (Cheng and Smyth 2016; Fridberg and Kangas 2008; Inglehart 2003; Rhodes-Purdy et al. 2023; Traunmuller 2011; van Oorschot and Arts 2005). The norm for social cohesion has buttressed sociality by strengthening civic engagement, community favor, financial help, institutional trust, political participation, and recourse and prevented violence (Z. Han et al. 2017; F. Lee 2012; Mitrut and Wolff 2011; Palmer et al. 2011; Su and Feng 2013; Whitham 2012; E. Wright et al. 2015). Social interaction has realized sociality by consolidating altruism, compliance, cooperation, donation, morality, political participation, reciprocity, social trust, and volunteering (Guillen et al. 2011; Dixon and McKeown 2021; Lucas and Livingston 2014; Musick 2000; Rodrigo-Gonzalez et al. 2019; Rubin and Step 2000). Social service adequacy has fostered sociality by buttressing government trust and the norm for donation (Bednall et al. 2013; Kumlin et al. 2025). The norm for social welfare has uplifted sociality by advancing neighboring, political participation, social capital, support for social welfare, and volunteering and diminishing migration and theft (Allard and Danziger 2000; J. Brown 2016; Musick and Wilson 2008; Portes and Vickstrom 2011; Rehm et al. 2012; Semino 2015). The norm for socialism has enhanced sociality by sustaining traditionalism and volunteering (Braun et al. 1994; Musick and Wilson 2008). The norm for trust has secured sociality by maintaining civic norm adherence, inclusive orientation, and institutional confidence (Delhey et al. 2011). The norm for organization has secured sociality regarding social cohesion (Milner 2002). Life satisfaction can benefit from the norm for social democracy (Radcliff 2001). The norm for social democracy sustains sociality by championing equality and solidarity (Andersson 2006). Volunteering has constituted sociality by raising altruism, charity orientation, civic motivation, donation, helping, moral responsibility, political participation, social integration, and social and government trust (Foster et al. 2001; Isham et al. 2006; Richey 2010; Richey and Ikeda 2009; Wiepking and Maas 2009).

Conversely, life satisfaction has stood on norms against corruption, crime, deprivation, problems, and risk to maintain sociality (Ciziceno and Travaglino 2019; Cramm et al. 2012; Manning et al. 2016; Zotti et al. 2016). The norm for corruption has eroded by undermining institutional and social trust and activating lying (Morris and Klesner 2010; van Hemert et al. 2002; J. You 2012). The norm for crime has eroded sociality by weakening community involvement, prosocial behavior, and social trust (Broadbent and Papadopoulos 2011; Zanin 2017; Zhong 2010). The norm for deprivation has worsened civic engagement, civility, community involvement, donation, relatedness, social trust, and volunteering and fomented cynicism, suicide, theft, violence, and victimization to impair sociality (Abascal 2015; Broadbent and Papadopoulos 2011; J. Brown 2016; Graddy and Wang 2009; Hagan et al. 2016; Krahe 2013; Nepal et al. 2011; Piatkowska 2020; C. Ross et al. 2000; Stoll 2001; Wuthnow 2004). The norm for problems has impaired sociality by jeopardizing civility, government and social trust, and political participation and breeding deviance (Backman and Nilsson 2011; Fahmy 2006; Marschall and Stolle 2004; Nicholls and Picou 2012). The norm for risk has impaired sociality by provoking protesting (Scafuto and La Barbera

2016). Moreover, the risk norm can hurt sociality by generating opposition to the establishment (P. Brown 2020). Life satisfaction can benefit from the norm against multiculturalism (Rhodes-Purdy et al. 2023). Multiculturalism espouses radicalism and unrest to accept deviance (Delanty 2009; Pehrson et al. 2011).

Current Findings

Factor analysis of experiences identified the five experience factors of economic hardship, neighbor nuisance, victimization, security, and family saving. Two additional well-being experiences were health and life satisfaction. These factors entered the regression analysis of social attitudes in the fourth or fifth step of stepwise selection. This selection entered predictors achieving the .001 level of significance (Table 4.1).

Based on existing knowledge, security, family saving, health, and life satisfaction are likely to buttress sociality. By contrast, economic hardship, neighborhood nuisance, and victimization are likely to erode sociality. Most of these expectations found support from regression analysis (see Table 4.2).

Most notably, confidence in institutions received a significant trivial positive effect from security ($\beta = .035$, see Table 4.3) and a significant trivial negative effect from economic hardship ($\beta = -.035$).

Justification for misdeeds received the strongest but weak negative effect from life satisfaction ($\beta = -.086$, see Table 4.4).

Justification for unconventional sexuality received the strongest but trivial negative effect from life satisfaction ($\beta = -.047$, see Table 4.5). Security gave the next strongest but trivial negative effect on justification for nonconventional sexuality ($\beta = -.040$).

Faith in religion received the strongest but trivial positive effect from economic hardship ($\beta = .017$, see Table 4.6). Health and neighborhood nuisance gave the next strongest but trivial negative effect on faith in religion ($\beta = -.016$).

Acceptance of outsiders received the strongest but trivial negative effect from life satisfaction ($\beta = -.060$, see Table 4.7). Health and neighborhood nuisance gave the next strongest but trivial negative effect on accepting outsiders ($\beta = -.044$).

Acceptance of deviants received the strongest but slight negative effect from life satisfaction ($\beta = -.070$, see Table 4.8). Health gave the next strongest but trivial negative effect on accepting deviants ($\beta = -.051$).

Trust in others received the trivial negative effect from victimization ($\beta = -.042$, see Table 4.9).

Contrary to expectation, confidence in institutions received a negative effect from health. With force theory enhancing the analytical functionalist framework, health generates a force of self-enhancement, whereas confidence in institutions reflects a force of compliance or submissiveness (Grimes 2006; Kazarian and Martin 2006). The force of self-enhancement thus opposes the force of submissiveness, producing a negative effect.

Table 4.1 Means, standard deviations, and factor loadings on experiences

Item	*M*	*SD*	hard	Nuisance	Victim	Family saving	Secure
Gone without medicine or medical treatment that you needed	22.7	30.6	.791	.120	.047	.057	.075
Gone without a cash income	27.1	32.9	.786	.116	.030	.134	– .005
Gone without enough food to eat	16.6	28.3	.749	.162	.013	.022	.118
Racist behavior in your neighborhood	16.3	27.0	.185	.781	.051	.114	.046
Police or military interfering with people's private life in your neighborhood	17.9	26.9	.232	.665	.052	.163	.141
Drug sale in streets in your neighborhood	24.0	34.5	.172	.615	.093	.381	.164
Robberies in your neighborhood	26.3	30.3	.164	.502	.111	.297	.392
Alcohol consumption in streets in your neighborhood	34.3	35.3	.140	.434	.083	.764	.169
Family saving money	46.9	34.8	.002	– .041	– .029	.002	– .003
Family as the crime victim	7.6	26.4	.026	.056	.996	.051	.024
You as the crime victim	6.6	24.8	.055	.102	.377	.035	.128
Feeling secure in your neighborhood	67.6	25.9	– .065	– .085	– .096	– .073	– .484
Felt unsafe from crime in your home	20.0	29.1	.563	.165	.115	.032	.462

Note % variance explained = 71.7
Hard = economic hardship, Nuisance = neighborhood nuisance, Victim = victimization, Secure = Security

Contrary to expectation, faith in religion received a negative effect from neighborhood nuisance. Based on force theory to enrich analytical functionalism, neighborhood nuisance engenders a force of disorder, whereas faith in religion denotes control, discipline, and strictness (Lindblad et al. 2013; Kay et al. 2008; Peifer 2010;

Table 4.2 Expected and actual effects of experiences on sociality

Predictor	Expected	Actual						
		Institution	Anti-misdeed	Anti-sex	Anti-faith	Anti-outsider	Anti-deviant	Other
Economic hardship	–	–			–			
Neighborhood nuisance	–			–	+			
Victimization	–	–						–
Security	+	+		+			–	
Family saving	+							
Health	+	–			+	+	+	
Life satisfaction	+		+	+		+	+	

Note Sociality unfolded in social attitudes in terms of confidence in institutions, refutation against misdeeds, refutation against unconventional sexuality, unfaith in religion, rejection of outsiders, rejection of deviants, and trust in others.
+ positive effect. – negative effect.

Table 4.3 Significant ($p <$ .001) standardized effects of experiences and practice on confidence in institutions

Predictor	(5)
Security	.035
Economic hardship	− .035
Health	− .022
Victimization	− .021
Life satisfaction	.010n
R^2	.401

n: $p > .001$

Table 4.4 Significant ($p <$ .001) standardized effects of experiences on justification for misdeeds

Predictor	(4)
Life satisfaction	− .086
Victimization	.015n
R^2	.069

n: $p > .001$

Table 4.5 Significant ($p <$ .001) standardized effects of experiences on justification for unconventional sexuality

Predictor	(5)
Life satisfaction	− .047
Security	− .040
Neighborhood nuisance	.022
Health	− .013n
R^2	.280

n: $p > .001$

Table 4.6 Significant ($p <$ .001) standardized effects of experiences on faith in religion

Predictor	(5)
Health	− .016
Economic hardship	.017
Neighborhood nuisance	− .016
R^2	.550

Table 4.7 Significant ($p <$ .001) standardized effects of experiences on acceptance of outsiders

Predictor	(5)
Life satisfaction	− .060
Health	− .044
R^2	.188

Table 4.8 Significant ($p < .001$) standardized effects of experiences on acceptance of deviants

Predictor	(5)
Life satisfaction	− .070
Health	− .051
Security	− .017
R^2	.179

n: $p > .001$

Table 4.9 Significant ($p < .001$) standardized effects of experiences on trust in others

Predictor	(5)
Victimization	− .042
R^2	.042

B. Turner 2009). The clash of forces from the two sides would underlie the negative effect.

Contrary to expectation, acceptance of deviants received a positive effect from security. Based on force theory to enrich analytical functionalism, the positive effect results from the compatibility of forces. On the one hand, security engenders the force of liberalism (Watson et al. 2021). On the other hand, acceptance of deviants stands on the force of liberalism (Orazani et al. 2020).

Despite the contrary findings, most of the significant effects supported the expectation that sociality arises from security, health, and life satisfaction and declines with economic hardship, neighborhood nuisance, and victimization. Nevertheless, family saving did not show a significant effect on sociality. Based on force theory, distance reduces the impact or susceptibility of force (Blauza et al. 2023). Hence, family saving is too remote to the person to demonstrate a significant effect on personal sociality.

Chapter 5
Functioning of National Norms for Social Attitudes

National norms are the national aggregates of averages of personal experiences and sociality attitudes. The experiences are economic hardship, neighborhood nuisance, victimization, security, family saving, health, and life satisfaction. The attitudes are confidence in institutions, refutation against misdeeds, refutation against unconventional sexuality, irreligion, rejection of outsiders, rejection of deviants, and trust in others. National norms affect personal attitudes with analytical functionalism's deterministic and voluntaristic mechanisms. The deterministic mechanism affects personal attitudes directly and indirectly through voluntaristic mechanisms. On the one hand, the direct deterministic mechanism operates when the national attitude affects the corresponding personal attitude. As such, national confidence in institutions determines personal confidence in institutions, national refutation against misdeeds determines personal refutations against misdeeds, and so on. The direct mechanism also operates privately and publicly or vicariously. Whereas the private mechanism means that the person takes up the national influence privately, the public or vicarious mechanism means that the person borrows the influence from others to take it as his or her own. An illustrative example of private determinism is that a person can easily pick up money when money abounds. By contrast, the corresponding instance of public or vicarious determinism is that a person benefits from affluent others when money abounds. The example of affluence can apply to social attitudes. On the other hand, the indirect deterministic mechanisms employ empowering, incentivizing, framing, and standardizing to trigger the voluntaristic mechanisms of power realization, utility optimization, ideal calibration, and norm conformity.

C.-k. Cheung, *Social Attitudes in the Early 21st Century*,
https://doi.org/10.1007/978-981-96-9705-2_5

Existing Knowledge

A norm means restriction to induce people's compliance (Y. Lin et al. 2021; Voss 2001). In analytical functionalism, a norm mainly enables the integration function to complement fulfilling, adaptation, and latency functions. Moreover, a norm exerts empowering, incentivizing, framing, and standardizing to influence indirectly through power realization, utility optimization, ideal calibration, and norm conformity. Empowering involves authority and institutions for arrangement, assignment, enforcement, institutionalization, and sanctioning to require compliance regarding norms (Chaney 2014; Navarra et al. 2018; Paraskevopoulos 2010; Smith and Hamon 2012; Stavrova 2014; S. Wong 2008). Incentivizing engages exchange and rewarding concerning recognition regarding norms, notably about reciprocity (Heitmeyer and Anhut 2008; Huesmann and Kirwil 2007; Lawler 2002). Framing or sensitizing provides categorizing, nudging, instigation, and reinforcement to invoke identification and similarity regarding norms (Arriaga et al. 2018; Hsee et al. 1999; Lahey and Waldman 2007; Uzumceker and Akfirat 2024; Zahnow et al. 2024). Standardizing features acculturation, cultivation, exposing, persuasion, socialization, and transmission to induce compliance, definition, empathy, imitation, learning, matching, meaning-making, and modeling regarding norms (Bjarnegard et al. 2019; Dolch 2003; Heitmeyer and Anhut 2008; Jensen 2007; Lahey and Waldman 2007; Markowitz 2001; Smith and Hamon 2012; Stavrova 2014; S. Wong 2008). Meanwhile, sociality evolves from power, utility, ideals, and norms received. Power from the norm accrues from adaptability, agency, attachment, coercion received, institutionalization received, intelligence, motivation, and signaling ability to shape sociality (Fowers 2015; Tuomela 2007). This power stands on the collective basis for the norm. Utility from the norm relies on exchange, interdependence, reward received, and stress experienced to induce sociality (Fowers 2015; Tomasello 2014). This utility resides in social approval, fitness, and recognition. Ideals from the norm stand on social categorization and identity to construct sociality (Fowers 2015). These ideals realize distinctiveness. Norms hinge on commonality, culture, homophily, and learning to assimilate sociality (Fowers 2015; Phithakkitnukoon and Smoreda 2016; Tuomela 2007). These norms uphold belongingness and integration. The fourteen norms underlying personal sociality attitudes cover economic hardship, neighborhood nuisance, victimization, security, family saving, health, life satisfaction, confidence in institutions, refutation against misdeeds, refutation against unconventional sexuality, irreligion, rejection of outsiders, rejection of deviants, and trust in others.

Norm for Economic Hardship

The norm for economic hardship or poverty is likely to obstruct sociality by withdrawing power, utility, ideals, and norms for sociality through the deterministic and voluntaristic mechanisms of analytical functionalism. The direct deterministic mechanisms produce or provide sociality privately and publicly, whereas the indirect deterministic mechanisms trigger voluntaristic mechanisms successively. The indirect determinisms activate empowering, incentivizing, framing, and standardizing involving power, utility, ideals, and norms. These determinisms activate the voluntaristic mechanisms of power realization, utility optimization, ideal calibration, and norm conformity to complete the influence.

Power for sociality reduced by the norm for economic hardship has stemmed from civility, education, family income, family intactness, and wealth (L. Hao 1996; Owens and Walker 2018; Roscigno 1999). Civility has constituted sociality by inducing fairness and trust (Vera-Toscano et al. 2013). Education has fostered sociality by raising civic engagement, civility, conformism, crime disapproval, equality support, morality, political discussion, political interest, political participation, socialism, and trust (Bullock 2021; E. Chan 2014; Djupe and Lewis 2015; Gilberbloom and Markham 1995; Kerrissey and Schofer 2013; Miyata et al. 2008; Norris 2011; Norris and Inglehart 2009; Ulbig 2002; Wilson and Dunham 2001). Conversely, education has sustained sociality by reducing political alienation, deviance, prostitution, resistance, and violence and its tolerance (Backman and Nilsson 2011; Coffe and Geys 2007; Lubbers et al. 2006; Michalski 2005; Simon et al. 2001; Swader and Vorobeva 2015). Family income has buttressed sociality by raising civility, civic engagement, community involvement, compliance, donation, friendliness, nationalism, political participation, social capital, social integration, social interaction, social support received, social trust (Alnsour and Meaton 2009; Crowder et al. 2006; Doff and Kleinhans 2011; Kleinhans et al. 2007; La Grange and Yip 2001; Lennartsson 2010; Norris and Inglehart 2009; Oliver 2003; Shin 2012; Wiepking and Maas 2009; Q. Xu et al. 2010). Conversely, family income has sustained sociality by preventing crime, discrimination experienced, sleeping, and social exclusion experienced (Cerin and Leslie 2008; Hamermesh 2019; Moore and Aweiss 2003; Stanley et al. 2011). Family intactness has elevated sociality by raising civic engagement (Hener et al. 2016). Wealth has safeguarded sociality by enhancing reciprocity experienced, social capital, social integration, and social trust and preventing migration and victimization (Angelusz and Tardos 2001; K. Chan et al. 2014; Crowder et al. 2006; Hackel and Zaki 2018; Reese et al. 2021; Uslaner 2008). Exactly, the norm for economic hardship has weakened power driving sociality (C. Ross et al. 2000). Power has enhanced sociality by raising attachment, empathy, giving, mimicking, punishment, trust received, and xenophobia (Barrera 2007; Campos-Castillo and Hitlin 2013; Molm 1997; Schwartz et al. 2014).

Conversely, the norm of economic hardship has fostered dysfunction, illness, and social welfare dependency to reduce power to uphold sociality (Hirschl and Rank 1999; B. Johnson et al. 2006; A. Jones et al. 2015). Dysfunction has weakened sociality by eroding social capital, social cohesion, social trust, and volunteering (Cornwall 2009; Granzin and Haggard 2000; Tang 2006; Zarin et al. 2013). Conversely, dysfunction has impeded sociality by instigating protesting and suicide (Van Vugt et al. 2003). Illness has eroded sociality by impeding volunteering (Wuthnow 2004). Welfare dependency has obstructed sociality by dampening caring, civic participation, government and social trust, political participation, and volunteering and breeding victimization (Andersen 1999; Bruch et al. 2010; Caputo 2010; Hyggen 2006; Knab et al. 2008; Sarasa 2008).

Utility attenuated by the norm for economic hardship has rested on neighborhood quality and satisfaction, relatedness, and security (Gaitan-Rossi and Shen 2018; Harris 2001; C. Ross et al. 2000; Sampson and Raudenbush 2004). Neighborhood quality has elevated sociality by building social capital, order, and cohesion (Rupp et al. 2020; Sampson and Raudenbush 2004). Neighborhood satisfaction has fostered sociality by enhancing attachment, community involvement, volunteering, and social capital (Cummins et al. 2003; Long and Perkins 2007; Xu 2007). Relatedness has consolidated sociality by raising sharing, social interaction, and relationship satisfaction (Downie et al. 2008; Frazer 1999; Wickham and Knee 2012). Security has buttressed sociality regarding civility, social capital, and trust (Curley 2010; Watson et al. 2021; Williamson 2002). Conversely, the norm for economic hardship has bred victimization as disutility against sociality (Nepal et al. 2011). Victimization experienced has impaired sociality by eroding social trust (Olivera 2015). Conversely, victimization experienced has hurt sociality by activating conflict and migration (Bar-Tal and Halperin 2013; Ramesh et al. 2019).

Ideals for sociality dismissed by the norm for economic hardship have valorized civic engagement, community involvement, donation, and social trust (Abascal 2015; Broadbent and Papadopoulos 2011; Graddy and Wang 2009; Stoll 2001). Civic engagement has propped sociality by strengthening attachment, civility, collective behavior, discussion, donation, neighboring, patriotism, prosociality, social capital, socialism, trust, and volunteering and impeding cheating and individualism (Coffe and Geys 2007; Gilberbloom and Markham 1995; Kerrissey and Schofer 2013; Mata and Pendakur 2014; Ozbay 2008; Pattie et al. 2004; Pena-Lopez and Sanchez-Santos 2016; Rahn 2008; Richey 2011; Tak 2017; M. Tang 2011; Taniguchi 2013; Yip et al. 2007). Community involvement has underlain sociality regarding cooperation, networking, and trust (Groves et al. 2000; Molitor et al. 2011; Rochelle 2015). Donation has constituted sociality by consolidating charity, service value, social capital, social trust, and volunteering (Bekkers 2010; Chang 2009; Foster et al. 2001; Uslaner 2000). Social trust has constituted sociality through donation, involvement, and volunteering (Uslaner 2000).

Conversely, the norm for economic hardship has fomented ideals for cynicism, suicide, theft, and violence to devalue sociality (Hagan et al. 2016; Krahe 2013; Piatkowska 2020). Cynicism has undermined sociality by eroding government and social trust, patriotism, and political participation and raising competition (Flanagan and Lee 2003; Guan et al. 2010; Uslaner 2002; van der Meer and van Ingen 2009). The ideal for suicide has impeded sociality by fomenting radicalism (Soliman et al. 2016). Theft has bred social avoidance to weaken sociality (Brayne 2014). Violence has undermined sociality by breeding antisociality, crime and recidivism, blaming, conflict, hostility, rejecting others, and impairing agreeableness, morality, and responsibility (Asendorpf et al. 2008; Del Bove et al. 2008; Morrison 2006; Scholte et al. 2009; Vitaro et al. 2007).

Norms for sociality dampened by the norm for economic hardship have popularized opportunity (Kingston et al. 2009). Opportunity has advanced sociality by enhancing cohesion, commitment received, and political participation (Bonaiuto et al. 1999; Emler and Frazer 1999; Q. Xu et al. 2018). Conversely, the norm for economic hardship has bred norms for anomie or normlessness, crime, disorder, inequality, and revolution against sociality (Kirk and Papachristos 2011; Teymoori et al. 2016; Mare 1996; McLeod et al. 2018; C. Ross et al. 2000). Anomie has impeded sociality by raising radicalism and support for violence (Troian et al. 2019). The norm for crime has eroded sociality by weakening community involvement, prosocial behavior, and social trust (Broadbent and Papadopoulos 2011; Zanin 2017; Zhong 2010). The norm for disorder has jeopardized sociality by erasing community attachment, neighborhood safety, social capital, and social trust (G. Brown et al. 2004; Congdon 2010; Kanan and Pruitt 2002; Ross and Mirowsky 2009). The norm for inequality has impeded sociality by eroding social capital, support for redistribution and welfare, sympathy, trust, and volunteering (Busemeyer 2013; Hitlin and Harkness 2018; Lipford and Yandle 2009; Oishi et al. 2011; Portes and Vickstrom 2011). Conversely, the norm for inequality has impaired sociality by provoking crime and violence (Ousey and Lee 2013; van Wilsem 2007). Revolution has impaired sociality by eroding solidarity and fomenting deviance (Foy et al. 2014; J. Williams 2011).

Norm for Neighborhood Nuisance

The norm for neighborhood nuisance or nuisance is likely to dampen power, utility, ideals, and norms to inhibit sociality through the deterministic and voluntaristic mechanisms of analytical mechanisms. These mechanisms engage empowering, incentivizing, framing, and standardizing to activate power realization, utility optimization, ideal calibration, and norm conformity.

Power for sociality weakened by the norm for nuisance has arisen from health (Franzini et al. 2005). Exactly, the norm for nuisance has weakened power for sociality (C. Ross et al. 2000). Health has uplifted sociality by boosting community sense, morality, popularity, social activity, social cohesion, social integration, social trust, social well-being, and volunteering (Huxhold et al. 2014; Jorgensen et al. 2010; Son and Wilson 2012; Tolsma et al. 2009; Yu and Chiu 2016). Conversely, health has sustained sociality by preventing loneliness (Koromeckyj-Cox et al. 2007). Exactly, the norm for economic hardship has weakened power for sociality (C. Ross et al. 2000). Power has enhanced sociality by raising attachment, empathy, giving, mimicking, punishment, trust received, and xenophobia (Barrera 2007; Campos-Castillo and Hitlin 2013; Molm 1997; Schwartz et al. 2014).

Utility for sociality reduced by the norm for nuisance has rested on police satisfaction (Y. Wu et al. 2019). Police satisfaction embraces compliance, cooperation, obedience, respect, and trust to enhance sociality (Hough 2012; Lowrey-Kinberg et al. 2020; Wahyurudhanto 2022). Conversely, the norm for nuisance has bred victimization as disutility against sociality (Like 2011). Victimization experienced has impaired sociality by eroding social trust (Olivera 2015). Conversely, victimization experienced has hurt sociality by activating conflict and migration (Bar-Tal and Halperin 2013; Ramesh et al. 2019).

Ideals for sociality dispelled by the norm for nuisance have accentuated social trust (Ross and Mirowsky 2009). Social trust has constituted sociality through donation, involvement, and volunteering (Uslaner 2000). Conversely, the norm for nuisance has fostered the ideal for avoidance to refute sociality (Brown and Zoorob 2022). Avoidance has hindered sociality by diminishing communication and prosociality and provoking radicalism (Collins and Feeney 2004; Makhanova and Shepherd 2020; Soliman et al. 2016).

Norms underlying the norm for nuisance have popularized disadvantage and impoverishment to withhold sociality (Franzini et al. 2005; Wilcox et al. 2004). The norm for disadvantage or impoverishment has worsened civic engagement, civility, community involvement, donation, relatedness, social trust, and volunteering and fomented cynicism, suicide, theft, violence, and victimization to impair sociality (Abascal 2015; Broadbent and Papadopoulos 2011; J. Brown 2016; Graddy and Wang 2009; Hagan et al. 2016; Krahe 2013; Nepal et al. 2011; Piatkowska 2020; C. Ross et al. 2000; Stoll 2001; Wuthnow 2004). Conversely, the norm for nuisance has reflected the norm against neighboring to obstruct sociality (Wilcox et al. 2004). The norm for neighboring has fostered sociality by facilitating association (Peyrot 2000).

Norm for Victimization

The norm for victimization, misdeeds, and deviance means the norm for crime, as victimization is the counterpart of crime (Price et al. 2019). Hence, the norm for crime is likely to weaken sociality by forbidding power, utility, ideals, and norms to run the deterministic and voluntaristic mechanisms of analytical functionalism.

Power for sociality eroded by the crime norm has stemmed from health (Stafford et al. 2005). Health has uplifted sociality by boosting community sense, morality, popularity, social activity, social cohesion, social integration, social trust, social well-being, and volunteering (Huxhold et al. 2014; Jorgensen et al. 2010; Son and Wilson 2012; Tolsma et al. 2009; Yu and Chiu 2016). Conversely, health has sustained sociality by preventing loneliness (Koromeckyj-Cox et al. 2007). The crime norm reduces solidarity as power consolidating sociality (Zhong 2009). Solidarity has constituted sociality by enhancing attachment and dampening tolerance for deviance (Stafford et al. 2005; Woosnam et al. 2018).

Utility for sociality impaired by the crime norm has resided in well-being, including life and neighborhood satisfaction (J. Jang et al. 2018; Manning et al. 2016; Parkes et al. 2002). Life satisfaction has incubated sociality regarding political participation, social cohesion, social trust, and volunteering (E. Chan 2014; Flavin and Keane 2011; Rochelle 2015). Neighborhood satisfaction has fostered sociality by enhancing attachment, community involvement, volunteering, and social capital (Cummins et al. 2003; Long and Perkins 2007; Xu 2007). More generally, well-being has uplifted sociality by consolidating altruism, conformism, cooperation, donation, liking for people, prosociality, sociability, and trust and social trust (Fetvadjiev and He 2019; A. Hu 2013; Lyubomirsky et al. 2006; Y. Pan et al. 2023; Wang and Graddy 2008). Additionally, well-being sustains sociality by enabling civilization, fairness, forgiveness, intimacy, kindness, love, loyalty, modesty, morality, open-mindedness, social intelligence, and societal functioning (Cummins 2016; D'raven and Pasha-Zaidi 2016; Meadows 2014). Conversely, the crime norm has bred death and victimization as disutility against sociality (Jacobs and Carmichael 2002; Kennedy et al. 1998). Dying can dampen sociality by fomenting aggression (Reeve 2021). Victimization experienced has impaired sociality by eroding social trust (Olivera 2015),

Ideals for sociality dampened by the crime norm have valorized community involvement, prosocial behavior, and social trust (Broadbent and Papadopoulos 2011; Zanin 2017; Zhong 2010). Community involvement has underlain sociality regarding cooperation, networking, and trust (Groves et al. 2000; Molitor et al. 2011; Rochelle 2015). Prosocial behavior has constituted sociality by civility, consolidating connectedness, cooperation, religiosity, responsibility, and volunteering (Hample 2018; Marsh and Dik 2021; Musick and Wilson 2008; Nelson-Coffey et al. 2023; Shahzalal and Adnan 2022). Moreover, prosocial behavior underlies sociality by enhancing citizenship, loyalty, social cohesion, socializing, and trust and diminishing self-interest (Dovidio et al. 2006; Hawley 2014; Kisliuk and WeiBmuller 2023; Music 2014). Social trust has constituted sociality through donation, involvement, and volunteering (Uslaner 2000).

The norm for sociality dismissed by the crime norm has popularized voluntary organizations (J. Wo 2018). The norm for voluntary organizations has espoused sociality by preventing accidents and suicide (Helliwell 2006). The crime norm has sprung from norms for deprivation, disadvantage, extremism, inequality, legal cynicism, poverty, racial heterogeneity, and unemployment to disrupt sociality (Hughes et al. 2015; Kirk and Papachristos 2011; Kubrin 2000; McVeigh and Cunningham 2012; Painter-Davis et al. 2010; Schulenberg 2003). Deprivation or disadvantage experienced erodes sociality by breeding conflict (J. Turner 2013b). Extremism has impeded sociality by provoking protesting (Moreira et al. 2018). Cynicism has undermined sociality by eroding government and social trust, patriotism, and political participation and raising competition (Flanagan and Lee 2003; Guan et al. 2010; Uslaner 2002; van der Meer and van Ingen 2009). Poverty has undermined sociality by reducing civic participation, trust, social connection, and volunteering (Caputo 2010; Stephens et al. 2014; R. Walker et al. 2010). The norm for racial heterogeneity has ruined sociality by undermining social capital and solidarity, including altruism, cooperation, friendship, and trust (Putnam 2007). Unemployment has impeded sociality by dissolving social capital, social cohesion, and trust (Espvall and Dellgren 2008; Manturuk et al. 2010; Reeskens and Vandecasteele 2017). Conversely, unemployment has hurt sociality by breeding conflict experienced, moving, protesting, threats experienced, and victimization (Bramley and Morgan 2003; Kaukinen 2004; Lewin-Epstein et al. 2003; Schneider 2007; Su and

Feng 2013). The crime norm has evolved from norms for conflict, disorganization, domination, hardship, immigration, social exclusion, strain, and threat to jeopardize sociality (Castells 2000; Herzog 2005; Hughes et al. 2015; Zhong 2009). Conflict has impeded sociality regarding donation and trust as opposed to violence (Farmer and Fedor 2001; Farrington 2018; Kunovich and Hodson 1999). The disorganization norm underlying the crime norm covers ethnic heterogeneity, family disruption, and residential instability as opposed to affluence, community cohesion, informal social control, opportunity, and sharing (Kingston et al. 2009; Quillian 2014; Schulenberg 2003). The norm for disorganization has jeopardized sociality by erasing community attachment, neighborhood safety, social capital, and social trust (G. Brown et al. 2004; Congdon 2010; Kanan and Pruitt 2002; Ross and Mirowsky 2009). Domination has impaired sociality by weakening social cohesion (E. Chan 2014). Meanwhile, domination experienced has worsened sociality by breeding violence (Felson and Outlaw 2007). The norm for hardship has worsened civic engagement, civility, community involvement, donation, relatedness, social trust, and volunteering and fomented cynicism, suicide, theft, violence, and victimization to impair sociality (Abascal 2015; Broadbent and Papadopoulos 2011; J. Brown 2016; Graddy and Wang 2009; Hagan et al. 2016; Krahe 2013; Nepal et al. 2011; Piatkowska 2020; C. Ross et al. 2000; Stoll 2001; Wuthnow 2004). Essentially, hardship has impaired sociality by dampening trust and fomenting social exclusion experienced, suicide, and victimization experienced (Economou et al. 2016; Reeskens and Vandecasteele 2017; Ross and Mirowsky 2009). The norm for immigration has inhibited sociality by activating relocation and dampening support for social welfare (Eger 2010; Permentier et al. 2009). Social exclusion has impeded sociality by fueling crime, doping, and violence (Barry and Hullett 1998). Meanwhile, social exclusion experienced has disturbed sociality by eroding closeness and prosocial behavior (Bockler et al. 2021; K. Lin et al. 2013). Strain has undermined sociality by fomenting resistance and impeding social capital and trust (Pulkkinen et al. 2009; Webber and Huxley 2007). Threat experienced has inhibited sociality by reducing cohesion and triggering conflict and resistance (Lubbers et al. 2006; B. Rick et al. 2006).

Conversely, the crime norm has created the norm of violence impairing sociality (Kwon and Baack 2005). The norm for violence has undermined sociality by engendering protesting and tolerance for violence (Douglas 2006; Smidt 2020). The crime norm has emerged from norms against Catholicism, civic engagement, employment, legality, opportunity, punishment, residential stability, and social spending to impede sociality (S. Cho et al. 2013; Herzog 2005; Kingston et al. 2009; Maume and Lee 2003; Munch 2012; Painter-Davis et al. 2010). Catholicism has enhanced sociality by raising conformity value and volunteering and dampening independence value and radicalism (Bekkers 2010; Devos et al. 2002; Fjellvang 2011). Catholicism has also safeguarded sociality by inculcating cooperation and interdependence (Bellah et al. 1991). Civic engagement has propped sociality by strengthening attachment, civility, collective behavior, discussion, donation, neighboring, patriotism, prosociality, social capital, socialism, trust, and volunteering and impeding cheating and individualism (Coffe and Geys 2007; Gilberbloom and Markham 1995; Kerrissey and Schofer 2013; Mata and Pendakur 2014; Ozbay 2008; Pattie et al. 2004; Pena-Lopez and Sanchez-Santos 2016; Rahn 2008; Richey 2011; Tak 2017; M. Tang 2011; Taniguchi 2013; Yip et al. 2007). Employment has facilitated sociality by elevating civic engagement, community involvement, donation, philanthropy value, political discussion, political participation, social capital, social functioning, social cohesion experienced, social interaction, and social trust (Anciaes et al. 2017; Fridberg and Kangas 2008b; Kerrissey and Schofer 2013; H. Lu et al. 2002; Ross and Mirowsky 2009; Tsai 2006). Conversely, employment has safeguarded sociality by lessening crime, relocation, and social exclusion experienced (Groot et al. 2007; Kleinhans 2009; Savolainen 2009). Legality has buttressed sociality by dismissing radicalism (Muthuswamy 2022). The norm for opportunity has upheld sociality by preventing crime (Kingston et al. 2009). The opportunity norm can also maintain sociality by fostering legality and social cohesion and prohibiting terrorism (Fox 1996; Olzak and Soule 2009; Maras 2013). Crucially, the opportunity norm can establish society (Swartz 2013). Punishment characterizes sociality (Fowers 2015). Relocation has impeded sociality by diminishing social integration (Kearns and Whitley 2015). The norm for social spending has secured sociality by boosting support for redistribution (Weisstanner 2023). The crime norm can arise from norms against affluence, civilization, government effectiveness, policing, state authority, and teaching to impair sociality (Quillian 2014; Zhong 2009). The norm for affluence has uplifted sociality by raising government support, nationalism, political participation, relationship quality, trust, volunteering, and xenophobia (Cheng and Smyth 2016; Fridberg and Kangas 2008; Inglehart 2003; Rhodes-Purdy et al. 2023; Traunmuller 2011; van Oorschot and Arts 2005). Civilization constitutes sociality by establishing civility, loyalty, social contact, and social identification (Collins 2001; Hudson 2023). Besides, civilization embraces legality, relational quality, social capital, social cohesion, and social quality and dismisses violence (Phillips 2006; Rindermann 2018; Szakolczai 2001). The norm for government effectiveness has upgraded sociality by advancing justice perceived, social harmony perceived, and institutional, political, and social trust and preventing suicide (Grimes 2006; Heatherington and Globetti 2002; Helliwell 2006; R. Taylor et al. 2015; Wong and Shik 2011; C. Wong et al. 2005). Moreover, the norm for government effectiveness can uphold sociality by preventing crime (Quillian 2014). The norm for government effectiveness also sustains sociality by cultivating civic literacy (Milner 2002). The norm for policing has maintained sociality by dampening protesting (Choi and Kim 2019). The norm for state authority has embraced communitarianism, coordination, institutionalism, and republicanism to uphold sociality (Chahboun 2024; Jessop 2016; Prokhovnik 2008). Teaching has strengthened collaboration and conformity to uphold sociality (Decuyper et al. 2023; Gursimsek and Goregenli 2005).

Norm for Security

The norm for security dismisses conflict, criminality, risk, terrorism, tolerance, and violence (Ganz 2023; Greco and Polli 2021; Loader and Walker 2007; Sheikh 2014). This norm features paternalism espousing bureaucracy, elitism, and technology (Loader and Walker 2007). The norm for security is likely to raise sociality by generating power, utility, ideals, and norms to achieve sociality functions. These functions are fulfillment based on power, adaptation based on utility, latency based on ideals, and integration based on norms.

Power for sociality afforded by the security norm has derived from health and networking (Curley 2010; Ziersch et al. 2005). Health has uplifted sociality by boosting community sense, morality, popularity, social activity, social cohesion, social integration, social trust, social well-being, and volunteering (Huxhold et al. 2014; Jorgensen et al. 2010; Son and Wilson 2012; Tolsma et al. 2009; Yu and Chiu 2016). Conversely, health has sustained sociality by preventing loneliness (Koromeckyj-Cox et al. 2007). Networking has fostered sociality regarding connectedness, friendship, giving, and social interaction (Eberl 2020; Liebler and Sandefur 2002; Nelson-Coffey et al. 2023; Phan et al. 2009).

Utility for sociality given by the security norm has resided in well-being (Ziersch et al. 2005). Well-being has buttressed sociality by securing intimacy, moral behavior, popularity, social cohesion, social well-being, and sociability, and preventing rejection experience, victimization experience, and violence (Dougherty 2006; Gallagher and Lopez 2007; Kayser et al. 2010; Lambert et al. 2009; Twenge et al. 2003; Yip and Martin 2006). Conversely, the security norm has lessened fear as disutility against sociality Chiricos et al. 2000). Fear has disrupted sociality by breeding interpersonal problems, loneliness, risking, suicide, and violence (Dutton et al. 2016; Gillath et al. 2005; Pulkkinen et al. 2009; Trumbo et al. 2008). Conversely, fear has undermined sociality by reducing donation, friendship, humor, political participation, prosocial behavior, and social well-being (Best and Krueger 2010; Hewstone et al. 2005; Litman et al. 2017; Kuiper and Nicholl 2004; Zhong 2010).

Ideals for sociality cultivated by the security norm have highlighted cohesion, neighboring, and trust (Grannis 2009; Rochelle 2015). Cohesion has constituted sociality by enhancing attachment and dampening tolerance for deviance (Stafford et al. 2005; Woosnam et al. 2018). Neighboring has elevated sociality by raising consulting and influencing (Hays and Kogl 2007). Trust has constituted sociality through donation, involvement, and volunteering (Uslaner 2000). Conversely, the security norm has diminished ideals for aggression and opposition to maintain sociality (Barbarin and Richter 2001). Aggression has undermined sociality by breeding antisociality, crime and recidivism, blaming, conflict, hostility, rejecting others, and impairing agreeableness, morality, and responsibility (Asendorpf et al. 2008; Del Bove et al. 2008; Morrison 2006; Scholte et al. 2009; Vitaro et al. 2007). Opposition has impaired sociality by eroding solidarity and fomenting deviance (Foy et al. 2014; J. Williams 2011).

The norm for sociality maintained by the security norm has popularized quality (Olson et al. 2016). The norm of quality has elevated donation, law abidance, and social trust and weakened lying to secure sociality (Fridberg and Kangas 2008b; van Hemert et al. 2002). The security norm sustains the norm for civilization to safeguard sociality (Loader and Walker 2007). Civilization constitutes sociality by establishing civility, loyalty, social contact, and social identification (Collins 2001; Hudson 2023). Besides, civilization embraces legality, relational quality, social capital, social cohesion, and social quality and dismisses violence (Phillips 2006; Rindermann 2018; Szakolczai 2001). The security norm has developed from the norm for socioeconomic status to enhance sociality (Frohlich et al. 2002). Socioeconomic status has enhanced sociality by raising help and the quality of interaction (Molana and Adams 2019). The security builds on norms for communitarianism, social contract or contractarianism to secure sociality (Loader and Walker 2007; Milstein 2021). Contractarianism prioritizes order, preservation, safety, and security rather than rights (Milstein 2021). As such, contractarianism enhances sociality by embracing attachment, civic engagement, civility, compliance, compromise, consent, cooperation, coordination, equality, fairness, morality, and trust (Bowker 2016; Dalbert 2001; Darwall 2003; de Jonge 2012; Ellis et al. 2006; Gardiner 2009; Irwin 2016; Jarvinen and Branders 2020; Kaurin 2020). The security norm rests on norms against cosmopolitanism and liberalism to sustain sociality (Loader and Walker 2007). Cosmopolitanism contradicts sociality by hailing autonomy, diversity, foreignness, fusion, individualism, and liberalism (Corstange and York 2018; Delanty 2009; Held 2010; Herrmann 2023). Cosmopolitanism has eroded sociality by raising liberalism and acceptance of deviants and outsiders (Costa et al. 2023; Motschenbacher 2013; Norris and Inglehart 2009). Liberalism has impeded sociality regarding morality, normativity, and social order (Feinberg et al. 2019).

Norm for Family Saving

The norm for family saving or saving is likely to buttress sociality by inducing power, utility, ideals, and norms for sociality through the deterministic and voluntaristic mechanisms of analytical functionalism. The deterministic mechanisms engage empowering, incentivizing, framing, and standardizing, whereas the voluntaristic mechanisms operate power realization, utility optimization, ideal calibration, and norm conformity.

Power enhanced by the norm for saving has rested on financial adequacy (van Praag and Ferrer-I-Carbonell 2004). Financial adequacy has enabled sociality by raising government trust (Li and Mayraz 2017).

Norms upheld by the norm for saving have populated civilization, investment, and prosperity to boost sociality (Gray 2010; Lee and Chang 2006; Malizia et al. 2021). Civilization constitutes sociality by establishing civility, loyalty, social contact, and social identification (Collins 2001; Hudson 2023). Besides, civilization embraces legality, relational quality, social capital, social cohesion, and social quality and dismisses violence (Phillips 2006; Rindermann 2018; Szakolczai 2001). The norm for investment has enhanced sociality by preventing protesting (Mesch 1996). The norm for prosperity has uplifted sociality by raising government support, nationalism, political participation, relationship quality, trust, volunteering, and xenophobia (Cheng and Smyth 2016; Fridberg and Kangas 2008; Inglehart 2003; Rhodes-Purdy et al. 2023; Traunmuller 2011; van Oorschot and Arts 2005). The norm for social security or welfare has underlain the norm for saving to standardize sociality (Lee and Chang 2006). The norm for conservatism has championed the norm for saving to develop sociality (Yoos 2007). The norm for social welfare has uplifted sociality by advancing neighboring, political participation, social capital, support for social welfare, and volunteering and diminishing migration, and theft (Allard and Danziger 2000; J. Brown 2016; Musick and Wilson 2008; Portes and Vickstrom 2011; Rehm et al. 2012; Semino 2015).

Norm for Health

The norm for health covers healthcare effectiveness, life expectancy, and non-mortality (Baldacci et al. 2003; J. Jiang 2023; T. Vu 2020). This norm is likely to induce sociality by providing power, utility, ideals, and norms to activate analytical functionalism's deterministic and voluntaristic mechanisms. These mechanisms comprise empowering, incentivizing, framing, and standardizing for determinism and power realization, utility optimization, ideal calibration, and norm conformity for voluntarism.

Power enhanced by the norm for health has sprung from social capital (Portes and Vickstrom 2011). Social capital has consolidated sociality by raising civic engagement, community involvement, donation, political involvement, social trust, and volunteering (Bekkers et al. 2008; Broadbent and Papadopoulos 2011; Brown and Ferris 2007; Chua et al. 2021; Narayan and Cassidy 2001). Conversely, social capital has strengthened sociality by erasing violence (Pulkkinen et al. 2009).

The norm raised by the norm for health has popularized well-being (El-Ghannam 2002). The norm for well-being has upgraded sociality by boosting donation, law abidance, social trust, and voting and dampening lying (Fridberg and Kangas 2008b; Norris 2002; van Hemert et al. 2002). The norm for health has stood on norms for prosperity, social capital, socioeconomic status, and trade to cultivate sociality (J. Jiang 2023; Bezo 2012; Rudra and Haggard 2005). The norm for prosperity or socioeconomic status has uplifted sociality by raising government support, nationalism, political participation, relationship quality, trust, volunteering, and xenophobia (Cheng and Smyth 2016; Fridberg and Kangas 2008; Inglehart 2003; Rhodes-Purdy et al. 2023; Traunmuller 2011; van Oorschot and Arts 2005). The norm for social capital or social cohesion has buttressed sociality by strengthening civic engagement, community favor, financial help, institutional trust, political participation, and recourse and prevented violence (Z. Han et al. 2017; F. Lee 2012; Mitrut and Wolff 2011; Palmer et al. 2011; Su and Feng 2013; Whitham 2012; E. Wright et al. 2015).

The norm for socioeconomic status has raised sociality by boosting sociability, volunteering, and satisfaction with the neighborhood and reducing mortality (Letki 2008; Sampson 1991; A. Williams et al. 2007; Ye and Aldrich 2019). The norm for trade has enhanced sociality by raising voting and diminishing victimization (Hellwig 2001; Schutte 2015).

Conversely, the norm for health has maintained the norm against inequality and unemployment to secure sociality (J. Jiang 2023). The norm for inequality has impeded sociality by eroding social capital, support for redistribution and welfare, sympathy, trust, and volunteering (Busemeyer 2013; Hitlin and Harkness 2018; Lipford and Yandle 2009; Oishi et al. 2011; Portes and Vickstrom 2011). Conversely, the norm for inequality has impaired sociality by provoking crime and violence (Ousey and Lee 2013; van Wilsem 2007). The norm for unemployment has jeopardized sociality by eroding legalism, social capital, social trust, and support for the market, and breeding protesting, radicalism, social exclusion experienced, and violence (L. Berger 2005; Buck 2001; Earl and Soule 2001; Gillham et al. 2019; Hayo 2004; Mitts 2019; Savelkoul et al. 2014; Smiley and Yang 2021).

Norm for Life Satisfaction

The norm for life satisfaction or satisfaction is likely to raise sociality by generating power, utility, ideals, and norms for sociality through the deterministic and voluntaristic mechanisms of analytical functionalism. These mechanisms activate empowering, incentivizing, framing, and standardizing to achieve determinism and power realization, utility optimization, ideal calibration, and norm conformity to embody voluntarism.

Norms for sociality upheld by the norm for satisfaction can popularize communitarianism, governance, and voting (Jackson and Miller 1995; Sciulli 2011; X. Zhu 2019). Communitarianism constitutes sociality by espousing caring, civility, collective identity, commonweal orientation, community, dutifulness or responsibility, education or socialization, equality, interdependence, loyalty, mentoring, patriotism, reciprocity, relatedness, self-discipline, servicing including volunteering, settlement, social construction, social participation, solidarity, and trust (Delanty 2009; Frazer 1999; Moore 2010; Speth 2012). The norm for governance quality can secure citizenship and social cohesion and prevent conflict, fragmentation, and threats experienced to install sociality (Bukenya and Golooba-Mutebi 2020; Rhodes-Purdy et al. 2021; Tang 1998; Taylor-Gooby 1991). The norm for voting has secured sociality by enabling government trust (Whiteley 2009). Conversely, the norm for satisfaction can erode the norm for conflict to secure sociality (J. Turner 2013b). The norm for conflict has impaired sociality by fomenting protesting and resistance (Schatzman 2005; Sorens 2011).

Norm for Confidence in Institutions

The norm for confidence in institutions or compliance with or obedience to authority is likely to uplift sociality by raising power, utility, ideals, and norms for sociality. Such raising applies the deterministic and voluntaristic mechanisms of analytical functionalism. The mechanisms activate empowering, incentivizing, framing, and standardizing for determinism and power realization, utility optimization, ideal calibration, and norm conformity for voluntarism. Among them, norms are the most pronounced fuel.

The norm for sociality strengthened by the norm for compliance can support governance (Swedlow 2017). The norm for governance has embraced communitarianism, coordination, institutionalism, and republicanism to uphold sociality (Chahboun 2024; Jessop 2016; Prokhovnik 2008). Norms for sociality underlying the norm for compliance popularize Christianity and notably Catholicism, conservatism, contractarianism, equality, fairness, Judaism, morality, pastoralism or caring, and paternalism (Basanez 2016; Biggar 2020; Ferrara 2022; Huemer 2013; Koven 2015; Linquiti 2023; Stalder 2018). Pastoralism characterizing compliance prizes confession, counseling, salvation, and workfare (Walters 2012). Christianity has buttressed sociality by securing conformity, donation, and morality and impeding cosmopolitanism (Hollinger 2017; Phillips and Smith 2008). Catholicism has enhanced sociality by raising conformity value and volunteering and dampening independence value and radicalism (Bekkers 2010; Devos et al. 2002; Fjellvang 2011). Catholicism has also safeguarded sociality by inculcating cooperation and interdependence (Bellah et al. 1991). The norm for conservatism has championed the norm for saving to develop sociality (Yoos 2007). Contractarianism enhances sociality by embracing attachment, civic engagement, civility, compliance, compromise, consent, cooperation, coordination, equality, fairness, morality, and trust (Bowker 2016; Dalbert 2001; Darwall 2003; de Jonge 2012; Ellis et al. 2006; Gardiner 2009; Irwin 2016; Jarvinen and Branders 2020; Kaurin 2020). Equality experienced can sustain sociality by preventing crime and illegality (Kyriacou 2020). The norm for fairness has upheld sociality by elevating morality and prosocial behavior (Barber 2004; McCaffoee 2016). Judaism safeguards sociality by upholding humanitarianism (H. Smith 1991). Republicanism upholds sociality regarding citizenship, the commonweal, interdependence, morality, nationalism, publicity, responsibility, social adaptation, and solidarity (Delanty 2009; Honohan 2002). The norm for morality has maintained sociality by developing morality and dampening self-interest (A. Liu et al. 2025; J. Wright et al. 2017). The norm for caring has supported sociality by enhancing civic engagement, community favor, government trust, political participation, and recourse and dampening violence (Z. Han et al. 2017; F. Lee 2012; Palmer et al. 2011; Pulkkinen et al. 2009; Su and Feng 2013; Whitham 2012). Paternalism underlies sociality featuring morality (Kullgen 1995).

Conversely, norms against sociality underlying the norm for compliance popularize anarchism and libertarianism (Huemer 2013). Anarchism has impeded sociality by fomenting criticalness, protesting, resistance, and terrorism experienced (Gans

1992; Roberts 2012; Shatz 2011). Libertarianism has dampened sociality by weakening cooperation and patriotism and championing cynicism, protesting, and tolerance for deviance (Eggert and Giugni 2015; Flanagan and Lee 2003; Kertzer et al. 2014).

Norms for Refutation Against Misdeeds and Rejection of Deviants

Norms for refutation against misdeeds and rejection of deviants originate from the norm against deviance. The norm against is likely to maintain sociality by securing power, utility, ideals, and norms to achieve the functional bases for sociality required in analytical functionalism. Such achievement stands on the deterministic mechanisms of empowering, incentivizing, framing, and standardizing and the voluntaristic mechanisms of power realization, utility optimization, ideal calibration, and norm conformity. These mechanisms hinge on bonding and learning (Hoffmann and Dufur 2018; Morris et al. 2015).

Power for sociality maintained by the norm against deviance has rested on self-efficacy (Soller et al. 2017). Self-esteem has buttressed sociality by raising attachment security, political participation, and prosociality and by preventing suicide (Kitayama and Markus 2000; Tracy et al. 2009). Power for sociality underlying the norm against deviance has evolved from agreeableness, employment, family intactness, intelligence, self-control, sociability, social bonding, and socioeconomic status (Barry and Wigfield 2002; Benda 2002; Costello and Vowell 1999; Jang 1999; Low and Shortt 2017; Menard and Mose 1984; Price et al. 2019). Agreeableness has fostered sociality by enhancing attachment (Fraley et al. 2011). Employment has facilitated sociality by elevating civic engagement, community involvement, donation, philanthropy value, political discussion, political participation, social capital, social functioning, social cohesion experienced, social interaction, and social trust (Anciaes et al. 2017; Fridberg and Kangas 2008b; Kerrissey and Schofer 2013; H. Lu et al. 2002; Ross and Mirowsky 2009; Tsai 2006). Conversely, employment has safeguarded sociality by lessening crime, relocation, and social exclusion experienced (Groot et al. 2007; Kleinhans 2009; Savolainen 2009). Family intactness has elevated sociality by raising civic engagement (Hener et al. 2016). Intelligence has raised sociality by facilitating donation and social capital and reducing criminality and protesting (Cornwall 2009; Feinstein and Bynner 2006; Paterson 2008; Piferi et al. 2006). Self-control has buttressed sociality by enhancing generativity and impeding crime, risking, and violence (Y. Cheung et al. 2014; Koegl and Day 2019; Peterson and Klohnen 1995; Welch et al. 2008). Sociability has enhanced sociality by raising civic engagement, civility, political participation, prosocial behavior, and social cohesion (Foschi and Lauriola 2014; Letki 2008). Social bonding has constituted sociality regarding connectedness, friendship, giving, and social interaction (Eberl 2020; Liebler and Sandefur 2002; Nelson-Coffey et al. 2023; Phan et al. 2009).

Socioeconomic status has enhanced sociality by increasing interaction quality and help (Molana and Adams 2019). Power against sociality underlying the norm for deviance has emanated from impulsivity, neuroticism, and social deficiency (Benda 2002; E. Smith et al. 2023; Wilhoit and Goodnight 2023). Impulsivity has impeded sociality by diminishing prosocial behavior and engendering protesting, radicalism, and violence (Breakwell 2007; Koehler and Fiebig 2019; Thielmann et al. 2020; Wright and DeLisi 2016). Neuroticism has impaired sociality by reducing attachment security, civic engagement, coordination, forgiveness, nationalism, relatedness, and socializing and generating crime and hostility (Bekkers 2005; Fraley et al. 2011; Hounkpatin et al. 2015; Kalish 2008; Marks 1996; Mullet et al. 2005; Pulkkinen et al. 2009; Schbley and McCauley 2005; Ward and Forney 2020). Social deficiency has impaired sociality by weakening reciprocity, social capital, and social cohesion and provoking suicide (C. Cheng et al. 2019; Espvall and Dellgren 2008).

Disutility against sociality reduced by the norm against deviance has emerged from victimization experienced (Bhochhibhoya et al. 2021). Victimization experienced has impaired sociality by eroding social trust (Olivera 2015). Disutility against sociality underlying the norm for deviance has rested on alienation experienced, anger, isolation experienced, and stigmatizing received (Gao et al. 2015; Menard and Mose 1984). Alienation experienced has eroded sociality regarding attachment (Bishop et al. 2002). Anger has jeopardized sociality by eroding social integration and fomenting protesting and violence and its tolerance (Krahe 2013; Molm 2008; Passini 2019; Tausch et al. 2011). Moreover, anger can dampen sociality by breeding crime and radicalism (Brant 2019; Larson et al. 2020). Distress has undermined sociality by fomenting resistance and impeding social capital and trust (Pulkkinen et al. 2009; Webber and Huxley 2007). Isolation experienced has disturbed sociality by eroding closeness and prosocial behavior (Bockler et al. 2021; K. Lin et al. 2013). Stigmatization received has eroded sociality by damping social cohesion (Walton and Cohen 2007). Utility for sociality underlying the norm against deviance has resided in achievement, relatedness, and self-esteem (Brendgen et al. 1998; Menard and Mose 1984; Paige et al. 2022). Achievement has induced sociality by enhancing love and trust (Nezlek et al. 2008; Rieger and Wang 2021). Relatedness has consolidated sociality by consolidating sharing, social interaction, and relationship satisfaction (Downie et al. 2008; Frazer 1999; Wickham and Knee 2012). Self-esteem has buttressed sociality by raising attachment security, political participation, and prosociality and preventing suicide (Kitayama and Markus 2000; Tracy et al. 2009).

Ideals for sociality upheld by the norm against deviance have championed conformity, prosocial behavior, and safety (Jackman and MacPhee 2017; H. Ma et al. 2007; Nivette et al. 2021). Conformity has constituted sociality by raising patriotism and impeding violence and acceptance of deviants and outsiders (Pulkkinen et al. 2009; Schwartz et al. 2014; Van Hootegem et al. 2000; Yeo and Chu 2018). Prosocial behavior underlying the norm against deviance has included altruism and compliance (Carlo et al. 2014). Prosocial behavior has constituted sociality by civility, consolidating connectedness, cooperation, religiosity, responsibility, and volunteering (Hample 2018; Marsh and Dik 2021; Musick and Wilson 2008; Nelson-Coffey et al. 2023; Shahzalal and Adnan 2022). Safety has buttressed sociality regarding civility, social capital, and trust (Curley 2010; Watson et al. 2021; Williamson 2002). Besides, the norm against deviance has strengthened sociality by distracting ideals for aggression, antisociality, delinquency, externalizing behavior, gang involvement, moving or relocation, recidivism, rejection, risking, theft, and violence (Carson 2013; Deptula and Cohen 2004; German et al. 2009; Grant et al. 2019; Holloway et al. 2022; Jackman and MacPhee 2017; Lenzi et al. 2015; Snyder et al. 2015; Walters 2020). Relocation has impeded sociality by diminishing social integration (Kearns and Whitley 2015). Aggression or violence has undermined sociality by breeding antisociality, crime and recidivism, blaming, conflict, hostility, rejecting others, and impairing agreeableness, morality, and responsibility (Asendorpf et al. 2008; Del Bove et al. 2008; Morrison 2006; Scholte et al. 2009; Vitaro et al. 2007). Antisociality has impeded sociality by impairing morality and triggering doping, recidivism, rejection received, and violence (Abbey et al. 2012; Bowen and Wretman 2014; Tsakpinoglou and Poulin 2017). Delinquency has undermined sociality by worsening attachment, empathy, helpfulness, morality, relational quality, sociability, and social capital (Cheung and Cheung 2006; Hoffmann et al. 2013; Keijsers et al. 2011). Conversely, delinquency has disrupted sociality by enhancing antisocial behavior, conflict, suicide, and victimization (Carson 2013; Cutler et al. 2001; P. Lau et al. 2005). Externalizing behavior has blocked sociality by raising antisocial behavior and conflict and dampening community participation and social support receipt (Crockett et al. 2018; Khamis 2006). Gang involvement has worsened sociality by breeding delinquency, prostitution, and violence and dampened social bonding (Barkin et al. 2001; Cusick 2002; Dukes and Stein 2003; Hutcherson 2012). Ideals for sociality underlying the norm against deviance have prized attachment, egalitarianism, family involvement, morality, and sociality (Benda 2002; Brezina and Piquero 2007; Garnier and Stein 2002; Prinstein and Wang 2005). Attachment has constituted sociality by boosting relationship satisfaction and social support received and dampening rejection expected (Arseth et al. 2009; Hand et al. 2013). Egalitarianism has underpinned sociality by enhancing empathy, support for welfare, and trust in government and impeding radicalism (Faricy and Ellis 2014; Lauriola et al. 2015; Lucas and Kteily 2018; Roosma et al. 2014). Family involvement has constituted sociality by enhancing cohesion and social support receipt (Espvall and Dellgren 2008; Rook and Ituarte 1999). Morality has constituted sociality by boosting volunteering and inhibiting violence (Piquero and Hickman 2002; Whitford et al. 2006). Ideals against sociality underlying the norm for deviance have boosted social withdrawal (J. Hong et al. 2017). Social withdrawal has inhibited sociality by breeding conflict (Debus et al. 2019).

Norms against sociality underlying the norm for deviance popularize coercion, dominance, and risking (Brendgen et al. 2000; Cairns et al. 1988; Low and Shortt 2017). Coercion or domination experienced has guided sociality regarding self-control and trust as opposed to violence (Gelfand and Lun 2013; Overall et al. 2020). The norm for risk has impaired sociality by provoking protesting (Scafuto and La Barbera 2016). Moreover, the risk norm can hurt sociality by generating opposition to the establishment (P. Brown 2020). The norm against sociality underlying the norm for deviance has popularized disorder (Vander Ven et al. 2001) The norm for disorder has jeopardized sociality by erasing community attachment, neighborhood safety, social capital, and social trust (G. Brown et al. 2004; Congdon 2010; Kanan and Pruitt 2002; Ross and Mirowsky 2009). Norms for sociality underlying the norm against deviance have popularized control and networking (Elliott and Wilson 1996). The norm for social control has enhanced sociality by raising civic engagement, government trust, political participation, and recourse (Su and Feng 2013; Z. Han et al. 2017; F. Lee 2012; Palmer et al. 2011). Conversely, the norm for social control has safeguarded sociality by dampening victimization and violence (Hansen-Nord et al. 2014; E. Wright et al. 2015). Furthermore, control received has secured sociality by enhancing institutional trust and patriotism (Overall et al. 2020). The norm for networking has buttressed sociality by strengthening civic engagement, community favor, financial help, institutional trust, political participation, and recourse and prevented violence (Z. Han et al. 2017; F. Lee 2012; Mitrut and Wolff 2011; Palmer et al. 2011; Su and Feng 2013; Whitham 2012; E. Wright et al. 2015).

Norm for Refuting Unconventional Sexuality

The norm for refuting unconventional sexuality features the norm against prostitution, which characterizes unconventional sexuality (Swami et al. 2017). Meanwhile, the norm against prostitution normalizes or standardizes disfavor against prostitution. As such, the norm against unconventional sexuality and the norm or disfavor against prostitution are likely to uphold sociality by generating power, utility, ideals, and norms to activate the deterministic and voluntaristic mechanisms of analytical functionalism. These mechanisms comprise empowering, incentivizing, framing, and standardizing for determinism and power realization, utility optimization, ideal calibration, and norm conformity for voluntarism.

Power for sociality underlying disfavor against prostitution has stemmed from marriage (Mancini et al. 2020). Marriage has consolidated sociality by enhancing community attachment, community evaluation, community involvement, civic engagement, closeness experienced, donation, friendship satisfaction, neighboring, political participation, prosocial behavior, reciprocity, relationship quality, social capital, social cohesion, social integration, social interaction, social support received, and trust (W. Chang 2009; Cornwall 2009; Degenne et al. 2004; Flavin and Keane 2011; Frye 2007; Kerrissey and Schofer 2013; Lizardo 2006; Louis and Zhao 2002; Mata and Pendakur 2014; McCabe 2014; Prezza et al. 2001; Ross and Mirowsky 2009; Sampson and Raudenbush 2004; Swaroop and Morenoff 2006; Tolsma et al. 2009). Conversely, marriage has upheld sociality by reducing crime, discrimination experienced, loneliness, social exclusion experienced, tolerance for deviance, and violence (Carr and Friedman 2005; Coffe and Geys 2007; Koromeckyj-Cox et al. 2007; Savolainen 2009; E. Wojcieszak and Mutz 2009; E. Wright et al. 2015).

Disutility against sociality represented by disfavor against prostitution emanates from danger, harm, and oppression experienced from prostitution (Mancini et al. 2020; D. May 1999). Danger has eroded sociality by weakening social integration and social trust (Hammer et al. 2009; Lindstrom and Rosvall 2015). Conversely, danger has dampened sociality by raising social exclusion (Hammer et al. 2009). Harm experienced has arisen from ideals for sexuality and weapon carrying to impair sociality (Krahe 2013; Wilcox 2002). Oppression experienced erodes sociality by fomenting violence (White et al. 2015).

The ideal for sociality favored by the norm against prostitution has valorized legality (Jonsson and Jakobsson 2017). Legality has buttressed sociality by dismissing radicalism (Muthuswamy 2022). Disfavor against prostitution refutes the ideal for promiscuity to secure sociality (Cao and Maguire 2013). Promiscuity can breed crime to hinder sociality (Walsh 2011). Disfavor against prostitution has rested on ideals for caring, conservatism, family, feminism, stability, and xenophobia to rationalize sociality (Cao and Stack 2010; H. Hsu et al. 2019; Jakobsson and Kotsadam 2011; Mancini et al. 2020). The ideal for a career has built sociality by increasing dependence and pleasing others (Willner et al. 2020). Conservatism sustains sociality by nurturing empathy, loyalty, prosocial behavior, religiousness, and sacrifice (Dutton and Rayner-Hilles 2022). Moreover, conservatism underpins sociality by maintaining allegiance or loyalty, attachment, civility, community, conformity, cooperation, discipline, ethnocentrism, honesty, humility, intimacy, legality, morality, nationalism, obedience, order, partnership, patriotism, peace, responsibility, sharing, trust, and xenophobia (Dutton and Rayner-Hilles 2022; Heilman and Kusev 2020; Hickson 2013; Lakoff 2009; Rhodes-Purdy et al. 2023; Scruton 2014; Yoos 2007; Zuk and Zuk 2020). Conversely, conservatism upholds sociality by condemning dehumanizing, evilness, revolution, sexuality, terrorism, and transgression (Dutton and Rayner-Hilles 2022; Malka and Soto 2011; Scruton 2014; Suhay 2015). Family involvement has constituted sociality by enhancing cohesion and social support receipt (Espvall and Dellgren 2008; Rook and Ituarte 1999). Feminism has also buttressed sociality regarding solidarity (van Breen et al. 2017). Stability has secured sociality, including civic engagement, cohesion, neighboring, and relational quality, as opposed to violence (Pulkkinen et al. 2009; C. Ross et al. 2000; Swaroop and Morenoff 2006; Villarreal and Silva 2006). Xenophobia has constituted sociality by boosting patriotism and social cohesion (Granzin and Olsen 1998; Wang and Chen 2004). Moreover, disfavor against prostitution stands on ideals for institutionalism, legalism, morality, paternalism, protectionism, social order, socialism, and universalism to rationalize sociality (Belliotti 1993; Brents 2016; Jakobsson and Kotsadam 2011; Primoratz 1999; Soble 2008). Institutionalism maintains sociality by emphasizing communication, relatedness, and social order (Jessop 2016). Legalism has maintained sociality by preventing radicalism (Muthuswamy 2022). Moralism has sustained sociality by boosting gratitude (Pohling et al. 2010). Paternalism underlying disfavor against prostitution condemns disease, exploitation, and violence and extols social status (Primoratz 1999). Hence, paternalism underlies sociality featuring morality (Kullgen 1995). The ideal for order fosters sociality by signifying cohesion, community, harmony, propriety or ritualism, and security or protection (C. Chung 2000; Heckscher 2015; P. Ip 2014; McGhee 2003; Peng 2003). Furthermore, the ideal for order constitutes sociality by espousing civility, cohesion, commitment, compliance, cooperation, harmony, protection, social interaction, and solidarity (Arat and Kerelian 2019; Kaurin 2020; Lawler et al. 2009; McGhee 2003; Mondak and Hurwitz 2012; Qin 2013). As such, the order ideal has upheld sociality by dampening deviance and its tolerance (Gibson 2013; Wright and DeLisi 2016). Socialism maintained in the community institution to frame sociality anticipates association, cooperation, equality, harmony, and mutuality as opposed to conflict (Powell 2007). Besides, socialism has enhanced sociality regarding cooperation and discussion as opposed to crime (Collier 2001; Lilly et al. 2011; Sanderson 2001). Universalism constitutes sociality by embodying morality (Mihailov 2023). Conversely, disfavor against prostitution has stood on ideals against deviance, liberalism, and religion to maintain sociality (Cao and Maguire 2013; Vlase and Grasso 2023). Deviance has ruined sociality by provoking social exclusion experienced (Backman and Nilsson 2011). Liberalism has impeded sociality regarding morality, normativity, and social order (Feinberg et al. 2019). The ideal for religion has hindered sociality by reducing nationalism, social interaction and engendering protesting, marginalization experienced, radicalism, and social distance (Ayalon et al. 1993; Kunovich 2009; Norris 2002; Pedahzur and Canetti-Nisim 2004; Wuthnow 2004). Moreover, disfavor against prostitution arises from the ideal against neoliberalism to endorse sociality (Brents 2016). Neoliberalism espouses atomization and silos and disregards ethics and social services to undermine sociality (Lobao et al. 2014; Lakoff 2009; Rhodes-Purdy et al. 2023; Smart 2003).

The norm against sociality inhibited by the norm against prostitution has popularized crime (S. Cho et al. 2013). The norm for crime has eroded sociality by weakening community involvement, prosocial behavior, and social trust (Broadbent and Papadopoulos 2011; Jakobsson and Kotsadam 2011; Zanin 2017; Zhong 2010). Moreover, the norm for sociality underlying the norm against prostitution can minimize decline or decay (B. Cohen 2019). Declines have hindered sociality by eroding compliance and government trust and fomenting suicide (Kirchler and Maciejovsky 2001; Nicholls and Picou 2012). The norm against prostitution secures sociality by grounding on the norm against patriarchy (Kochak 2022). The norm for patriarchy can underlie norms for crime and sadomasochism (Cross and Matheson 2006; Sammons and Putwain 2019). The norm for crime has eroded sociality by weakening community involvement, prosocial behavior, and social trust (Broadbent and Papadopoulos 2011; Zanin 2017; Zhong 2010). The norm for sadomasochism represents norms for victimization and violence. The norm for victimization disrupts sociality by triggering revolution (Seoighe 2016). The norm for violence has undermined sociality by engendering protesting and tolerance for violence (Douglas 2006; Smidt 2020). The norm against prostitution maintains sociality by representing norms against dehumanization, harm, and liberalism (Gao and Petrova 2022; Vicente 2016). Furthermore, the norm for dehumanization or harm disrupts sociality by triggering revolution (Seoighe 2016). The norm for liberalism impairs sociality by dismissing punishment (Vicente 2016).

Norm for Unfaith in Religion

The norm for unfaith in religion or irreligion dismisses the afterlife, control over faith, sacred, salvation, supernatural, and utopism (Garrod and Jones 2009; Pelters and Wijma 2016; Turner and Maryanski 2008; J. Turner et al. 2018). As such, the irreligion norm rejects antagonism and patriarchy and champions social conformity (Garrod and Jones 2009). The irreligion norm is likely to foster sociality by enabling power, utility, ideals, and norms as bases for sociality. This fostering builds on the deterministic and voluntaristic mechanisms of analytical functionalism.

The ideal for sociality enhanced by the irreligion norm has prized voting (DeLeon and Naff 2004). Voting has engendered sociality by boosting civic and community participation and neighboring (Djupe and Lewis 2015; Dorff 2017; Hays and Kogl 2007).

The norm for sociality strengthened by the irreligion norm has popularized punishment (Meier 1994). Punishment characterizes sociality (Fowers 2015). Furthermore, the norm for sociality embraced by the irreligion norm popularizes social conformity (Garrod and Jones 2009). Conformity has constituted sociality by raising patriotism and impeding violence and acceptance of deviants and outsiders (Pulkkinen et al. 2009; Schwartz et al. 2014; Van Hootegem et al. 2000; Yeo and Chu 2018). The irreligion norm has benefitted from norms for education and prosperity to enhance sociality (Kelley and De Graaf 1997). Education has fostered sociality by raising civic engagement, civility, conformism, crime disapproval, equality support, morality, political discussion, political interest, political participation, socialism, and trust (Bullock 2021; E. Chan 2014; Djupe and Lewis 2015; Gilberbloom and Markham 1995; Kerrissey and Schofer 2013; Miyata et al. 2008; Norris 2011; Norris and Inglehart 2009; Ulbig 2002; Wilson and Dunham 2001). Conversely, education has sustained sociality by reducing political alienation, deviance, prostitution, resistance, and violence and its tolerance (Backman and Nilsson 2011; Coffe and Geys 2007; Lubbers et al. 2006; Michalski 2005; Simon et al. 2001; Swader and Vorobeva 2015). The norm for prosperity has uplifted sociality by raising government support, nationalism, political participation, relationship quality, trust, volunteering, and xenophobia (Cheng and Smyth 2016; Fridberg and Kangas 2008; Inglehart 2003; Rhodes-Purdy et al. 2023; Traunmuller 2011; van Oorschot and Arts 2005).

Conversely, the irreligion norm rejects norms for antagonism and patriarchy to assimilate sociality (Garrod and Jones 2009). Antagonism has impaired sociality by eroding solidarity and fomenting deviance (Foy et al. 2014; J. Williams 2011). The norm for patriarchy can underlie norms for crime and sadomasochism (Cross and Matheson 2006; Sammons and Putwain 2019). The norm for crime has eroded sociality by weakening community involvement, prosocial behavior, and social trust (Broadbent and Papadopoulos 2011; Zanin 2017; Zhong 2010). The norm for sadomasochism represents norms for victimization and violence. The norm for victimization disrupts sociality by triggering revolution (Seoighe 2016). The norm for violence has undermined sociality by engendering protesting and tolerance for violence (Douglas 2006; Smidt 2020).

Norm for Rejection of Outsiders

The norm for rejecting outsiders or xenophobia represents the norm of societalization or social cohesion (Alexander and Adams 2023; Hayashi 2022). Societalization features communication, cooperation, coordination, production, reproduction, and sociability (Schmidt 2020). As such, the norm is likely to create sociality by furnishing power, utility, ideals, and norms for sociality through the deterministic and voluntaristic mechanisms of analytical functionalism. Empowering, incentivizing, framing, and standardizing constitute deterministic mechanisms, and power realization, utility optimization, ideal calibration, and norm conformity constitute voluntaristic mechanisms.

Power for sociality raised by the norm for social cohesion has rested on health (Fujisawa et al. 2009). Health has uplifted sociality by boosting community sense, morality, popularity, social activity, social cohesion, social integration, social trust, social well-being, and volunteering (Huxhold et al. 2014; Jorgensen et al. 2010; Son and Wilson 2012; Tolsma et al. 2009; Yu and Chiu 2016). Conversely, health has sustained sociality by preventing loneliness (Koromeckyj-Cox et al. 2007). Meanwhile, the norm for social cohesion has reduced illness to retain power for sociality (M. Wen et al. 2010). Illness has eroded sociality by impeding volunteering (Wuthnow 2004).

Utility for sociality created by the norm for social cohesion has derived from life satisfaction, neighborhood quality and satisfaction, and success (Cramm et al. 2012; Furstenberg and Hughes 1995; Olson et al. 2016). Life satisfaction has incubated sociality regarding political participation, social cohesion, social trust, and volunteering (E. Chan 2014; Flavin and Keane 2011; Rochelle 2015). Neighborhood quality has elevated sociality by building social capital, order, and cohesion (Rupp et al. 2020; Sampson and Raudenbush 2004). Neighborhood satisfaction has fostered sociality by enhancing attachment, community involvement, volunteering, and social capital (Cummins et al. 2003; Long and Perkins 2007; Xu 2007). Success has induced sociality by enhancing love and trust (Nezlek et al. 2008; Rieger and Wang 2021).

Conversely, disutility against sociality diminished by the norm for social cohesion has emanated from depression and distress (Gary et al. 2007; E. Wright et al. 2015). Depression has eroded sociality by breeding conflict, hate, hostility perceived, loneliness, revenge, risking, suicide, and violence (Cacioppo and Hawkley 2009; Economou et al. 2016; Haner et al. 2020; Morokoff et al. 2009; Mullet et al. 2005; Proulx et al. 2004; H. Smith et al. 2016; E. Wright et al. 2015). Conversely, depression has attenuated sociality by impeding benevolence, closeness experienced, fairness, forgiveness, gratitude, honesty, leadership, love, social integration, teamwork, and volunteering (Blanchard et al. 2021; Cornwall 2009; Holzel et al. 2011; Mancini et al. 2011; Mullet et al. 2005; Thoits and Hewitt 2001). Distress has undermined sociality by fomenting resistance and impeding social capital and trust (Pulkkinen et al. 2009; Webber and Huxley 2007).

Ideals for sociality touted by the norm for social cohesion have favored civic engagement, community, government trust, political participation, recourse, and transfer or financial help (Z. Han et al. 2017; F. Lee 2012; Mitrut and Wolff 2011; Palmer et al. 2011; Whitham 2012). Civic engagement has propped sociality by strengthening attachment, civility, collective behavior, discussion, donation, neighboring, patriotism, prosociality, social capital, socialism, trust, and volunteering and impeding cheating and individualism (Coffe and Geys 2007; Gilberbloom and Markham 1995; Kerrissey and Schofer 2013; Mata and Pendakur 2014; Ozbay 2008; Pattie et al. 2004; Pena-Lopez and Sanchez-Santos 2016; Rahn 2008; Richey 2011; Tak 2017; M. Tang 2011; Taniguchi 2013; Yip et al. 2007). The ideal for community constitutes sociality (Fowers 2015). Government trust has constituted sociality by sustaining compliance, conformity, nationalism, political participation, and preventing protesting (Rhodes-Purdy et al. 2023; Ulbig 2002; van der Meer and van Ingen 2009; V. Vu 2021). Political participation has buttressed civility to reject deviance (J. Berry et al. 1993). Recourse reflects sociality regarding affiliation and social support received (Ledbetter et al. 2013; Sullivan 2001). Transferring has raised sociality by facilitating donation (Piferi et al. 2006).

Norms for sociality popularized by the norm for social cohesion have spread association, education, happiness, income, organizational participation, prosperity, and voting (Carpiano 2008; Kampen 2010; D. Lee et al. 2011; Semenova et al. 2020). Association has fostered sociality regarding connectedness, friendship, giving, and social interaction (Eberl 2020; Liebler and Sandefur 2002; Nelson-Coffey et al. 2023; Phan et al. 2009). The norm for education has fostered sociality by boosting civic participation, government and social trust, social capital, volunteering, and xenophobia and dampening violence (Cohen and Bolt 2005; Lipford and Yandle 2009; Portes and Vickstrom 2011; Poveda 2011; Rupasingha et al. 2006; Uslaner and Brown 2005). The norm for happiness has upgraded sociality by boosting donation, law abidance, social trust, and voting and dampening lying (Fridberg and Kangas 2008b; Norris 2002; van Hemert et al. 2002). The norm for income has uplifted sociality by raising government support, nationalism, political participation, relationship quality, trust, volunteering, and xenophobia (Cheng and Smyth 2016; Fridberg and Kangas 2008; Inglehart 2003; Rhodes-Purdy et al. 2023; Traunmuller 2011; van Oorschot and Arts 2005). The norm for organizational participation has secured sociality regarding social cohesion (Milner 2002). Life satisfaction can benefit from the norm for social democracy (Radcliff 2001). The norm for prosperity has uplifted sociality by raising government support, nationalism, political participation, relationship quality, trust, volunteering, and xenophobia (Cheng and Smyth 2016; Fridberg and Kangas 2008; Inglehart 2003; Rhodes-Purdy et al. 2023; Traunmuller 2011; van Oorschot and Arts 2005). The norm for social cohesion upholds sociality by advancing norms for contribution, production, and resilience (Foster et al. 2001; Milner 2002; Ungar 2011). Contribution has constituted sociality by enhancing attachment and dampening tolerance for deviance (Stafford et al. 2005; Woosnam et al. 2018). Production has enabled sociality by preventing crime (Tanner-Smith et al. 2013). Resilience has attracted sociality by raising bonding and inhibiting crime and violence (Fields and McNamara 2003; Hoffman 2003; Solomon and Roloff

2018). Furthermore, resilience sustains sociality by embodying or fostering adaptation and legality (Hoffman 2003; Ungar 2012). Resilience also underlies sociality by demonstrating altruism, attractiveness, communication or conversation, community, compassion, empathy or perspective-taking, negotiation, peacefulness, relationality, relatedness, social capital or resourcefulness, social cohesion, and social competence (Elfers et al. 2024; Hjemdal et al. 2015; Jones and d'Errico 2019; Kelley et al. 2019; Kent and Davis 2010; Ungar 2010; Zautra 2014). The norm for social cohesion has developed from norms for bridging, cultural continuity, government quality, inclusiveness, political interest, and union participation to popularize sociality (Cummings 2000; Hileman et al. 2018; Norris 2002; Petro 2001; Puntscher et al. 2016). Bridging has constituted sociality by strengthening agreeableness, empathy, morality, and social capital (Halevy et al. 2019). Continuity has secured sociality, including civic engagement, cohesion, neighboring, and relational quality, as opposed to violence (Pulkkinen et al. 2009; C. Ross et al. 2000; Swaroop and Morenoff 2006; Villarreal and Silva 2006). The norm for government quality has upgraded sociality by advancing justice perceived, social harmony perceived, and institutional, political, and social trust and preventing suicide (Grimes 2006; Heatherington and Globetti 2002; Helliwell 2006; R. Taylor et al. 2015; Wong and Shik 2011; C. Wong et al. 2005). Inclusiveness can constitute sociality regarding loving (Aron et al. 2006). Political interest has elevated sociality by raising civic engagement, civic and social motivation, civility, and discussion as opposed to protesting (Gil de Zuniga et al. 2017; Lee and Chan 2011; Pattie et al. 2004). Moreover, gender stereotyping represents traditionalism (Yeh et al. 2013). Union participation embraces social capital to build sociality (Nissen and Jarley 2005). The norm for social cohesion has reflected the norm for cooperation to constitute sociality (Graeff and Svendsen 2013). Cooperation has constituted sociality regarding attachment and trustworthiness as opposed to argument (Gerbasi and Cook 2008; Hample 2018; Tak 2017). Ideologically, the norm for social cohesion stands on the norm for statism to spread sociality (Munch 2012). The norm for statism has embraced communitarianism, coordination, institutionalism, and republicanism to uphold sociality (Chahboun 2024; Jessop 2016; Prokhovnik 2008).

Conversely, the norm for social cohesion has strengthened ideals against liberalism, mortality, and violence to maintain sociality (Brody and Lovrich 2002; D. Lee et al. 2011; E. Wright et al. 2015). The norm for liberalism has disrupted sociality by standardizing radicalism (Norrander and Wilcox 2001). Mortality risk can dampen sociality by fomenting aggression (Reeve 2021). The norm for violence has weakened sociality by boosting antisocial behavior and victimization (Ehrensuft et al. 2003; Krahe 2013). The norm for social cohesion can maintain sociality by boosting the norm against delinquency (Munch 2012). Delinquency has undermined sociality by worsening attachment, empathy, helpfulness, morality, relational quality, sociability, and social capital (Cheung and Cheung 2006; Hoffmann et al. 2013; Keijsers et al. 2011). Conversely, delinquency has disrupted sociality by enhancing antisocial behavior, conflict, suicide, and victimization (Carson 2013; Cutler et al. 2001; P. Lau et al. 2005). The norm for social cohesion secures sociality by dampening norms for competition, exclusion, and privatization (Fukuyama 1999; Mannion 2003;

Munch 2012). Competition has impeded sociality by eroding volunteering (Martinez and McMullin 2004). The norm for exclusion has obstructed sociality by diminishing political participation and breeding inequality (Dawson 2021; Dorling 2010). Privatization opposes sociality (Karger et al. 2007). The norm for social cohesion has arisen from norms against nationality diversity, stigmatization, and migration to secure sociality (Coffe and Geys 2006; Tauber 2018). The norm for diversity has ruined sociality by undermining social capital and solidarity, including altruism, cooperation, friendship, and trust (Putnam 2007). Stigmatization received has eroded sociality by damping social cohesion (Walton and Cohen 2007). Ideologically, the norm for social cohesion stands on norms against individualism to achieve sociality (Munch 2012). The norm for individualism inhibits sociality by featuring competition, deintegration, disembeddedness, disengagement, independence, inequality, risk, and self-indulgence (Bauman 2001; Beck and Beck-Gernsheim 2002; Burgess 2018; Dannreuther and Perren 2013; Krys et al. 2019; Stankov et al. 2014).

Norm for Trust in Others

The norm for trust in others characterizes the norm for trust (Inoguchi 2017). The norm for social trust or trust generally is likely to advance sociality by furnishing power, utility, ideals, and norms to run the deterministic and voluntaristic mechanisms of analytical functionalism. These mechanisms hinge on social capital and urbanization to activate empowering and power realization (X. Chen 2011; Schulenberg 2003). The mechanisms set games to afford incentivizing and utility optimization (Deng 2011). The mechanisms engage the culture to trigger framing, standardizing, and ideal calibration (J. Stein 2013). The mechanisms employ networking to popularize standardizing and norm conformity (W. Jackson 2019).

Power for sociality enhanced by the trust norm has rested on health (Herian et al. 2014). Health has uplifted sociality by boosting community sense, morality, popularity, social activity, social cohesion, social integration, social trust, social well-being, and volunteering (Huxhold et al. 2014; Jorgensen et al. 2010; Son and Wilson 2012; Tolsma et al. 2009; Yu and Chiu 2016). Conversely, health has sustained sociality by preventing loneliness (Koromeckyj-Cox et al. 2007). Meanwhile, the trust norm has prevented mortality, thus maintaining power to drive sociality (Lochner et al. 2003). Mortality risk can dampen sociality by fomenting aggression (Reeve 2021).

Utility attracting sociality afforded by the trust norm has arisen from life satisfaction (Knight and Rosa 2011). Life satisfaction has incubated sociality regarding political participation, social cohesion, social trust, and volunteering (E. Chan 2014; Flavin and Keane 2011; Rochelle 2015).

Ideals rationalizing sociality fostered by the trust norm have prized charity, civic engagement and norms, institutional confidence, social inclusion, and volunteering (Ayob 2019; Delhey et al. 2011; Graddy and Wang 2009; Delhey et al. 2011; Uslaner and Brown 2005). The ideal for charity upholds sociality by embracing altruism, compassion, mercy, and volunteering (Apinunmahakul and Devlin 2008; Eggemeier and Fritz 2020; Musick and Wilson 2008; Pommier et al. 2020). Civic engagement has propped sociality by strengthening attachment, civility, collective behavior, discussion, donation, neighboring, patriotism, prosociality, social capital, socialism, trust, and volunteering and impeding cheating and individualism (Coffe and Geys 2007; Gilberbloom and Markham 1995; Kerrissey and Schofer 2013; Mata and Pendakur 2014; Ozbay 2008; Pattie et al. 2004; Pena-Lopez and Sanchez-Santos 2016; Rahn 2008; Richey 2011; Tak 2017; M. Tang 2011; Taniguchi 2013; Yip et al. 2007). Institutional confidence has constituted sociality by enhancing civic engagement, civility, compliance, legalism, political participation, prosocial behavior, responsibility, and social trust (Coffe and van der Lippe 2010; Grimes 2006; Jakobsen 2010; Seifert 2018; Stagnaro et al. 2017; Stolle and Micheletti 2013). Conversely, institutional confidence has maintained sociality by preventing risking (Ehrke et al. 2023). Social inclusion can constitute sociality regarding loving (Aron et al. 2006). Volunteering has constituted sociality by raising altruism, charity orientation, civic motivation, donation, helping, moral responsibility, political participation, social integration, and social and government trust (Foster et al. 2001; Isham et al. 2006; Richey 2010; Richey and Ikeda 2009; Wiepking and Maas 2009). Conversely, the trust norm has secured sociality by consolidating the ideal against suicide (Helliwell 2006). Suicide jeopardizes the function of goal attainment by defying the authority, thus abandoning duties to the authority and raising oneself above the authority (Lewis 2001; W. Siu 2008).

Norms for sociality strengthened by the trust norm have spread governance (Kyriacon 2020). The norm for governance has embraced communitarianism, coordination, institutionalism, and republicanism to uphold sociality (Chahboun 2024; Jessop 2016; Prokhovnik 2008). The trust norm can foster norms for economic growth and prosperity to uplift sociality (Bjornskow 2009; Fukuyama 1995). The norm for economic growth has raised sociality by buttressing government and institutional trust and preventing protesting (Grasso and Giugni 2016; Nicholson et al. 2002; Yang and Tang 2010). The norm for prosperity has uplifted sociality by raising government support, nationalism, political participation, relationship quality, trust, volunteering, and xenophobia (Cheng and Smyth 2016; Fridberg and Kangas 2008; Inglehart 2003; Rhodes-Purdy et al. 2023; Traunmuller 2011; van Oorschot and Arts 2005). The trust norm has benefitted from norms for intelligence to boost sociality (Dutton and Rayner-Hilles 2022). Intelligence has raised sociality by facilitating donation and social capital and reducing criminality and protesting (Cornwall 2009; Feinstein and Bynner 2006; Paterson 2008; Piferi et al. 2006). The trust norm arises from norms for civic culture and civil society to advance sociality (Edwards 2004). The norm for civil society has espoused sociality by preventing accidents and suicide (Helliwell 2006). The trust norm stands on norms for caring, Catholicism, communitarianism, conservatism, nationalism, republicanism, and social democracy to induce sociality (Abizadeh 2002; Frazer 1999; Held 2008; O'Hara 2011). The norm for caring has supported sociality by enhancing civic engagement, community favor, government trust, political participation, and recourse and dampening violence (Z. Han et al. 2017; F. Lee 2012; Palmer et al. 2011; Pulkkinen et al. 2009; Su and Feng 2013;

Whitham 2012). Catholicism promulgated by the cultural institution fosters sociality by emphasizing consensus, groupness, obedience, and teamwork (Basanez 2016). Moreover, Catholicism has enhanced sociality by raising conformity value and volunteering and dampening independence value and radicalism (Bekkers 2010; Devos et al. 2002; Fjellvang 2011). Catholicism has also safeguarded sociality by inculcating cooperation and interdependence (Bellah et al. 1991). Communitarianism constitutes sociality by espousing caring, civility, collective identity, commonweal orientation, community, dutifulness or responsibility, education or socialization, equality, interdependence, loyalty, mentoring, patriotism, reciprocity, relatedness, self-discipline, servicing including volunteering, settlement, social construction, social participation, solidarity, and trust (Delanty 2009; Frazer 1999; Moore 2010; Speth 2012). Conservatism sustains sociality by nurturing empathy, loyalty, prosocial behavior, religiousness, and sacrifice (Dutton and Rayner-Hilles 2022). Nationalism has underpinned sociality by fostering attachment, intolerance against deviance, patriotism, political participation, religiousness, social inclusion, trust in government, and xenophobia, and diminishing protesting (N. Chen 2012; Flanagan and Lee 2000; Huddy et al. 2021; Li and Brewer 2004; Osborne et al. 2017; Pinto et al. 2020; Rippl et al. 2010). Republicanism upholds sociality regarding citizenship, the commonweal, interdependence, morality, nationalism, publicity, responsibility, social adaptation, and solidarity (Delanty 2009; Honohan 2002). The norm for social democracy sustains sociality by championing equality and solidarity (Andersson 2006). The trust norm represents norms for agreeableness, civility, partnership, resiliency, social capital, solidarity, and virtue to enable sociality (Cochrane 2007; Elliott and Turner 2012; Farrelly 2007; Hall and Zautra 2010; McCrae 2009; Shin 2012; Von Mulmborg 2003). Agreeableness has fostered sociality by enhancing attachment (Fraley et al. 2011). Moreover, agreeableness constitutes sociality by featuring communion, compliance, cooperation, empathy, helping, intimacy, morality, politeness, prosociality, respect, solidarity, sympathy, understanding, warmth, and unity (Dinic and Bodroza 2021; Graziano and Tobin 2009; J. Sun et al. 2018). The norm for civility has constituted sociality by enhancing political trust (Mutz and Reeves 2005). Partnership has constituted sociality by preventing victimization (Jones and Ferguson 2009). Moreover, partnership establishes sociality by maintaining equality and responsibility (Harvie and Manzis 2011; Waiton 2008). Resiliency has facilitated sociality by raising bonding and inhibiting crime and violence (Fields and McNamara 2003; Hoffman 2003; Solomon and Roloff 2018). Furthermore, resiliency sustains sociality by embodying or fostering adaptation and legality (Hoffman 2003; Ungar 2012). Resiliency also buttresses sociality by demonstrating altruism, attractiveness, communication or conversation, community, compassion, empathy or perspective-taking, negotiation, peacefulness, relationality, relatedness, social capital or resourcefulness, social cohesion, and social competence (Elfers et al. 2024; Hjemdal et al. 2015; Jones and d'Errico 2019; Kelley et al. 2019; Kent and Davis 2010; Ungar 2010; Zautra 2014). The norm for social capital has buttressed sociality by strengthening civic engagement, community favor, financial help, institutional trust, political participation, and recourse and prevented violence (Z. Han et al. 2017; F. Lee 2012; Mitrut and Wolff 2011; Palmer et al. 2011; Su and Feng 2013; Whitham 2012; E.

Wright et al. 2015). Solidarity has constituted sociality by enhancing attachment and dampening tolerance for deviance (Stafford et al. 2005; Woosnam et al. 2018). The norm for virtue has maintained sociality by developing morality and dampening self-interest (A. Liu et al. 2025; J. Wright et al. 2017). Morality has constituted sociality by boosting volunteering and inhibiting violence (Piquero and Hickman 2002; Whitford et al. 2006).

Conversely, the trust norm has uplifted sociality by strengthening the norm against inequality (Inglehart 1997). The norm for inequality has impeded sociality by eroding social capital, support for redistribution and welfare, sympathy, trust, and volunteering (Busemeyer 2013; Hitlin and Harkness 2018; Lipford and Yandle 2009; Oishi et al. 2011; Portes and Vickstrom 2011). Conversely, the norm for inequality has impaired sociality by provoking crime and violence (Ousey and Lee 2013; van Wilsem 2007). The trust norm can maintain norms against crime, repression, and war to facilitate sociality (Deng 2011; J. Stein 2013). The norm for crime has eroded sociality by weakening community involvement, prosocial behavior, and social trust (Broadbent and Papadopoulos 2011; Zanin 2017; Zhong 2010). The norm for repression has eroded sociality by fomenting conflict, opposition, protesting, and resistance and dampening political participation and voting (Aytac and Stokes 2019; Booth and Richard 1998; Schatzman 2005; Sexton and Benson 2006). The norm for war has weakened sociality by fostering religiousness (Immerzeel and van Tubergen 2013). Furthermore, the norm for war has consolidated the norm for conflict (Bebber 1995). The norm for conflict has impaired sociality by fomenting protesting and resistance (Schatzman 2005; Sorens 2011). The trust norm has arisen from norms against corruption and diversity to sustain sociality (Graeff and Svendsen 2013; Dutton and Rayner-Hilles 2022). The norm for corruption has undermined sociality by disrupting institutional trust (Morris and Klesner 2010). The norm for diversity has ruined sociality by undermining social capital and solidarity, including altruism, cooperation, friendship, and trust (Putnam 2007). The trust norm stands on the norm against neoliberalism to maintain sociality (Olssen et al. 2004). Neoliberalism espouses atomization and silos and disregards ethics and social services to undermine sociality (Lobao et al. 2014; Lakoff 2009; Rhodes-Purdy et al. 2023; Smart 2003). The trust norm represents norms against anarchy, postmodernity, and problems to secure sociality (Dandaneau 2001; Heinze and Jolliff 2011; Inglehart 2000). Anarchism has impeded sociality by fomenting criticalness, protesting, resistance, and terrorism experienced (Gans 1992; Roberts 2012; Shatz 2011). The norm for postmodernity has eroded norms for fairness, traditionalism, and xenophobia (Jacques 1998; Yeganeh 2017). The norm for fairness has upheld sociality by elevating morality and prosocial behavior (Barber 2004; McCaffoee 2016). Traditionalism in community involvement upholds dependency, dutifulness, groupness, loyalty, obedience, order, and religiosity to foster sociality (Heckscher 2015). Additionally, traditionalism has buttressed sociality by enhancing patriotism and faith in religion and discouraging protesting and accepting deviants and outsiders (Costa et al. 2023; Datler et al. 2013; Meuleman et al. 2019; Schwartz et al. 2014). Xenophobia has constituted sociality by boosting patriotism and social cohesion (Granzin and Olsen 1998; Wang and Chen

2004). Moreover, xenophobia represents sociality by upholding nationalism (Biggs and Knauss 2012).

Current Findings

Regression analysis continued to examine the effects of national norms on personal sociality, indicated by confidence in institutions, refutations against misdeeds and unconventional sexuality, unfaith in religion, rejections of deviants and outsiders, and trust in others. National norms were the averages of personal experiences and attitudes in corresponding countries. Adding to the previous steps of regression analysis, Steps 4 and 5 showed the net effects without and with the control for personal experiences, respectively. Effects retained in Step 4 by the stepwise procedure were significant at the .001 level. Most effects of national norms were significant in expected ways (see Table 5.1).

Confidence in institutions received significant positive effects from national security and life satisfaction ($\beta = .123$ and .057, see Table 5.2). Meanwhile, such confidence received significant negative effects from national health and acceptance of deviants ($\beta = -.097$ and $-.098$). After controlling for personal experiences, national neighborhood nuisance emerged to manifest a significant negative effect on confidence in institutions ($\beta = -.090$).

Justification for unconventional sexuality received significant positive effects from national justification for misdeeds ($\beta = .059$, see Table 5.3). Meanwhile, such justification received significant negative effects from national acceptance of deviants, life satisfaction, and neighborhood nuisance ($\beta = -.193$, $-.113$, and $-.059$).

Faith in religion received significant positive effects from national economic hardship and health ($\beta = .146$ and .093, see Table 5.4). Meanwhile, such faith received significant negative effects from national justification for misdeeds and life satisfaction ($\beta = -.034$ and $-.015$).

Acceptance of outsiders received significant negative effects from national health, life satisfaction, and misdeeds ($\beta = -.102$, $-.100$, and $-.020$, see Table 5.5). Notably, the negative effect of national justification for misdeeds on acceptance of outsiders was negligible.

Acceptance of deviants received a significant positive effect from national acceptance of deviants ($\beta = .084$, see Table 5.6).

Trust in others received a significant negative effect from national justification for misdeeds ($\beta = -.032$, see Table 5.7).

Contrary to expectation, confidence in institutions received a negative effect from the national norm for health. According to force theory as an enhancement of analytical functionalism, the negative effect stems from the contradiction of forces between the norm for health and confidence in institutions. On the one hand, the force of the health norm represents individualistic power, thus capable of caring for oneself

Table 5.1 Expected and actual effects of national norms on sociality

Predictor	Expected	Actual						
		Institution	Anti-misdeed	Anti-sex	Anti-faith	Anti-outsider	Anti-deviant	Other
Economic hardship	–				–			
Neighborhood nuisance	–	–		+				
Victimization	–							
Security	+	+						
Family saving	+							
Health	+	–			+	+		
Life satisfaction	+	+		+	+	+		
Confidence in institutions	+							
Refutation against misdeeds	+			+	–	–		+
Refutation against unconventional sexuality	+							
Unfaith in religion	+							
Rejection of outsiders	+							
Rejection of deviants	+	+		–				
Trust in others	+							

Note. Sociality unfolded in social attitudes in terms of confidence in institutions, refutation against misdeeds, refutation against unconventional sexuality, unfaith in religion, rejection of outsiders, rejection of deviants, and trust in others
+ positive effect. – negative effect

Table 5.2 Significant ($p <$ .001) standardized effects of norms on confidence in institutions

Predictor	(4)	(5)
National security	.123	.086
National health	− .097	− .095
National life satisfaction	.057	.068
National neighborhood nuisance		− .090
National acceptance of deviants	− .098	− .078
R^2	.386	.401

n: $p > .001$

Table 5.3 Significant ($p <$ .001) standardized effects of norms on justification for unconventional sexuality

Predictor	(4)	(5)
National life satisfaction	− .113	− .098
National neighborhood nuisance	− .059	− .078
National acceptance of deviants	− .193	− .190
National justification for misdeeds	.059	.058
R^2	.275	.280

n: $p > .001$

Table 5.4 Significant ($p <$ .001) standardized effects of norms on faith in religion

Predictor	(4)	(5)
National economic hardship	.146	.145
National health	.093	.094
National life satisfaction	− .015	− .013
National justification for misdeeds	− .034	− .035
R^2	.544	.550

n: $p > .001$

Table 5.5 Significant ($p <$ .001) standardized effects of norms on acceptance of outsiders

Predictor	(4)	(5)
National health	− .102	− .097
National life satisfaction	− .100	− .082
National justification for misdeeds	− .020	− .017
R^2	.182	.188

n: $p > .001$

Table 5.6 Significant ($p <$ .001) standardized effects of norms on acceptance of deviants

Predictor	(4)	(5)
National acceptance of deviants	.084	.075
R^2	.170	.179

n: $p > .001$

Table 5.7 Significant ($p <$ .001) standardized effects of norms on trust in others

Predictor	(4)	(5)
National justification for misdeeds	– .032	– .032
R^2	.040	.042

n: $p > .001$

(S. Miller 2010). On the other hand, the force of confidence in institutions represents collective power and relative personal powerlessness, thus relying on institutional protection (Edlund 2006). That is, such confidence contradicts individualism (Lowndes and Roberts 2013).

Contrary to expectation, refutation against unconventional sexuality received a negative effect from the national norm for rejection of deviants. According to force theory as an enhancement of analytical functionalism, the negative effect originates from the contradiction of forces between the norm against deviance and refutation against unconventional sexuality. On the one hand, the norm against deviance indicates the force of safety and denies the force of risk (Patterson and Keefe 2008). On the other hand, refutation against unconventional sex suggests the force of risk or unsafety in unconventional sex (Contrary to expectation, unfaith in religion received a negative effect from the national norm for refutation against misdeeds. According to force theory as an enhancement of analytical functionalism, the negative effect originates from the contradiction of forces between the norm against deviance and refutation against unconventional sexuality. On the one hand, the norm against misdeeds indicates the force against misdeeds. On the other hand, unfaith in religion accepts a force for misdeeds prohibited by religion (Muluk et al. 2013). That is, unfaith in religion represents tolerance for religiously prohibited misdeeds or profanity (Harris et al. 2018). Religiously prohibited misdeeds include homosexuality, oppression, promiscuity, suicide, and violence (Horell 2014). Hence, the norm against misdeeds contradicts the unfaith tolerating misdeeds.

Contrary to expectation, rejecting outsiders received a negative effect from the national norm for refutation against misdeeds. According to force theory, the negative effect resulted from the contradiction between the rejection and national norm. On the one hand, the national norm emits a force against misdeeds. On the other hand, refutation against outsiders represents a misdeed and its force (Huntington 2004). That is, xenophobia is a misdeed even though it registers sociality. Thus, the national norm contradicts the refutation.

Chapter 6
Functioning of National Performance for Social Attitudes

National performance encompasses 15 indicators: population size and per capita phone subscription, land, technology publication, bank credit, prosperity, income inequality, globalization, government effectiveness, democracy, liberty, human development, human capital, carbon dioxide emission, and rule of law. They manifest development or modernization in political, economic, cultural, and communal aspects (Steinhardt and Delhey 2020). These performances are likely to influence personal sociality regarding seven social attitudes: confidence in institutions, refutation against misdeeds, refutation against unconventional sexuality, unfaith in religion, rejection of outsiders, rejection of deviants, and trust in others. The influence builds on the deterministic and voluntaristic mechanisms of analytical functionalism. Deterministic mechanisms work directly and indirectly. Direct deterministic mechanisms comprise private and public provision and taking. Public provision and taking involve sharing and taking vicariously such that one takes others' possession as one's possession. Indirect deterministic mechanisms employ power, utility, ideals, and norms to activate empowering, incentivizing, framing, and standardizing, respectively. These mechanisms complete their influences by triggering the voluntaristic mechanisms of power realization, utility optimization, ideal calibration, and norm conformity.

Existing Knowledge

The 15 national performances represent modernization to influence personal sociality. This influence is likely generally positive by exercising analytical functionalism's deterministic and voluntaristic mechanisms. These mechanisms run with power, utility, ideals, and norms generated by the national performances.

Power against sociality reduced by modernization has rested on freedom (Moller and Skaaning 2013). Freedom opposes communality and embeddedness (Loewy

C.-k. Cheung, *Social Attitudes in the Early 21st Century*,
https://doi.org/10.1007/978-981-96-9705-2_6

1993). As such, freedom has undermined sociality by fomenting crime (Costello 2013).

Norms for sociality increased by modernization have popularized fairness, pacification, and prosperity (Dioale and Seda 2001; (P. Smith 1991; Yeganeh 2017). The norm for fairness of justice has upheld sociality by elevating morality and prosocial behavior (Barber 2004; McCaffoee 2016). Pacification exhibits morality and legality as opposed to conflict (Arat and Kerelian 2019; G. Zhang 2006). The norm for prosperity has uplifted sociality by raising government support, nationalism, political participation, relationship quality, trust, volunteering, and xenophobia (Cheng and Smyth 2016; Fridberg and Kangas 2008; Inglehart 2003; Rhodes-Purdy et al. 2023; Traunmuller 2011; van Oorschot and Arts 2005). Modernization can raise norms for civility and feminization to standardize sociality (Heaphy 2007; Inglehart 2018). The norm for civility has enhanced political trust to champion sociality (Mutz and Reeves 2005). Feminization embraces generativity, nurturance, and politeness to boost sociality (Gutmann 1997). Modernization has benefitted from the norm for Confucianism to standardize sociality (Inglehart and Baker 2000). Confucianism has championed sociality regarding association, civility, and collectivism as opposed to violence (Y. Lin et al. 2021; Shin 2012; Stotzer 2014). Furthermore, modernization can benefit from norms for adaptation, humanism, social inclusion or integration, and trade to standardize sociality (Bickel 2018; Martinelli 2005). Adaptation has secured sociality regarding partnership and social adjustment and satisfaction as opposed to discord (Chow et al. 2014; Mitchell 2005). Humanism bolsters sociality by highlighting attachment, caring, collectivity, community, cooperation, friendship, helpfulness, institutions, loving, order, respect, relatedness, responsibility, and sharing (Browning and Cooper 2004; Fuchs 2020; Selznick 2008; Stefanski and Jach 2022; Visher 1997; Waterman 2013). Conversely, humanism sustains sociality by rejecting alienation, conflict, and individualization (Fuchs 2020; Selznick 2008). Social inclusion or integration has constituted sociality by strengthening cooperation and preventing suicide (Duberstein et al. 2004; Lepkowski and Couper 2002). The norm for trade has enhanced sociality by raising voting and diminishing victimization (Hellwig 2001; Schutte 2015). Modernization embraces norms for citizenship, commonality, communication, employment, equality, friendship, harmony, health, justice, legality, morality, mutuality, nation-building, nationality, networking, organization, policing, rationality, security, societalization, and unity to standardize sociality (Andreeva et al. 2017; Beck et al. 1994; Dioale and Seda 2001; He and Wang 2024; Kroneberg and Wimmer 2012; Martinelli 2005; Mouzelis 2012; Rindermann 2018; Scaff 2000; Sorensen and Christiansen 2013; Venkatesh 1999; R. Walker et al. 2018; W. Zhang 1999; Zhang and Zhao 2023). Citizenship underlies sociality regarding confidence in public institutions (Vera-Toscano et al. 2013). Commonality or unity has raised sociality by facilitating donating (Piferi et al. 2006). Communication has incubated sociality regarding social cohesion, participation, and trust (Miyata et al. 2008; Rothstein and Uslaner 2005). The norm for employment has elevated sociality by reducing migration, victimization, and violence and raising prosocial behavior (DiMaggio and Garip 2011; Hampton 2016; Nepal et al. 2011; Poveda 2011). The norm for equality has fostered sociality by championing cohesion and its experience, fairness, justice, social capital, sympathy, trust, and volunteering (Eriksson et al. 2015; Green et al. 2003; Hitlin and Harkness 2018; Musick and Wilson 2008; Oishi et al. 2011; Portes and Vickstrom 2011; van Oorschot and Arts 2005). The norm for friendship has consolidated sociality by reducing protesting (Sampson et al. 2005). Harmoniousness has buttressed compliance to maintain sociality (Braithwaite and Ahmed 2005). Furthermore, harmony experienced has induced sociality characterized by adjustment, attunement, civility, compromise, connectedness, interdependency, order, peace, relatedness, respect, sacrifice, selflessness, solidarity, and sympathy as opposed to competition and conflict (Arat and Kerelian 2019; Cheung and Ma 2011; P. Ip 2014; Kjell et al. 2016; Peck 2002; G. Zhang 2006). The norm for health has created social capital to enable sociality (Portes and Vickstrom 2011). Legality has buttressed sociality by dismissing radicalism (Muthuswamy 2022). The norm for morality has maintained sociality by developing morality and dampening self-interest (A. Liu et al. 2025; J. Wright et al. 2017). Mutuality has constituted sociality by fostering prosocial behavior (Thielmann et al. 2020). Nationalism has underpinned sociality by fostering attachment, intolerance against deviance, patriotism, political participation, religiousness, social inclusion, trust in government, and xenophobia, and diminishing protesting (N. Chen 2012; Flanagan and Lee 2000; Huddy et al. 2021; Li and Brewer 2004; Osborne et al. 2017; Pinto et al. 2020; Rippl et al. 2010). The norm for networking has buttressed sociality by strengthening civic engagement, community favor, financial help, institutional trust, political participation, and recourse and prevented violence (Z. Han et al. 2017; F. Lee 2012; Mitrut and Wolff 2011; Palmer et al. 2011; Su and Feng 2013; Whitham 2012; E. Wright et al. 2015). The norm for organization has secured sociality regarding social cohesion (Milner 2002). The norm for policing has maintained sociality by dampening protesting (Choi and Kim 2019). Rationality has championed sociality by dampening aggression and antisociality (DiGiuseppe et al. 2017). The norm for security has enhanced sociality by maintaining neighboring, social cohesion, and trust and reducing aggression and opposition (Barbarin and Richter 2001; Grannis 2009; Rochelle 2015). The norm for societalization constitutes sociality regarding commonality, community, cooperation, coordination, contracting, networking, and solidarity (Turner and Maryanski 2008).

Conversely, norms against sociality reduced by modernization have normalized ethnic fractionalization and repression (Kukreja and Miley 1989; Powell 1982). The norm for ethnic fractionalization has ruined sociality by undermining social capital and solidarity, including altruism, cooperation, friendship, and trust (Putnam 2007). The norm for repression has eroded sociality by fomenting conflict, opposition, protesting, and resistance and dampening political participation and voting (Aytac and Stokes 2019; Booth and Richard 1998; Schatzman 2005; Sexton and Benson 2006). Modernization can elevate norms against religion and violence to standardize sociality (Inglehart 2018). The norm for religion has eroded sociality by reducing voting (DeLeon and Naff 2004). The norm for violence has weakened sociality by boosting antisocial behavior and victimization (Ehrensuft et al. 2003; Krahe 2013). Modernization embraces norms against extremity and stratification to standardize sociality (Scaff 2000; W. Zhang 1999). Extremism has impeded sociality by provoking protesting (Moreira et al. 2018). The norm for stratification has impeded sociality by eroding social capital, support for redistribution and welfare, sympathy, trust, and volunteering (Busemeyer 2013; Hitlin and Harkness 2018; Lipford and Yandle 2009; Oishi et al. 2011; Portes and Vickstrom 2011). Conversely, the norm for stratification has impaired sociality by provoking crime and violence (Ousey and Lee 2013; van Wilsem 2007).

Population Size

National population size is likely to sustain sociality by providing power, utility, ideals, and norms to activate analytical functionalism's deterministic and voluntaristic mechanisms. These mechanisms wield empowering, incentivizing, framing, and standardizing for determinism and power realization, utility optimization, ideal calibration, and norm conformity for voluntarism.

Power for sociality raised by population size has rested on wages (Glaeser and Gottlieb 2009). Wages constitute income (Lavrijsen and Nicaise 2017). Income has upheld sociality by boosting civic engagement, community attachment and involvement, civic dutifulness, civility, conformity value, neighboring, political interest and participation, political and social trust, prosocial behavior, social capital, social integration, social interaction, social support received, social well-being, and volunteering (Bjornberg and Latta 2007; Chang 2009; Djupe and Lewis 2015; Frei et al. 2009; Kerrissey and Schofer 2013; Letki 2006; McCabe 2014; Patulny and Morris 2012; Son and Wilson 2012; Sun and Wang 2012; Swaroop and Morenoff 2006; Ulbig 2002). Conversely, income has maintained sociality by dampening alienation, discrimination experienced, migration, protesting, relocation, social deprivation experienced, social exclusion experienced, victimization, and violence (Broom et al. 2013; Brown and Connell 2004; Buck 2001; Rijken and Groenewegen 2008; V. Taylor et al. 2009; Weakliem and Borch 2006). Conversely, population size has diminished immigration status to maintain power driving sociality (Morenoff and Sampson 1997). Immigration status has impeded sociality by weakening civic engagement, egalitarianism, political participation, social capital, social cohesion, social contact, social trust, volunteering, voting, and neighborhood social control experienced (Brayne 2014; K. Brown et al. 2014; Fanning et al. 2011; Lien 1994; Lilly et al. 2011; Ravanera et al. 2003; Saunders and Wong 2012; Sonderskov 2011; Stromblad and Myrberg 2013). Moreover, immigrant status has diminished sociality by heightening migration, sleeping, social exclusion experienced, and suicide (Bask 2005; Gurak and Kritz 2000; Hamermesh 2019; Hassan 1995).

Ideals for sociality boosted by population size have espoused social welfare and xenophobia (Iida and Matsubayashi 2010; Paxton and Knack 2012). Social welfare support has sustained sociality by enhancing government trust (U. Kim et al. 2002). Xenophobia has constituted sociality by boosting patriotism and social cohesion (Granzin and Olsen 1998; Wang and Chen 2004). Conversely, population size has fostered ideals against migration to maintain sociality (Beinc et al. 2001). Migration has impeded sociality by diminishing social integration (Kearns and Whitley 2015).

Norms for sociality enhanced by population size have popularized economic growth, punishment, resources, social interaction, well-being, and government spending (Frey and Song 1997; Havinga 2002; Obschonk et al. 2016; Pattie et al. 2004; J. Turner 2003). The norm for economic growth has raised sociality by buttressing government and institutional trust and preventing protesting (Grasso and Giugni 2016; Nicholson et al. 2002; Yang and Tang 2010). Punishment characterizes sociality (Fowers 2015). Resources can facilitate sociality by raising social integration and obstructing crime, risking, social exclusion received, and violence (Agnew 2007; Figueredo et al. 2018; Gallie 2004; Lilly et al. 2011; Tsai 2006). Social interaction has realized sociality by consolidating altruism, compliance, cooperation, donation, morality, political participation, reciprocity, social trust, and volunteering (Guillen et al. 2011; Dixon and McKeown 2021; Lucas and Livingston 2014; Musick 2000; Rodrigo-Gonzalez et al. 2019; Rubin and Step 2000). The norm for well-being has upgraded sociality by boosting donation, law abidance, social trust, and voting and dampening lying (Fridberg and Kangas 2008b; Norris 2002; van Hemert et al. 2002). The norm for government spending has uplifted sociality by raising voting and preventing unemployment (Hobolt and Klemmensen 2005; White and Smith 1994).

Conversely, norms against sociality reduced by population size have popularized crime, liberty, neoliberalism, rights or entitlement, and violence (Abouharb and Cingranelli 2007; Browning et al. 2004; Hughes et al. 2015; Lobao et al. 2014). The norm for crime has eroded sociality by weakening community involvement, prosocial behavior, and social trust (Broadbent and Papadopoulos 2011; Jakobsson and Kotsadam 2011; Zanin 2017; Zhong 2010). Freedom has undermined sociality by fomenting crime (Costello 2013). Neoliberalism espouses atomization and silos and disregards ethics and social services to undermine sociality (Lobao et al. 2014; Lakoff 2009; Rhodes-Purdy et al. 2023; Smart 2003). Entitlement has undermined sociality by fomenting domination motivation, envy, hostility, liberalism, narcissism, selfish behavior, war support, wronging received and eroding compliance, humanitarianism, and relationship quality (Griffin and Bollen 2009; Lange et al. 2019; Moeller et al. 2009; Piff 2014; Rosler and Branscombe 2020; Zitek and Jordan 2019). The norm for violence has weakened sociality by boosting antisocial behavior and victimization (Ehrensuft et al. 2003; Krahe 2013).

Phone Subscription

National phone subscription represents the norm for communication. Remarkably, communication embodies sociality (Tan 2003). Hence, the norm for communication is likely to boost sociality by providing power, utility, ideals, and norms to run the deterministic and voluntaristic mechanisms of analytical functionalism. Deterministic mechanisms feature empowering, incentivizing, framing, and standardizing to activate the voluntaristic mechanisms of power realization, utility optimization, ideal calibration, and norm conformity. Notably, these mechanisms activate modernization (Basanez 2016). Among the mechanisms, those engaging norms are predominant.

The norm for sociality enhanced by the norm for communication popularizes normativity (Turner 2013). Normativity has countenanced sociality by raising civic engagement, donation, prosocial behavior, punishment, support for policy, volunteering, and voting and eroding cheating, violence, and tolerance for violence (Brown and Ferris 2007; Hennessy et al. 2015; Huesmann 2018; B. Liu et al. 2023; Opp 2002; Pavlova and Silbereisen 2015; Wade-Benzoni and Tost 2009; Waterman et al. 2022; Wenzel 2004). Norms for sociality upheld by the norm for communication can propagate prosperity and well-being (Peet and Hatwick 2009; J. Turner 2013b). The norm for prosperity has uplifted sociality by raising government support, nationalism, political participation, relationship quality, trust, volunteering, and xenophobia (Cheng and Smyth 2016; Fridberg and Kangas 2008; Inglehart 2003; Rhodes-Purdy et al. 2023; Traunmuller 2011; van Oorschot and Arts 2005). The norm for well-being has upgraded sociality by boosting donation, law abidance, social trust, and voting and dampening lying (Fridberg and Kangas 2008b; Norris 2002; van Hemert et al. 2002). The norm for communication has arisen from norms for development and population to foster sociality (J. James 2010; Sultanov et al. 2016). The norm for development has secured sociality by raising donation, legality, responsibility, social trust, and voting (Fridberg and Kangas 2008b; Jakobsen 2010; Norris 2002). Conversely, the norm for development has safeguarded sociality by lessening extremity and lying (J. He et al. 2014; van Hemert et al. 2002). Population size has sustained sociality by raising support for welfare and reducing immigration (Iida and Matsubayashi 2010; Morenoff and Sampson 1997). The norm for communication benefits from norms for education and social interaction to enable sociality (J. Turner 2003). The norm for education has fostered sociality by boosting civic participation, government and social trust, social capital, volunteering, and xenophobia and dampening violence (Cohen and Bolt 2005; Lipford and Yandle 2009; Portes and Vickstrom 2011; Poveda 2011; Rupasingha et al. 2006; Uslaner and Brown 2005). Social interaction has realized sociality by consolidating altruism, compliance, cooperation, donation, morality, political participation, reciprocity, social trust, and volunteering (Guillen et al. 2011; Dixon and McKeown 2021; Lucas and Livingston 2014; Musick 2000; Rodrigo-Gonzalez et al. 2019; Rubin and Step 2000). Ideologically, the norm for communication emanates from norms for humanism, institutionalism, interconnectedness, and nurturance to uplift sociality (Cooper 2016; Lakoff 2002; Saurugger 2013; Sirgy et al. 2004). Humanism bolsters sociality by highlighting attachment, caring, collectivity, community, cooperation, friendship, helpfulness, institutions, loving, order, respect, relatedness, responsibility, and sharing (Browning and Cooper 2004; Fuchs 2020; Selznick 2008; Stefanski and Jach 2022; Visher 1997; Waterman 2013). Conversely, humanism sustains sociality by rejecting alienation, conflict, and individualization (Fuchs 2020; Selznick 2008). Institutionalism maintains sociality by emphasizing communication, relatedness, and social order (Jessop 2016). Interconnectedness has constituted sociality by enhancing attachment and dampening tolerance for deviance (Stafford et al. 2005; Woosnam et al. 2018). The norm for nurturance has supported sociality by enhancing civic engagement, community favor, government trust, political participation, and recourse and dampening violence (Z. Han et al. 2017; F. Lee 2012; Palmer et al. 2011; Pulkkinen et al. 2009; Su and Feng 2013; Whitham 2012). The norm for communication represents norms for flexibility, knowledge, and organizing to constitute sociality. Flexibility advances sociality by facilitating adaptation and representing acceptance and staying (Pyszkowska 2020; Pyszkowska and Ronnlund 2021). Knowledge has maintained sociality by promoting civic engagement, civility, community involvement, compliance, cooperation, intimacy, leadership, marital satisfaction, political interest participation, politician favor, prosocial behavior, social cohesion, social trust, unification support, volunteering, and xenophobia (Barker and Tinnick 2006; de Groot and Steg 2009; Hunter et al. 2013; Kentmen 2010; Lepkowski and Couper 2002; Mikulincer et al. 2003; Moore et al. 2017; Norris 2011; Pattie et al. 2004; Rose and Pettersen 2000; Sarkheyli et al. 2012; Simon-Bemd and Steffens 2000; Stokman et al. 2013; Volker et al. 2007; Wernet et al. 2005). Organizing has constituted sociality by strengthening agreeableness, empathy, morality, and social capital (Halevy et al. 2019). Conversely, the norm for communication represents the norm against hierarchy to activate sociality (A. Kim 2004). The norm for hierarchy has worsened sociality by raising loneliness and lying (van Hemert et al. 2002; K. Yang 2019).

Land

Land per capita or the land share is the reciprocal of crowding. The land share is likely to dampen sociality by diminishing power, utility, ideals, and norms for sociality. This diminishing results from the deterministic and voluntaristic mechanisms of analytical functionalism. These mechanisms engage empowering, incentivizing, framing, and standardizing for determinism and power realization, utility optimization, ideal calibration, and norm conformity for voluntarism.

Utility for sociality reduced by the land share has resided in life satisfaction, neighborhood quality, and satisfaction (Oliver 2003; Whitham 2012). Life satisfaction has incubated sociality regarding political participation, social cohesion, social trust, and volunteering (E. Chan 2014; Flavin and Keane 2011; Rochelle 2015). Neighborhood quality has elevated sociality by building social capital, order, and cohesion (Rupp et al. 2020; Sampson and Raudenbush 2004). Neighborhood satisfaction has fostered sociality by enhancing attachment, community involvement, volunteering, and social capital (Cummins et al. 2003; Long and Perkins 2007; Xu 2007).

Ideals for sociality dampened by the land share have prized civic engagement, collectivism, donation, neighboring, political participation, and prosocial behavior (Graddy and Wang 2009; Nai et al. 2018; Pattie et al. 2004; Swaroop and Morenoff 2006; Triandis 1995). Civic engagement has propped sociality by strengthening attachment, civility, collective behavior, discussion, donation, neighboring, patriotism, prosociality, social capital, socialism, trust, and volunteering and impeding cheating and individualism (Coffe and Geys 2007; Gilberbloom and Markham 1995;

Kerrissey and Schofer 2013; Mata and Pendakur 2014; Ozbay 2008; Pattie et al. 2004; Pena-Lopez and Sanchez-Santos 2016; Rahn 2008; Richey 2011; Tak 2017; M. Tang 2011; Taniguchi 2013; Yip et al. 2007). Collectivism has constituted sociality by securing civility, cooperation, prosocial behavior, and religiousness and preventing extremism (Hample 2018; Harzing 2006; Oyserman et al. 1998; Saucier and Skrzypinska 2006; Thielmann et al. 2020). Donation has constituted sociality by consolidating charity, service value, social capital, social trust, and volunteering (Bekkers 2010; Chang 2009; Foster et al. 2001; Uslaner 2000). Neighboring has elevated sociality by raising consulting and influencing (Hays and Kogl 2007). Political participation has buttressed sociality regarding civility (Campbell 2003). Prosocial behavior has constituted sociality by civility, consolidating connectedness, cooperation, religiosity, responsibility, and volunteering (Hample 2018; Marsh and Dik 2021; Musick and Wilson 2008; Nelson-Coffey et al. 2023; Shahzalal and Adnan 2022). Moreover, prosocial behavior underlies sociality by enhancing citizenship, loyalty, social cohesion, socializing, and trust and diminishing self-interest (Dovidio et al. 2006; Hawley 2014; Kisliuk and WeiBmuller 2023; Music 2014).

Norms for sociality inhibited by the land share have popularized economic growth and government spending (Obschonk et al. 2016; Pattie et al. 2004). The norm for government spending has uplifted sociality by raising voting and preventing unemployment (Hobolt and Klemmensen 2005; White and Smith 1994). The norm for economic growth has raised sociality by buttressing government and institutional trust and preventing protesting (Grasso and Giugni 2016; Nicholson et al. 2002; Yang and Tang 2010).

Technology

Technology, in terms of its journal publication, is likely to prop sociality by furnishing power, utility, ideals, and norms to activate the deterministic and voluntaristic mechanisms of analytical functionalism. These mechanisms hinge on empowering, incentivizing, framing, and standardizing for determinism and power realization, utility optimization, ideal calibration, and norm conformity for voluntarism. Specifically, the mechanisms activate aligning, mobilizing, representing, resolving, and solidifying (Matthewman 2011). Among them, standardizing and norm conformity employing norms are predominant.

Norms for sociality buttressing technology have upheld business emphasis, Confucianism, cultural amenities, legalism, prosperity, security, and talent or university education (Collins 1998; Florida 2005; Schofer 2004; Welzel 2013). Business emphasis has sustained sociality regarding morality (Patwardhan et al. 2012). Confucianism has championed sociality regarding association, civility, and collectivism as opposed to violence (Y. Lin et al. 2021; Shin 2012; Stotzer 2014). Cultural involvement has fostered sociality regarding organizational involvement and social trust (Freitag 2003b; Guillen et al. 2011). Legalism has maintained sociality by preventing radicalism (Muthuswamy 2022). The norm for prosperity has uplifted sociality by raising government support, nationalism, political participation, relationship quality, trust, volunteering, and xenophobia (Cheng and Smyth 2016; Fridberg and Kangas 2008; Inglehart 2003; Rhodes-Purdy et al. 2023; Traunmuller 2011; van Oorschot and Arts 2005). The norm for security has enhanced sociality by maintaining neighboring, social cohesion, and trust and reducing aggression and opposition (Barbarin and Richter 2001; Grannis 2009; Rochelle 2015). The norm for talent has uplifted sociality by boosting support for redistribution (Busemeyer 2013). The norm for education has fostered sociality by promoting civic participation, government and social trust, social capital, volunteering, and xenophobia and dampening violence (Cohen and Bolt 2005; Lipford and Yandle 2009; Portes and Vickstrom 2011; Poveda 2011; Rupasingha et al. 2006; Uslaner and Brown 2005). Technology also features norms for sociality by popularizing civic virtue, communication and informing, education, intelligence or superintelligence, and social capital (C. Chen 2008; Elliott 2022; Goetz et al. 2011; G. Sun 2019). Civic engagement has propped sociality by strengthening attachment, civility, collective behavior, discussion, donation, neighboring, patriotism, prosociality, social capital, socialism, trust, and volunteering and impeding cheating and individualism (Coffe and Geys 2007; Gilberbloom and Markham 1995; Kerrissey and Schofer 2013; Mata and Pendakur 2014; Ozbay 2008; Pattie et al. 2004; Pena-Lopez and Sanchez-Santos 2016; Rahn 2008; Richey 2011; Tak 2017; M. Tang 2011; Taniguchi 2013; Yip et al. 2007). Communication has incubated sociality regarding social cohesion, participation, and trust (Miyata et al. 2008; Rothstein and Uslaner 2005). Intelligence has raised sociality by facilitating donation and social capital and reducing criminality and protesting (Cornwall 2009; Feinstein and Bynner 2006; Paterson 2008; Piferi et al. 2006). The norm for social capital has buttressed sociality by strengthening civic engagement, community favor, financial help, institutional trust, political participation, and recourse and prevented violence (Z. Han et al. 2017; F. Lee 2012; Mitrut and Wolff 2011; Palmer et al. 2011; Su and Feng 2013; Whitham 2012; E. Wright et al. 2015).

Bank Credit

Bank credit characterizes financialization (Barthold 2018). Financialization secures capital and thus capitalism (Barthold 2018; Haiven 2014). As such, financialization is likely to buttress sociality by furnishing power, utility, ideals, and norms for sociality through the deterministic and voluntaristic mechanisms of analytical functionalism. Among these norms, those handling norms are predominant.

A norm for sociality created by financialization has popularized economic growth. The norm for economic growth has raised sociality by buttressing government and institutional trust and preventing protesting (Grasso and Giugni 2016; Nicholson et al. 2002; Yang and Tang 2010). Financialization can enhance the norm for circulation to strengthen sociality (Harvey 2016). Circulation has constituted sociality by improving leadership and neighboring (Dubois et al. 2020; Grannis 2009). Moreover, circulation constitutes sociality regarding friendship (Launay and Dunbar 2015).

Circulation can also underlie sociality by boosting morality, punishment, and social cohesion (N. Duncan 2017; Delton and Krasnow 2017). Financialization has built on the norm against inflation to secure sociality (Asongu 2013). The norm for inflation has hindered sociality by weakening social integration, support for welfare, and trust in government and fueling protesting (Bahry and Lipsmeyer 2001; Mishler and Willerton 2003; Naveed and Wang 2021; Page and Shapiro 1992).

Prosperity

Prosperity features consumption, fulfillment, and income, as opposed to inflation and poverty (Bandelj and Sowers 2010; Peet and Hatwick 2009; Wilkinson and Pickett 2017; Wolff and Resnick 2012). As such, prosperity in terms of gross domestic product per capita is likely to facilitate sociality. Such facilitation hinges on the deterministic and voluntaristic mechanisms in analytical functionalism to apply power, utility, ideals, and norms to activate empowering, incentivizing, framing, and standardizing for determinism and power realization, utility optimization, ideal calibration, and norm conformity for voluntarism.

Power for sociality enhanced by prosperity has resided in health and self-efficacy (Corcoran et al. 2011; S. Miller 2015). Health has uplifted sociality by boosting community sense, morality, popularity, social activity, social cohesion, social integration, social trust, social well-being, and volunteering (Huxhold et al. 2014; Jorgensen et al. 2010; Son and Wilson 2012; Tolsma et al. 2009; Yu and Chiu 2016). Conversely, health has sustained sociality by preventing loneliness (Koromeckyj-Cox et al. 2007). Self-efficacy has sustained sociality by raising civic engagement, donation, government and social trust, leadership, political participation, prosocial behavior, and social activity (Bednall et al. 2013; Frye 2007; Gnambs and Batinic 2012; Huber et al. 2022; Mangum 2012; Rahn 2008; Pei and Pan 2018; Yao and Enright 2019). Conversely, prosperity has prevented illness, thus retaining power for sociality (Fridberg and Kangas 2008). Illness has eroded sociality by impeding volunteering (Wuthnow 2004).

Utility for sociality afforded by prosperity has resided in relationship quality and satisfaction with democracy and life (Fridberg and Kangas 2008; Helliwell et al. 2010; Norris 2011). Relationship quality features attachment, closeness, friendship, security, and sharing (Hample 2018; Koerner 2018; Mikulincer and Shaver 2018; Van Lear et al. 2006). Satisfaction with democracy has boosted sociality by uplifting civility, political participation, government, legislature, and social trust and curbing protesting (Cais et al. 2021; E. Chi and Kwon 2016; Finkel and Lim 2021; Giugni and Grasso 2019; Norris 2011). Life satisfaction has incubated sociality regarding political participation, social cohesion, social trust, and volunteering (E. Chan 2014; Flavin and Keane 2011; Rochelle 2015). Conversely, disutility against sociality reduced by prosperity has stemmed from economic hardship (Fridberg and Kangas 2008). Economic hardship has impaired sociality by dampening trust and fomenting social exclusion experienced, suicide, and victimization experienced (Economou et al. 2016; Reeskens and Vandecasteele 2017; Ross and Mirowsky 2009).

Ideals for sociality upheld by prosperity have hailed institutional trust, political participation, social trust, volunteering, and xenophobia (Cheng and Smyth 2016; Inglehart 2003; Norris 1999a; Traunmuller 2011; van Oorschot and Arts 2005). Institutional trust has constituted sociality by enhancing civic engagement, civility, compliance, legalism, political participation, prosocial behavior, responsibility, and social trust (Coffe and van der Lippe 2010; Grimes 2006; Jakobsen 2010; Seifert 2018; Stagnaro et al. 2017; Stolle and Micheletti 2013). Political participation has buttressed sociality regarding civility (Campbell 2003). Social trust has constituted sociality through donation, involvement, and volunteering (Uslaner 2000). Volunteering has constituted sociality by raising altruism, charity orientation, civic motivation, donation, helping, moral responsibility, political participation, social integration, and social and government trust (Foster et al. 2001; Isham et al. 2006; Richey 2010; Richey and Ikeda 2009; Wiepking and Maas 2009). Conversely, volunteering has safeguarded sociality by preventing deviance and its tolerance, delinquency, and loneliness (Gillath et al. 2005; J. Wilson 2000; Woolley 2003). Xenophobia has constituted sociality by boosting patriotism and social cohesion (Granzin and Olsen 1998; Wang and Chen 2004). Moreover, xenophobia represents sociality by upholding nationalism (Biggs and Knauss 2012). Conversely, prosperity has reduced the ideal against sociality based on religiousness (Fjellvang 2011). Religiousness has hindered sociality by reducing nationalism, social interaction and engendering protesting, marginalization experienced, radicalism, and social distance (Ayalon et al. 1993; Kunovich 2009; Norris 2002; Pedahzur and Canetti-Nisim 2004; Wuthnow 2004).

Norms for sociality enhanced by prosperity have spread government effectiveness, government social spending, justice, legality and legal quality, trade, and universalism (Bjornskov 2005; Guisan 2009; Kang and Powell 2010; Minkov 2011; Oneal et al. 2003; Rindermann 2008). The norm for government effectiveness has upgraded sociality by advancing justice perceived, social harmony perceived, and institutional, political, and social trust and preventing suicide (Grimes 2006; Heatherington and Globetti 2002; Helliwell 2006; R. Taylor et al. 2015; Wong and Shik 2011; C. Wong et al. 2005). Moreover, the norm for government effectiveness can uphold sociality by preventing crime (Quillian 2014). The norm for government effectiveness also sustains sociality by cultivating civic literacy (Milner 2002). The norm for government social spending has secured sociality by boosting support for redistribution (Weisstanner 2023). The norm for justice has upheld sociality by elevating morality and prosocial behavior (Barber 2004; McCaffoee 2016). Legality has buttressed sociality by dismissing radicalism (Muthuswamy 2022). The norm for trade has enhanced sociality by raising voting and diminishing victimization (Hellwig 2001; Schutte 2015). Universalism constitutes sociality by embodying morality (Mihailov 2023).

Conversely, norms against sociality diminished by prosperity have popularized anomie, homicide, inequality, risk, segregation, theft, and threat (Moller and Li 2009; Schneider 2007; Schwartz and Melech 2000; Teymoori et al. 2016; van Wilsem 2004;

Weakliem et al. 2005). Anomie has impeded sociality by raising radicalism and support for violence (Troian et al. 2019). Homicide represents crime (L. Cao et al. 2016). The norm for crime has eroded sociality by weakening community involvement, prosocial behavior, and social trust (Broadbent and Papadopoulos 2011; Zanin 2017; Zhong 2010). The norm for inequality has impeded sociality by eroding social capital, support for redistribution and welfare, sympathy, trust, and volunteering (Busemeyer 2013; Hitlin and Harkness 2018; Lipford and Yandle 2009; Oishi et al. 2011; Portes and Vickstrom 2011). Conversely, the norm for inequality has impaired sociality by provoking crime and violence (Ousey and Lee 2013; van Wilsem 2007). The norm for risk has impaired sociality by provoking protesting (Scafuto and La Barbera 2016). Segregation characterizes social exclusion (Smets and Salman 2008). Social exclusion has impeded sociality by fueling crime, doping, and violence (Barry and Hullett 1998). Theft has bred social avoidance to weaken sociality (Brayne 2014). Threats received have inhibited sociality by reducing cohesion and triggering conflict and resistance (Lubbers et al. 2006; B. Rick et al. 2006). Prosperity has developed from norms for education, human development, population size, security, and talent to induce sociality (X. Chen 2011; Lee and Chang 2006; Ranis and Zhao 2013; Farla 2015). The norm for education has fostered sociality by boosting civic participation, government and social trust, social capital, volunteering, and xenophobia and dampening violence (Cohen and Bolt 2005; Lipford and Yandle 2009; Portes and Vickstrom 2011; Poveda 2011; Rupasingha et al. 2006; Uslaner and Brown 2005). The norm for human development has maintained donation, legalism, and social trust to secure sociality (Fridberg and Kangas 2008b). The norm for population size has sustained sociality by raising welfare support and xenophobia and dampening migration (Beinc et al. 2001; Iida and Matsubayashi 2010; Paxton and Knack 2012). The norm for security has enhanced sociality by maintaining neighboring, social cohesion, and trust and reducing aggression and opposition (Barbarin and Richter 2001; Grannis 2009; Rochelle 2015). The norm for talent has uplifted sociality by boosting support for redistribution (Busemeyer 2013).

Prosperity can develop from norms for citizenship, civic society, communitarianism, egalitarianism, employment, integration, nationalism, networking, organizational attachment and commitment, patriotism, sharing, sociability, redistribution, secularism, social order, social welfare, and stability to establish sociality (Brett 2009; Fukuyama 1995; Ghosh 2001; Haque 1999; Hunt 1989; Jaffee 1990; Peet and Hatwick 2009; Wolff and Resnick 2012). Citizenship underlies sociality regarding confidence in public institutions (Vera-Toscano et al. 2013). The norm for civil society has espoused sociality by preventing accidents and suicide (Helliwell 2006). Communitarianism constitutes sociality by espousing caring, civility, collective identity, commonweal orientation, community, dutifulness or responsibility, education or socialization, equality, interdependence, loyalty, mentoring, patriotism, reciprocity, relatedness, self-discipline, servicing including volunteering, settlement, social construction, social participation, solidarity, and trust (Delanty 2009; Frazer 1999; Moore 2010; Speth 2012). Egalitarianism has underpinned sociality by enhancing empathy, support for welfare, and trust in government and impeding radicalism (Faricy and Ellis 2014; Lauriola et al. 2015; Lucas and Kteily 2018;

Roosma et al. 2014). The norm for employment has elevated sociality by reducing migration, victimization, and violence and raising prosocial behavior (DiMaggio and Garip 2011; Hampton 2016; Nepal et al. 2011; Poveda 2011). Social integration has constituted sociality by strengthening cooperation and preventing suicide (Duberstein et al. 2004; Lepkowski and Couper 2002). Nationalism has underpinned sociality by fostering attachment, intolerance against deviance, patriotism, political participation, religiousness, social inclusion, trust in government, and xenophobia, and diminishing protesting (N. Chen 2012; Flanagan and Lee 2000; Huddy et al. 2021; Li and Brewer 2004; Osborne et al. 2017; Pinto et al. 2020; Rippl et al. 2010). The norm for networking has buttressed sociality by strengthening civic engagement, community favor, financial help, institutional trust, political participation, and recourse and prevented violence (Z. Han et al. 2017; F. Lee 2012; Mutrut and Wolff 2011; Palmer et al. 2011; Su and Feng 2013; Whitham 2012; E. Wright et al. 2015). Organizational involvement has fostered sociality by enhancing attachment, civility, political participation, social integration, socialism (favor), and trust (Geys 2012; Guillen et al. 2011; Pattie et al. 2004; Tak 2017). Patriotism has constituted sociality by raising government trust, nationalism, prosocial behavior or prosociality, social cohesion, volunteering, and xenophobia (Beyerlein and Sikkink 2008; Gross et al. 2004; Ishii 2009; Straume and Odeen 2010). Sharing has constituted sociality by strengthening leadership and neighboring (Dubois et al. 2020; Grannis 2009). Moreover, sharing constitutes sociality regarding friendship (Launay and Dunbar 2015). Sharing can also underlie sociality by boosting morality, punishment, and social cohesion (N. Duncan 2017; Delton and Krasnow 2017). Sociability has enhanced sociality by raising civic engagement, civility, political participation, prosocial behavior, and social cohesion (Foschi and Lauriola 2014; Letki 2008). The norm for social order has prevented the norm of protesting (Fuller 2006). Protesting has impaired sociality by escalating distancing and radicalism and dampening moral motivation (Kutlaca et al. 2020; Vestergren et al. 2017). The norm for redistribution or social welfare has uplifted sociality by advancing neighboring, political participation, social capital, support for social welfare, and volunteering and diminishing migration, and theft (Allard and Danziger 2000; J. Brown 2016; Musick and Wilson 2008; Portes and Vickstrom 2011; Rehm et al. 2012; Semino 2015). The norm for secularism has induced sociality by promoting volunteering and voting (DeLeon and Naff 2004; Lim and MacGregor 2012). The norm for stability has propped sociality, including civic engagement, cohesion, neighboring, and relational quality, as opposed to violence (Pulkkinen et al. 2009; C. Ross et al. 2000; Swaroop and Morenoff 2006; Villarreal and Silva 2006). Prosperity has arisen from norms against conflict and dependence to induce sociality (Bornschier et al. 2005; Lim and Montes 2000). The norm for conflict has impaired sociality by fomenting protesting and resistance (Schatzman 2005; Sorens 2011). Dependence has impaired sociality by hindering social capital, social cohesion, social trust, and equality value, and engendering protesting and suicide (Cornwall 2009; Granzin and Haggard 2000; Konarska 2005; Van Vugt et al. 2003; Zanin et al. 2013).

Prosperity can develop from norms against classism, contradiction, corruption, differentiation, exploitation, hierarchy, liberalism, multiculturalism, nepotism, polarization, privatization, self-interest, and unemployment (Fukuyama 1995; Hunt 1989; Lichtenstein 2016; Milward 2000; Munch 1988; Peet and Hatwick 2009; Wolff and Resnick 2012). Classism has impeded sociality by dampening support for redistribution (Sainz and Jimenez-Moya 2023). Contradiction has impeded sociality regarding donation and trust as opposed to violence (Farmer and Fedor 2001; Farrington 2018; Kunovich and Hodson 1999). The norm for corruption has undermined sociality by disrupting institutional trust (Morris and Klesner 2010). Differentiation has diminished sociality by provoking protesting (Badea et al. 2021). Exploitation experienced erodes sociality by breeding conflict (J. Turner 2013b). The norm for hierarchy has eroded sociality by boosting loneliness and lying and reducing moderation (Harzing 2006; van Hemert et al. 2002; K. Yang 2019). The norm for liberalism impairs sociality by dismissing punishment (Vicente 2016). Multiculturalism obstructs sociality by denouncing assimilation, embracing unrest, and standing on independence (Pehrson et al. 2011; Verkuyten 2005). Nepotism can impair sociality by breeding conflict (Y. Kim 2013). The norm for polarization has hindered sociality by dampening support for unification and fanning protesting (Kleiner 2018; Lahusen 2021). Self-interest impairs sociality by weakening deontology or duty and strengthening egocentrism (Beauregard and Dunning 1998; Rocha and Ghoshal 2006). Privatization opposes sociality (Karger et al. 2007). The norm for unemployment has jeopardized sociality by eroding legalism, social capital, social trust, and support for the market, and breeding protesting, radicalism, social exclusion experienced, and violence (L. Berger 2005; Buck 2001; Earl and Soule 2001; Gillham et al. 2019; Hayo 2004; Mitts 2019; Savelkoul et al. 2014; Smiley and Yang 2021).

Income Inequality

Income or economic inequality represents class, diversity, hierarchy, and stratification (Fein 2012; S. Smith 2011; Themelis 2008). Contrariwise, income inequality defies democracy, fairness, and justice (Diefenbach 2013). As such, income inequality is likely to hurt sociality by weakening power, utility, ideals, and norms for sociality and generating power, utility, ideals, and norms against sociality through the deterministic and voluntaristic mechanisms of analytical functionalism. These mechanisms engage empowering, incentivizing, framing, and standardizing for determinism and power realization, utility optimization, ideal calibration, and norm conformity for voluntarism. Specifically, these mechanisms activate conflict, construction, friction, segregation, and struggle as opposed to cooperation (Alessio 2011; Baldus 2017; J. Brown 2019).

Power for sociality weakened by income inequality has rested on health, social capital, and sympathy (Hitlin and Harkness 2018; Kim and Kawachi 2007; Portes and Vickstrom 2011). Health has uplifted sociality by boosting community sense, morality, popularity, social activity, social cohesion, social integration, social trust, social well-being, and volunteering (Huxhold et al. 2014; Jorgensen et al. 2010; Son and Wilson 2012; Tolsma et al. 2009; Yu and Chiu 2016). Conversely, health has sustained sociality by preventing loneliness (Koromeckyj-Cox et al. 2007). Social capital has consolidated sociality by raising civic engagement, community involvement, donation, political involvement, social trust, and volunteering (Bekkers et al. 2008; Broadbent and Papadopoulos 2011; Brown and Ferris 2007; Chua et al. 2021; Narayan and Cassidy 2001). Conversely, social capital has strengthened sociality by erasing violence (Pulkkinen et al. 2009). Sympathy has constituted sociality by securing religiosity and volunteering (Barr et al. 2005). Income inequality has induced disability, illness, mortality, and poverty to eliminate power for sociality (A. Jones et al. 2015; Kawachi et al. 1997; Kim and Kawachi 2007). Disability has weakened sociality by eroding social capital, social cohesion, social trust, and volunteering (Cornwall 2009; Granzin and Haggard 2000; Tang 2006; Zanin et al. 2013). Conversely, disability has impeded sociality by instigating protesting and suicide (Van Vugt et al. 2003). Illness has eroded sociality by impeding volunteering (Wuthnow 2004). Mortality risk can dampen sociality by fomenting aggression (Reeve 2021). Poverty has undermined sociality by reducing civic participation, trust, social connection, and volunteering (Caputo 2010; Stephens et al. 2014; R. Walker et al. 2010). Conversely, poverty has disrupted sociality by creating isolation, relationship problems, and social exclusion experienced (Dhal et al. 2008; Stephens et al. 2014; R. Walker et al. 2010).

Utility for sociality reduced by income inequality has transpired in financial satisfaction (Winkelmann and Winkelmann 2010). Financial satisfaction has upheld sociality by diminishing hostility (Rhodes-Purdy et al. 2023). Conversely, income inequality has bred disutility against sociality based on disadvantages, problems, and social exclusion experienced (Reardon and Bischoff 2011; Portes and Vickstrom 2011; Wilkinson and Pickett 2009). Disadvantages or problems have undermined sociality by eroding civility, forgiveness, generativity, relationship quality and satisfaction, social integration, social support received, and trust and heightening conflict, maltreatment, substance abuse, suicide, and violence (Atkinson et al. 2005; Dutton et al. 2016; Gelles 2007; Grzywacz and Almeida 2008; Jackson et al. 2006; Sobeck et al. 2020; Toussaint et al. 2016). Shame can erode sociality by breeding suicide and violence (Kral 2019; J. Turner 2007). Social exclusion experienced has disturbed sociality by eroding closeness and prosocial behavior (Bockler et al. 2021; K. Lin et al. 2013).

Ideals for sociality hampered by income inequality have supported social cohesion, social welfare, trust, volunteering, and voting (Gelissen 2002; Green et al. 2003; Lipford and Yandle 2009; Lister 2007; Oishi et al. 2011). Social cohesion has constituted sociality by enhancing attachment and dampening tolerance for deviance (Stafford et al. 2005; Woosnam et al. 2018). The ideal for social welfare has championed sociality by consolidating government trust (U. Kim et al. 2002). Trust has constituted sociality through donation, involvement, and volunteering (Uslaner 2000). Volunteering has constituted sociality by raising altruism, charity orientation, civic motivation, donation, helping, moral responsibility, political participation, social integration, and social and government trust (Foster et al. 2001; Isham et al. 2006; Richey 2010; Richey and Ikeda 2009; Wiepking and Maas 2009). Voting has engendered sociality by boosting civic and community participation and neighboring (Djupe and Lewis 2015; Dorff 2017; Hays and Kogl 2007). Trust weakened by income inequality covers government, institutional, and social trust (Lundasen et al. 2013; van Oorschot and Arts 2005; Zmerli and Castillo 2015). Government trust has constituted sociality by sustaining compliance, conformity, nationalism, political participation, and preventing protesting (Rhodes-Purdy et al. 2023; Ulbig 2002; van der Meer and van Ingen 2009; V. Vu 2021). Institutional trust has constituted sociality by enhancing civic engagement, civility, compliance, legalism, political participation, prosocial behavior, responsibility, and social trust (Coffe and van der Lippe 2010; Grimes 2006; Jakobsen 2010; Seifert 2018; Stagnaro et al. 2017; Stolle and Micheletti 2013). Conversely, institutional trust has maintained sociality by preventing risking (Ehrke et al. 2023). Social trust has benefited from agreeableness, familiarity, friendship, knowledge, language proficiency, moderateness, self-efficacy, and sociability to provide power to drive sociality (Freitag and Bauer 2016; Halvorsen 2007; Kende et al. 2022; Lancee and Dronkers 2011; McCabe 2012; Pattie et al. 2004; Rahn 2008).

Conversely, income inequality has diminished ideals against crime, education, and violence to impair sociality (Ousey and Lee 2013; Maurer 2011; van Wilsem 2007). Crime has impaired sociality by reducing community involvement, prosocial behavior, and social trust and fomenting avoidance, protesting, risking, victimization, and violence (Brayne 2014; McNeeley and Yuan 2017; Broadbent and Papadopoulos 2011; Sun and Wang 2012; Wittebrood and Nieuwbeerta 2000; Zhong 2010). Education has fostered sociality by raising civic engagement, civility, conformism, crime disapproval, equality support, morality, political discussion, political interest, political participation, socialism, and trust (Bullock 2021; E. Chan 2014; Djupe and Lewis 2015; Gilberbloom and Markham 1995; Kerrissey and Schofer 2013; Miyata et al. 2008; Norris 2011; Norris and Inglehart 2009; Ulbig 2002; Wilson and Dunham 2001). Conversely, education has sustained sociality by reducing political alienation, deviance, prostitution, resistance, and violence and its tolerance (Backman and Nilsson 2011; Coffe and Geys 2007; Lubbers et al. 2006; Michalski 2005; Simon et al. 2001; Swader and Vorobeva 2015). Violence has undermined sociality by breeding antisociality, crime and recidivism, blaming, conflict, hostility, rejecting others, and impairing agreeableness, morality, and responsibility (Asendorpf et al. 2008; Del Bove et al. 2008; Morrison 2006; Scholte et al. 2009; Vitaro et al. 2007).

Norms for sociality eroded by income inequality have popularized civic participation, fairness, justice, and trust (Eriksson et al. 2015; Oishi et al. 2011; Wilkinson and Pickett 2017; Uslaner 2002). Civic participation has propped sociality by strengthening attachment, civility, collective behavior, discussion, donation, neighboring, patriotism, prosociality, social capital, socialism, trust, and volunteering and impeding cheating and individualism (Coffe and Geys 2007; Gilberbloom and Markham 1995; Kerrissey and Schofer 2013; Mata and Pendakur 2014; Ozbay 2008; Pattie et al. 2004; Pena-Lopez and Sanchez-Santos 2016; Rahn 2008; Richey 2011; Tak 2017; M. Tang 2011; Taniguchi 2013; Yip et al. 2007). The norm for fairness or justice has upheld sociality by elevating morality and prosocial behavior (Barber 2004; McCaffoee 2016). The norm for trust has secured sociality by maintaining civic norm adherence, inclusive orientation, and institutional confidence (Delhey et al. 2011). Income inequality has risen with norms against education, employment, prosperity, and well-being to obstruct sociality (Inglehart 1997; Lobao and Hooks 2003; Sun 2011; Weakliem et al. 2005). The norm for education has fostered sociality by boosting civic participation, government and social trust, social capital, volunteering, and xenophobia and dampening violence (Cohen and Bolt 2005; Lipford and Yandle 2009; Portes and Vickstrom 2011; Poveda 2011; Rupasingha et al. 2006; Uslaner and Brown 2005). The norm for employment has elevated sociality by reducing migration, victimization, and violence and raising prosocial behavior (DiMaggio and Garip 2011; Hampton 2016; Nepal et al. 2011; Poveda 2011). The norm for prosperity has uplifted sociality by raising government support, nationalism, political participation, relationship quality, trust, volunteering, and xenophobia (Cheng and Smyth 2016; Fridberg and Kangas 2008; Inglehart 2003; Rhodes-Purdy et al. 2023; Traunmuller 2011; van Oorschot and Arts 2005). The norm for well-being has upgraded sociality by boosting donation, law abidance, social trust, and voting and dampening lying (Fridberg and Kangas 2008b; Norris 2002; van Hemert et al. 2002). Income inequality can rise with norms against alliances, citizenship, coordination, social welfare, unionization, and universalism to hinder sociality (Edlund and Gronlund 2010; Guenther et al. 2016; Navarro 2002; Tomaskovic-Devey and Avent-Holt 2019). Alliances constitute sociality by realizing equality and responsibility and opposing conflict (Harvie and Manzis 2011; Mills and Taht 2010; Waiton 2008). Citizenship has constituted sociality by inducing fairness and trust (Vera-Toscano et al. 2013). The norm for social welfare has uplifted sociality by advancing neighboring, political participation, social capital, support for social welfare, and volunteering and diminishing migration and theft (Allard and Danziger 2000; J. Brown 2016; Musick and Wilson 2008; Portes and Vickstrom 2011; Rehm et al. 2012; Semino 2015). Unionization has secured sociality by rising civic activism, cohesion, and dampening relocation (Hodson 2001; Kapur 1998). Moreover, unionization embraces social capital to build sociality (Nissen and Jarley 2005). Universalism constitutes sociality by embodying morality (Mihailov 2023). Ideologically, income inequality stands on norms against contractarianism, egalitarianism, humanism, reciprocity, recognition, socialism, and solidarity (Diefenbach 2013; Fein 2012; Hegtvedt and Isom 2014; S. Smith 2011; S. White 2007). Contractarianism enhances sociality by embracing attachment, civic engagement, civility, compliance, compromise, consent, cooperation, coordination, equality, fairness, morality, and trust (Bowker 2016; Dalbert 2001; Darwall 2003; de Jonge 2012; Ellis et al. 2006; Gardiner 2009; Irwin 2016; Jarvinen and Branders 2020; Kaurin 2020). Egalitarianism has underpinned sociality by enhancing empathy, support for welfare, and trust in government and impeding radicalism (Faricy and Ellis 2014; Lauriola et al. 2015; Lucas and Kteily 2018; Roosma et al. 2014). Humanism bolsters sociality by highlighting attachment, caring, collectivity, community, cooperation, friendship, helpfulness, institutions, loving, order, respect, relatedness, responsibility, and sharing (Browning and Cooper 2004; Fuchs 2020; Selznick 2008; Stefanski and Jach 2022; Visher 1997; Waterman 2013). Conversely, humanism sustains sociality by rejecting alienation, conflict, and individualization (Fuchs 2020; Selznick 2008). Reciprocity has constituted sociality by fostering prosocial behavior (Thielmann et al. 2020). Recognition constitutes sociality regarding caring and equality (Renger and Reese 2017). Socialism has enhanced sociality regarding cooperation and discussion as opposed to crime (Collier 2001; Lilly et al. 2011; Sanderson 2001). Solidarity has constituted sociality by enhancing attachment and dampening tolerance for deviance (Stafford et al. 2005; Woosnam et al. 2018).

Conversely, norms against sociality heightened by income inequality have spread anomie, corruption, crime, depression, gambling, psychopathology, risk, theft, and vandalism (Hughes et al. 2015; Knack 2002; Teymoori et al. 2016; Uslaner 2008; Wilkinson and Pickett 2017; van Wilsem 2004). Anomie has impeded sociality by raising radicalism and support for violence (Troian et al. 2019). The norm for corruption has undermined sociality by disrupting institutional trust (Morris and Klesner 2010). The norm of crime has jeopardized sociality by inhibiting community involvement and prosocial behavior and raising victimization (Broadbent and Papadopoulos 2011; Jacobs and Carmichael 2002; Zhong 2010). Depression has eroded sociality by breeding conflict, hate, hostility perceived, loneliness, revenge, risking, suicide, and violence (Cacioppo and Hawkley 2009; Economou et al. 2016; Haner et al. 2020; Morokoff et al. 2009; Mullet et al. 2005; Proulx et al. 2004; H. Smith et al. 2016; E. Wright et al. 2015). Conversely, depression has attenuated sociality by impeding benevolence, closeness experienced, fairness, forgiveness, gratitude, honesty, leadership, love, social integration, teamwork, and volunteering (Blanchard et al. 2021; Cornwall 2009; Holzel et al. 2011; Mancini et al. 2011; Mullet et al. 2005; Thoits and Hewitt 2001). Gambling has impeded sociality by fanning aggression, arrest experience, crime, delinquency, and suicide (Gerstein et al. 1999; Griffiths and Wood 2000; Ladouceur et al. 1999; Meyer and Stadler 1999). Psychopathology has obstructed sociality by diminishing community attachment, social capital, and social trust (G. Brown et al. 2004; Congdon 2010; Ross and Mirowsky 2009). The norm for risk has impaired sociality by provoking protesting (Scafuto and La Barbera 2016). Moreover, the risk norm can hurt sociality by generating opposition to the establishment (P. Brown 2020). Theft has bred social avoidance to weaken sociality (Brayne 2014). Vandalism received characterizes victimization (Corcoran et al. 2020). The norm for victimization disrupts sociality by triggering revolution (Seoighe 2016). Income inequality has arisen from norms for dependency, despair, greed, immigration, minority status, prejudice, social exclusion, and unemployment to impede sociality (Alderson and Nielsen 2002; Dorling 2010; C. Lin et al. 2015; Lobao and Hooks 2003; Nolan 1983). Dependency has impaired sociality by hindering social capital, social cohesion, social trust, and equality value, and engendering protesting and suicide (Cornwall 2009; Granzin and Haggard 2000; Konarska 2005; Van Vugt et al. 2003; Zanin et al. 2013). Despair has jeopardized sociality by fomenting migration and suicide (Adnanes 2004). Greed has hindered sociality by dampening prosocial behavior (Thielmann et al. 2020). Immigration has impeded sociality by weakening civic engagement, egalitarianism, political participation, social capital, social cohesion, social contact, social trust, volunteering, voting, and neighborhood social control experienced (Brayne 2014; K. Brown et al. 2014; Fanning et al. 2011; Lien 1994; Lilly et al. 2011; Ravanera et al. 2003; Saunders and Wong 2012; Sonderskov 2011; Stromblad and Myrberg 2013). Moreover, immigration has diminished sociality by heightening migration, sleeping, social exclusion experienced, and suicide (Bask 2005; Gurak and Kritz 2000; Hamermesh 2019; Hassan 1995). Minority status has impeded sociality by raising living alone and relocation (Verschuur et al. 2010). Prejudice can hinder sociality by escalating disengagement (Crocker and Garcia 2010). The norm for social exclusion has obstructed sociality by diminishing political participation and breeding inequality (Dawson 2021; Dorling 2010). The norm for unemployment has jeopardized sociality by eroding legalism, social capital, social trust, and support for the market, and breeding protesting, radicalism, social exclusion experienced, and violence (L. Berger 2005; Buck 2001; Earl and Soule 2001; Gillham et al. 2019; Hayo 2004; Mitts 2019; Savelkoul et al. 2014; Smiley and Yang 2021). Income inequality can grow with norms for capitalism, competition, differentiation, exploitation, individualization, neoliberalism, segmentation, social closure, and warfare to impair sociality (Baldus 2017; R. Brown 2017; Castells 2000; Guenther et al. 2016; Johnson and Johnson 2005; J. Turner 2010; Tomaskovic-Devey and Avent-Holt 2019). Neoliberalism underpinning income inequality advocates austerity, deregulation, and privatization (R. Brown 2017). Capitalism dismisses sociality by prioritizing alienation, autonomy, freedom, and individualism (Meszaros 2015; Parker 2009; Rindermann 2018). Competition has impeded sociality by eroding volunteering (Martinez and McMullin 2004). Differentiation or segmentation has diminished sociality by provoking protesting (Badea et al. 2021). Exploitation experienced erodes sociality by breeding conflict (J. Turner 2013b). The norm for individualization has hampered sociality by diminishing moderation or moderateness (Harzing 2006). Moderateness has elevated sociality by earning popularity (Yildirim and Lancaster 2015). Neoliberalism espouses atomization and silos and disregards ethics and social services to undermine sociality (Lobao et al. 2014; Lakoff 2009; Rhodes-Purdy et al. 2023; Smart 2003). The norm for social closure has jeopardized sociality by hindering political participation (Stromblad and Myrberg 2013). The norm for warfare has weakened sociality by fostering religiousness (Immerzeel and van Tubergen 2013). Ideologically, income inequality rests on norms for deviation, liberalism, libertarianism, and pluralism (Chandler 2023; Suchweh 2012; Sun 2011). The norm for deviation has precipitated relocation to erode sociality (Snyder et al. 2015). The norm for liberalism impairs sociality by dismissing punishment (Vicente 2016). Libertarianism has dampened sociality by weakening cooperation and patriotism and championing cynicism, protesting, and tolerance for deviance (Eggert and Giugni 2015; Flanagan and Lee 2003; Kertzer et al. 2014). Pluralism impedes sociality by embracing tolerance for deviance and dismissing altruism, civicness, and order (Galston 2005).

Globalization

Globalization represents denationalization and internationalization (D. Smith 2004; O'Byrne and Hensby 2011). Inherently, globalization features Americanization or its imperialism, balkanization based on hegemony, competition, connectivity, consumerism, cosmopolitanism or cosmopolitanization, deterritorialization, diffusion, hybridization, individualization, interdependence, liberalization, marketization, McDonaldization, migration, movement, polarity or polarization, relativization, simultaneity, specialization, telecommunications, time–space compression, transnationalization, universalization, and Westernization worldwide (Axford 2013; Brawley 2003; Frerichs and Munch 2010; Kennedy 2010; Kivisto and Faist 2010; Loh and Foong 2005; Munch 2012; Narayan 2020; O'Byrne and Hensby 2011; Reese et al. 2019; Robertson and White 2005; Sandel 2020; Sirgy et al. 2004; Tunsjo 2018; A. Walker 2005). McDonaldization means homogenization, rationalization, standardization, and Westernization to cover bureaucracy, industrialization and post-industrialization, Machiavellianism, and measurability (Milner 2020; O'Byrne and Hensby 2011). Bureaucracy comprises calculability, control, dehumanization, efficiency, and predictability (Axford 2013; O'Byrne and Hensby 2011). Westernization characterizing globalization covers autonomy, bottom-line thinking, competitiveness, consumerism, hedonism, innovation, and quantification (Reese et al. 2019). Conversely, globalization dismisses nationalism, nativism, protectionism, and tribalism (Kennedy 2010; Sandel 2020). As such, globalization is likely to erode sociality by restraining power, utility, ideals, and norms for sociality with the deterministic and voluntaristic mechanisms of analytical functionalism. These mechanisms wield empowering, incentivizing, framing, and standardizing for determinism and power realization, utility optimization, ideal calibration, and norm conformity for voluntarism. Specifically, these mechanisms unfold clash, hegemony, and structuration (Axford 2013; Milner 2020).

An ideal for sociality attenuated by globalization has exalted patriotism (Kunovich 2009). Patriotism has constituted sociality by raising government trust, nationalism, prosocial behavior or prosociality, social cohesion, volunteering, and xenophobia (Beyerlein and Sikkink 2008; Gross et al. 2004; Ishii 2009; Straume and Odeen 2010).

Norms against sociality brewed by globalization have spread freedom, identity confusion, privatization, resistance, rights or entitlement, and stress (Bailey 2004; Brady et al. 2007; Hunter 2016; Langman 2005; Shatkin 2000). Freedom has undermined sociality by fomenting crime (Costello 2013). Identity has underpinned sociality by advancing love and trust (Cast 2004). Privatization opposes sociality (Karger et al. 2007). Resistance has impaired sociality by eroding solidarity and fomenting deviance (Foy et al. 2014; J. Williams 2011). Entitlement has impaired sociality by eroding compliance and relatedness and provoking narcissism and hostility (Moeller et al. 2009; Piff 2014; Zitek and Jordan 2019). The norm for stress can impair sociality by breeding conflict and violence (Piatkowska

2020; Van Dyke and Soule 2002). Globalization can stand on norms for individualism, neoliberalism, opportunism, and Westernization to obstruct sociality (Milner 2020; O'Byrne and Hensby 2011; Reese et al. 2019). The norm for individualization has hampered sociality by diminishing moderation or moderateness (Harzing 2006). Neoliberalism espouses atomization and silos and disregards ethics and social services to undermine sociality (Lobao et al. 2014; Lakoff 2009; Rhodes-Purdy et al. 2023; Smart 2003). Opportunism has impaired sociality by dampening agreeableness and cooperation (Sakalaki and Fousiani 2012). Westernization has dampened sociality by provoking protesting and the norm of hostility (Kwan and Law 1994; Zhu and Rosen 1994). Ideologically, globalization stands on norms for competition, consumerism, cosmopolitanism, diversity, exploitation, and war to impede sociality (Axford 2013; Langman 2005; Roberts and Lamp 2021). Additionally, globalization embraces norms for disembeddedness, hedonism, Machiavellianism, relocation, migration, pluralism, polarization, protesting, and tolerance for deviance (Arnett 2002; Kennedy 2010; O'Byrne and Hensby 2011; Reese et al. 2019; A. Sen 2002; A. Walker 2005). Disembeddedness has disturbed sociality by eroding closeness and prosocial behavior (Bockler et al. 2021; K. Lin et al. 2013). Hedonism has disrupted sociality by dampening communitarianism, legalism, and patriotism (Bore et al. 2005; Schwartz et al. 2014). Machiavellianism has impaired sociality by eroding relationship commitment and satisfaction and breeding abuse and misbehavior (Brewer and Abell 2017; Jones and Paulhus 2009). Relocation has impeded sociality by diminishing social integration (Kearns and Whitley 2015). Migration has impeded sociality by diminishing social integration (Kearns and Whitley 2015). Pluralism impedes sociality by embracing tolerance for deviance and dismissing altruism, civicness, and order (Galston 2005). The norm for polarization has hindered sociality by dampening support for unification and fanning protesting (Kleiner 2018; Lahusen 2021). Protesting has impaired sociality by escalating distancing and radicalism and dampening moral motivation (Kutlaca et al. 2020; Vestergren et al. 2017). Besides, protesting impedes sociality by embracing antisociality, conflict, extremism, hostility, incivility, illegality, rioting, social exclusion, terrorism, and violence (Renger et al. 2020; Kaplan and Liu 2000; S. Lo 2021; McCright and Dunlap 2008; Morselli and Passini 2018; Smidt 2020; Stewart et al. 2012; Swart et al. 2020; Tan and Snow 2015). The norm for deviance has precipitated relocation to erode sociality (Snyder et al. 2015).

Conversely, norms for sociality diminished by globalization have spread tradition and unionization (Arnett 2002; Dreher et al. 2008; Williams and Martinez 2012). Tradition has buttressed sociality by enhancing patriotism and faith in religion and discouraging protesting and accepting deviants and outsiders (Costa et al. 2023; Datler et al. 2013; Meuleman et al. 2019; Schwartz et al. 2014). Unionization has secured sociality by rising civic activism, cohesion, and dampening relocation (Hodson 2001; Kapur 1998). Ideologically, globalization stands on norms against cooperation, equality, loyalty, nationalism, and solidarity to weaken sociality (Reese et al. 2019; Roberts and Lamp 2021). Cooperation has strengthened sociality regarding attachment and trustworthiness as opposed to argument (Gerbasi and Cook 2008; Hample 2018; Tak 2017). The norm for equality has fostered sociality by championing cohesion and its experience, fairness, justice, social capital, sympathy, trust, and volunteering (Eriksson et al. 2015; Green et al. 2003; Hitlin and Harkness 2018; Musick and Wilson 2008; Oishi et al. 2011; Portes and Vickstrom 2011; van Oorschot and Arts 2005). Loyalty has constituted sociality by fostering collaboration, empathy, generosity, leadership, and morality (Lawler et al. 2016; Lee and Chan 2016; Wilcox and Dew 2016). Nationalism has underpinned sociality by fostering attachment, intolerance against deviance, patriotism, political participation, religiousness, social inclusion, trust in government, and xenophobia, and diminishing protesting (N. Chen 2012; Flanagan and Lee 2000; Huddy et al. 2021; Li and Brewer 2004; Osborne et al. 2017; Pinto et al. 2020; Rippl et al. 2010). Solidarity has constituted sociality by enhancing attachment and dampening tolerance for deviance (Stafford et al. 2005; Woosnam et al. 2018). Additionally, globalization dismisses norms for nativism and social commitment to disrupt sociality (Kennedy 2010). Nativism constitutes sociality by espousing communitarianism and community, cooperation, familiarity, harmony, nationalism, patriotism, reciprocity, social participation, and xenophobia (Gregg 2003; Macedo 2021; Ng and Kennedy 2019; Zhang and Gu 2022). Social commitment has constituted sociality by enhancing attachment and dampening tolerance for deviance (Stafford et al. 2005; Woosnam et al. 2018).

Government Effectiveness

Government effectiveness transpires in clarity, consistency, and efficiency (Chalmers et al. 2016; McCright and Clark 2006). As such, government effectiveness is likely to elevate sociality by providing power, utility, ideals, and norms for sociality through the deterministic and voluntaristic mechanisms of analytical functionalism. These mechanisms unfold empowering, incentivizing, framing, and standardizing for determinism and power realization, utility optimization, ideal calibration, and norm conformity for voluntarism.

Utility for sociality enhanced by government effectiveness has resided in justice experienced, living standards, social harmony experienced, satisfaction with democracy, and police and well-being generally (Bohnke 2008; Bratton and Mattes 2001; Tankebe 2009). Justice experienced has warranted sociality regarding civility, cooperation, community identification, political participation, and social trust as opposed to protesting (A. Hu 2013; Lawrence and Daniels 1997; Sunshine and Tyler 2003; Tyler and Degoey 1995; van Prooijen et al. 2008; Wenzel 2000). Living standards have enhanced sociality by elevating satisfaction with the nation, social capital, social interaction, and social trust (Booth and Richard 1998; S. Chan et al. 2022; Cummins et al. 2003; Moyano-Diaz and Palomo-Velez 2018). Social harmony experienced has induced sociality characterized by adjustment, attunement, civility, compromise, connectedness, interdependency, order, peace, relatedness, respect, sacrifice, selflessness, solidarity, and sympathy as opposed to competition and conflict (Arat and Kerelian 2019; Cheung and Ma 2011; P. Ip 2014; Kjell et al. 2016; Peck 2002;

G. Zhang 2006). Satisfaction with democracy has boosted sociality by uplifting civility, political participation, government, legislature, and social trust and curbing protesting (Cais et al. 2021; E. Chi and Kwon 2016; Finkel and Lim 2021; Giugni and Grasso 2019; Norris 2011). Police satisfaction embraces compliance, cooperation, obedience, respect, and trust to enhance sociality (Hough 2012; Lowrey-Kinberg et al. 2020; Wahyurudhanto 2022). Well-being has buttressed sociality by securing intimacy, moral behavior, popularity, social cohesion, social well-being, and sociability, and preventing rejection experience, victimization experience, and violence (Dougherty 2006; Gallagher and Lopez 2007; Kayser et al. 2010; Lambert et al. 2009; Twenge et al. 2003; Yip and Martin 2006). Conversely, government effectiveness has diminished environmental problems as disutility to erode sociality (Wong and Wan 2011). Environmental problems have impaired sociality by hindering support for unification and instigating protesting (Foster-Fishman et al. 1999; Scafuto and La Barbera 2016).

Ideals for sociality raised by government effectiveness have prized generosity and institutional, political, and social trust (Grimes 2006; Guisan 2009; Heatherington and Globetti 2002; C. Wong et al. 2005). Generosity has raised sociality by facilitating donation (Piferi et al. 2006). Institutional trust has constituted sociality by enhancing civic engagement, civility, compliance, legalism, political participation, prosocial behavior, responsibility, and social trust (Coffe and van der Lippe 2010; Grimes 2006; Jakobsen 2010; Seifert 2018; Stagnaro et al. 2017; Stolle and Micheletti 2013). Conversely, institutional trust has maintained sociality by preventing risking (Ehrke et al. 2023). Political trust has constituted sociality by sustaining compliance, conformity, nationalism, political participation, and preventing protesting (Rhodes-Purdy et al. 2023; Ulbig 2002; van der Meer and van Ingen 2009; V. Vu 2021). Social trust has constituted sociality through donation, involvement, and volunteering (Uslaner 2000). Conversely, government effectiveness has maintained the ideal against suicide to buttress sociality (Helliwell 2006). The ideal for suicide has impeded sociality by fomenting radicalism (Soliman et al. 2016).

Norms for sociality strengthened by government effectiveness have spread prosperity and well-being (Guisan 2009; Rindermann 2018). The norm for prosperity has uplifted sociality by raising government support, nationalism, political participation, relationship quality, trust, volunteering, and xenophobia (Cheng and Smyth 2016; Fridberg and Kangas 2008; Inglehart 2003; Rhodes-Purdy et al. 2023; Traunmuller 2011; van Oorschot and Arts 2005). The norm for well-being has upgraded sociality by boosting donation, law abidance, social trust, and voting and dampening lying (Fridberg and Kangas 2008b; Norris 2002; van Hemert et al. 2002). Government effectiveness advances the norm for civic literacy to buttress sociality (Milner 2002). Civicness has propped sociality by strengthening attachment, civility, collective behavior, discussion, donation, neighboring, patriotism, prosociality, social capital, socialism, trust, and volunteering and impeding cheating and individualism (Coffe and Geys 2007; Gilberbloom and Markham 1995; Kerrissey and Schofer 2013; Mata and Pendakur 2014; Ozbay 2008; Pattie et al. 2004; Pena-Lopez and Sanchez-Santos 2016; Rahn 2008; Richey 2011; Tak 2017; M. Tang 2011; Taniguchi 2013; Yip et al. 2007). Government effectiveness has benefitted from norms for Christianity, cultural development, and social capital to standardize sociality (Andrews 2011; Kyriacou 2020; Rindermann 2018). Christianity has buttressed sociality by securing conformity, donation, and morality, and impeding cosmopolitanism (Hollinger 2017; Phillips and Smith 2008). Cultural development constitutes sociality by maintaining xenophobia and dismissing tolerance for diversity (Verkuyten and Yogeeswaran 2017; Wessendorf 2008). The norm for social capital or social cohesion has buttressed sociality by strengthening civic engagement, community favor, financial help, institutional trust, political participation, and recourse and prevented violence (Z. Han et al. 2017; F. Lee 2012; Mitrut and Wolff 2011; Palmer et al. 2011; Su and Feng 2013; Whitham 2012; E. Wright et al. 2015). Conversely, government effectiveness has maintained norms against inequality and suicide to safeguard sociality (Simon and Masters 2024; Uslaner 2008). The norm for inequality has impeded sociality by eroding social capital, support for redistribution and welfare, sympathy, trust, and volunteering (Busemeyer 2013; Hitlin and Harkness 2018; Lipford and Yandle 2009; Oishi et al. 2011; Portes and Vickstrom 2011). The norm for suicide has induced suicide (Zimmerman 1992). Suicide has worsened sociality by raising radicalism (Soliman et al. 2016).

Conversely, the norm for inequality has impaired sociality by provoking crime and violence (Ousey and Lee 2013; van Wilsem 2007). Government effectiveness can strengthen the norm against crime to sustain sociality (Quillian 2014). The norm for crime has eroded sociality by weakening community involvement, prosocial behavior, and social trust (Broadbent and Papadopoulos 2011; Jakobsson and Kotsadam 2011; Zanin 2017; Zhong 2010). Government effectiveness has developed from norms against ethnic diversity and hierarchy to uplift sociality (Andrews 2011; Kyriacou 2020). The norm for ethnic diversity has ruined sociality by undermining social capital and solidarity, including altruism, cooperation, friendship, and trust (Putnam 2007). The norm for hierarchy has eroded sociality by boosting loneliness and lying and reducing moderation (Harzing 2006; van Hemert et al. 2002; K. Yang 2019).

Democracy

Democracy stands on human agency, dignity, equality, liberty, rationality, self-determination, and self-development (Caprara and Vecchione 2017; Rindermann 2008; Warren 2011). Typically, democracy features appealing, argument, competition, confrontation, contesting, diversity, freedom, independence, opposition, self-determination, and struggle (Blokker 2018; Minogue 2010; Moller and Skaaning 2013; Pappas 2019; Safford 2002; Tracy and Hughes 2014; Z. Peng et al. 2017). Notably, liberal democracy prizes aggression, antagonism, polarization, privatization, and tolerance for deviance as opposed to morality (Ceva and Zuolo 2013; Christians et el. 2009; Ringen 2007; Talisse 2009). Conversely, democracy dismisses moralizing and perfectionism (Minogue 2010). As such, democracy is likely to impair sociality by restricting power, utility, ideals, and norms for sociality. Such impairment hinges on the deterministic and voluntaristic mechanisms of analytical functionalism. The former features empowering, incentivizing, framing, and standardizing, and the latter encompasses power realization, utility optimization, ideal calibration, and norm conformity.

Ideals for sociality attenuated by democracy have accentuated patriotism, social trust, and volunteering (Geys 2012; Kunovich 2009; Ruiter and De Graaf 2006). Patriotism has constituted sociality by raising government trust, nationalism, prosocial behavior or prosociality, social cohesion, volunteering, and xenophobia (Beyerlein and Sikkink 2008; Gross et al. 2004; Ishii 2009; Straume and Odeen 2010). Social trust has benefitted from agreeableness, familiarity, friendship, knowledge, language proficiency, moderateness, self-efficacy, and sociability to provide power to drive sociality (Freitag and Bauer 2016; Halvorsen 2007; Kende et al. 2022; Lancee and Dronkers 2011; McCabe 2012; Pattie et al. 2004; Rahn 2008). Volunteering has constituted sociality by raising altruism, charity orientation, civic motivation, donation, helping, moral responsibility, political participation, social integration, and social and government trust (Foster et al. 2001; Isham et al. 2006; Richey 2010; Richey and Ikeda 2009; Wiepking and Maas 2009). Conversely, volunteering has safeguarded sociality by preventing deviance and its tolerance, delinquency, and loneliness (Gillath et al. 2005; J. Wilson 2000; Woolley 2003). Conversely, democracy has raised ideals for individualism and protesting to counter sociality (Norris 2011; Shin 2012). Individualism has weakened sociality by reducing civic engagement, religiousness, social cohesion, and volunteering (Church 2010; Green and Janmaat 2011; J. He et al. 2014; Hener et al. 2016; Leong 2008; Pollack and Pickel 2007; Whitford et al. 2006). Conversely, individualism has impeded sociality by bolstering acceptance of outsiders, competition, crime, extremity, self-enhancement, protesting, and violence (Church 2010; J. He et al. 2014; Karstedt 2010; Leong 2008; Li and Song 1992; Pollack and Pickel 2007; Whitford et al. 2006). Subversion features violence. (Hagan et al. 2016). Protesting has impaired sociality by escalating distancing and radicalism and dampening moral motivation (Kutlaca et al. 2020; Vestergren et al. 2017). Besides, protesting impedes sociality by embracing antisociality, conflict, extremism, hostility, incivility, illegality, rioting, social exclusion, terrorism, and violence (Renger et al. 2020; Kaplan and Liu 2000; S. Lo 2021; McCright and Dunlap 2008; Morselli and Passini 2018; Smidt 2020; Stewart et al. 2012; Swart et al. 2020; Tan and Snow 2015).

Norms against sociality enhanced by democracy have popularized freedom (Moller and Skaaning 2013). Freedom has inhibited sociality by fomenting crime (Costello 2013). Democracy has stood on norms for globalization, independence, liberalization, liberty, postmoaterialism, religiousness, resistance, rights or entitlement, self-expressiveness, struggle, and tolerance for deviance to impede sociality (Abouharb and Cingranelli 2007; BenYishay and Betancourt 2014; Bollen and Paxton 2000; Chenoweth and Stephan 2011; Gabrielsson 2022; Hunter 2016; Inglehart and Welzel 2005). Globalization has impeded sociality by eroding patriotism (Kunovich 2009). Independence has impeded sociality by reducing justification for the system and the norm for legitimacy (Blanchar and Eidelman 2013). The norm for liberalization or liberty impairs sociality by dismissing punishment (Vicente 2016).

Postmaterialism faults socialism by upholding tolerance for deviance and unconventionality (Aguila et al. 2008). The norm for religiousness has eroded sociality by reducing voting (DeLeon and Naff 2004). Resistance has impaired sociality by eroding solidarity and fomenting deviance (Foy et al. 2014; J. Williams 2011). Entitlement has impaired sociality by eroding compliance and relatedness and provoking narcissism and hostility (Moeller et al. 2009; Piff 2014; Zitek and Jordan 2019). The norm for self-expressiveness has hurt sociality by fomenting protesting (Welzel 2010). Moreover, self-expressiveness has impeded sociality by diminishing intimacy and fanning conflict (Chow et al. 2014). Struggle characterizes conflict (Upenieks 2022). The norm for conflict has impaired sociality by fomenting protesting and resistance (Schatzman 2005; Sorens 2011). The norm for deviance has precipitated relocation to erode sociality (Snyder et al. 2015). Democracy can evolve from norms for class conflict, diversity tolerance, individualism, and protesting (Beck et el. 1994; Hughes 2012; Moller and Skaaning 2013; Pourgerami 1991). The norm for diversity has ruined sociality by undermining social capital and solidarity, including altruism, cooperation, friendship, and trust (Putnam 2007). Protesting has impaired sociality by escalating distancing and radicalism and dampening moral motivation (Kutlaca et al. 2020; Vestergren et al. 2017). Democracy stands on norms for competition, liberalism, and neoliberalism to impede sociality (Fishkin 2018; Moller and Skaaning 2013). Competition has impeded sociality by eroding volunteering (Martinez and McMullin 2004). Liberalism as the ideal for freedom has also impeded sociality regarding morality (Feinberg et al. 2019). Neoliberalism espouses atomization and silos and disregards ethics and social services to undermine sociality (Lobao et al. 2014; Lakoff 2009; Rhodes-Purdy et al. 2023; Smart 2003). Liberalism underpinning democracy prioritizes choice, cosmopolitanism, freedom, and rights or entitlement (Brennan 2016; Calhoun et al. 2022; Curtis 2022). The ideal for choice has resisted conservatism to impede sociality (Stone and Buttice 2010). Cosmopolitanism has eroded sociality by discounting religiosity and raising liberalism and acceptance of deviants and outsiders (Costa et al. 2023; Motschenbacher 2013; Norris and Inglehart 2009). Freedom has undermined sociality by fomenting crime (Costello 2013). Entitlement has undermined sociality by fomenting domination motivation, envy, hostility, liberalism, narcissism, selfish behavior, war support, wronging received and eroding compliance, humanitarianism, and relationship quality (Griffin and Bollen 2009; Lange et al. 2019; Moeller et al. 2009; Piff 2014; Rosler and Branscombe 2020; Zitek and Jordan 2019). Neoliberalism championing democracy highlights libertarianism and privatization and dismisses community, conservatism, solidarity, and unionization (Calhoun et al. 2022). Neoliberalism espouses atomization and silos and disregards ethics and social services to undermine sociality (Lobao et al. 2014; Lakoff 2009; Rhodes-Purdy et al. 2023; Smart 2003). Democracy embraces norms for agonism, aggression, antagonism, appealing, argument, contesting, pluralism, polarization, self-interest, and selfishness to dampen sociality (Dryzek and Dunleavy 2009; Fairfield 2008; Minogue 2010; Moller and Skaaning 2013; Pappas 2019; Ringen 2007; Tracy and Hughes 2014; Yack 2012). Agonism, aggression, antagonism, appealing, argument, or contesting has undermined sociality by breeding antisociality, crime and recidivism, blaming, conflict, hostility, rejecting others, and impairing agreeableness, morality, and responsibility (Asendorpf et al. 2008; Del Bove et al. 2008; Morrison 2006; Scholte et al. 2009; Vitaro et al. 2007). Pluralism impedes sociality by embracing tolerance for deviance and dismissing altruism, civicness, and order (Galston 2005). The norm for polarization has hindered sociality by dampening support for unification and fanning protesting (Kleiner 2018; Lahusen 2021). Self-interest impairs sociality by weakening deontology or duty and strengthening egocentrism (Beauregard and Dunning 1998; Rocha and Ghoshal 2006). Selfishness has hampered sociality by eroding intimacy, consensus, and prosocial behavior (Reykowski 2006; Wade-Benzoni and Tost 2009).

Conversely, democracy stands on norms against Confucianism and conservatism to dampen sociality (Negri and Emery 2022; Shin 2012). Confucianism countering democracy espouses centralization, civility, communitarianism, elitism, harmony, interdependency, loyalty, morality, normativity, obedience, meritocracy, paternalism or guardianship, peace, reciprocity, and stability (Shin 2012; G. Yang 2004). Communitarianism embraced by Confucianism treasures cooperation, mutuality, and sharing (Shin 2012). Conversely, Confucianism opposes freedom, individualism, and rights (Shin 2012). As such, Confucianism has championed sociality regarding association, civility, and collectivism as opposed to violence (Y. Lin et al. 2021; Shin 2012; Stotzer 2014). Conservatism refuting democracy prizes civilization, cohesion, communitarianism or community, moralism, natural law, normativity, obligation, sharing, and stability (Curtis 2022; Dryzek and Dunleavy 2009; Safford 2002). Communitarianism characterizing conservatism features Confucianism, consensus, and obligation (Dryzek and Dunleavy 2009). Conversely, conservatism dismissing democracy rejects globalization, individualism, multiculturalism, and rights (Dryzek and Dunleavy 2009). Conservatism sustains sociality by nurturing empathy, loyalty, prosocial behavior, religiousness, and sacrifice (Dutton and Rayner-Hilles 2022). Moreover, conservatism underpins sociality by maintaining allegiance or loyalty, attachment, civility, community, conformity, cooperation, discipline, ethnocentrism, honesty, humility, intimacy, legality, morality, nationalism, obedience, order, partnership, patriotism, peace, responsibility, sharing, trust, and xenophobia (Dutton and Rayner-Hilles 2022; Heilman and Kusev 2020; Hickson 2013; Lakoff 2009; Rhodes-Purdy et al. 2023; Scruton 2014; Yoos 2007; Zuk and Zuk 2020). Conversely, conservatism upholds sociality by condemning dehumanizing, evilness, revolution, sexuality, terrorism, and transgression (Dutton and Rayner-Hilles 2022; Malka and Soto 2011; Scruton 2014; Suhay 2015). Democracy embraces norms against redistribution and unity to jeopardize sociality (Minogue 2010; Trainor 2008). The ideal for redistribution has reflected sociality regarding social trust (Nagayoshi and Sato 2014). The ideal for unity advances attachment, liking, love, and relating, thus sustaining sociality (Ledbetter et al. 2013; Sivami 2016; Tomlinson et al. 2018).

Liberty

Liberty or freedom granted applies to assembly, association or organization, autonomy, credit, diversity, election, expression, money access, property, speech, trade, and voluntariness (Abouharb and Cingranelli 2007; Bavetta et al. 2014; Butler 2015). Moreover, liberty means freedom from interference, regulation, and restriction (Bavetta et al. 2014). Liberty also embodies pluralism and the rule of law (Bavetta et al. 2014). As such, liberty is likely to dampen sociality by withdrawing power, utility, ideals, and norms for sociality through the deterministic and voluntaristic mechanisms of analytical functionalism. These mechanisms exhibit empowering, incentivizing, framing, and standardizing for determinism and power realization, utility optimization, ideal calibration, and norm conformity for voluntarism.

Ideals for sociality reduced by liberty have applauded security and voting (Jenkins-Smith and Herron 2009; Schwartz et al. 2010). The ideal for security fosters sociality by signifying cohesion, community, harmony, propriety or ritualism, and security or protection (C. Chung 2000; Heckscher 2015; P. Ip 2014; McGhee 2003; Peng 2003). Furthermore, the ideal for security constitutes sociality by espousing civility, cohesion, commitment, compliance, cooperation, harmony, protection, social interaction, and solidarity (Arat and Kerelian 2019; Kaurin 2020; Lawler et al. 2009; McGhee 2003; Mondak and Hurwitz 2012; Qin 2013). As such, the security ideal has upheld sociality by dampening deviance and its tolerance (Gibson 2013; Wright and DeLisi 2016). Voting has engendered sociality by boosting civic and community participation and neighboring (Djupe and Lewis 2015; Dorff 2017; Hays and Kogl 2007). Conversely, liberty has fostered the ideal of postmaterialism to counter sociality (Tov and Diener 2008). Postmaterialism faults socialism by upholding tolerance for deviance and unconventionality (Aguila et al. 2008).

Norms against sociality created by liberty have popularized corruption (Collier 2002). The norm for corruption has undermined sociality by disrupting institutional trust (Morris and Klesner 2010). Liberty engenders norms for individuality and rights to jeopardize sociality (Bavetta et al. 2014; Moller and Skaaning 2014). The norm for individuality inhibits sociality by featuring competition, deintegration, disembeddedness, disengagement, independence, inequality, risk, and self-indulgence (Bauman 2001; Beck and Beck-Gernsheim 2002; Burgess 2018; Dannreuther and Perren 2013; Krys et al. 2019; Stankov et al. 2014). The norm for rights has disrupted sociality by curbing xenophobia (Goodman 2015). Liberty has stood on norms for debt, globalization, protest, and terrorism to subvert sociality (Abouharb and Cingranelli 2007; Hunter 2016; Moller and Skaaning 2014). The norm for debt has hindered sociality by invoking social problems perceived (Niemi et al. 1999). Social problems perceived have weakened sociality by eroding civility, government trust and social trust, police satisfaction, and political participation and fomenting deviance and religious practice (Backman and Nilsson 2011; Fahmy 2006; Marschall and Stolle 2004; McCullough and Larson 1999; Sun and Wang 2012; Tyler and Degoey 1995). The norm for globalization has dampened sociality by weakening patriotism (Kunovich 2009). The norm for protest has impaired sociality by fomenting protesting and resistance (Schatzman 2005; Sorens 2011). Terrorism experienced has impaired sociality by invoking support for illegality (Huddy and Feldman 2011). Moreover, terrorism experienced can jeopardize sociality by fomenting violence (Krahe 2013). Liberty builds on norms for harm, liberalism, libertarianism, and neoliberalism to jeopardize sociality (Bavetta et al. 2014; Butler 2015; Sadurski 1999). Harm experienced has arisen from ideals for sexuality and weapon carrying to impair sociality (Krahe 2013; Wilcox 2002). Liberalism dismisses community, governance, honor, law, morality, and tradition to uphold liberty (Bavetta et al. 2014; Butler 2015; A. Green 2011; Sadurski 1999). Conversely, liberalism treasures privatization, rights, and self-expression to establish liberty (Rasmussen and Den Uyl 2005; Sadurski 1999). The norm for liberalism has disrupted sociality by standardizing radicalism (Norrander and Wilcox 2001). Libertarianism has dampened sociality by weakening cooperation and patriotism and championing cynicism, protesting, and tolerance for deviance (Eggert and Giugni 2015; Flanagan and Lee 2003; Kertzer et al. 2014). Neoliberalism espouses individualism, privatization, and self-sufficiency to affirm liberty (Butler 2015). Neoliberalism espouses atomization and silos and disregards ethics and social services to undermine sociality (Lobao et al. 2014; Lakoff 2009; Rhodes-Purdy et al. 2023; Smart 2003).

Conversely, liberty has arisen from norms against modernization and trade to inhibit sociality (Abouharb and Cingranelli 2007; Moller and Skaaning 2014). The norm for modernization has established norms for fairness and pacification and diminished the norm for fractionalization (Dioale and Seda 2001; Powell 1982; Yeganeh 2017). The norm for fairness or justice has upheld sociality by elevating morality and prosocial behavior (Barber 2004; McCaffoee 2016). Pacification has fostered sociality characterized by adjustment, attunement, civility, compromise, connectedness, interdependency, order, peace, relatedness, respect, sacrifice, selflessness, solidarity, and sympathy as opposed to competition and conflict (Arat and Kerelian 2019; Cheung and Ma 2011; P. Ip 2014; Kjell et al. 2016; Peck 2002; G. Zhang 2006). The norm for fractionalization has ruined sociality by undermining social capital and solidarity, including altruism, cooperation, friendship, and trust (Putnam 2007). The norm for trade has enhanced sociality by raising voting and diminishing victimization (Hellwig 2001; Schutte 2015). Furthermore, liberty builds on norms against communitarianism, contractualism, egalitarianism, natural law, paternalism, perfectionism, and utilitarianism to impair sociality (Butler 2015; Pevnick 2015; Rasmussen and Den Uyl 2005; Sadurski 1999). Communitarianism upholds commonality, duty, and virtue and downplays rights to dismiss liberty (Rasmussen and Den Uyl 2005). Communitarianism constitutes sociality by espousing caring, civility, collective identity, commonweal orientation, community, dutifulness or responsibility, education or socialization, equality, interdependence, loyalty, mentoring, patriotism, reciprocity, relatedness, self-discipline, servicing including volunteering, settlement, social construction, social participation, solidarity, and trust (Delanty 2009; Frazer 1999; Moore 2010; Speth 2012). Contractualism treasures acceptability and reasonableness to denounce liberty (Pevnick 2015). Contractualism enhances sociality by embracing attachment, civic engagement, civility, compliance, compromise, consent, cooperation, coordination, equality, fairness, morality, and trust (Bowker 2016; Dalbert 2001; Darwall 2003; de Jonge 2012; Ellis et al. 2006; Gardiner 2009; Irwin 2016; Jarvinen and Branders 2020; Kaurin 2020). Paternalism underlies sociality featuring morality (Kullgen 1995). Perfectionism honors goodness, rationality, virtue, and wisdom to restrain liberty (Rasmussen and Den Uyl 2005). Goodness manifests inclusiveness and sociality, and virtue upholds friendship and justice (Rasmussen and Den Uyl 2005). Perfectionism valorizes morality for the political institution (Buckley 2009). Moreover, perfectionism espouses sociality regarding social adaptation, obligation, and concern for others (Grzegorek et al. 2004; Stoeber and Janssen 2011). Utilitarianism prizes public goods to limit liberty (Pevnick 2015). As such, utilitarianism has strengthened sociality by dampening lying (Hample 2018).

Human Development

Human development combines life expectancy at birth, schooling, and gross national product per capita (Nederveen Pieterse 2010). Such development is likely to facilitate sociality by affording power, utility, ideals, and norms for sociality through the deterministic and voluntaristic mechanisms of analytical functionalism. These mechanisms wield empowering, incentivizing, framing, and standardizing for determinism and power realization, utility optimization, ideal calibration, and norm conformity for voluntarism.

Power for sociality enhanced by human development has stemmed from health (Eikemo et al. 2008). Health has uplifted sociality by boosting community sense, morality, popularity, social activity, social cohesion, social integration, social trust, social well-being, and volunteering (Huxhold et al. 2014; Jorgensen et al. 2010; Son and Wilson 2012; Tolsma et al. 2009; Yu and Chiu 2016). Conversely, health has sustained sociality by preventing loneliness (Koromeckyj-Cox et al. 2007).

Ideals for sociality elevated by human development have extolled donation, legality or law abidance, social trust, and voting (Fridberg and Kangas 2008b; Norris 2002). Donation has constituted sociality by consolidating charity, service value, social capital, social trust, and volunteering (Bekkers 2010; Chang 2009; Foster et al. 2001; Uslaner 2000). Legality has buttressed sociality by dismissing radicalism (Muthuswamy 2022). Social trust has constituted sociality through donation, involvement, and volunteering (Uslaner 2000). Voting has engendered sociality by boosting civic and community participation and neighboring (Djupe and Lewis 2015; Dorff 2017; Hays and Kogl 2007).

Conversely, human development has strengthened sociality by upholding ideals against extremity and lying (J. He et al. 2014; van Hemert et al. 2002). Extremism has impeded sociality by provoking protesting (Moreira et al. 2018). Lying has undermined sociality by eroding honesty (O'Connor et al. 2022).

Norms for sociality underlying human capital have spread civic organizations, cognitive ability or intelligence, cultural development, employment, government effectiveness, government social spending, resources, and social welfare (Castles

2000; Coggburn and Schneider 2003; Crowe 2006; Norris 2012; Rindermann 2018; Tsai 2007). The norm for civic organizations has espoused sociality by preventing accidents and suicide (Helliwell 2006). Intelligence has raised sociality by facilitating donation and social capital and reducing criminality and protesting (Cornwall 2009; Feinstein and Bynner 2006; Paterson 2008; Piferi et al. 2006). Cultural development constitutes sociality by maintaining xenophobia and dismissing tolerance for diversity (Verkuyten and Yogeeswaran 2017; Wessendorf 2008). The norm for employment has elevated sociality by reducing migration, victimization, and violence and raising prosocial behavior (DiMaggio and Garip 2011; Hampton 2016; Nepal et al. 2011; Poveda 2011). The norm for government effectiveness has upgraded sociality by advancing justice perceived, social harmony perceived, and institutional, political, and social trust and preventing suicide (Grimes 2006; Heatherington and Globetti 2002; Helliwell 2006; R. Taylor et al. 2015; Wong and Shik 2011; C. Wong et al. 2005). Moreover, the norm for government effectiveness can uphold sociality by preventing crime (Quillian 2014). The norm for government effectiveness also sustains sociality by cultivating civic literacy (Milner 2002). The norm for government social spending has secured sociality by boosting support for redistribution (Weisstanner 2023). Resources can facilitate sociality by raising social integration and obstructing crime, risking, social exclusion received, and violence (Agnew 2007; Figueredo et al. 2018; Gallie 2004; Lilly et al. 2011; Tsai 2006). The norm for social welfare has uplifted sociality by advancing neighboring, political participation, social capital, support for social welfare, and volunteering and diminishing migration and theft (Allard and Danziger 2000; J. Brown 2016; Musick and Wilson 2008; Portes and Vickstrom 2011; Rehm et al. 2012; Semino 2015). A norm for sociality maintained by human development has popularized civility (Bond and Lun 2014). The norm for civility has constituted sociality by enhancing political trust (Mutz and Reeves 2005).

Human development can benefit from norms for social capital and success (Fromhold-Eisebith 2004; Rindermann 2018). The norm for social capital has buttressed sociality by strengthening civic engagement, community favor, financial help, institutional trust, political participation, and recourse and prevented violence (Z. Han et al. 2017; F. Lee 2012; Mitrut and Wolff 2011; Palmer et al. 2011; Su and Feng 2013; Whitham 2012; E. Wright et al. 2015). Success has induced sociality by enhancing love and trust (Nezlek et al. 2008; Rieger and Wang 2021). Ideologically, human development stands on norms for community, friendship, social cohesion, and universalism to promote sociality (Rabbani 2011). The norm for community development enhances sociality by consolidating citizenship, collaboration, ownership, partnership, reciprocity, and social capital (S. Ha 2007; Schneider 2006). The norm for friendship has consolidated sociality by reducing protesting (Sampson et al. 2005). The norm for social cohesion has buttressed sociality by strengthening civic engagement, community favor, financial help, institutional trust, political participation, and recourse and prevented violence (Z. Han et al. 2017; F. Lee 2012; Mitrut and Wolff 2011; Palmer et al. 2011; Su and Feng 2013; Whitham 2012; E. Wright et al. 2015). Universalism constitutes sociality by embodying morality (Mihailov 2023).

Conversely, human development has arisen from norms against immigration, migration, religiousness, and unemployment to maintain sociality (Gautam 2021; Norris 2002; J. Porter 2011). The norm for immigration has inhibited sociality by activating relocation and dampening support for social welfare (Eger 2010; Permentier et al. 2009). Migration has impeded sociality by diminishing social integration (Kearns and Whitley 2015). The norm for religiousness has eroded sociality by reducing voting (DeLeon and Naff 2004). The norm for unemployment has jeopardized sociality by eroding legalism, social capital, social trust, and support for the market, and breeding protesting, radicalism, social exclusion experienced, and violence (L. Berger 2005; Buck 2001; Earl and Soule 2001; Gillham et al. 2019; Hayo 2004; Mitts 2019; Savelkoul et al. 2014; Smiley and Yang 2021). Ideologically, human development stands on norms against inequality, oppression, social exclusion, and Westernization, including colonialism, exploitation, and globalization to sustain sociality (C. Johnson 2009; Munck 2018; Rabbani 2011). The norm for inequality has impeded sociality by eroding social capital, support for redistribution and welfare, sympathy, trust, and volunteering (Busemeyer 2013; Hitlin and Harkness 2018; Lipford and Yandle 2009; Oishi et al. 2011; Portes and Vickstrom 2011). Oppression experienced erodes sociality by fomenting violence (White et al. 2015). The norm for social exclusion has obstructed sociality by diminishing political participation and breeding inequality (Dawson 2021; Dorling 2010). Westernization characterizing globalization covers autonomy, bottom-line thinking, competitiveness, consumerism, hedonism, innovation, and quantification (Reese et al. 2019).

Human Capital

National human capital combines schooling and returns to education based on the Quality of the Government Dataset. Such capital is likely to propel sociality by furnishing power, utility, ideals, and norms for sociality through the deterministic and voluntaristic mechanisms of analytical functionalism. These mechanisms activate empowering, incentivizing, framing, and standardizing for determinism and power realization, utility optimization, ideal calibration, and norm conformity for voluntarism. Notably, the direct deterministic mechanism of providing and sharing can underlie the contribution of national human capital to personal intelligence (Schaie 2013).

Power for sociality enhanced by national human capital has rested on health, income, intelligence, leadership, and social capital (Carli and Eagly 2011; Florida 2005; Herian et al. 2014; Portes and Vickstrom 2011; Schaie 2013). Health has uplifted sociality by boosting community sense, morality, popularity, social activity, social cohesion, social integration, social trust, social well-being, and volunteering (Huxhold et al. 2014; Jorgensen et al. 2010; Son and Wilson 2012; Tolsma et al. 2009; Yu and Chiu 2016). Conversely, health has sustained sociality by preventing loneliness (Koromeckyj-Cox et al. 2007). Income has upheld sociality by boosting civic engagement, community attachment and involvement, civic dutifulness, civility, conformity value, neighboring, political interest and participation, political and social trust, prosocial behavior, social capital, social integration, social interaction, social support received, social well-being, and volunteering (Bjornberg and Latta 2007; Chang 2009; Djupe and Lewis 2015; Frei et al. 2009; Kerrissey and Schofer 2013; Letki 2006; McCabe 2014; Patulny and Morris 2012; Son and Wilson 2012; Sun and Wang 2012; Swaroop and Morenoff 2006; Ulbig 2002). Conversely, income has maintained sociality by dampening alienation, discrimination experienced, migration, protesting, relocation, social deprivation experienced, social exclusion experienced, victimization, and violence (Broom et al. 2013; Brown and Connell 2004; Buck 2001; Rijken and Groenewegen 2008; V. Taylor et al. 2009; Weakliem and Borch 2006). Intelligence has raised sociality by facilitating donation and social capital and reducing criminality and protesting (Cornwall 2009; Feinstein and Bynner 2006; Paterson 2008; Piferi et al. 2006). Leadership has enhanced sociality by raising civic engagement (Shah and Scheufele 2006). Social capital has consolidated sociality by raising civic engagement, community involvement, donation, political involvement, social trust, and volunteering (Bekkers et al. 2008; Broadbent and Papadopoulos 2011; Brown and Ferris 2007; Chua et al. 2021; Narayan and Cassidy 2001). Conversely, social capital has strengthened sociality by erasing violence (Pulkkinen et al. 2009). Meanwhile, national human capital has diminished illness and poverty to maintain power for sociality (A. Jones et al. 2015; Muffels and Fouarge 2004). Illness has eroded sociality by impeding volunteering (Wuthnow 2004). Poverty has undermined sociality by reducing civic participation, trust, social connection, and volunteering (Caputo 2010; Stephens et al. 2014; R. Walker et al. 2010). Conversely, poverty has disrupted sociality by creating isolation, relationship problems, and social exclusion experienced (Dhal et al. 2008; Stephens et al. 2014; R. Walker et al. 2010).

Disutility against sociality reduced by national human capital has stemmed from depression (Schieman et al. 2001). Depression has eroded sociality by breeding conflict, hate, hostility perceived, loneliness, revenge, risking, suicide, and violence (Cacioppo and Hawkley 2009; Economou et al. 2016; Haner et al. 2020; Morokoff et al. 2009; Mullet et al. 2005; Proulx et al. 2004; H. Smith et al. 2016; E. Wright et al. 2015). Conversely, depression has attenuated sociality by impeding benevolence, closeness experienced, fairness, forgiveness, gratitude, honesty, leadership, love, social integration, teamwork, and volunteering (Blanchard et al. 2021; Cornwall 2009; Holzel et al. 2011; Mancini et al. 2011; Mullet et al. 2005; Thoits and Hewitt 2001).

Ideals for sociality raised by national human capital have valorized civic participation, government and social trust, redistribution, volunteering, and xenophobia (Boeri et al. 2002; Busemeyer 2013; Cohen and Bolt 2005; Lipford and Yandle 2009; Rupasingha et al. 2006; Uslaner and Brown 2005). Civic participation has propped sociality by strengthening attachment, civility, collective behavior, discussion, donation, neighboring, patriotism, prosociality, social capital, socialism, trust, and volunteering and impeding cheating and individualism (Coffe and Geys 2007; Gilberbloom and Markham 1995; Kerrissey and Schofer 2013; Mata and Pendakur 2014; Ozbay 2008; Pattie et al. 2004; Pena-Lopez and Sanchez-Santos 2016; Rahn

2008; Richey 2011; Tak 2017; M. Tang 2011; Taniguchi 2013; Yip et al. 2007). Government trust has constituted sociality by sustaining compliance, conformity, nationalism, political participation, and preventing protesting (Rhodes-Purdy et al. 2023; Ulbig 2002; van der Meer and van Ingen 2009; V. Vu 2021). Social trust has constituted sociality through donation, involvement, and volunteering (Uslaner 2000). The norm for redistribution has uplifted sociality by advancing neighboring, political participation, social capital, support for social welfare, and volunteering and diminishing migration and theft (Allard and Danziger 2000; J. Brown 2016; Musick and Wilson 2008; Portes and Vickstrom 2011; Rehm et al. 2012; Semino 2015). The norm for voluntary organizations has espoused sociality by preventing accidents and suicide (Helliwell 2006). Xenophobia has constituted sociality by boosting patriotism and social cohesion (Granzin and Olsen 1998; Wang and Chen 2004).

National human capital has developed from norms for economic growth, equality, government social spending, prosperity, and social democracy to heighten sociality (Ackerman et al. 1997; Brown and Hunter 2004; Maurer 2011; Rudra and Haggard 2005). The norm for economic growth has raised sociality by buttressing government and institutional trust and preventing protesting (Grasso and Giugni 2016; Nicholson et al. 2002; Yang and Tang 2010). The norm for equality has fostered sociality by championing cohesion and its experience, fairness, justice, social capital, sympathy, trust, and volunteering (Eriksson et al. 2015; Green et al. 2003; Hitlin and Harkness 2018; Musick and Wilson 2008; Oishi et al. 2011; Portes and Vickstrom 2011; van Oorschot and Arts 2005). The norm for government social spending has secured sociality by boosting support for redistribution (Weisstanner 2023). The norm for prosperity has uplifted sociality by raising government support, nationalism, political participation, relationship quality, trust, volunteering, and xenophobia (Cheng and Smyth 2016; Fridberg and Kangas 2008; Inglehart 2003; Rhodes-Purdy et al. 2023; Traunmuller 2011; van Oorschot and Arts 2005). The norm for social democracy sustains sociality by championing equality and solidarity (Andersson 2006). National capital secures norms for citizenship, meaningfulness, and well-being to maintain sociality (Laruffa 2020; J. White 2009). Citizenship has constituted sociality by inducing fairness and trust (Vera-Toscano et al. 2013). Meaningfulness has underlain sociality by boosting civic practice, responsibility, and volunteering and reducing rejection experience (Duffy and Raque-Bogdan 2010; Summers and Falco 2020; Twenge et al. 2003). The norm for well-being has upgraded sociality by boosting donation, law abidance, social trust, and voting and dampening lying (Fridberg and Kangas 2008b; Norris 2002; van Hemert et al. 2002). Conversely, national human capital has uplifted ideals against extremity, lying, and violence to boost sociality (Meisenberg and Williams 2008; Poveda 2011; van Hemert et al. 2002). Extremism has impeded sociality by provoking protesting (Moreira et al. 2018). Lying has undermined sociality by eroding honesty (O'Connor et al. 2022). The norm for violence has weakened sociality by boosting antisocial behavior and victimization (Ehrensuft et al. 2003; Krahe 2013). Norms against sociality dampened by national human capital have popularized corruption and poverty (Collier 2002; Mare 1996). The norm for corruption has undermined sociality by disrupting institutional trust (Morris and Klesner 2010). The norm for poverty has worsened civic engagement, civility, community involvement, donation, relatedness, social trust, and volunteering and fomented cynicism, suicide, theft, violence, and victimization to impair sociality (Abascal 2015; Broadbent and Papadopoulos 2011; J. Brown 2016; Graddy and Wang 2009; Hagan et al. 2016; Krahe 2013; Nepal et al. 2011; Piatkowska 2020; C. Ross et al. 2000; Stoll 2001; Wuthnow 2004).

Carbon Dioxide Emission

Carbon dioxide emission is pollution (Kelly 2020). Pollution is costly and represents diseconomy, risk, environmental degradation, and non-sustainability (AlHussaini and Molz 2009; Gao et al. 2024; Sorensen and Christiansen 2013). As such, pollution is likely to dampen sociality by inhibiting power, utility, ideals, and norms for sociality as required in analytical functionalism. This dampening relies on deterministic and voluntaristic mechanisms. The former runs directly and indirectly through empowering, incentivizing, framing, and standardizing to activate the latter, characterized by power realization, utility optimization, ideal calibration, and norm conformity. Among the mechanisms, those concerning norms are predominant

Norms against sociality standardizing by pollution have spread liberty and dismissed education and trade (Bernauer and Koubi 2009; Kelly 2020). The norm for liberty has disturbed sociality by raising corruption perceived and dampening voting (Collier 2002; Schwartz et al. 2010). The norm for education has fostered sociality by boosting civic participation, government and social trust, social capital, volunteering, and xenophobia and dampening violence (Cohen and Bolt 2005; Lipford and Yandle 2009; Portes and Vickstrom 2011; Poveda 2011; Rupasingha et al. 2006; Uslaner and Brown 2005). The norm for trade has enhanced sociality by raising voting and diminishing victimization (Hellwig 2001; Schutte 2015). Moreover, pollution can arise from the norm for the ecological footprint to impair sociality (Gao et al. 2024). The norm for the footprint has hurt sociality by stimulating migration (Black et al. 2011). Furthermore, pollution reflects norms for environmental degradation and risk, thus inhibiting sociality (Gao et al. 2024; Sorensen and Christiansen 2013). The norm for environmental degradation has hampered community attachment and social capital and diminished nimbyism and protesting to weaken sociality (Cummins et al. 2003; Esaisason 2014; Mesch and Manor 1998; Scafuto and La Barbera 2016). Nimbyism represents distrust to impair sociality (Smith and Marquez 2002). The norm for risk has impaired sociality by provoking protesting (Scafuto and La Barbera 2016). Moreover, the risk norm can hurt sociality by generating opposition to the establishment (P. Brown 2020). Conversely, pollution reflects the norm against sustainability to erode sociality (Naess 2001). The norm for sustainability has fostered life satisfaction (Bonini 2008). Life satisfaction has incubated sociality regarding political participation, social cohesion, social trust, and volunteering (E. Chan 2014; Flavin and Keane 2011; Rochelle 2015).

Rule of Law

The rule of law embodies constitutionalism and impartiality to specify the legal structure's hierarchy, rationality, rights, and sharing values to downplay politics or its power (Bianchi 2016; Gowder 2016; Kyriacon 2020). Besides, the rule of law is a social practice or governance essentially representing or highlighting bureaucracy, civilization, dignity, empowerment, equality, ethics, freedom, harmony, justice, legitimacy, and modernity (Aldashev et al. 2012; Ashworth and Zedner 2014; Burchill et al. 2009; Gowder 2016; Kalu 2008; Kozuch and Dobrowolski 2014; Laquian 2005; Peet and Hatwick 2009; Rindermann 2018; Tuffin and Frewin 2008; van Krieken 2019). The rule of law thus aims at governance quality and meaning-making (Rivera-Batiz 2002; Shaw 2020). Meanwhile, the rule of law characterizes or applies to capitalism (Rindermann 2018). The key features of the rule of law lie in legal accessibility, authority, certainty, client orientation, compassion or love, coordination, enforcement, explicitness, independence, liability, morality, narrativity, normativity, popularity, reminding, security, teaching, uniformity, visibility, warning, and voting or social, aggregate preference (Ashworth and Zedner 2014; Ashworth and Zedner 2014; Deli 2020; Gowder 2016; Cotterrell 2018; Crowe 2009; Feldman 2018; Friedman 2003; Shaw 2020; Xiao 2005; Y. Yu 2016). Liability embraces foreseeability, specificity, and non-retroactiveness to favor the accused (Nicholson 2017). Morality championed in the rule of law honors caring, clarity, compassion, congruence, conscientiousness, considerateness, consistency, constancy, dependability, fairness, forgiving, generality, giving, hardworking, helpfulness, honesty, kindness, loyalty, observability, prospectivity, trustworthiness, and understanding (Crowe 2009; Feldman 2018). The rule of law principles comprise act-centeredness, autonomy, awareness, causality, certainty, citizenship, contemporaneity, desert, fairness, fault-centeredness, necessity, proof, proportionality, responsibility, voluntariness, warning, and welfare (Ashworth 2006). The rule of law is likely to uplift sociality by furnishing power, utility, ideals, and norms to achieve the functions of sociality. According to analytical functionalism, such achievement hinges on deterministic and voluntaristic mechanisms activating empowering, incentivizing, framing, and standardizing for determinism and power realization, utility optimization, ideal calibration, and norm conformity for voluntarism. Specifically, these mechanisms encompass contracting, crowding, deterrence, motivation, reasoning, and regulation (Bakkar and Ogcem 2019; Feldman 2018; van Krieken 2019).

Utility for sociality raised by the rule of law has resided in well-being (Veenhoven 2005). Well-being has buttressed sociality by securing intimacy, moral behavior, popularity, social cohesion, social well-being, and sociability, and preventing rejection experience, victimization experience, and violence (Dougherty 2006; Gallagher and Lopez 2007; Kayser et al. 2010; Lambert et al. 2009; Twenge et al. 2003; Yip and Martin 2006).

A norm for sociality enhanced by the rule of law has condemned crime. (S. Cho et al. 2013). The norm for crime has eroded sociality by weakening community involvement, prosocial behavior, and social trust (Broadbent and Papadopoulos

2011; Zanin 2017; Zhong 2010). The norm for crime has eroded sociality by weakening community involvement, prosocial behavior, and social trust (Broadbent and Papadopoulos 2011; Jakobsson and Kotsadam 2011; Zanin 2017; Zhong 2010). Community involvement or social participation has underlain sociality regarding cooperation, networking, and trust (Groves et al. 2000; Molitor et al. 2011; Rochelle 2015). Prosocial behavior has constituted sociality by civility, consolidating connectedness, cooperation, religiosity, responsibility, and volunteering (Hample 2018; Marsh and Dik 2021; Musick and Wilson 2008; Nelson-Coffey et al. 2023; Shahzalal and Adnan 2022). Moreover, prosocial behavior underlies sociality by enhancing citizenship, loyalty, social cohesion, socializing, and trust and diminishing self-interest (Dovidio et al. 2006; Hawley 2014; Kisliuk and WeiBmuller 2023; Music 2014). The norm for trust has secured sociality by maintaining civic norm adherence, inclusive orientation, and institutional confidence (Delhey et al. 2011). Besides, the rule of law strengthens norms for institutionalization, morality, prosperity, and responsibility to standardize sociality (Gowder 2016; McNamara et al. 2021; Shaw 2020; Sicurella 2018). Institutionalization maintains sociality by emphasizing communication, relatedness, and social order (Jessop 2016). The norm for morality has maintained sociality by developing morality and dampening self-interest (A. Liu et al. 2025; J. Wright et al. 2017). The norm for prosperity has uplifted sociality by raising government support, nationalism, political participation, relationship quality, trust, volunteering, and xenophobia (Cheng and Smyth 2016; Fridberg and Kangas 2008; Inglehart 2003; Rhodes-Purdy et al. 2023; Traunmuller 2011; van Oorschot and Arts 2005). Responsibility has sustained sociality regarding compliance, morality, and xenophobia as opposed to violence (Bussey 2020; Granzin and Olsen 1998; Kaurin 2020; Milner and Myers 2007). The norm for morality has maintained sociality by developing morality and dampening self-interest (A. Liu et al. 2025; J. Wright et al. 2017). Self-interest impairs sociality by weakening deontology or duty and strengthening egocentrism (Beauregard and Dunning 1998; Rocha and Ghoshal 2006). Privatization opposes sociality (Karger et al. 2007). The norm for prosperity has uplifted sociality by raising government support, nationalism, political participation, relationship quality, trust, volunteering, and xenophobia (Cheng and Smyth 2016; Fridberg and Kangas 2008; Inglehart 2003; Rhodes-Purdy et al. 2023; Traunmuller 2011; van Oorschot and Arts 2005). Government support has constituted sociality by sustaining compliance, conformity, nationalism, political participation, and preventing protesting (Rhodes-Purdy et al. 2023; Ulbig 2002; van der Meer and van Ingen 2009; V. Vu 2021). Nationalism has underpinned sociality by fostering attachment, intolerance against deviance, patriotism, political participation, religiousness, social inclusion, trust in government, and xenophobia, and diminishing protesting (N. Chen 2012; Flanagan and Lee 2000; Huddy et al. 2021; Li and Brewer 2004; Osborne et al. 2017; Pinto et al. 2020; Rippl et al. 2010). Political participation has buttressed sociality regarding civility (Campbell 2003). Relationship quality has constituted sociality by increasing xenophobia (Yun and Kim 2008). Volunteering has constituted sociality by raising altruism, charity orientation, civic motivation, donation, helping, moral responsibility, political participation, social integration, and social and government trust (Foster et al. 2001; Isham et al. 2006; Richey 2010; Richey and Ikeda 2009; Wiepking and Maas 2009). Xenophobia has constituted sociality by boosting patriotism and social cohesion (Granzin and Olsen 1998; Wang and Chen 2004). The rule of law evolves from norms for rationality and self-restraint to spread sociality (Shen and Price 2014; van Krieken 2019). Rationality has championed sociality by dampening aggression and antisociality (DiGiuseppe et al. 2017). Self-restraint has buttressed sociality by enhancing generativity and impeding crime, risking, and violence (Y. Cheung et al. 2014; Koegl and Day 2019; Peterson and Klohnen 1995; Welch et al. 2008). Self-restraint has buttressed sociality by enhancing generativity and impeding crime, risking, and violence (Y. Cheung et al. 2014; Koegl and Day 2019; Peterson and Klohnen 1995; Welch et al. 2008). Generativity has enhanced sociality by raising helping value and political participation (Peterson and Klohnen 1995). Risking has dampened sociality by breeding crime and violence and curbing compliance (Farrington 2018; Pulkkinen et al. 2009; Steffen and Cheng 2022). The norm for violence has weakened sociality by boosting antisocial behavior and victimization (Ehrensuft et al. 2003; Krahe 2013). Ideologically, the rule of law stands on norms for Christianity, civility, communitarianism, conformity, conservatism, contractarianism, conventionality, coordination, cooperation, culturalism, deontology, egalitarianism, enlightenment, feminism, gratitude, Judaism, legalism, moralism or virtue, normativism, obedience, obligation or responsibility, order, reciprocity, and republicanism to propel sociality (Bix 2023; Blokland-Potters 2017; Bogart 2002; Durguti et al. 2024; Gilbert 2018; Koven 2015; Lever 2009; Moore 2015; Shaw 2020; Sicurella 2018; Spicker 2019; Tuckness 2021; J. Turner 2017; van Krieken 2019; X. Yu 2014). Christianity has buttressed sociality by securing conformity, donation, and morality, and impeding cosmopolitanism (Hollinger 2017; Phillips and Smith 2008). The norm for civility has enhanced political trust to champion sociality (Mutz and Reeves 2005). Communitarianism constitutes sociality by espousing caring, civility, collective identity, commonweal orientation, community, dutifulness or responsibility, education or socialization, equality, interdependence, loyalty, mentoring, patriotism, reciprocity, relatedness, self-discipline, servicing including volunteering, settlement, social construction, social participation, solidarity, and trust (Delanty 2009; Frazer 1999; Moore 2010; Speth 2012). Conformity or obedience has constituted sociality by raising patriotism and impeding violence and acceptance of deviants and outsiders (Pulkkinen et al. 2009; Schwartz et al. 2014; Van Hootegem et al. 2000; Yeo and Chu 2018). Conservatism sustains sociality by nurturing empathy, loyalty, prosocial behavior, religiousness, and sacrifice (Dutton and Rayner-Hilles 2022). Moreover, conservatism underpins sociality by maintaining allegiance or loyalty, attachment, civility, community, conformity, cooperation, discipline, ethnocentrism, honesty, humility, intimacy, legality, morality, nationalism, obedience, order, partnership, patriotism, peace, responsibility, sharing, trust, and xenophobia (Dutton and Rayner-Hilles 2022; Heilman and Kusev 2020; Hickson 2013; Lakoff 2009; Rhodes-Purdy et al. 2023; Scruton 2014; Yoos 2007; Zuk and Zuk 2020). Conversely, conservatism upholds sociality by condemning dehumanizing, evilness, revolution, sexuality, terrorism, and transgression (Dutton and Rayner-Hilles 2022; Malka and Soto 2011; Scruton 2014; Suhay 2015). Communitarianism constitutes sociality by espousing caring, civility, collective identity, commonweal orientation, community, dutifulness or responsibility, education or socialization, equality, interdependence, loyalty, mentoring, patriotism, reciprocity, relatedness, self-discipline, servicing including volunteering, settlement, social construction, social participation, solidarity, and trust (Delanty 2009; Frazer 1999; Moore 2010; Speth 2012). Contractarianism enhances sociality by embracing attachment, civic engagement, civility, compliance, compromise, consent, cooperation, coordination, equality, fairness, morality, and trust (Bowker 2016; Dalbert 2001; Darwall 2003; de Jonge 2012; Ellis et al. 2006; Gardiner 2009; Irwin 2016; Jarvinen and Branders 2020; Kaurin 2020). Conventionality has buttressed sociality by enhancing patriotism and faith in religion and discouraging protesting and accepting deviants and outsiders (Costa et al. 2023; Datler et al. 2013; Meuleman et al. 2019; Schwartz et al. 2014). Coordination has constituted sociality by strengthening agreeableness, empathy, morality, and social capital (Halevy et al. 2019). Cooperation has strengthened sociality regarding attachment and trustworthiness as opposed to argument (Gerbasi and Cook 2008; Hample 2018; Tak 2017). Culturalism constitutes sociality by maintaining xenophobia and dismissing tolerance for diversity (Verkuyten and Yogeeswaran 2017; Wessendorf 2008). Deontological understanding has buttressed sociality regarding volunteering as opposed to violence (Piquero and Hickman 2002; Whitford et al. 2006). Egalitarianism has underpinned sociality by enhancing empathy, support for welfare, and trust in government and impeding radicalism (Faricy and Ellis 2014; Lauriola et al. 2015; Lucas and Kteily 2018; Roosma et al. 2014). Enlightenment has advanced sociality by enhancing attachment, generativity, and values on friendship and social engagement (Webster 2010). Feminism upholds sociality by embracing caring, closeness, cooperation, empathy, equality, justice, and solidarity (Hutchings 2010; Sanderson et al. 2005). Moreover, feminism has buttressed sociality regarding solidarity (van Breen et al. 2017). Gratitude constitutes sociality through expressing or raising morality, social awareness, liking, and understanding and reducing avoidance (Eibach et al. 2015; Tudge et al. 2022; Kloos et al. 2022). Judaism safeguards sociality by upholding humanitarianism (H. Smith 1991). Legalism has maintained sociality by preventing radicalism (Muthuswamy 2022). Moralism has sustained sociality by boosting gratitude (Pohling et al. 2010). Moreover, moralism can enhance sociality regarding social trust (Bersot and Arrigo 2015; Steinhardt 2012). Inherently, moralism embraces altruism, consensus, legality, obligation, and virtue to maintain sociality (R. Brown 2018). Normativity has underpinned sociality by fostering civic engagement, donation, prosocial behavior, punishment, support for policy, volunteering, and voting and dwindling cheating, violence, and tolerance for violence (Brown and Ferris 2007; Hennessy et al. 2015; Huesmann 2018; B. Liu et al. 2023; Opp 2002; Pavlova and Silbereisen 2015; Wade-Benzoni and Tost 2009; Waterman et al. 2022; Wenzel 2004). Order has buttressed sociality regarding civility, social capital, and trust (Curley 2010; Watson et al. 2021; Williamson 2002). Reciprocity has constituted sociality by fostering prosocial behavior (Thielmann et al. 2020). Republicanism upholds sociality regarding citizenship, the commonweal, interdependence, morality, nationalism, publicity, responsibility, social adaptation, and solidarity (Delanty 2009; Honohan 2002). The rule of law represents norms for civilization, harmony, and government quality to nurture sociality (Rivera-Batiz 2002; van Krieken 2019; Yu et al. 2010). Civilization constitutes sociality by establishing civility, loyalty, social contact, and social identification (Collins 2001; Hudson 2023). Harmony perceived has fostered sociality characterized by adjustment, attunement, civility, compromise, connectedness, interdependency, order, peace, relatedness, respect, sacrifice, selflessness, solidarity, and sympathy as opposed to competition and conflict (Arat and Kerelian 2019; Cheung and Ma 2011; P. Ip 2014; Kjell et al. 2016; Peck 2002; G. Zhang 2006). The norm for governance quality can secure citizenship and social cohesion and prevent conflict, fragmentation, and threats experienced to install sociality (Bukenya and Golooba-Mutebi 2020; Rhodes-Purdy et al. 2021; Tang 1998; Taylor-Gooby 1991).

The rule of law features norms for accommodation, altruism, caring, citizenship, the commonweal, compassion, compliance, connection, conscientiousness, education, forgiving, friendship, honesty, humanity or humaneness, interdependence, life, love, loyalty, opportunity, peace, relatedness, respect, sociability, stability, and trustworthiness to uplift sociality (Ashworth 2006; Bianchi 2016; Bix 2023; Cotterrell 2018; Crowe 2009; Feldman 2018; Ratnapala 2013; Shaw 2020; Shen and Price 2014; Zeng 2021). Accommodation can sustain sociality by raising loving (Aron et al. 2006). Moreover, accommodation experienced has constituted sociality by strengthening cooperation and preventing suicide (Duberstein et al. 2004; Lepkowski and Couper 2002). Altruism has constituted sociality by boosting attachment, civic engagement, friendship quality, likability, moral behavior, popularity, relatedness and diminishing loneliness and violence (Bond and Kwan 2000; W. Chen et al. 2022; Layous et al. 2012; Markiewicz et al. 2001; Martela and Ryan 2016; Mesch 2009; Na and Paternoster 2019; L. Taylor et al. 2018; Wright and Li 2011). The norm for caring has supported sociality by enhancing civic engagement, community favor, government trust, political participation, and recourse and dampening violence (Z. Han et al. 2017; F. Lee 2012; Palmer et al. 2011; Pulkkinen et al. 2009; Su and Feng 2013; Whitham 2012). Citizenship underlies sociality regarding confidence in public institutions (Vera-Toscano et al. 2013). The commonweal has constituted sociality by strengthening leadership and neighboring (Dubois et al. 2020; Grannis 2009). Compassion has underlain sociality by securing religiosity and volunteering (Barr et al. 2005). Connection or relatedness has consolidated sociality by consolidating sharing, social interaction, and relationship satisfaction (Downie et al. 2008; Frazer 1999; Wickham and Knee 2012). Conscientiousness has elevated sociality by consolidating attachment, compliance, order value, responsibility, social desirability, and volunteering and reducing deviance, violence, and justification for unconventional sexuality (Bekkers 2005; de Jong et al. 2012; Fraley et al. 2011; Gotzsche-Astrup 2020; Mondak and Hurwitz 2012; Mullet et al. 2005; Saucier and Skrzypinska 2006; Twardawski et al. 2021; Wright and DeLisi 2016). The norm for education has fostered sociality by boosting civic participation, government and social trust, social capital, volunteering, and xenophobia and dampening violence (Cohen and Bolt 2005; Lipford and Yandle 2009; Portes and Vickstrom 2011; Poveda 2011; Rupasingha et al. 2006; Uslaner and Brown 2005). Forgiving has consolidated sociality by raising government trust (Choi and David

2012). The norm for friendship has consolidated sociality by reducing protesting (Sampson et al. 2005). Honesty has built sociality by raising compliance and prosocial behavior and eschewing crime (Jolley et al. 2019; Thielmann et al. 2020; Twardawski et al. 2021). Humanity or humanness has enhanced sociality by activating political participation (Foschi and Lauriola 2014). Interdependence has buttressed sociality by securing attachment, donation, prosocial behavior, social inclusion, and social interaction (Feeney and Collins 2001; Uskul et al. 2004; Z. Xin et al. 2017). Living or survival can develop sociality by engendering morality (Narvaez 2014). Love sustains sociality by enhancing adaptation and dampening aloneness, conflict, and loneliness (Jeffries 2000; Rokach 2019; Sanderson 2001; Soble 2008). Loyalty has constituted sociality by fostering collaboration, empathy, generosity, leadership, and morality (Lawler et al. 2016; Lee and Chan 2016; Wilcox and Dew 2016). Opportunity has advanced sociality by enhancing cohesion, commitment received, and political participation (Bonaiuto et al. 1999; Emler and Frazer 1999; Q. Xu et al. 2018). Peace has fostered sociality characterized by adjustment, attunement, civility, compromise, connectedness, interdependency, order, peace, relatedness, respect, sacrifice, selflessness, solidarity, and sympathy as opposed to competition and conflict (Arat and Kerelian 2019; Cheung and Ma 2011; P. Ip 2014; Kjell et al. 2015; Peck 2002; G. Zhang 2006). Respect constitutes sociality regarding caring and equality (Renger and Reese 2017). Sociability has enhanced sociality by raising civic engagement, civility, political participation, prosocial behavior, and social cohesion (Foschi and Lauriola 2014; Letki 2008). The norm for stability has propped sociality, including civic engagement, cohesion, neighboring, and relational quality, as opposed to violence (Pulkkinen et al. 2009; C. Ross et al. 2000; Swaroop and Morenoff 2006; Villarreal and Silva 2006). Trustworthiness underlies sociality by establishing attachment, intimacy, social capital, and trust (X. Chen et al. 2015; Harvey and Wenzel 2006).

Conversely, the rule of law can build on norms against anomie and violence (Galavis 2020). Anomie has impeded sociality by raising radicalism and support for violence (Troian et al. 2019). The norm for violence has weakened sociality by boosting antisocial behavior and victimization (Ehrensuft et al. 2003; Krahe 2013). Ideologically, the rule of law stands on norms against populism, postmodernism, and war to secure sociality (Bix 2023; Cotterrell 2018; van Krieken 2019). Populism has undermined sociality by provoking separatism (Norris and Inglehart 2019). Postmodernism dampens sociality by embracing individualism or individualization, resistance, self-sufficiency, and skepticism and dismissing coordination (Beardsworth 2011; Fine 2007; Harambam and Aupers 2015; Hollinger 2017; Zukin and Maguire 2004). Conversely, postmodernism rejects sociality by dismissing cohesion and coordination (Elliott 2003; Weissman 2000). The rule of law embraces norms against class or inequality, discrimination, bullying, domination, greed, harm, interference, and revenge to maintain sociality (Bianchi 2016; Bogart 2002; Deli 2020; Ratnapala 2013; Sabia and Bass 2017). The norm for inequality has impeded sociality by eroding social capital, support for redistribution and welfare, sympathy, trust, and volunteering (Busemeyer 2013; Hitlin and Harkness 2018; Lipford and Yandle 2009; Oishi et al. 2011; Portes and Vickstrom 2011). The norm for inequality has impeded sociality by eroding social capital, support for redistribution and welfare, sympathy, trust, and volunteering (Busemeyer 2013; Hitlin and Harkness 2018; Lipford and Yandle 2009; Oishi et al. 2011; Portes and Vickstrom 2011). Bullying has dampened sociality by raising aggressiveness, antisociality, blaming, conflict, crime and recidivism, hostility, and social rejection (Asendorpf et al. 2008; Morrison 2006; Del Bove et al. 2008; Vitaro et al. 2007). Conversely, bullying has impeded sociality by inhibiting agreeableness and morality (Del Bove et al. 2008; Scholte et al. 2009). Domination has impaired sociality by weakening social cohesion (E. Chan 2014). Meanwhile, domination experienced has worsened sociality by breeding violence (Felson and Outlaw 2007). Greed has hindered sociality by dampening prosocial behavior (Thielmann et al. 2020). Harm experienced has arisen from ideals for sexuality and weapon carrying to impair sociality (Krahe 2013; Wilcox 2002). Interference obstructs sociality by mispresenting kindness (Qin 2013). Revenge has impeded sociality by breeding radicalism (Stankov et al. 2018).

Time: Global Development

Time on a global scale represents global development generally and zeitgeist culturally (Puohiniemi and Verkasalo 2020). Remarkably, time or global development features individualization, neoliberalization, secularization, and urbanization (Cole et al. 2023; de Graaf et al. 2001; M. Smith et al. 2001). Time is likely to advance sociality by affording power, utility, ideals, and norms for sociality through the deterministic and voluntaristic mechanisms of analytical functionalism. These mechanisms activate empowering, incentivizing, framing, and standardizing for determinism and power realization, utility optimization, ideal calibration, and norm conformity for voluntarism.

Power for sociality rising with time has stemmed from friendliness, helpfulness, income, knowledge, prosociality, and survival (Beckfield 2004; Hamermesh 2019; Ramarajan et al. 2017; Singer et al. 1999; M. Smith et al. 2001). Friendliness has enabled sociality regarding prosocial behavior (Foschi and Lauriola 2014). Helpfulness or prosociality has constituted sociality by boosting attachment, civic engagement, friendship quality, likability, moral behavior, popularity, and relatedness and diminishing loneliness and violence (Bond and Kwan 2000; W. Chen et al. 2022; Layous et al. 2012; Markiewicz et al. 2001; Martela and Ryan 2016; Mesch 2009; Na and Paternoster 2019; L. Taylor et al. 2018; Wright and Li 2011). Income has upheld sociality by boosting civic engagement, community attachment and involvement, civic dutifulness, civility, conformity value, neighboring, political interest and participation, political and social trust, prosocial behavior, social capital, social integration, social interaction, social support received, social well-being, and volunteering (Bjornberg and Latta 2007; Chang 2009; Djupe and Lewis 2015; Frei et al. 2009; Kerrissey and Schofer 2013; Letki 2006; McCabe 2014; Patulny and Morris 2012; Son and Wilson 2012; Sun and Wang 2012; Swaroop and Morenoff 2006; Ulbig 2002). Conversely, income has maintained sociality by dampening alienation, discrimination experienced, migration, protesting, relocation, social deprivation experienced, social exclusion experienced, victimization, and violence (Broom et al. 2013; Brown and Connell 2004; Buck 2001; Rijken and Groenewegen 2008; V. Taylor et al. 2009; Weakliem and Borch 2006). Knowledge has maintained sociality by facilitating civic engagement, civility, community involvement, compliance, cooperation, intimacy, leadership, marital satisfaction, political interest participation, politician favor, prosocial behavior, social cohesion, social trust, unification support, volunteering, and xenophobia (Barker and Tinnick 2006; de Groot and Steg 2009; Hunter et al. 2013; Kentmen 2010; Lepkowski and Couper 2002; Mikulincer et al. 2003; Moore et al. 2017; Norris 2011; Pattie et al. 2004; Rose and Pettersen 2000; Sarkheyli et al. 2012; Simon-Bemd and Steffens 2000; Stokman et al. 2013; Volker et al. 2007; Wernet et al. 2005). Survival can sustain morality and social commitment to uplift sociality (Narvaez 2014; Ogolsky and Monk 2018)

Conversely, power against sociality declining with time has resided in anomie or normlessness, poverty, and unemployment (Bulmahn 2000; Dekkers 2008; Francesconi and Golsch 2005). Anomie or normlessness has impeded sociality by raising radicalism and support for violence (Troian et al. 2019). Poverty has undermined sociality by reducing civic participation, trust, social connection, and volunteering (Caputo 2010; Stephens et al. 2014; R. Walker et al. 2010). Unemployment has impeded sociality by dissolving social capital, social cohesion, and trust (Espvall and Dellgren 2008; Manturuk et al. 2010; Reeskens and Vandecasteele 2017).

Utility for sociality rising with time has resided in financial satisfaction, justice perceived, relational quality, safety, and welfare satisfaction (Hsieh 2002; Logan and Cobb 2013; Malahy et al. 2009; Y. Wong et al. 2010). Financial or welfare satisfaction has upheld sociality by diminishing hostility (Rhodes-Purdy et al. 2023). Justice perceived has warranted sociality regarding civility, cooperation, community identification, political participation, and social trust as opposed to protesting (A. Hu 2013; Lawrence and Daniels 1997; Sunshine and Tyler 2003; Tyler and Degoey 1995; van Prooijen et al. 2008; Wenzel 2000). Relational quality has consolidated sociality by raising sharing, social interaction, and relationship satisfaction (Downie et al. 2008; Frazer 1999; Wickham and Knee 2012). Safety has buttressed sociality regarding civility, social capital, and trust (Curley 2010; Watson et al. 2021; Williamson 2002).

Conversely, disutility against sociality diminishing with time has resided in fear and threat (M. Smith et al. 2001; Sahar 2008). Fear has disrupted sociality by breeding interpersonal problems, loneliness, risking, suicide, and violence (Dutton et al. 2016; Gillath et al. 2005; Pulkkinen et al. 2009; Trumbo et al. 2008). Conversely, fear has undermined sociality by reducing donation, friendship, humor, political participation, prosocial behavior, and social well-being (Best and Krueger 2010; Hewstone et al. 2005; Litman et al. 2017; Kuiper and Nicholl 2004; Zhong 2010). Threats experienced have inhibited sociality by reducing cohesion and triggering conflict and resistance (Lubbers et al. 2006; B. Rick et al. 2006).

Ideals for sociality rising with time have favored birth, cohesion, conservatism, neighboring, security, social interaction, traditionalism, trust , volunteering, and working (Adsera 2003; de Beer and Kostere 2009; Gershuny 2000; Pazhoohi and Kingstone 2021; Puohiniemi and Verkasalo 2020; Saracino 2010; M. Smith et al. 2001). Birth has raised sociality by enhancing civic engagement, community involvement, conformism, donation, social capital, social cohesion, social integration, social interaction, social support received, and volunteering (Apinunmahakul and Devlin 2008; Bjornberg and Ekbrand 2008; Frei et al. 2009; Ghimire 2021a; Kleinhans et al. 2007; Magdol and Bessel 2003; Taniguichi and Thomas 2011; Wilkinson 2008; Xiao 2000; Xu and Lai 2002). Cohesion has constituted sociality by enhancing attachment and dampening tolerance for deviance (Stafford et al. 2005; Woosnam et al. 2018). Conservatism sustains sociality by nurturing empathy, loyalty, prosocial behavior, religiousness, and sacrifice (Dutton and Rayner-Hilles 2022). Moreover, conservatism underpins sociality by maintaining allegiance or loyalty, attachment, civility, community, conformity, cooperation, discipline, ethnocentrism, honesty, humility, intimacy, legality, morality, nationalism, obedience, order, partnership, patriotism, peace, responsibility, sharing, trust, and xenophobia (Dutton and Rayner-Hilles 2022; Heilman and Kusev 2020; Hickson 2013; Lakoff 2009; Rhodes-Purdy et al. 2023; Scruton 2014; Yoos 2007; Zuk and Zuk 2020). Conversely, conservatism upholds sociality by condemning dehumanizing, evilness, revolution, sexuality, terrorism, and transgression (Dutton and Rayner-Hilles 2022; Malka and Soto 2011; Scruton 2014; Suhay 2015). Neighboring has elevated sociality by raising consulting and influencing (Hays and Kogl 2007). The ideal for security fosters sociality by signifying cohesion, community, harmony, propriety or ritualism, and security or protection (C. Chung 2000; Heckscher 2015; P. Ip 2014; McGhee 2003; Peng 2003). Furthermore, the ideal for security constitutes sociality by espousing civility, cohesion, commitment, compliance, cooperation, harmony, protection, social interaction, and solidarity (Arat and Kerelian 2019; Kaurin 2020; Lawler et al. 2009; McGhee 2003; Mondak and Hurwitz 2012; Qin 2013). As such, the security ideal has upheld sociality by dampening deviance and its tolerance (Gibson 2013; Wright and DeLisi 2016). Social interaction has realized sociality by consolidating altruism, compliance, cooperation, donation, morality, political participation, reciprocity, social trust, and volunteering (Guillen et al. 2011; Dixon and McKeown 2021; Lucas and Livingston 2014; Musick 2000; Rodrigo-Gonzalez et al. 2019; Rubin and Step 2000). Traditionalism in community involvement upholds dependency, dutifulness, groupness, loyalty, obedience, order, and religiosity to foster sociality (Heckscher 2015). Trust has constituted sociality through donation, involvement, and volunteering (Uslaner 2000). Volunteering has constituted sociality by raising altruism, charity orientation, civic motivation, donation, helping, moral responsibility, political participation, social integration, and social and government trust (Foster et al. 2001; Isham et al. 2006; Richey 2010; Richey and Ikeda 2009; Wiepking and Maas 2009). Working has facilitated sociality by elevating civic engagement, community involvement, donation, philanthropy value, political discussion, political participation, social capital, social functioning, social cohesion experienced, social interaction, and social trust (Anciaes et al. 2017; Fridberg and Kangas 2008b; Kerrissey and Schofer 2013; H. Lu et al. 2002; Ross and Mirowsky 2009; Tsai 2006).

Conversely, ideals against sociality declining with time have hailed capitalism, liberalism, mobility, protesting, religiosity, resistance, violence, and war (Bjornskov and Paldam 2012; Brynin et al. 2009; Cheung and Yip 2010; Kaufmann et al.

2012; Norris and Inglehart 2009; Pinker 2011; Sahar 2008). The ideal for capitalism impedes sociality by boosting narcissism and disrupting mutuality (De Vos 2010; Young and Reynolds 2017). Moreover, the ideal for capitalism undermines sociality by embracing competition, conflict, and egoism (Bernstein 2012; S. Hall 2014; LaMothe 2012). Conversely, the ideal for capitalism weakens sociality by dispelling collectivism, reciprocity, socialism, and statism (Beardsworth 2011; Bernstein 2012). Liberalism has impeded sociality regarding morality, normativity, and social order (Feinberg et al. 2019). Mobility or relocation has impeded sociality by diminishing social integration (Kearns and Whitley 2015). Protesting has impaired sociality by escalating distancing and radicalism and dampening moral motivation (Kutlaca et al. 2020; Vestergren et al. 2017). Religiosity has hindered sociality by reducing nationalism, social interaction and engendering protesting, marginalization experienced, radicalism, and social distance (Ayalon et al. 1993; Kunovich 2009; Norris 2002; Pedahzur and Canetti-Nisim 2004; Wuthnow 2004). Resistance has impaired sociality by eroding solidarity and fomenting deviance (Foy et al. 2014; J. Williams 2011). Violence has undermined sociality by breeding antisociality, crime and recidivism, blaming, conflict, hostility, rejecting others, and impairing agreeableness, morality, and responsibility (Asendorpf et al. 2008; Del Bove et al. 2008; Morrison 2006; Scholte et al. 2009; Vitaro et al. 2007). War dampens sociality by triggering crime and religiousness (Immerzeel and van Tubergen 2013; Reiner 2016).

Norms for sociality rising with time have propagated human development, prosperity, social integration, survival or life expectancy, sympathy, and welfare (Hamermesh 2019; Lee and Coleman 2014; Norris 2012). The norm for human development has maintained donation, legalism, and social trust to secure sociality (Fridberg and Kangas 2008b). The norm for prosperity has uplifted sociality by raising government support, nationalism, political participation, relationship quality, trust, volunteering, and xenophobia (Cheng and Smyth 2016; Fridberg and Kangas 2008; Inglehart 2003; Rhodes-Purdy et al. 2023; Traunmuller 2011; van Oorschot and Arts 2005). Social integration has constituted sociality by strengthening cooperation and preventing suicide (Duberstein et al. 2004; Lepkowski and Couper 2002). Survival can sustain morality and social commitment to uplift sociality (Narvaez 2014; Ogolsky and Monk 2018). Sympathy has constituted sociality by securing religiosity and volunteering (Barr et al. 2005). The norm for welfare has uplifted sociality by advancing neighboring, political participation, social capital, support for social welfare, and volunteering and diminishing migration and theft (Allard and Danziger 2000; J. Brown 2016; Musick and Wilson 2008; Portes and Vickstrom 2011; Rehm et al. 2012; Semino 2015). Ideologically, norms for sociality rise with time to propagate Christianity and humanism (Lemon 2003). Christianity has buttressed sociality by securing conformity, donation, and morality and impeding cosmopolitanism (Hollinger 2017; Phillips and Smith 2008). Humanism bolsters sociality by highlighting attachment, caring, collectivity, community, cooperation, friendship, helpfulness, institutions, loving, order, respect, relatedness, responsibility, and sharing (Browning and Cooper 2004; Fuchs 2020; Selznick 2008; Stefanski and Jach 2022; Visher 1997; Waterman 2013). Conversely, humanism sustains sociality by rejecting alienation, conflict, and individualization (Fuchs 2020; Selznick 2008).

Conversely, norms against sociality declining with time have dwelled on conflict, independence, and inequality (Diez-Nicolas 2002; Lange and Dawson 2009). The norm for conflict has impaired sociality by fomenting protesting and resistance (Schatzman 2005; Sorens 2011). Independence has impeded sociality by reducing justification for the system and the norm for legitimacy (Blanchar and Eidelman 2013). The norm for inequality has obstructed sociality by eroding social capital, support for redistribution and welfare, sympathy, trust, and volunteering (Busemeyer 2013; Hitlin and Harkness 2018; Lipford and Yandle 2009; Oishi et al. 2011; Portes and Vickstrom 2011).

Current Findings

Waves 5 and 6 World Values Survey data shows that time or the survey wave represented global development through correlations with national performance: population size ($r = .047$) and per capita phone subscription ($r = -\ .052$), land ($r = -\ .026$), technology publication ($r = .032$), bank credit ($r = .069$), prosperity ($r = .075$), income inequality ($r = .050$), globalization ($r = .142$), government effectiveness ($r = .044$), democracy ($r = .025$), liberty ($r = .034$), human development ($r = .136$), human capital ($r = .062$), carbon dioxide emission ($r = .041$), and rule of law ($r = -\ .042$). Hence, national performance grew with time, except for the land share and the rule of law. Nevertheless, the correlations were very weak, except for that with human development, suggesting relative independence between national and global development as indicated by time. This independence reflected the variation in performance across nations at the same time.

Regression analysis exhibited the effects of global and national performances on personal sociality from Step 1 to Step 5 of the analysis. Step 1 solely showed the time or global performance effect. Step 2 added national performances as predictors. Steps 3 to 5 additionally entered personal characteristics, national norms, and personal experiences as predictors to reveal the effects of national performance net of the added effects. The analysis applied stepwise selection to retain significant effects. Most national and time or global effects were significant in expected ways (see Table 6.1).

Confidence in institutions received a moderate positive effect from national population size and weak negative effects ($\beta = .255$, see Table 6.2) from national democracy and land per capita ($\beta = -\ .103$ to $-\ .142$). The effect of national globalization on confidence in institutions, albeit significant, was negligible ($\beta = -\ .028$). The time effect was nonsignificant initially ($\beta = .004$). Nevertheless, it became significantly positive after controlling for national and personal predictors ($\beta = .111$). This net effect on confidence in institutions revealed the contribution of global development that did not pass through national and personal development.

Justification for misdeeds declined with time ($\beta = -\ .060$, see Table 6.3). Besides time or global development, national inequality and technology manifested positive weak effects on justification for misdeeds ($\beta = .202$ to $.130$). The effects of

Table 6.1 Expected and actual effects of national performance on sociality

Predictor	Expected	Actual						
		Institution	Anti-misdeed	Anti-sex	Anti-faith	Anti-outsider	Anti-deviant	Other
Wave	+		+		+	+	–	
Population	+	+		+	+	–		
Phone	+							
Land	–	–				–		
Technology	+		–		+		+	
Credit	+		+		+		–	
Prosperity	+						+	
Inequality	–		–	–		+	+	
Globalization	–	–				+		
Government effectiveness	+							+
Democracy	–				–	–		
Liberty	–		+	–				
Human development	+				+			–
Human capital	+			–				
CO_2	–		–					
Rule of law	–							

Note. Sociality unfolded in social attitudes in terms of confidence in institutions, refutation against misdeeds, refutation against unconventional sexuality, unfaith in religion, rejection of outsiders, rejection of deviants, and trust in others
+ positive effect. – negative effect

Table 6.2 Significant ($p < .001$) standardized effects of national performance on confidence in institutions

Predictor	(1)	(2)	(3)	(4)	(5)
Wave 6 vs. Wave 5	.004n	– .002n	.084	.112	.111
National population		.255	.236	.222	.223
National democracy		– .142	– .227	– .287	– .257
National land		– .103	– .073	– .107	– .092
National globalization		– .028	.100	.060	.047
R^2	.000	.163	.364	.386	.401

n: $p > .001$

national liberty, bank credit, and CO_2 emission on the justification were slight, albeit significant.

Justification for unconventional sexuality received a moderate positive effect from natural human capital ($\beta = .362$, see Table 6.4). By contrast, national population size displayed a weak negative effect on the justification ($\beta = -.124$). The effects of national liberty and income inequality on the justification were slight, albeit significant.

Faith in religion declined with time ($\beta = -.130$, see Table 6.5). Besides time or global development, national democracy demonstrated a strong positive effect on faith in religion ($\beta = .397$). By contrast, national technology displayed a moderate negative effect on religious faith ($\beta = -.346$). Besides, national population size, bank credit, and human development unfolded weak negative effects on religious faith ($\beta = -.102$ to $-.181$).

Acceptance of outsiders diminished with time ($\beta = -.071$, see Table 6.6). Besides time or global development, national globalization exhibited a moderate negative effect on such acceptance ($\beta = -.284$). By contrast, national democracy displayed a weak positive effect on this acceptance ($\beta = .234$). Besides, the effects of national

Table 6.3 Significant ($p < .001$) standardized effects of national performance on justification for misdeeds

Predictor	(1)	(2)	(3)	(4)
Wave 6 vs. Wave 5	– .050	– .060	– .011n	– .006n
National income inequality		.202	.189	.192
National technology		.130	.153	.165
National liberty		– .074	– .121	– .129
National CO_2 emission		.067	.106	.113
National bank credit		– .060	– .044	– .042
R^2	.002	.021	.062	.069

n: $p > .001$

Table 6.4 Significant ($p < .001$) standardized effects of national performance on justification for unconventional sexuality

Predictor	(1)	(2)	(3)	(4)	(5)
Wave 6 vs. Wave 5	− .013n	− .037	− .009n	.042	.039
National human capital		.362	.300	.308	.310
National liberty		.069	.120	.060	.067
National population		− .124	− .169	− .153	− .156
National income inequality		.090	.116	.119	.118
R^2	.000	.180	.238	.275	.280

n: $p > .001$

Table 6.5 Significant ($p < .001$) standardized effects of national performance on faith in religion

Predictor	(1)	(2)	(3)	(4)	(5)
Wave 6 vs. Wave 5	− .130	− .115	− .102	− .125	− .126
National bank credit		− .121	.033	.004	.002
National democracy		.397	.134	.076	.080
National technology		− .346	− .210	− .119	− .118
National population		− .181	− .125	− .044	− .040
National human development		− .102	− .015	.055	.056
R^2	.017	.385	.524	.544	.550

n: $p > .001$

population size, income inequality, and land on this acceptance were slight, albeit significant.

Acceptance of deviants grew with time ($\beta = .075$, see Table 6.7). Besides time or global development, national prosperity indicated a moderate negative effect on such acceptance ($\beta = -.284$). By contrast, national bank credit displayed a weak

Table 6.6 Significant ($p < .001$) standardized effects of national performance on acceptance of outsiders

Predictor	(1)	(2)	(3)	(4)	(5)
Wave 6 vs. Wave 5	− .071	− .037	.022	.041	.042
National globalization		− .284	− .217	− .126	− .121
National democracy		.234	.189	.181	.180
National population		.086	.058	.017n	.019n
National income inequality		− .052	− .090	− .046	− .047
National land		.024	.060	− .032	− .032
R^2	.005	.111	.166	.182	.188

n: $p > .001$

positive effect on this acceptance ($\beta = .185$). Besides, the effects of national income inequality and technology on this acceptance were slight, albeit significant.

Trust in others received a moderate positive effect from national government effectiveness ($\beta = .251$, see Table 6.8). By contrast, national human development indicated a negative weak effect on trust in others ($\beta = -.198$).

Effects that contradicted expectations were those of national technology and liberty on refutation against misdeeds, national human capital on refutation against unconventional sexuality, national population size, inequality, and globalization on the rejection of outsiders, national bank credit, inequality, and time on the rejection of deviants, and national human development on trust in others. These contradictory effects were explicable with force theory as a higher-level explanation focusing on forces transmitted from the input and accepted by the outcome. When the forces are consonant, a positive effect holds, and vice versa. These forces cover power, utility, ideals, and norms for transmitting and receiving sociality and others.

Contrary to expectation, refutation against misdeeds received a negative effect from national technology. This negative effect is due to the clash between the forces of national technology and refutation against misdeeds. On the one hand, national technology rests on the forces of anti-humanism, Bohemianism, and liberalism (Florida 2005; Matthewman 2011; G. Sun 2019). On the other hand, refutation against misdeeds stands on the forces of anti-liberalism, conscientiousness,

Table 6.7 Significant ($p < .001$) standardized effects of national performance on acceptance of deviants

Predictor	(1)	(2)	(3)	(4)
Wave 6 vs. Wave 5	.075	.094	.154	.162
National prosperity		– .360	– .370	– .372
National bank credit		.185	.227	.239
National income inequality		– .061	– .076	– .074
National technology		– .058	– .031	– .023n
R^2	.008	.090	.182	.192

n: $p > .001$

Table 6.8 Significant ($p < .001$) standardized effects of national performance on trust in others

Predictor	(1)	(2)	(3)	(4)	(5)
Wave 6 vs. Wave 5	– .009n	.007n	.001n	– .003n	– .003n
National government effectiveness		.251	.225	.221	.219
National human development		– .198	– .184	– .184	– .181
R^2	.000	.020	.039	.040	.042

n: $p > .001$

conservatism, humanism, humanitarianism, regulation, responsibility, and temperance (Boer and Fischer 2013; N. Duncan 2017; McCaffoee 2016; Narvaez 2014; Rosler and Branscombe 2020; Stichter 2018; Warburton 2005).

Contrary to expectation, refutation against misdeeds received a positive effect from national liberty. This positive effect is due to the compatibility between the forces of national liberty and refutation against misdeeds. National education embraces the forces of education and the rule of law (Bogart 2002; C. Martin 2020). Likewise, refutation against misdeeds stands on the forces of education and legality (de Jonge 2012; Stavrova and Siegers 2014).

Contrary to expectation, refutation against unconventional sexuality received a negative effect from national liberty. This negative effect is due to the clash between the forces of national liberty and refutation against unconventional sexuality. On the one hand, national liberty espouses the forces of change, homosexuality, prostitution, and radicalism and downplays the force of the establishment (Cole et al. 2023; Fein 2015; Norrander and Wilcox 2001; Vicente 2016; Wilson 2007). On the other hand, refutation against unconventional sexuality safeguards the forces of conservatism, heterosexuality, normativity, regulation, and tradition and denounces the forces of homosexuality, prostitution, and unconventionality (Conde Dias et al. 2012; de Jong et al. 2012; Jackson and Scott 2010; Kirsch 2000; Primoratz 1999; Rival et al. 1998; Soble 2008; Swami et al. 2017).

Contrary to expectation, refutation against unconventional sexuality received a negative effect from national human capital. This negative effect is due to the clash between the forces of national human capital and refutation against unconventional sexuality. On the one hand, human capital furnishes or stands on the forces of individualism and sexuality (Beauvais and Higham 2016; C. Liu 2000). On the other hand, refutation against unconventional sexuality downplays the forces of self-determination and sexuality (Jackson and Scott 2010; Shim 2001).

Contrary to expectation, rejection of outsiders received a negative effect from national population size. This negative effect is due to the clash between the forces of national population size and the rejection of outsiders. On the one hand, population size dismisses the forces of cohesion and participation and breeds the forces of conflict, crime, and revolution (S. Cho et al. 2013; Coffe and Geys 2006; Collier and Hoeffler 2004; Fridberg and Kangas 2008b; Yagci 2017). On the other hand, rejection of outsiders or xenophobia stands on the forces of assimilation, community, conformity, groupism, homogeneity, localism, nationalism, participation, and patriotism and dismisses the forces of conflict and multiculturalism (Amin 2012; Elias and Feagin 2016; Greve 2019; Macedo 2021; Marotta 2017; Zienkowski 2017).

Contrary to expectation, the rejection of outsiders received a positive effect from national inequality. This positive effect is due to the compatibility between the forces of national inequality and the rejection of outsiders. National inequality stands on the forces of conservatism, exclusion, hierarchy, and sacrifice and rejects the forces of friction, multiculturalism, protest, and struggle (Baldus 2017; R. Brown 2017; Chandler 2023; Diefenbach 2013; Dodson 2016; Fein 2012; Sun 2011; S. White 2007). Similarly, rejection of outsiders or xenophobia cherishes the forces of authoritarianism, cohesion, conformity, conservatism, cooperation, differentiation, exclusion, dominance, favoritism, hierarchy, nationalism, status, subordination, superiority and opposes the forces of multiculturalism (Amin 2012; de Figueiredo and Elins 2003; Elias and Feagin 2016; Greve 2019; Husband and Alam 2011; Jolly and DiGiusto 2014; Licata and Klein 2002; Nijs et al. 2022; Norris and Inglehart 2019; Sidanius and Kurzban 2013; Wojcieszak and Garrett 2018; Zienkowski 2017). Most pertinently, xenophobia embraces the force of inequality (Dunn et al. 2004).

Contrary to expectation, the rejection of outsiders received a positive effect from national globalization. This positive effect is due to the compatibility between the forces of national globalization and the rejection of outsiders. National globalization displays the forces of commonality, conservatism, cooperation, homogenization, inequality, peace, and security and refutes the forces of antagonism and war (Axford 2013; Brady et al. 2007; Dryzek 2006; Meszaros 2015; Milner 2020; Roberts and Lamp 2021; Sandel 2020). Essentially, rejection of outsiders or xenophobia arises from the force of globalization (Marotta 2017). Moreover, rejection of outsiders or xenophobia embraces the forces of assimilation, cohesion, conformity, conservatism, cooperation, groupism, hierarchy, homogeneity, inequality, superiority, and unity and resists the forces of confrontation, diversity, multiculturalism, oppression, and pluralism (Amin 2012; Burchianti and Zapata-Barrero 2014; Dunn et al. 2004; Elias and Feagin 2016; Feinberg et al. 2012; Hartmann et al. 2017; Jolly and DiGiusto 2014; Olatunji and Adamis 2025; Pride 2000; Szekeres et al. 2019; Uygur et al. 2024; Zienkowski 2017).

Contrary to expectation, the rejection of deviants received a negative effect from national bank credit. This negative effect is due to the clash between the forces of national bank credit and the rejection of deviants. On the one hand, national bank credit or financialization espouses the forces of autonomy, deregulation, freedom, and individuality and withholds the force of regulation (Barthold 2018; Haiven 2014). On the other hand, the rejection of deviants cherishes the forces of attachment, bonding, communitarianism, compliance, conformity, consensus, control, cooperation, discipline, regulation, self-control, and social integration (S. Henry 2009; Herman-Kinney 2003; Iacobucci and Frieh 2018; Kaplan et al. 2013; Vauclair and Fischer 2011; J. Williams 2011; Wright and DeLisi 2016; Y. Yau 2014).

Contrary to expectation, the rejection of deviants received a positive effect from national inequality. This positive effect is due to the compatibility between the forces of national inequality and the rejection of deviants. Crucially, national inequality rejects the force of deviation, disintegration, or separation (Suchweh 2012). Furthermore, national inequality exhibits the force of self-enhancement and abandons the forces of individualism, individualization, and protest (Diefenbach 2013; Dodson 2016; Uslaner 2002; Wilkinson and Pickett 2017). Likewise, rejection of deviants treasures the forces of attachment, bonding, communitarianism, compliance, conformity, and social integration and resists the forces of rebellion, resistance, and self-derogation (S. Henry 2009; Herman-Kinney 2003; Kaplan et al. 2013; J. Williams 2011; Wright and DeLisi 2016; Y. Yau 2014).

Contrary to expectation, the rejection of deviants received a negative effect from time or global development. This negative effect is due to the clash between the forces of time and the rejection of deviants. On the one hand, time displays the forces of disconnection, individualization, liberalization, radicalism, and social exclusion and withholds the forces of conformity, control, government, social capital, social integration, and suicide (S. Chang et al. 2009; de Graaf et al. 2001; Demant and de Graaf 2010; Grenier and Wright 2006; Hertzog et al. 2019; Loftus 2001; Puohiniemi and Verkasalo 2020; McPherson et al. 2006; T. Smith 2005; Wang and You 2016). On the other hand, the rejection of deviants accepts the forces of attachment, bonding, community, compliance, control, discipline, governmentality, normativity, regulation, self-control, social integration and resists the forces of disintegration and resistance (S. Henry 2009; Herman-Kinney 2003; Iacobucci and Frieh 2018; Kaplan et al. 2013; J. Williams 2011; Wright and DeLisi 2016; Y. Yau 2014).

Contrary to expectation, trust in others received a negative effect from national human development. This negative effect is due to the clash between the forces of national human development and trust in others. On the one hand, national human development exhibits the forces of bargaining, conflict, precaution, privatization, regulation, struggle, and voicing and discounts the forces of communitarianism and tradition (Davis and Robinson 2006; Gautam 2021; Hoekstra 2019; Jakobsen 2010; C. Johnson 2009; Norris 2012; Quah 2003). On the other hand, trust in others embraces the forces of agreeableness, attachment, cohesion or cohesiveness, collaboration, collectivity, communitarianism, community, cooperation or cooperativeness, fraternity, openness, permissiveness, sharing, tolerance, and tradition and resists the forces of caution, conflict, obtrusion, self-culture, and surveillance (Abascal 2015; Burke and Stets 1999; Freitag and Bauer 2016; Jarvinen and Branders 2020; Kramer 1999; McCabe 2012; Miller and Mitamura 2003; Newton 1999; Rahn 2008; B. Six 2014; Taylor-Gooby 2005; Uslaner 2002; Vera-Toscano et al. 2013).

Contrary to the expectation for the positive effect, the rule of law failed to indicate an effect on any sociality indicators. This failure may reflect the neutralization of positive and negative effects. The negative effects have applied when the rule of law has raised control experienced, corruption perceived, and violence (You and Khagram 2005). Control experienced has worsened sociality by breeding violence (Felson and Outlaw 2007). Corruption perceived has impaired sociality regarding civic relatedness and social trust (Seligson 2005). Violence has undermined sociality by breeding antisociality, crime and recidivism, blaming, conflict, hostility, rejecting others, and impairing agreeableness, morality, and responsibility (Asendorpf et al. 2008; Del Bove et al. 2008; Morrison 2006; Scholte et al. 2009; Vitaro et al. 2007). Moreover, the rule of law conveys the forces of norms for individualization and liberty (Gowder 2016; Sorensen and Christiansen 2013). The norm for individualization inhibits sociality by featuring competition, deintegration, disembeddedness, disengagement, independence, inequality, risk, and self-indulgence (Bauman 2001; Beck and Beck-Gernsheim 2002; Burgess 2018; Dannreuther and Perren 2013; Krys et al. 2019; Stankov et al. 2014). The norm for liberaty impairs sociality by dismissing punishment (Vicente 2016). Meanwhile, sociality resists the force of individualism and accepts the force of coercion (Fowers 2015; Tuomela 2007).

Chapter 7
Functioning of Superpowers for Social Attitudes

China and the United States of America are two global superpowers whose impacts on social attitudes are noteworthy. These attitudes are confidence in institutions, refutations against misdeeds and unconventional sexuality, unfaith in religion, rejection of outsiders and deviants, and trust in other people. Essentially, they represent sociality featuring altruism, attachment, bonding, caring, community, conformity, conscientiousness, conservation, consulting, cooperation, extraversion, fairness or justice, friendship, gifting, gregariousness, group focus, group membership, guilt, helping, honesty, honoring, imitation, institutionalism, laughter, leadership, learning, liking, morality, networking, normativity, organization, participation, punishment, rapport, reciprocity, relatedness, role-taking, self-expansion, shame, sharing, social interaction, socialization, socializing, sympathy, support, teaching, togetherness, trust, trustworthiness, and xenophobia (Boer and Fischer 2013; Capraro 2024; Cottrell et al. 2007; Christophers et al. 2020; Fenwick 2008; Fowers 2015; Hughes et al. 2017; Koster 2013; M. Ma 2021; Marres 2017; Provine 2000; Ratner et al. 2023; Rogers et al. 2014; Tomasello 2014). Conversely, sociality dismisses aggression, defection, individualism, independence, misanthropy, privatization, risking, self-interest, stealing, and violence (Bissell 2010; Christophers et al. 2020; Fowers 2015; Hughes et al. 2017; Schinkel 2010; Tuomela 2007). Intrinsically, sociality represents friendship, humanity, morality, and sociotropy (de Vries and Megathlin 2009; Fowers 2015; Marres 2017). Extinsically, sociality benefits institutionalization, morality, socializability, solidarity, and well-being (Fenwick 2008; Ratner et al. 2023; Sunar 2009; Tuomela 2007). Meanwhile, China and the United States are global superpowers (Kachiga 2021; Rollo 2023). China's superpower transpires in its putative global colonialization, competition, disruption, entanglement, globalization, growth or rise, hegemony, share, and threat (Evans 2006; 2009; Kachiga 2021; Kang 2005; Lai and Tao 2006; Meng 2011; X. Qi 2013; Yu and Chiu 2016). Similarly, the United States's superpower unfolds in its alleged global Americanization, expansionism, imperialism or imperium, intervention, mass, militarism, share, and triumphalism (Narayan 2020; Nowlin and Stupak 1998; Rollo 2023; Speth 2012; F. Wang 2024).

C.-k. Cheung, *Social Attitudes in the Early 21st Century*,
https://doi.org/10.1007/978-981-96-9705-2_7

Existing Knowledge

China and the United States are likely to sustain higher sociality than others with the deterministic and voluntaristic mechanisms of analytical functionalism. These mechanisms employ power, utility, ideals, and norms to run empowering, incentivizing, framing, and standardizing for determinism and power realization, utility optimization, ideal calibration, and norm conformity for voluntarism. These mechanisms achieve the requisite functions of fulfillment or goal attainment, adaptation, latency, and integration underlying sociality. Particularly, integration by norms from communal or community, cultural or culture, and political or polity realms is remarkable.

China

China features differential order, networking, and parenting in terms of guanxi communally; Buddhism, collectivism, Confucianism, dialecticism, nationalism, patriotism, relationism, socialism, and traditionalism culturally; and authoritarianism, education, globalization, harmony, peace, pragmatism, and realism politically (X. Chen et al. 2005; Gao 2018; Genevaz 2019; Y. Hu 2005; Kachiga 2021; H. Li 2021; Miles and Wang 2018; F. Wang 2024; Willis and Guan 2009; Xiong et al. 2022; Zee 2022; S. Zhang 2003; Zhang and Mo 2005; Zhong 2009). Differential order in China means a preference for close relations (Y. Hu 2005). Guanxi relies on ethical, familial, geographical, and work-relatedness or similarity with flexibility and unclear boundaries (Y. Hu 2005). Moreover, guanxi can be asymmetric and extend beyond the core family and network (Zhong 2009). Parenting in China is coercive rather than affectionate, authoritative, and inductive (X. Chen et al. 2005). Buddhism in China exalts altruism, compassion, emptiness, forbearance, and transcendence (S. Zhang 2003). Collectivism in China boosts community, conformity, connection, cooperation, dependence, group interest, harmony, hierarchy, humility, loyalty, obedience, relatedness, responsiveness, simplicity, togetherness, as opposed to heroism and rights (Sun and Bitter 2012; Xiong et al. 2022). Confucianism or scholarism in China preaches benevolence, civility, classism, collectivism, deliberation, diligence, education, effort, familism, filiality, forgiveness, harmony, honesty, hierarchy, humanism, interdependence, learning, magnanimity, meritocracy, loyalty, male dominance, moderation, modesty, moralism, morality, order, peacefulness, persistence, propriety, quietness, rationalism, righteousness, ritual, self-consciousness, self-cultivation, statism, teamwork, virtue, and work as opposed to freedom and rights (S. Chan et al. 2022; Xiong et al. 2022). Dialecticism based on the Classic of Change extols balance, contradiction, dynamics in cycling, equality, fusion, harmony, hiddenness, holism, matching, moderation, morality, perseverance, self-discipline, softness, symmetry, and trustworthiness as opposed to arrogance, autonomy, independence, outstanding, pride, risking, and urgency (Spencer-Rodgers et al. 2009; Zhang and Mo 2005). Relationalism in China embraces collectivism, comparison, differential order, embeddedness, face, familism, heteronomy, interdependence, parentalism, promise, reciprocity, reighteousness, and shame as opposed to individualism, self-esteem, and self-reliance (D. Ho et al. 2006; Miles and Wang 2018). Socialism in China embodies construction, contribution, cooperation, equality, labor, mutuality, productivity, and win–win benefits as opposed to exploration and hegemony (Gao 2018; Y. Yang et al. 2014). Traditionalism preserves achievement, balance, benevolence, Buddhism, collectivism, and Confucianism. Daoism, empathy, face, Filiality, guanxi, harmony, Maoism, life, moderation, morality, naturalness, optimism, perfection, perseverance, propriety, self-control, self-discipline, stability, submission, thrift, tolerance, tranquility, and unity, as opposed to impulsivity (Gao 2018; Willis and Guan 2009). Authoritarianism or totalitarianism foregrounds bureaucracy, Confucianism, dictatorship, indoctrination, legality, militarism, nationalism, policing, and surveillance as opposed to civil society, democracy, and freedom (S. Lo 2021; Naftali 2021; F. Wang 2024). Education in China cultivates collectivism, differentiation, equalizing, gratitude, health, hierarchy, morality, and patriotism (Genevaz 2019). Globalization in China prioritizes complementarity, connectivity, coordination, facility, friendship, infrastructure, integration, investment, multilateralism, trade, and trust (Kachiga 2021; Zee 2022). Pragmatism in China treasures application, approximation, Confucianism, contradiction, flexibility, muddling, relationism, and syncretism (Kachiga 2021). Realism in China favors defense, force, materialism, power, security, and stability (Dai and Luqiu 2024; Kachiga 2021).

China generates power, utility, ideals, and norms to enhance sociality and effectiveness. According to the voluntaristic mechanism of analytical functionalism, effectiveness hinges on action based on commitment, persistence, and repetition (Schwirian et al. 2001). As such, effectiveness builds on power, utility, ideals, and norms for an action to activate the action. Power balancing is a notable mechanism of China's influence (Kachiga 2021).

Sociality

Power for sociality maintained by China has stemmed from reduced mortality risk (Lassey et al. 1997). Mortality risk can dampen sociality by fomenting aggression (Reeve 2021).

Ideals for sociality enhanced by China have favored civic engagement, cooperation, egalitarianism, familism, government and social trust, modesty, punishing, reciprocity, recourse, and volunteering (Buchan et al. 2002; Chen and Mak 2008; Hitlin and Harkness 2018; Houser and Xiao 2015; Y. Pan et al. 2023; Shin 2012; G. Walker et al. 2001; Wang and Han 2023; X. Wu 2009; Y. Zhou 2024). Civic engagement has propped sociality by strengthening attachment, civility, collective behavior, discussion, donation, neighboring, patriotism, prosociality, social capital, socialism, trust, and volunteering and impeding cheating and individualism (Coffe and Geys 2007; Gilberbloom and Markham 1995; Kerrissey and Schofer 2013; Mata and Pendakur 2014; Ozbay 2008; Pattie et al. 2004; Pena-Lopez and Sanchez-Santos 2016; Rahn 2008; Richey 2011; Tak 2017; M. Tang 2011; Taniguchi 2013; Yip et al. 2007). Cooperation has strengthened sociality regarding attachment and trustworthiness as opposed to argument (Gerbasi and Cook 2008; Hample 2018; Tak 2017). Egalitarianism has underpinned sociality by enhancing empathy, support for welfare, and trust in government and impeding radicalism (Faricy and Ellis 2014; Lauriola et al. 2015; Lucas and Kteily 2018; Roosma et al. 2014). Familism benefits sociality regarding the commonweal and community duty (Edwards and Gillies 2004). Government trust has constituted sociality by sustaining compliance, conformity, nationalism, political participation, and preventing protesting (Rhodes-Purdy et al. 2023; Ulbig 2002; van der Meer and van Ingen 2009; V. Vu 2021). Social trust has constituted sociality through donation, involvement, and volunteering (Uslaner 2000). Modesty has advanced sociality by enhancing altruism, connectedness, cooperation, egalitarianism, forgiveness, gratitude, perspective-taking, responsibility, and social evaluation as opposed to dominance and stigmatizing (Angelis and Pensini 2024; Bowes et al. 2022; Hilbig et al. 2013; Krumrei-Mancuso 2017; Ryu et al. 2023; Schmitt and Huyuh 2024). Punishing characterizes sociality (Fowers 2015). Reciprocity has constituted sociality by fostering prosocial behavior (Thielmann et al. 2020). Recourse reflects sociality regarding affiliation and social support received (Ledbetter et al. 2013; Sullivan 2001). Volunteering has constituted sociality by raising altruism, charity orientation, civic motivation, donation, helping, moral responsibility, political participation, social integration, and social and government trust (Foster et al. 2001; Isham et al. 2006; Richey 2010; Richey and Ikeda 2009; Wiepking and Maas 2009). Conversely, China has dampened ideals for liberalism and religiousness to buttress sociality (Shin 2012; Tang 2001). Liberalism has impeded sociality regarding morality, normativity, and social order (Feinberg et al. 2019). Religiousness has hindered sociality by reducing nationalism, social interaction and engendering protesting, marginalization experienced, radicalism, and social distance (Ayalon et al. 1993; Kunovich 2009; Norris 2002; Pedahzur and Canetti-Nisim 2004; Wuthnow 2004).

Communal norms for sociality embraced by China popularize collective functioning, control, connection, cooperation, exchange, familization, filiality, gifting, harmony, health, homogeneity, indebtedness, moral cultivation, networking, reciprocity, relatedness, role modeling, sacrifice, and visitation (Bian et al. 2005; J. Chen 2013; Chua 2002; Fallman 2010; X. Gu 2022; Y. Guo et al. 2023; Leung and Nann 1995; J. Li 2003; Reed 1995; Sun et al. 2013; Wang et al. 2010; Zhong 2009). The norm for collectivism has strengthened sociality by raising intimacy and institutional trust (Georgas et al. 1997; McAllister 1999). The norm for familization sustains sociality (Jin and Liu 1993). Filiality has uplifted sociality by boosting family cohesion and relational quality through enhancing sensitivity to need (Hwang et al. 2022; Mair et al. 2016). The norm for social control has enhanced sociality by raising civic engagement, government trust, political participation, and recourse (Su and Feng 2013; Z. Han et al. 2017; F. Lee 2012; Palmer et al. 2011). Conversely, the norm for social control has safeguarded sociality by dampening victimization and violence (Hansen-Nord et al. 2014; E. Wright et al. 2015). Connection or relatedness has consolidated sociality by consolidating sharing, social interaction, and relationship satisfaction (Downie et al. 2008; Frazer 1999; Wickham and Knee 2012). Cooperation has constituted sociality regarding attachment and trustworthiness as opposed to argument (Gerbasi and Cook 2008; Hample 2018; Tak 2017). Exchange has sustained sociality regarding compliance, cooperation, morality, social cohesion, social commitment, social integration, social interaction, social participation, trust, and volunteering (Bagherior et al. 2009; Carter 2016; Drollinger 2010; Lawler et al. 2016; Skopek et al. 2011; Yoon et al. 2013; Zhang and Zhou 2018). Conversely, exchange has maintained sociality by dampening resistance and violence (Foy et al. 2014; Hattery and Smith 2012). Gifting has constituted sociality regarding sociability (d'Astous and Mouakhar-Klouz 2022). Harmony experienced has induced sociality characterized by adjustment, attunement, civility, compromise, connectedness, interdependency, order, peace, relatedness, respect, sacrifice, selflessness, solidarity, and sympathy as opposed to competition and conflict (Arat and Kerelian 2019; Cheung and Ma 2011; P. Ip 2014; Kjell et al. 2016; Peck 2002; G. Zhang 2006). The norm for health has created social capital to enable sociality (Portes and Vickstrom 2011). Homogeneity constitutes sociality by embracing discussion and friendship (Brundidge and Rice 2009; Seder and Oishi 2009). Gratitude constitutes sociality through expressing or raising morality, social awareness, liking, and understanding, and reducing avoidance (Eibach et al. 2015; Tudge et al. 2022; Kloos et al. 2022). The norm for morality has maintained sociality by developing morality and dampening self-interest (A. Liu et al. 2025; J. Wright et al. 2017). The norm for networking has buttressed sociality by strengthening civic engagement, community favor, financial help, institutional trust, political participation, and recourse and prevented violence (Z. Han et al. 2017; F. Lee 2012; Mitrut and Wolff 2011; Palmer et al. 2011; Su and Feng 2013; Whitham 2012; E. Wright et al. 2015). Reciprocity has constituted sociality by fostering prosocial behavior (Thielmann et al. 2020). Role modeling has strengthened collaboration and conformity to uphold sociality (Decuyper et al. 2023; Gursimsek and Goregenli 2005). Sacrifice has upheld sociality by raising donating and leadership (Dubois et al. 2020; Piferi et al. 2006). Visitation has secured sociality by enhancing attachment and social capital (Navarra et al. 2018; Tsaur et al. 2014).

Cultural norms for sociality espoused by China propagate adaptation, altruism, atheism, belonging, benevolence, brotherhood, civility or civilization, collectivism or collectivity, the commonweal, compassion, compliance, contribution, deference, duty, equality, familism, flexibility, forgiveness or magnanimity, government trust, group orientation, harmony, honesty, human orientation, integrity, interdependence, interpersonal trust, learning, moralism, morality, nationalism, order, patriotism, peacefulness, relationalism, self-discipline, socialism, societal well-being, submission, teamwork, tradition or traditionalism, trustworthiness, and welfare (Butler 2008; S. Chen 1996; Cheung and Pomerantz 2011; Gao 2018; Hirono 2013; Inglehart 1997; Leung and Nann 1995; H. Li 2021; S. Li et al. 2024; C. Lin 2003; Luk 2001; Nevis 1983; Y. Jin 2003; J. Liu et al. 2005; Miles and Wang 2018; Reed 1995; Rolandsen 2008; Steinhardt 2012; Szalay et al. 1994; Wang and Zhu 1996; D. Wang et al. 2010; Yang and Zhang 2001; Y. Yang et al. 2010; S. Zhang 2003; Zhang and

Mo 2005; Zhang with Stening 2010; Zhou and Yan 2002). Adaptation has secured sociality regarding partnership and social adjustment and satisfaction as opposed to discord (Chow et al. 2014; Mitchell 2005). Altruism has constituted sociality by boosting attachment, civic engagement, friendship quality, likability, moral behavior, popularity, relatedness, and diminishing loneliness and violence (Bond and Kwan 2000; W. Chen et al. 2022; Layous et al. 2012; Markiewicz et al. 2001; Martela and Ryan 2016; Mesch 2009; Na and Paternoster 2019; L. Taylor et al. 2018; Wright and Li 2011). The norm for atheism has buttressed sociality by inducing voting (DeLeon and Naff 2004). Belongingness constitutes sociality (Fowers 2015). Benevolence has upheld sociality by enhancing government trust and likability (Patricio et al. 2022). The norm for brotherhood characterizes the norm for civilization (Szakolczai 2001). The norm for civilization constitutes sociality regarding civility and loyalty (Hudson 2023; Tester 2020). Collectivism espoused by China covers community, conformity, connection, cooperation, harmony, humility, loyalty, obedience, relatedness, responsiveness, and togetherness as opposed to individualism (S. Li et al. 2024; Peterson et al. 2006). The commonweal has constituted sociality by strengthening leadership and neighboring (Dubois et al. 2020; Grannis 2009). Compassion has underlain sociality by securing religiosity and volunteering (Barr et al. 2005). Compliance or submission has constituted sociality by raising patriotism and impeding violence and acceptance of deviants and outsiders (Pulkkinen et al. 2009; Schwartz et al. 2014; Van Hootegem et al. 2000; Yeo and Chu 2018). Contribution has constituted sociality by enhancing attachment and dampening tolerance for deviance (Stafford et al. 2005; Woosnam et al. 2018). Deference constitutes sociality regarding caring and equality (Renger and Reese 2017). Dutifulness has fostered sociality regarding compliance, morality, and xenophobia as opposed to violence (Bussey 2020; Granzin and Olsen 1998; Kaurin 2020; Milner and Myers 2007). The norm for equality has fostered sociality by championing cohesion and its experience, fairness, justice, social capital, sympathy, trust, and volunteering (Eriksson et al. 2015; Green et al. 2003; Hitlin and Harkness 2018; Musick and Wilson 2008; Oishi et al. 2011; Portes and Vickstrom 2011; van Oorschot and Arts 2005). Flexibility advances sociality by facilitating adaptation and representing acceptance and staying (Pyszkowska 2020; Pyszkowska and Ronnlund 2021). Forgiveness has consolidated sociality by raising government trust (Choi and David 2012). Government trust has constituted sociality by sustaining compliance, conformity, nationalism, political participation, and preventing protesting (Rhodes-Purdy et al. 2023; Ulbig 2002; van der Meer and van Ingen 2009; V. Vu 2021). Grouping has fostered sociality regarding cohesion, common identity, and identification (Fischer et al. 2007). Honesty has built sociality by raising compliance and prosocial behavior and eschewing crime (Jolley et al. 2019; Thielmann et al. 2020; Twardawski et al. 2021). Human orientation has enhanced sociality by activating political participation (Foschi and Lauriola 2014). Integrity has buttressed sociality by boosting volunteering and inhibiting violence (Piquero and Hickman 2002; Whitford et al. 2006). Interdependence has buttressed sociality by securing attachment, donation, prosocial behavior, social inclusion, and social interaction (Feeney and Collins 2001; Uskul et al. 2004; Z. Xin et al. 2017). Interpersonal trust has constituted sociality through donation, involvement, and volunteering

(Uslaner 2000). Learning constitutes sociality (Fowers 2015). Moreover, learning has buttressed sociality by enhancing attachment, political interest and participation, social integration, voting, and welfare support and reducing threatening (Roosma et al. 2016; Glanville 1999; Gundert and Hohendanner 2015; Howe 2010; Schneider 2007; van Riper et al. 2019). Moralism has sustained sociality by boosting gratitude (Pohling et al. 2010). Moreover, moralism can enhance sociality regarding social trust (Bersot and Arrigo 2015; Steinhardt 2012). Nationalism has underpinned sociality by fostering attachment, intolerance against deviance, patriotism, political participation, religiousness, social inclusion, trust in government, and xenophobia, and diminishing protesting (N. Chen 2012; Flanagan and Lee 2000; Huddy et al. 2021; Li and Brewer 2004; Osborne et al. 2017; Pinto et al. 2020; Rippl et al. 2010). The norm for order has supported sociality by enhancing civic engagement, community favor, government trust, political participation, and recourse and dampening violence (Z. Han et al. 2017; F. Lee 2012; Palmer et al. 2011; Pulkkinen et al. 2009; Su and Feng 2013; Whitham 2012). Patriotism has consolidated sociality by uplifting prosociality, social cohesion, volunteering, and xenophobia (Granzin and Olsen 1998; Ishii 2009; Straume and Odeen 2010; Vida and Reardon 2008; Y. Yang et al. 2010). Peacefulness has fostered sociality characterized by adjustment, attunement, civility, compromise, connectedness, interdependency, order, peace, relatedness, respect, sacrifice, selflessness, solidarity, and sympathy as opposed to competition and conflict (Arat and Kerelian 2019; Cheung and Ma 2011; P. Ip 2014; Kjell et al. 2016; Peck 2002; G. Zhang 2006). Relationalism normalized by China covers collectivism, embeddedness, face, order, familism, interdependence, parentalism, promise, reciprocity, and shame as opposed to individualism (D. Ho et al. 2006; Luk 2001; Nevis 1983). Self-discipline has buttressed sociality by enhancing generativity and impeding crime, risking, and violence (Y. Cheung et al. 2014; Koegl and Day 2019; Peterson and Klohnen 1995; Welch et al. 2008). Socialism exalted by China encompasses the commonweal, contribution, cooperation, equality, mutuality, and win–win benefit as exposed to exploitation (Gao 2018; Leung and Nann 1995; Zhou 2000). The norm for socialism has enhanced sociality by sustaining traditionalism and volunteering (Braun et al. 1994; Musick and Wilson 2008). The norm for well-being has upgraded sociality by boosting donation, law abidance, social trust, and voting and dampening lying (Fridberg and Kangas 2008b; Norris 2002; van Hemert et al. 2002). Teamwork has boosted sociality by raising organizational commitment and social cohesion (Carter et al. 2024; Gould-Williams 2005). Traditionalism inherited by China cherishes benevolence, harmony, morality, prosperity, self-control or self-discipline, submissiveness, and unity (Chu 2001; Gao 2018). Tradition or traditionalism has buttressed sociality by enhancing patriotism and faith in religion and discouraging protesting and accepting deviants and outsiders (Costa et al. 2023; Datler et al. 2013; Meuleman et al. 2019; Schwartz et al. 2014). Trustworthiness underlies sociality by establishing attachment, intimacy, social capital, and trust (X. Chen et al. 2015; Harvey and Wenzel 2006). The norm for welfare has uplifted sociality by advancing neighboring, political participation, social capital, support for social welfare, and volunteering and diminishing migration and theft (Allard and Danziger 2000; J. Brown 2016; Musick and Wilson 2008; Portes and Vickstrom

2011; Rehm et al. 2012; Semino 2015). Besides, welfare support has upheld sociality by elevating government trust (U. Kim et al. 2002). China can elevate the norm for social integration to secure sociality (Schlevogt 2002). Social integration has constituted sociality by strengthening cooperation and preventing suicide (Duberstein et al. 2004; Lepkowski and Couper 2002).

Political norms for sociality propagated by China spread anti-foreignism, atheism, befriending, bridging, civilization, collectivism, communism, communitarianism, Confucianism, consultation, cooptation, cooperation, equalizing, forgiveness, gratitude, group interest, harmony, helping, humaneness or humanity, legalism, moderation, morality or ethocracy, multilateralism, mutuality, nationalism, patriotism, peace, sharing, socialism, socialization, solidarity, unity, and win–win benefit (S. Chen 1996; Dai and Luqiu 2024; Dickson 2001; Genevaz 2019; W. Hou et al. 2003; J. Hu et al. 2018; Kachiga 2021; S. Lo 2021; Lu and Treiman 2008; Nai et al. 2020; Rosen 2009; Vickers 2024; F. Wang 2024; Zee 2022). Anti-foreignism or xenophobia has constituted sociality by boosting patriotism and social cohesion (Granzin and Olsen 1998; Wang and Chen 2004). Befriending has enabled sociality regarding prosocial behavior (Foschi and Lauriola 2014). Bridging has constituted sociality by strengthening agreeableness, empathy, morality, and social capital (Halevy et al. 2019). The norm for communism has enhanced sociality by sustaining traditionalism and volunteering (Braun et al. 1994; Musick and Wilson 2008). Communitarianism constitutes sociality by espousing caring, civility, collective identity, commonweal orientation, community, dutifulness or responsibility, education or socialization, equality, interdependence, loyalty, mentoring, patriotism, reciprocity, relatedness, self-discipline, servicing including volunteering, settlement, social construction, social participation, solidarity, and trust (Delanty 2009; Frazer 1999; Moore 2010; Speth 2012). Confucianism cherished by China accentuates benevolence, brotherhood, community, duty, familism, harmony, inclusion, ingroup trust, morality or virtue, obedience, order, outgroup distrust, prosperity, pacificism, paternalism, and respect as opposed to antagonism, belligerence, conflict, hegemony, rights, selfishness (X. Chen 2002; Kachiga 2021; Moore 2017). Confucianism has championed sociality regarding association, civility, and collectivism as opposed to violence (Y. Lin et al. 2021; Shin 2012; Stotzer 2014). Consulting enhances sociality by representing community involvement and consent (Ball 2004; Holbig 2011). The norm for cooptation has maintained sociality by curbing revolution (Ferwerda and Miller 2014). Forgiveness has consolidated sociality by raising government trust (Choi and David 2012). The norm for helping has raised responsibility to enhance sociality (Shahzalal and Adnan 2022). Legalism has maintained sociality by preventing radicalism (Muthuswamy 2022). Moderation has elevated sociality by earning popularity (Yildirim and Lancaster 2015). The norm for multilateralism sustains sociality by embracing reciprocity (Malone and Medhora 2020). Mutuality has constituted sociality by fostering prosocial behavior (Thielmann et al. 2020). Sharing has constituted sociality by strengthening leadership and neighboring (Dubois et al. 2020; Grannis 2009). Moreover, sharing constitutes sociality regarding friendship (Launay and Dunbar 2015). Sharing can also underlie sociality by boosting morality, punishment, and social cohesion (N. Duncan 2017; Delton and Krasnow 2017). Socialization has constituted sociality by impeding violence (Pulkkinen et al. 2009). Unity has constituted sociality by strengthening leadership and neighboring (Dubois et al. 2020; Grannis 2009). The norm for the win–win champions sociality by registering cooperation and harmony (Z. Peng et el. 2017).

Conversely, China has opposed the norm for capitalism, thus maintaining sociality (F. Wang 2024). China upholds norms against aggression, competition, deprivation, extremism, fragmentation, freedom, imperialism or hegemony, individualism, queer theory, religion, rights, separatism, struggle, and terrorism to sustain sociality (J. Chen 2013; Chen and Lees 2018; Davey and Rato 2011; Jeffreys 2012; Kachiga 2021; W. Ho and Li 2022; S. Lo 2021; F. Wang 2024; Zee 2022). The norm for aggression has weakened sociality by boosting antisocial behavior and victimization (Ehrensuft et al. 2003; Krahe 2013). Competition has impeded sociality by eroding volunteering (Martinez and McMullin 2004). The norm for deprivation has worsened civic engagement, civility, community involvement, donation, relatedness, social trust, and volunteering and fomented cynicism, suicide, theft, violence, and victimization to impair sociality (Abascal 2015; Broadbent and Papadopoulos 2011; J. Brown 2016; Graddy and Wang 2009; Hagan et al. 2016; Krahe 2013; Nepal et al. 2011; Piatkowska 2020; C. Ross et al. 2000; Stoll 2001; Wuthnow 2004). Extremism has impeded sociality by provoking protesting (Moreira et al. 2018). The norm for fragmentation has worsened sociality by inciting suicide and eroding social trust (Alesina and La Ferrara 2002; O'Farrell et al. 2016). The norm for freedom has disturbed sociality by raising corruption perceived and dampening voting (Collier 2002; Schwartz et al. 2010). The norm for imperialism hurts sociality by registering coercion and oppression as opposed to reciprocity (Deutsch 2006; Fukuyama 1992; Pass 2019). The norm for individualism inhibits sociality by featuring competition, deintegration, disembeddedness, disengagement, independence, inequality, risk, and self-indulgence (Bauman 2001; Beck and Beck-Gernsheim 2002; Burgess 2018; Dannreuther and Perren 2013; Krys et al. 2019; Stankov et al. 2014). Queering impedes sociality by cherishing anarchy, antisociality, conflict, and struggle and resisting assimilation, compassion, morality, and normativity (K. Johnson 2015; Nicholas 2014; Smith and Windes 2000; Wiegman 2017; Zanghellini 2020). The norm for separatism erodes sociality by inciting or registering insurgency, revolution, and war (Bukit 2022; Seoighe 2016). The norm for religion has eroded sociality by reducing voting (DeLeon and Naff 2004). The norm for rights has disrupted sociality by curbing xenophobia (Goodman 2015). Struggle characterizes conflict (Upenieks 2022). The norm for conflict has impaired sociality by fomenting protesting and resistance (Schatzman 2005; Sorens 2011). Terrorism experienced has impaired sociality by invoking support for illegality (Huddy and Feldman 2011).

Effectiveness

Age is likely more effective in China because of the norm that social status has increased with age, and thus, the norm for age benefits there (Ikels 1989). Moreover, age is likely more effective in China because of the norm for age worth there (Niblett 2024). Hence, the norms would increase the effectiveness of age in raising sociality.

Gender is likely more effective in China because of the norm for gender inequality (He and Wu 2006). Moreover, gender is likely more effective in China because of the norm for sexism there (Tan 1996). Hence, the norms would increase the effectiveness of female gender in raising sociality and the effectiveness of male gender in dampening sociality.

Education is likely more effective in China because of norms for education and learning values there (C. Lin 2003; Edney 2012). Hence, the norms would increase the effectiveness of education in raising sociality.

Marriage and non-marriage are likely more effective in China because of norms for familism and familization there (Chua 2002; X. Gu 2022). Hence, the norms would increase the effectiveness of marriage and non-marriage in raising sociality.

The number of children is likely more effective in China because of the norm for fertility control to raise fertility value there (Lau and Li 2011). Hence, the norm would increase the effectiveness of the number of children in raising sociality.

Employment and work are likely more effective in China because of norms for Confucianism and socialism there, which valorize production and working (S. Chan et al. 2022; Gao 2018). Hence, the norms would increase the effectiveness of employment and work in raising sociality.

Public employment is likely more effective in China because of norms for public ownership and service and its advertising there (D. Bell 1999; H. Gu 2018; Landsberger 2009). Hence, the norms would increase the effectiveness of public employment in raising sociality.

Creative work is likely less effective in China because of the norm against creativity support there (Rudowicz and Yue 2002). Hence, the norms would decrease the effectiveness of creativity in reducing sociality.

Independent work is likely more effective in China because of the norm for independence there (Xiong et al. 2022). Hence, the norm would increase the effectiveness of independent work in raising sociality.

Intellectual work is likely more effective in China because of the norm for respect for intellectuals there (D. Bell 1999). Hence, the norm would increase the effectiveness of intellectual work in reducing sociality.

Economic hardship is likely more effective in China because of the norm against poverty or anti-poverty policy, which makes economic hardship a crucial concern (Li and Walker 2018). Hence, the norm would increase the effectiveness of economic hardship in impairing sociality.

Neighborhood nuisance is likely more effective in China because of norms for communitarianism, Confucianism, and collectivism, which emphasize the community (Kachiga 2021; S. Li et al. 2024; Zee 2022). Hence, the norm would increase the effectiveness of neighborhood nuisance and its norm in diminishing sociality.

Religious faith or irreligion is likely more effective in China because of the norm for atheism, which marks the concern for religion there (W. Ho and Li 2022). Notably, atheism, like religionism, indicates the importance of religion in the absolute sense.

Hence, the norm would increase the effectiveness of religious faith or irreligion in reducing sociality.

Life satisfaction is likely less effective in China as happiness value or importance has been lower, and thus, the ideal for life satisfaction would be lower there (Cummins 1996; J. Zhang et al. 2009). In addition, life satisfaction is likely less effective in China because of the norm against promoting happiness there (Davey 2012). Hence, the ideals would increase the effectiveness of life satisfaction in raising sociality.

United States

The United States of America features consumerism, cost-effectiveness, exceptionalism, individualism, neoconservatism, and Protestantism (Cullen and Jonson 2017; Kruse 2015; Schroeder 2013; Speth 2012). Consumerism in the United States accentuates advertising, comparison, hedonism, identity, and meaning as opposed to need (Speth 2012). Cost-effectiveness or efficiency in the United States realizes accountability, commodification or pricing, and rationality (Cullen and Jonson 2017; Epstein 1997). Exceptionalism in the United States particularizes inequality, patriotism, religiousness, and voluntarism (Cullen and Jonson 2017). Individualism in the United States applauds autonomy, competence, competition, consumption, dignity, heroism, initiative, rehabilitation, privatization, rationality, and success (Kruse 2015). Neoconservatism hails aggression, democracy, exceptionalism, hierarchy, hegemony, idealism, imperialism, liberty, moralism, and unilateralism (Pan and Turner 2017; Rollo 2023). Protestantism in the United States cherishes bureaucracy, conquering, individualism, law-abidance, and loyalty (Braun 2011).

The United States of America can shape sociality and the effectiveness of factors in achieving sociality based on the deterministic and voluntaristic mechanisms of analytical functionalism. These mechanisms employ power, utility, ideals, and norms to activate empowering, incentivizing, framing, and standardizing for determinism and power realization, utility optimization, ideal calibration, and norm conformity for voluntarism. Among them, norms are paramount in representing the functions of the United States. These norms buttress sociality. The influences of the United States reflect the American century (Chiozza 2023). Alternatively, a norm enhances the effectiveness of a factor's influence on sociality by boosting the factor's action, including commitment, strength, and others, to raise the effectiveness. This enhancement can benefit from the direct deterministic mechanisms of sharing privately and publicly and the indirect deterministic mechanism of standardizing coupled with the voluntaristic mechanism of norm conformity. For instance, the norm for a factor's importance or effectiveness engenders the factor's importance or effectiveness personally.

Sociality

Norms for sociality upheld by the United States popularize compromise, conformity, equality or egalitarianism, fame or recognition, harmony, humanitarianism, justice, legality, loyalty, moralism, morality, nationalism, Protestantism, punishment, and sympathy (J. Barry 2011; Braun 2011; Epstein 1997; Garrett et al. 2014; Kruse 2015; Moore 2017; Rollo 2023; J. Turner 2011, 2015; F. Wang 2024). Compromise constitutes sociality by representing harmony (G. Zhang 2006). Conversely, compromise maintains sociality by espousing reconciliation and dismissing conflict and radicalism (J. Berger 2018; Auerbach 2009). The norm for equality has fostered sociality by championing cohesion and its experience, fairness, justice, social capital, sympathy, trust, and volunteering (Eriksson et al. 2015; Green et al. 2003; Hitlin and Harkness 2018; Musick and Wilson 2008; Oishi et al. 2011; Portes and Vickstrom 2011; van Oorschot and Arts 2005). Fame has buttressed sociality by enhancing compliance and trust experienced and diminishing relocation (Kas et al. 2022; Permentier et al. 2009; G. Wang et al. 2020). Recognition constitutes sociality regarding caring and equality (Renger and Reese 2017). The norm for harmony has supported sociality by enhancing civic engagement, community favor, government trust, political participation, and recourse and dampening violence (Z. Han et al. 2017; F. Lee 2012; Palmer et al. 2011; Pulkkinen et al. 2009; Su and Feng 2013; Whitham 2012). Humanitarianism has enhanced sociality by activating political participation (Foschi and Lauriola 2014). Moreover, humanitarianism sustains sociality by favoring altruism, caring, civility, empathy, groupness, other orientation, pity, prosociality, and solidarity (Angelis and Pensini 2024; Bendixsen 2018; Chouliaraki 2013; Regilme 2020). The norm for justice has upheld sociality by elevating morality and prosocial behavior (Barber 2004; McCaffoee 2016). The norm for legality has sustained sociality by resisting radicalism (Muthuswamy 2022). Loyalty has constituted sociality by fostering collaboration, empathy, generosity, leadership, and morality (Lawler et al. 2016; Lee and Chan 2016; Wilcox and Dew 2016). Moralism has sustained sociality by boosting gratitude (Pohling et al. 2010). Moreover, moralism can enhance sociality regarding social trust (Bersot and Arrigo 2015; Steinhardt 2012). Inherently, moralism embraces altruism, consensus, legality, obligation, and virtue to maintain sociality (R. Brown 2018). The norm for morality has maintained sociality by developing morality and dampening self-interest (A. Liu et al. 2025; J. Wright et al. 2017). Nationalism has underpinned sociality by fostering attachment, intolerance against deviance, patriotism, political participation, religiousness, social inclusion, trust in government, and xenophobia, and diminishing protesting (N. Chen 2012; Flanagan and Lee 2000; Huddy et al. 2021; Li and Brewer 2004; Osborne et al. 2017; Pinto et al. 2020; Rippl et al. 2010). Protestantism has uplifted sociality by elevating civic voluntarism, institutional trust, legalism, morality, patriotism, political participation, social cohesion, social contact, social trust, volunteering, and voting and diminishing aggression and multiculturalism (Bekkers and Boisman 2009; Iceland et al. 2023; E. Kim and Cohen 2017; Lim and MacGregor 2012; Stavrova and Siegers 2014; Stolle and Micheletti 2013; Timberlake et al. 2003; Tolsma et al. 2009; Traunmuller 2011; Verkuyten 2004;

Woolley 2003; Wuthnow 2004). Multiculturalism obstructs sociality by denouncing assimilation, embracing unrest, and standing on independence (Pehrson et al. 2011; Verkuyten 2005). Punishment characterizes sociality (Fowers 2015). Sympathy has constituted sociality by securing religiosity and volunteering (Barr et al. 2005).

Conversely, norms against sociality downplayed by the United States spread imperialism and inequality (Brady and Leicht 2008; J. Cheng 2016). The norm for imperialism obstructs sociality by favoring norms for aggression, colonialism, cosmopolitanism, diversity, and migration (Baik 2019; Chhachhi and Herrera 2007; Khomyakov 2020). Cosmopolitanism has eroded sociality by discounting religiosity and raising liberalism and acceptance of deviants and outsiders (Costa et al. 2023; Motschenbacher 2013; Norris and Inglehart 2009). The norm for inequality has impeded sociality by eroding social capital, support for redistribution and welfare, sympathy, trust, and volunteering (Busemeyer 2013; Hitlin and Harkness 2018; Lipford and Yandle 2009; Oishi et al. 2011; Portes and Vickstrom 2011).

Effectiveness

Age is likely more effective in the United States because of the cultural norm for youth regarding malleability there (Cullen and Jonson 2017). The norm would increase the effectiveness of or difference due to age in raising sociality. Notably, the importance of youth means age effectiveness.

Employment and work are likely more effective in the United States because of the norm for work ethics there (Kruse 2015). That is, the norm would increase the effectiveness of employment and work in raising sociality.

Independent work is likely more effective in the United States because of norms for individualism and voluntarism and thus self-reliance and self-responsibility there (Hitlin and Pinkston 2013; Kruse 2015). That is, the norms would increase the effectiveness of independent work in raising sociality.

Marriage and non-marriage are likely more effective in the United States because of the norm for familialism (Oyserman et al. 2002). That is, the norm would increase the effectiveness of marriage in raising sociality and the effectiveness of non-marriage in diminishing sociality.

Immigration is likely less effective in the United States because of the norm for cosmopolitanism there (Vucetic 2011). Cosmopolitanism weakens the concern for immigration and, thus, its impact (Delanty 2009). That is, the norm would reduce the effectiveness of immigration in dampening sociality.

Religious faith is likely more effective in the United States because of the norm for Protestantism as a religion (Kruse 2015). That is, the norm would increase the effectiveness of religious faith in eroding sociality.

Economic hardship is likely more effective in the United States because of the norm for success ideology (Garrett et al. 2014). Here, economic hardship or poverty represents failure (Rank et al. 2003). Meanwhile, success ideology raises the concern for failure and success. That is, the norm would increase the effectiveness of economic hardship in obstructing sociality.

Family saving is likely less effective in the United States because of the norm against family value there (Vlaicu 2002). That is, the norm would reduce the effectiveness of family saving in raising sociality.

Security is likely more effective in the United States because of norms for realism and its emphasis on security (Kachiga 2021). That is, the norms would increase the effectiveness of security in raising sociality.

Current Findings

Regression analyses of Waves 5 and 6 World Values Survey data examined the effects of China and the United States of America and their interactions in the second and sixth steps of the analyses. The second step included time and the national indicators of China and the United States to show the crude differences due to China and the United States. Furthermore, the sixth step additionally included all significant personal characteristics, personal and national experiences, national social attitudes, and interactions between national indicators and personal characteristics and experiences. This step also showed the net differences due to China and the United States when the analyses employed standard scores to compute interaction terms. The analyses tested the hypotheses that China and the United States exhibit higher sociality than others (see Table 7.1). Statistically significant findings distilled from the analyses generally supported the hypotheses.

Essentially, China, the United States, and the superpower generally exhibited personal and national conditions. China displayed strong and strongest negative correlations with democracy ($r = -.891$, see Table 7.2), liberty ($r = -.812$), faith in religion ($r = -.543$), neighborhood nuisance ($r = -.411$). By contrast, China showed strong and strongest positive correlations with irreligion ($r = .730$), population size ($r = .630$), and bank credit per capita ($r = .527$). Meanwhile, the United States displayed strong and strongest positive correlations with carbon dioxide emission per capita ($r = .818$), gross domestic product per capita ($r = .782$), government effectiveness ($r = .713$), human capital ($r = .654$), globalization ($r = .616$), phone subscription per capita ($r = .601$), human development ($r = 596$), bank credit per capita ($r = .576$), the rule of law ($r = .549$), and liberty ($r = .494$). The superpower, China or the United States, exhibited strong and strongest positive correlations with bank credit per capita ($r = .813$), irreligion ($r = .678$), carbon dioxide emission per capita ($r = .483$), phone subscription per capita ($r = .481$), population size ($r = .449$), and globalization ($r = .431$). By contrast, the superpower indicated strong and strongest negative correlations with democracy ($r = -.668$), liberty ($r = -.512$), faith in religion ($r = -.493$), and neighborhood nuisance ($r = -.415$). These correlates represented some of the crude differences due to China, the United States, and the superpower in general.

Confidence in institutions was moderately higher in China than in the non-superpower ($\beta = .318$, see Table 7.3). Meanwhile, this confidence was weakly higher in the United States than in the non-superpower based on the crude difference ($\beta =$

Table 7.1 Expected and actual effects of superpowers on sociality

Predictor	Expected	Actual						
		Institution	Anti-misdeed	Anti-sex	Anti-faith	Anti-outsider	Anti-deviant	Other
China	+	+	–	+	+	+	–	
US	+	–	+	–	+	+	+	+

Note. Sociality unfolded in social attitudes regarding confidence in institutions, refutation against misdeeds, refutation against unconventional sexuality, unfaith in religion, rejection of outsiders, rejection of deviants, and trust in others
+ positive effect. – negative effect.

Table 7.2 Correlations with superpowers

Correlate	China	US	China or US
Wave	− .002	.002	− .001
Population	.630***	− .286***	.449***
Phone	.166***	.601***	.481***
Land	− .199***	.220***	− .073***
Technology	.010*	.329***	.186***
Credit	.527***	.576***	.813***
GDP	− .249***	.782***	.181***
Gini	− .131***	− .319***	− .296***
Globalization	.106***	.616***	.431***
Government effectiveness	− .088***	.713***	.299***
Democracy	− .891***	.345***	− .668***
Liberty	− .812***	.494***	− .512***
Human development	.042***	.596***	.360***
Human capital	− .063***	.654***	.290***
CO_2	.047***	.818***	.483***
Rule of law	− .316***	.549***	− .007
Acquiescence	− .303***	− .069***	− .327***
Female	.012**	.019***	.022***
Age	− .006***	.089***	.042***
Education	.028***	.195***	.132***
Graduation age	− .169***	.138***	− .085***
Irreligious	.730***	− .039***	.678***
Family income	− .057***	.080***	− .011*
Age squared	− .067***	.077***	− .023***
Married	.154***	− .111***	.088***
Cohabited	− .116***	.008	− .107***
Divorced	− .049***	.168***	.044***
Separated	− .044***	.042***	− .019***
Widowed	− .037***	.016***	− .027***
Kid	− .178***	− .033***	− .188***
Mother immigrant	-	.056***	.056***
Father immigrant	-	.061***	.061***
Living with parents	− .054***	− .144***	− .128***
Full-time employment	.216***	.025***	.220***
Part-time employment	− .088***	− .070***	− .122***
Self-employment	− .060***	.037***	− .037***
Retired	− .145***	− .012**	− .145***

(continued)

Table 7.2 (continued)

Correlate	China	US	China or US
Homemaking	– .033***	– .001	– .032***
Student	– .156***	– .042***	– .172***
Unemployed	– .079***	– .027***	– .091***
Public employment	– .038***	.021***	– .025***
Private business employment	– .109***	.063***	– .070***
Nonprofit organization employment	– .018***	– .082***	– .061***
Intellectual work	– .062***	.107***	– .002***
Creative work	– .103***	.080***	– .055***
Independent work	– .119***	.081***	– .070***
Supervision	– .071***	.080***	– .022***
Earner status	.020***	.064***	0.054***
Earner employed	.081***	.005	.081***
Survey interest	– .201***	-	– .201***
Economic hardship	– .261***	– .034***	– .268***
Neighborhood nuisance	– .411***	– .046***	– .415***
Victimization	– .086***	.045***	– .057***
Security	.047***	.043***	.068***
Family saving	.095***	.037***	.111***
Health	– .003	.063***	.031***
Life satisfaction	.027***	.078***	.068***
Confidence in institutions	.304***	– .166***	.200***
Justification for misdeeds	.024***	– .032***	.005
Justification for unconventional sexuality	– .153***	.251***	– .009
Faith in religion	– .543***	.047***	– .493***
Acceptance of outsiders	– .213***	– .122***	– .270***
Acceptance of deviants	.170***	– .158***	.078***
Trust in others	– .033***	.122***	.035***

$^{*}p < .05$; $^{**}p < .01$; $^{***}p < .001$

– .110). The strongest substantive interaction effect was the slight negative effect of education in China on confidence in institutions ($\beta = -.050$).

Justification for misdeeds was slightly higher in China and slightly lower in the United States than in the non-superpower, based on crude differences ($\beta = .017$ and – .028, see Table 7.4). The strongest substantive interaction effect was the slight negative effect of economic hardship in China on justification for misdeeds ($\beta = -$ .045).

Table 7.3 Additional significant ($p < .001$) standardized effects of superpowers on confidence in institutions

Predictor	(2)	(6)
China	.276	.318
US	− .110	− .020
China × Education		− .050
China × Acquiescence		− .064
China × Age		.032
China × Public employment		− .033
China × Security		.033
US × Acquiescence		− .028
China × Full-time employment		.026
China × Living with parents		.024
China × Private business employment		− .016
US × Age		− .019
China × Kid		.023
China × Female		− .016
China × Part-time employment		− .014
US × Part-time employment		− .013
R^2	.100	.415

Table 7.4 Additional significant ($p < .001$) standardized effects of superpowers on justification for misdeeds

Predictor	(2)	(5)
China	.017	.045
US	− .028	.060
China × Economic hardship		− .045
China × Separated		− .028
China × Earner employed		− .031
US × Earner employed		− .027
R^2	.004	.073

Justification for unconventional sexuality was weakly lower in China than in the non-superpower based on the crude difference ($\beta = -\ .102$, see Table 7.5). Meanwhile, this justification was weakly higher in the United States than in the non-superpower based on the crude difference ($\beta = -\ .226$). The strongest substantive interaction effect was the slight positive effect of irreligion in the United States on the justification ($\beta = .039$).

Faith in religion was strongly lower in China than in the non-superpower country ($\beta = -\ .492$, see Table 7.6). Meanwhile, this faith was slightly lower in the United States than in the non-superpower based on the crude difference ($\beta = -\ .061$). The

Table 7.5 Additional significant ($p < .001$) standardized effects of superpowers on justification for unconventional sexuality

Predictor	(2)	(6)
China	− .102	− .090
US	.226	− .022
US × Irreligious		.039
US × Security		.034
China × Nonprofit organization employment		− .029
China × Health		− .019
US × Cohabited		.017
China × Separated		− .022
US × Divorced		− .019
US × Kid		− .017
China × Family income		− .016
China × Female		− .016
China × Full-time employment		− .017
China × Economic hardship		.016
US × Separated		− .015
R^2	.071	.286

strongest substantive interaction effect was the slight negative effect of irreligion in China on confidence in the faith ($\beta = -.088$).

Acceptance of outsiders was weakly lower in China and the United States than in the non-superpower based on crude differences ($\beta = -.245$ and $-.170$, see Table 7.7). The strongest substantive interaction effect was the slight positive effect of irreligion in China on such acceptance ($\beta = .044$).

Acceptance of deviants was weakly higher in China than in the non-superpower based on the crude difference ($\beta = .143$, see Table 7.8). Meanwhile, this acceptance was weakly lower in the United States than in the non-superpower based on the crude difference ($\beta = -.129$). The strongest substantive interaction effect was the negligible positive effect of health in China on this acceptance ($\beta = .025$).

Trust in others was weakly higher in the United States than in the non-superpower ($\beta = .133$, see Table 7.9). The strongest substantive interaction effect was the slight positive effect of age in the United States on such trust ($\beta = .050$).

The significant interaction effects showed that China elevated the effectiveness of age, education, full-time employment, irreligion, and marriage (see Table 7.10). By contrast, China diminished the effectiveness of acquiescence, female gender, health, and nonprofit organization employment. Meanwhile, the United States reduced the effectiveness of divorce and time. Besides, the United States showed mixed effects on the effectiveness of acquiescence and age.

The effect of the interaction between China and time indicated that China remarkably increased more or decreased less than other countries in nonprofit organization

Table 7.6 Additional significant ($p < .001$) standardized effects of superpowers on faith in religion

Predictor	(2)	(6)
China	− .546	− .492
US	− .061	.282
China × Irreligious		− .088
US × Wave		.054
China × Life satisfaction		− .041
China × Victimization		.029
China × Economic hardship		.035
China × Intellectual work		.026
China × Security		.027
China × Student		− .020
China × Public employment		− .017
US × Acquiescence		.019
US × Father immigrant		− .016
China × Neighborhood nuisance		.017
China × Divorced		− .012
R^2	.305	.557

Table 7.7 Additional significant ($p < .001$) standardized effects of superpowers on acceptance of outsiders

Predictor	(2)	(6)
China	− .245	− .391
US	− .170	− .043
US × Acquiescence		− .038
China × Irreligious		.044
China × Married		.028
China × Full-time employment		.021
R^2	.077	.191

Table 7.8 Additional significant ($p < .001$) standardized effects of superpowers on acceptance of deviants

Predictor	(2)	(5)
China	.143	.020
US	− .129	.064
China × Health		.025
China × Victimization		.025
China × Homemaking		− .022
R^2	.050	.194

Table 7.9 Additional significant ($p < .001$) standardized effects of superpowers on trust in others

Predictor	(2)	(6)
China	− .009n	− .060
US	.119	.133
US × Age		.050
China × Intellectual work		− .042
US × Neighborhood nuisance		− .025
R^2	.015	.047

n: $p > .001$

employment ($\beta = .318$, see Table 7.11), justification for misdeeds ($\beta = .147$), justification for unconventional sexuality ($\beta = .147$), family saving ($\beta = .135$), carbon dioxide emission per capita ($\beta = .104$), and self-employment ($\beta = .101$), earner employment ($\beta = .101$). Conversely, China remarkably decreased more or increased less than other countries in neighborhood nuisance ($\beta = -.296$), economic hardship ($\beta = -.187$), faith in religion ($\beta = -.181$), acquiescence ($\beta = -.141$), independent work ($\beta = -.135$), creative work ($\beta = -.126$), part-time employment ($\beta = -.117$), and survey interest ($\beta = -.113$). Meanwhile, the United States notably increased more or decreased less than other countries in student status ($\beta = .097$), cohabitation ($\beta = .090$), supervisory work ($\beta = .080$, education ($\beta = .075$), and justification for unconventional sexuality ($\beta = .073$). By contrast, the United States notably decreased more or increased less than other countries in retirement ($\beta = -.113$), neighborhood nuisance ($\beta = -.091$), phone subscription per capita ($\beta = -.075$), and technology publication per capita ($\beta = -.074$). Hence, the declining effectiveness of the United States in reducing religious faith more likely reflected the relative reduction in retirement and neighborhood nuisance and the relative increase in student status and cohabitation there.

Contrary to expectation, China showed less refutation against misdeeds and less rejection of deviants than the non-superpower. According to force theory as an enhancement of analytical functionalism, the negative effects reflected the clash between forces emitted by China and forces accepted by such refutation and rejection. On the one hand, forces emitted by China are atheism, forgiveness, magnanimity, and irreligion (W. Ho and Li 2022; Inglehart 1997; Zhou and Yan 2002). On the other hand, forces accepted by refuting misdeeds and rejecting deviants are non-forgiving, religiousness, and stigmatization (Cerulo and Ruane 2014; van der Leun and Koemans 2013; Vauclair and Fischer 2011).

Contrary to expectation, China did not reveal higher trust in other people than the non-superpower. According to force theory as an enhancement of analytical functionalism, the null effect reflected the neutralization of compatible and contradictory forces between China and trust in other people. On the one hand, contradictory forces delivered by China embrace battling, challenge, competition, conflict, defense, discrimination, involution, polarization, and stigmatizing (Heung and Zweig 2011; Jeffreys 2012; Kachiga 2021; L. Li 2010; Shambaugh 2007; Sun et al. 2013; Wang

Table 7.10 Significant moderation effects of superpowers on the effects on attitudes

Interaction	(1)	(2)	(3)	(4)	(5)	(6)	(7)
China × Acquiescence	− .064↓						
China × Age	.032↑						
China × Divorced				− .012			
China × Earner employed		− .031					
China × Economic hardship		− .045	.016	.035			
China × Education	− .050↑						
China × Family income			− .016				
China × Female	− .016↓		− .016↓				
China × Full-time employment	.026↑		− .017↑		.021		
China × Health			− .019			.025↓	
China × Homemaking						− .022	
China × Intellectual work				.026			− .042
China × Irreligious				− .088↑	.044		
China × Kid	.023						
China × Life satisfaction				− .041			
China × Living with parents	.024						
China × Married					.028↑		
China × Neighborhood nuisance				.017			
China × Nonprofit organization employment			− .029↓				
China × Part-time employment	− .014						
China × Private business employment	− .016						
China × Public employment	− .033			− .017			
China × Security	.033			.027			

(continued)

Table 7.10 (continued)

Interaction	(1)	(2)	(3)	(4)	(5)	(6)	(7)
China × Separated		− .028	− .022				
China × Student				− .020			
China × Victimization				.029		.025	
US × Acquiescence	− .028↓			.019↑	− .038↓		
US × Age	− .019↓						.050↑
US × Cohabited			.017				
US × Divorced			− .019↓				
US × Earner employed		− .027					
US × Father immigrant				− .016			
US × Irreligious			.039				
US × Kid			− .017				
US × Neighborhood nuisance							− .025
US × Part-time employment	− .013						
US × Security			.034				
US × Separated			− .015				
US × Wave				.054↓			

Note. Attitudinal outcomes were (1): confidence in institutions. (2): justification for misdeeds. (3): justification for unconventional sexuality. (4): faith in religion. (5): acceptance of outsiders. (6): acceptance of deviants. (7): trust in others
↑: China/US strengthening the significant main effect
↓: China/US weakening the significant main effect

and VanderWeele 2011; G. Zhao et al. 2022). On the other hand, contradictory forces underlying trust in others espouse agreeableness, civility, cohesiveness, considerateness, cooperation, communitarianism, discrimination, fraternity, neighboring, sociability, and social integration and resist competition, conflict, cynicism, ostracism, surveillance, threatening, and victimization (Abascal 2015; Dinesen and Sønderskov 2015; Freitag and Bauer 2016; Gundelach and Manatschal 2017; Halvorsen 2007; Kramer 1999; Newton 1999; Olivera 2015; Ross and Jang 2000; Rothstein and Uslaner 2005; Shao et al. 2021; B. Six 2014; Uslaner 2002; Vera-Toscano et al. 2013). Notably, China also emits forces compatible with those underlying trust in others. This compatibility would offset contradiction to erase China's influence on trust in others.

Contrary to expectation, the United States exhibited less confidence in institutions and refutation against unconventional sexuality than the non-superpower. According to force theory as an enhancement of analytical functionalism, the negative effects reflected the clash between forces emitted by the United States and forces accepted by such confidence and refutation. On the one hand, forces emitted by the United

Table 7.11 Effects of interactions between China and time and between the US and time

Outcome	China X Time	US X Time
Population	– .013*	– .012*
Phone	.010	– .075*
Land	.015*	.001
Technology	.090*	– .074*
Credit	– .011*	.000
GDP	.017*	.036*
Gini	– .015*	.000
Globalization	– .053*	– .069*
Government effectiveness	.043*	– .063*
Democracy	– .018*	– .010*
Liberty	– .025*	– .014*
Human development	.074*	– .009
Human capital	– .002	.000
CO_2	.104*	– .066*
Rule of law	.034*	.019*
Acquiescence	– .141*	– .063*
Female	.001	– .001
Age	.027*	.000
Education	.071*	.075*
Graduation age	– .050*	– .016*
Irreligious	– .021*	.024*
Family income	– .001	– .014*
Age squared	.000	.001
Married	– .009	– .015*
Cohabited	.045*	.090*
Divorced	– .008	– .032*
Separated	– .014	– .009
Widowed	.016*	– .001
Kid	– .039*	– .023*
Mother immigrant	.007	.018*
Father immigrant	– .003	.007
Living with parents	– .031*	.001
Full-time employment	– .085*	– .058*
Part-time employment	– .117*	– .013
Self-employment	.101*	.069*
Retired	– .117*	– .113*
Homemaking	– .005	.002

(continued)

Table 7.11 (continued)

Outcome	China X Time	US X Time
Student	.088*	.097*
Unemployed	−.024*	.005
Public employment	−.017*	.037*
Private business employment	.052*	−.025*
Nonprofit organization employment	.318*	.069*
Intellectual work	−.077*	.066*
Creative work	−.126*	.029*
Independent work	−.135*	.031*
Supervision	.063*	.080*
Earner status	−.016*	−.019*
Earner employed	.101*	.040*
Survey interest	−.113*	−.033*
Economic hardship	−.187*	−.061*
Neighborhood nuisance	−.296*	−.091*
Victimization	−.055*	.021*
Security	.039*	.038*
Family saving	.135*	.008
Health	−.023*	−.017*
Life satisfaction	−.034*	−.021*
Confidence in institutions	−.014	−.006
Justification for misdeeds	.147*	.038
Justification for unconventional sexuality	.143*	.073*
Faith in religion	−.181*	−.013
Acceptance of outsiders	−.002	.026*
Acceptance of deviants	−.141*	.061*
Trust in others	.015*	−.013

*$p < .001$

States favor autonomy, freedom, individualism, liberalism, neoliberalism, rights, and voluntarism and oppose government (J. Barry 2011; Hitlin and Pinkston 2013; Kruse 2015; J. Martin 2014; Narayan 2020; Rollo 2023; J. Turner 2011). On the other hand, forces accepted by confidence in institutions safeguard authoritarianism, collectivism, conservatism, government, and social cohesion and dismiss neoliberalism and rights (Bolger et al. 2020; Janmaat 2011; McAllister 1999; Mingo and Faggiano 2020; Pernia 2022; Zuckerman 2021). Similarly, forces underlying refuting unconventional sexuality cherish asceticism, authoritarianism, conservatism, discipline, interference, interdependence, regulation, repression, solidarity, temperance, tradition, and traditionalism and dismiss autonomy, freedom, individualism, independence, liberalism, rights, self-determination, self-expression (Alparone et al. 2024; Belliotti 1993; Conde Dias et al. 2012; de Jong et al. 2012; Jackson and Scott 2010; Jakobsson and Kotsadam 2011; Jung 2016; Kirsch 2000; Rival et al. 1998; Shim 2001; Soble 2008; Treger and Schmitt 2019; Vauclair and Fischer 2011).

The higher effectiveness of age, education, full-time employment, irreligion, and marriage in China than in the non-superpower supports hypotheses based on existing work. Accordingly, norms for age worth, atheism, familism, learning emphasis in Confucianism, and work emphasis in Confucianism and socialism in China are influential.

Contrary to or deviating from expectation, the effectiveness of female gender, health, and nonprofit organization employment was lower in China than in the non-superpower. According to the enhancement of analytical functionalism by force theory, the deviation reflects the clash of forces between effectiveness or importance and gender, health, and nonprofit organization employment in China.

The lower effectiveness of gender in China than in others registers the clash between forces emitted from China and forces driving gender effectiveness or importance. The former forces flow from gender and sex revolution and gender unbiasedness to diminish gender and sexual inequality or its impact there (Short et al. 2001; Xiao et al. 2011; J. Zhang et al. 2011). Moreover, China upholds the forces of authoritarianism, conservatism, and traditionalism (Gao 2018; Z. Su et al. 2019; Zheng 1994). Meanwhile, gender importance benefits from feminism (Mulinari and Sandell 2009). Feminism has declined with the forces of authoritarianism, conservatism, and traditionalism (Bettencourt et al. 2011; Duncan 1999).

The lower effectiveness of gender in China than in others registers the clash between forces arising from China and forces underlying health effectiveness or importance. On the one hand, China engenders forces about security culture, health confusion, and risk management and forces against autonomy, freedom, liberalism, neoliberalism, and religious culture (Chen and Mak 2008; Gilley and Holbig 2009; W. Ho and Li 2022; Liu and Berkowitz 2014; Shin 2012; Spencer-Rodgers et al. 2009; F. Wang 2024; Xie and Shen 2020; Zhang and Mo 2005). On the other hand, health effectiveness, importance, or value stands on the forces of autonomy, freedom, insecurity, liberalism, neoliberalism, religiousness, and risk society (Harrington and Fullagar 2013; Jaye et al. 2018; MacGregor et al. 2021; Pelters and Wijma 2016; Wiest et al. 2015).

The lower effectiveness of nonprofit organization employment in China than in others registers the clash between forces emanating from China and forces buttressing such employment. On the one hand, China dismisses the forces of civil society and nonprofit organizations and prizes the force of bureaucracy (C. Lee et al. 2006; S. Lo 2021; Naftali 2021; K. Yu 2002). On the other hand, the effectiveness or importance of nonprofit organization employment stands on the forces of civil society and resists the force of bureaucracy (Perotin 2001; Sanyal 2006).

The effectiveness of age in raising trust in others was higher in the United States than in others. This American edge supported the hypothesis grounded on the compatibility between the forces of the United States and the forces of age's effectiveness based on enhancing analytical functionalism by force theory. Accordingly, the United States highlights the force of youth culture to amplify the age difference or effectiveness (Cullen and Jonson 2017). Specifically, the United States displays the forces of autonomy, future focus, and religiosity (Garrett et al. 2014; Schroeder 2013; Solomon 2006). Meanwhile, age involves the forces of privacy and religiosity and dismisses the force of future orientation (Goerres 2007; Penningroth and Scott 2012; Van den Broeck et al. 2015). Hence, age effectiveness in raising social trust benefits from the forces toward autonomy and religiosity and the force against future orientation (Cais et al. 2021; Uslaner 2002).

By contrast, the effectiveness of age in raising confidence in institutions in others was lower in the United States than in others. This American deficit reflects the contradiction between the forces of the United States and the forces of age effectiveness in raising institutional confidence. Specifically, the United States favors the force of liberalism (Kruse 2015). Liberalism opposes conservatism (Lane and Sulikowski 2017). Meanwhile, age upholds the force of conservatism (Cornelis et al. 2009). Hence, age effectiveness in raising institutional confidence benefits from the force of conservatism (Bolger et al. 2020).

The effectiveness of divorce in the United States was lower in others. While contradicting the hypothesis, this deficit reflects the contradiction between the forces of the United States and forces accepted by divorce or marriage effectiveness. On the one hand, the United States displays the force of immigration or minority (Gottschalk 2014). On the other hand, divorce or marriage effectiveness or value resists the force of minority (Ovadia 2001).

The effectiveness of time in reducing faith in religion was lower in the United States than in others. This American deficit reflects the clash of forces between the United States and time effectiveness. On the one hand, the United States cherishes the force of religion (Schroeder 2013). On the other hand, time effectiveness in reducing religious faith embodies the force of secularization (Harper and Leicht 2011).

Chapter 8
Conclusions

Analytical functionalism enhanced by force theory secures the understanding of sociality regarding seven social attitudes. These attitudes are confidence in institutions, refutations against misdeeds and unconventional sexuality, unfaith in religion, rejection of outsiders and deviants, and trust in others. Principally, functionalism highlights the contribution to functioning as the basis for influence (Parsons 1968; Tetlock 2002). To represent functioning, analytical functionalism differentiates the requisite functions of fulfillment or goal attainment, adaptation, latency, and integration (Kral 2019; Munch 1987; Parsons 1968). Specifically, the fulfillment function is the externally consummatory function; the adaptation function is the externally instrumental function; the latency function is the internally instrumental function; and the integration is the internally consummatory function. Fulfillment or goal attainment covers achievement, conduciveness, fertility, reproduction, and restoration as opposed to discrepancy (Andrews et al. 1991; Crossley 2012; Klandermans and van Stekelenburg 2013; Malesevic 2022; Steel et al. 2012; Tetlock 2002). Adaptation covers affluence, availability, benefit, complementarity equilibrium, safety, satisfaction, and social status experienced as opposed to blaming, chaos, difficulty, precarity, and strain (Adamus et al. 2024; Brennan et al. 2001; Hattery and Smith 2012; Jackson and Scott 2010; Rojek 2005; Herman-Kinney 2003; Jenkins and Form 2005; Klandermans and van Stekelenburg 2013; Osberg and Smeeding 2006; S. Morgan 2021; Steel et al. 2012). Latency covers belief, ideology, mindset, and morality formation as opposed to inconsistency (Crossley 2012; Jenkins and Form 2005; S. Morgan 2021; Simpson et al. 2019; Skitka et al. 2014). Integration covers association, collaboration, coordination, institutionalization, interdependence, normativity, organicity, regulation, and socialization as opposed to anomie, conflict, normlessness, deregulation, destructuring, disintegration, disjuncture, independence, individualism, and individualization (Abrutyn and Lizardo 2023; Adamus et al. 2024; Brennan et al. 2001; Cote 2014; Crow 2002; Gordon 2009; Herman-Kinney 2003; Kral 2019; Skitka et al. 2014; Jackson and Scott 2010; J. Williams 2011). To achieve these functions, the voluntaristic mechanisms of analytical functionalism activate power realization

C.-k. Cheung, *Social Attitudes in the Early 21st Century*,
https://doi.org/10.1007/978-981-96-9705-2_8

for driving, utility optimization for attracting, ideal calibration for rationalizing, and norm conformity for assimilating. Furthermore, the deterministic mechanisms of analytical functionalism run directly through sharing privately and publicly and indirectly through empowering, incentivizing, framing, and standardizing. The indirect mechanisms eventually trigger the voluntaristic mechanisms. Hence, these mechanisms hinge on the forces of power, utility, ideals, and norms generalized in force theory. Force theory posits that a positive effect arises from the compatibility between input and outcome forces or their components, and a negative effect arises from the contradiction between input and outcome forces or their components. Here, a force engenders diverse components toward different directions or vectors. The component's strength is proportional to the correlation between the vectors of the component and its parent or generative force. Hence, the voluntaristic mechanisms of analytical functionalism engage a positive personal predictor of sociality to provide power to drive, utility to attract, ideals to rationalize, and/or norms to assimilate sociality. The deterministic mechanisms of analytical functionalism engage a positive national predictor to share sociality directly and/or empower, incentivize, frame, and/or standardize to advance sociality indirectly through activating voluntaristic mechanisms. Besides, force theory adds that the forces of the positive predictor and sociality need to be compatible.

Sociality embraces the four requisite functions. Its fulfillment function rests on conscientiousness, extraversion, gregariousness, guilt, honesty, leadership, morality, normativity, open-mindedness, shame, stability, togetherness, and trustworthiness as opposed to autonomy, misanthropy (Bissell 2010; Capraro 2024; Cottrell et al. 2007; Fowers 2015; Hughes et al. 2017; Tomasello 2014, 2020). Its adaptation function resides in altruism, attachment, bonding, caring, conformity, conservation, consulting, cooperation, dependence, honoring, fairness, gifting, helping, imitation, interaction, investment, justice, laughter, learning, liking, phone use, participation, punishment, reciprocity, role-taking, self-expansion, sharing, socializing, support, teaching, tolerance, and trust as opposed to aggression, discrimination, forfeiting, raging, risking, trolling, and violence (Boer and Fischer 2013; Capraro 2024; Cottrell et al. 2007; Fenwick 2008; Fowers 2015; Hughes et al. 2017; Koster 2013; Marres 2017; Phithakkitnukoon and Smoreda 2016; Provine 2000; Ratner et al. 2023). Its latency function lies in collective identification, group focus, and xenophobia as opposed to individual identity, individualism, and self-interest (Fowers 2015). Its integration function registers in community, friendship, institutionalization, membership, networking, organization, and rapport (Couldry and Hepp 2017; Fowers 2015; Hughes et al. 2017; Marres 2017; Rogers et al. 2014).

Sociality stands on the four functional bases. Its fulfillment or power functional bases are adaptability, agency, attachment, authenticity, belongingness, fitness, flexibility, friendship, homophily, intelligence, rationality, and trustworthiness (Fowers 2015; Phithakkitnukoon and Smoreda 2016). Its adaptation or utility functional bases are caring received, commonality, harmony, interdependence, predictability as opposed to alienation, and uncertainty (Fowers 2015; Tomasello 2014). Its latency or idealistic functional bases are actualization, categorization, collaboration, communitarianism, coordination, devotion, humanism, interaction, learning, reciprocity, republicanism, and socialism as opposed to individualism, instrumentalism or treating people as instruments, self-interest, and separation (Dean 2020; Fowers 2015; Tuomela 2007). Its integration or normative functional bases coercion, institutionalization, group living, manipulation, membership, and promotion experienced as opposed to hierarchy experienced (Fowers 2015; Tuomela 2007; Tomasello 2014).

Sociality unfolds as confidence or trust in institutions and other people, refutation or rejection of misdeeds, unconventional sexuality, outsiders, and deviants, and unfaith in religion. As such, sociality entails the separation of the inside and outside, encompassing misdeeds, unconventionality, outsiders, deviance, religion, or the supernatural or unnatural. This separation is an axis in analytical functionalism (Munch 1987; Parsons 1968). Meanwhile, sociality exhibits constructive and destructive approaches, with the former covering confidence and trust in the inside and the latter covering rejection of the outside (Hughes et al. 2017; Koster 2013). More specifically, the latter engages discrimination, punishment, and xenophobia to prohibit antisociality, defection, destruction, misanthropy, risk, and violence (Bissell 2010; Cottrell et al. 2007; Fowers 2015; Hughes et al. 2017; M. Ma 2021; Paasonen et al. 2023; Schinkel 2010; Tuomela 2007). Hence, sociality defines its boundary for functioning to stand on collectivism, communitarianism, conservatism, and socialism as opposed to cosmopolitanism, individualism, liberalism, radicalism, and reductionism (Fowers 2015; M. Ma 2021; Tuomela 2007; Winter and Feixas 2019).

Sociality is thus social living based on confidence and trust in insiders, rejection of deviants and outsiders, and refutation of their misdeeds and unconventionality (Cottrell et al. 2007; Fowers 2015; Tomasello 2014). Such living thrives on the functions of power, utility, ideals, and norms to achieve fulfillment, adaptation, latency, and integration. Power blaze from adaptability, agency, commonality, executive function, fitness, flexibility, morality, normativity, signaling ability, social intelligence, and trustworthiness as opposed to isolation (Fowers 2015; Tuomela 2007). Hence, health empowers or drives sociality. Utility derives from care, exchange, interdependence, and reward received as opposed to stress and uncertainty experienced, particularly iterated (Boer and Fischer 2013; Fowers 2015; Tuomela 2007). Hence, life satisfaction, prosperity, and security as opposed to economic hardship incentivizes or attracts sociality. Ideals evolve from collaboration, homophily, learning, reciprocity, social categorization, social identity, and social interaction, espousing social goals, language, and mentalizing (Fowers 2015; Phithakkitnukoon and Smoreda 2016; Tomasello 2020; Tuomela 2007). Norms accrue from culture and inheritance, propagating coordination, intuition, and predictability (Capraro 2024; Fowers 2015; Tuomela 2007). Hence, China or its collectivist norm, nonprofit organization employment, and population or human availability standardize or assimilate sociality.

Appreciable Effects

Understanding Waves 5 and 6 data of the World Values Survey revealed that appreciable ($|\beta| > .10$) effects emanated from some personal and national predictors. Positive predictors were time, the superpowers of China and the United States of America, national population size, national prosperity, national globalization, national government effectiveness, independent work, national security, national health, and national life satisfaction (see Table 8.1). Negative predictors were national democracy, national land per capita, national human capital, national income inequality, irreligion, national economic hardship, and national rejection of deviants. Nevertheless, these predictors did not apply to all seven social attitudes of sociality. Besides, national technology, national bank credit, national human development, and nonprofit organizational employment showed mixed effects on some social attitudes representing sociality.

Time

Time reflects global development to afford power, utility, ideals, and norms to grow sociality with analytical-functionalist mechanisms. Power for sociality rising with time has stemmed from friendliness, helpfulness, income, knowledge, prosociality, and survival (Beckfield 2004; Hamermesh 2019; Ramarajan et al. 2017; Singer et al. 1999; M. Smith et al. 2001). Utility for sociality rising with time has resided in financial satisfaction, justice perceived, relational quality, safety, and welfare satisfaction (Hsieh 2002; Logan and Cobb 2013; Malahy et al. 2009; Y. Wong et al. 2010). Conversely, disutility against sociality diminishing with time has resided in fear and threat (M. Smith et al. 2001; Sahar 2008). Ideals for sociality rising with time have favored birth, cohesion, conservatism, neighboring, security, social interaction, traditionalism, trust, volunteering, and working (Adsera 2003; de Beer and Kostere 2009; Gershuny 2000; Pazhoohi and Kingstone 2021; Puohiniemi and Verkasalo 2020; Sarracino 2010; M. Smith et al. 2001). Conversely, ideals against sociality declining with time have hailed capitalism, liberalism, mobility, protesting, religiosity, resistance, violence, and war (Bjornskov and Paldam 2012; Brynin et al. 2009; Cheung and Yip 2010; Kaufmann et al. 2012; Norris and Inglehart 2009; Pinker 2011; Sahar 2008). Norms for sociality rising with time have propagated human development, prosperity, social integration, survival or life expectancy, sympathy, and welfare (Hamermesh 2019; Lee and Coleman 2014; Norris 2012). Conversely, norms against sociality declining with time have dwelt on conflict, independence, and inequality (Diez-Nicolas 2002; Lange and Dawson 2009).

Nevertheless, time only raised sociality regarding unfaith in religion. According to force theory, the time effect of secularization reflects the match of forces between global development and religious unfaith. The forces emitted with time or by global development are secularization and individualization, reflecting empiricism or value

Table 8.1 Appreciable ($|\beta| > .10$) effects on sociality

Predictor	Institution	Anti-misdeed	Anti-sex	Anti-faith	Anti-outsider	Anti-deviant	Other
Time				.130			
China	.276		.102	.546	.245	–.143	
US	–.110		–.226		.170	.129	.119
National population	.255		.124	.181			
National democracy	–.142			–.397	–.234		
National land	–.103						
National prosperity						.360	
National technology		–.130		.346			
National bank credit				.121		–.185	
National human capital			–.362				
National human development				.102			–.198
National globalization					.284		
National income inequality		–.202					
National government effectiveness							.251
National economic hardship				–.146			
National security	.123						
National health					.102		
National life satisfaction			.113		.100		
National rejection of deviants			–.193				
Irreligious			–.156				

(continued)

Table 8.1 (continued)

Predictor	Institution	Anti-misdeed	Anti-sex	Anti-faith	Anti-outsider	Anti-deviant	Other
Nonprofit organization employment		–.126	–.139	.414		.105	
Independent work		.104					

Note Sociality unfolded in social attitudes in terms of confidence in institutions, refutation against misdeeds, refutation against unconventional sexuality, unfaith in religion, rejection of outsiders, rejection of deviants, and trust in others
+ positive effect. – negative effect

on experience, humanism, and rationalism, and reducing religiousness (de Graaf et al. 2001; Lemon 2003; Requena and Stanek 2014). Meanwhile, religious unfaith accepts forces favoring enlightenment, humanism, individualization, modernization, positivism or value on facticity, rationality, scientification, and secularization (Grayling 2013; Requena and Stanek 2014; Spilka et al. 2003; W. Tang 2014; von Stuckrad 2013).

China

China sustained sociality more than others by affording power, utility, ideals, and norms to activate analytical-functionalist mechanisms. Power for sociality maintained by China has stemmed from reduced mortality risk (Lassey et al. 1997). Ideals for sociality enhanced by China have favored civic engagement, cooperation, egalitarianism, familism, government and social trust, modesty, punishing, reciprocity, recourse, and volunteering (Buchan et al. 2002; Chen and Mak 2008; Hitlin and Harkness 2018; Houser and Xiao 2015; Y. Pan et al. 2023; Shin 2012; G. Walker et al. 2001; Wang and Han 2023; X. Wu 2009; Y. Zhou 2024). Communal norms for sociality embraced by China popularize collective functioning, control, connection, cooperation, exchange, familization, filiality, gifting, harmony, health, homogeneity, indebtedness, moral cultivation, networking, reciprocity, relatedness, role modeling, sacrifice, and visitation (Bian et al. 2005; J. Chen 2013; Chua 2002; Fallman 2010; X. Gu 2022; Y. Guo et al. 2023; Leung and Nann 1995; J. Li 2003; Reed 1995; Sun et al. 2013; D. Wang et al. 2010; Zhong 2009). Cultural norms for sociality espoused by China propagate adaptation, altruism, atheism, belonging, benevolence, brotherhood, civility or civilization, collectivism or collectivity, the commonweal, compassion, compliance, contribution, deference, duty, equality, familism, flexibility, forgiveness or magnanimity, government trust, group orientation, harmony, honesty, human orientation, integrity, interdependence, interpersonal trust, learning, moralism, morality, nationalism, order, patriotism, peacefulness, relationalism, self-discipline, socialism, societal well-being, submission, teamwork, tradition or traditionalism, trustworthiness, and welfare (Butler 2008; S. Chen 1996; Cheung and Pomerantz 2011; Gao 2018; Hirono 2013; Inglehart 1997; Leung and Nann 1995; H. Li 2021; S. Li et al. 2024; C. Lin 2003; Luk 2001; Nevis 1983; Y. Jin 2003; J. Liu et al. 2005; Miles and Wang 2018; Reed 1995; Rolandsen 2008; Steinhardt 2012; Szalay et al. 1994; Wang and Zhu 1996; D. Wang et al. 2010; Yang and Zhang 2001; Y. Yang et al. 2010; S. Zhang 2003; Zhang and Mo 2005; Zhang with Stening 2010; Zhou and Yan 2002). Adaptation has secured sociality regarding partnership and social adjustment and satisfaction as opposed to discord (Chow et al. 2014; Mitchell 2005). Political norms for sociality propagated by China spread anti-foreignism, atheism, befriending, bridging, civilization, collectivism, communism, communitarianism, Confucianism, consultation, cooptation, cooperation, equalizing, forgiveness, gratitude, group interest, harmony, helping, humaneness or humanity, legalism, moderation, morality or ethocracy, multilateralism, mutuality, nationalism, patriotism, peace, sharing, socialism, socialization, solidarity, unity, and win–win benefit (S. Chen 1996; Dai and Luqiu 2024; Dickson 2001; Genevaz 2019; W. Hou et al. 2003; J. Hu et al. 2018; Kachiga 2021; S. Lo 2021; Lu and Treiman 2008; Nai et al. 2020; Rosen 2009; Vickers 2024; F. Wang 2024; Zee 2022). Anti-foreignism or xenophobia has constituted sociality by boosting patriotism and social cohesion (Granzin and Olsen 1998; Wang and Chen 2004). Conversely, China has opposed the norm for capitalism, thus maintaining sociality (F. Wang 2024).

However, China showed less refutation against misdeeds and less rejection of deviants than the non-superpower. According to force theory as an enhancement of analytical functionalism, the negative effects reflected the clash between forces emitted by China and forces accepted by such refutation and rejection. On the one hand, forces emitted by China are atheism, forgiveness, magnanimity, and irreligion (W. Ho and Li 2022; Inglehart 1997; Zhou and Yan 2002). On the other hand, forces accepted by refuting misdeeds and rejecting deviants are non-forgiving, religiousness, and stigmatization (Cerulo and Ruane 2014; van der Leun and Koemans 2013; Vauclair and Fischer 2011).

United States of America

The United States of America raised sociality more than others by distributing norms to activate analytical-functionalist mechanisms. Norms for sociality upheld by the United States popularize compromise, conformity, equality or egalitarianism, fame or recognition, harmony, humanitarianism, justice, legality, loyalty, moralism, morality, nationalism, Protestantism, punishment, and sympathy (J. Barry 2011; Braun 2011; Epstein 1997; Garrett et al. 2014; Kruse 2015; Moore 2017; Rollo 2023; J. Turner 2011, 2015; F. Wang 2024). Conversely, norms against sociality downplayed by the United States spread imperialism and inequality (Brady and Leicht 2008; J. Cheng 2016).

However, the United States exhibited less confidence in institutions and refutation against unconventional sexuality than the non-superpower. According to force theory as an enhancement of analytical functionalism, the negative effects reflected the clash between forces emitted by the United States and forces accepted by such confidence and refutation. On the one hand, forces emitted by the United States favor autonomy, freedom, individualism, liberalism, neoliberalism, rights, and voluntarism and oppose government (J. Barry 2011; Hitlin and Pinkston 2013; Kruse 2015; J. Martin 2014; Narayan 2020; Rollo 2023; J. Turner 2011). On the other hand, forces accepted by confidence in institutions safeguard authoritarianism, collectivism, conservatism, government, and social cohesion and dismiss neoliberalism and rights (Bolger et al. 2020; Janmaat 2011; McAllister 1999; Mingo and Faggiano 2020; Pernia 2022; Zuckerman 2021). Similarly, forces underlying refuting unconventional sexuality cherish asceticism, authoritarianism, conservatism, discipline, interference, interdependence, regulation, repression, solidarity, temperance, tradition, and traditionalism and dismiss autonomy, freedom, individualism, independence, liberalism, rights, self-determination, self-expression (Alparone et al. 2024; Belliotti 1993; Conde Dias et al. 2012; de Jong et al. 2012; Jackson and Scott 2010; Jakobsson and Kotsadam 2011; Jung 2016; Kirsch 2000; Rival et al. 1998; Shim 2001; Soble 2008; Treger and Schmitt 2019; Vauclair and Fischer 2011).

National Population Size

National population size enhanced sociality by evolving power, utility, ideals, and norms to leverage analytical-functionalist mechanisms. Power for sociality raised by population size has rested on wages (Glaeser and Gottlieb 2009). Ideals for sociality boosted by population size have espoused social welfare and xenophobia (Iida and Matsubayashi 2010; Paxton and Knack 2012). Norms for sociality enhanced by population size have popularized economic growth, punishment, resources, social interaction, well-being, and government spending (Frey and Song 1997; Havinga 2002; Obschonk et al. 2016; Pattie et al. 2004; J. Turner 2003). Conversely, norms against sociality reduced by population size have popularized crime, liberty, neoliberalism, rights or entitlement, and violence (Abouharb and Cingranelli 2007; Browning et al. 2004; Hughes et al. 2015; Lobao et al. 2014).

National Prosperity

National prosperity based on gross domestic product per capita uplifted sociality by engendering power, utility, ideals, and norms to leverage analytical-functionalist mechanisms. Power for sociality enhanced by prosperity has resided in health and self-efficacy (Corcoran et al. 2011; S. Miller 2015). Utility for sociality afforded by prosperity has resided in relationship quality and satisfaction with democracy and life (Fridberg and Kangas 2008a; Helliwell et al. 2010; Norris 2011). Ideals for sociality upheld by prosperity have hailed institutional trust, political participation, social trust, volunteering, and xenophobia (Cheng and Smyth 2016; Inglehart 2003; Norris 1999a; Traunmuller 2011; van Oorschot and Arts 2005). Norms for sociality enhanced by prosperity have spread government effectiveness, government social spending, justice, legality and legal quality, trade, and universalism (Bjornskov 2005; Guisan 2009; Kang and Powell 2010; Minkov 2011; Oneal et al. 2003; Rindermann 2008). Conversely, norms against sociality diminished by prosperity have popularized anomie, homicide, inequality, risk, segregation, theft, and threat (Moller and Li 2009; Schneider 2007; Schwartz and Melech 2000; Teymoori et al. 2016; van Wilsem 2004; Weakliem et al. 2005).

Particularly, national prosperity raised sociality based on the rejection of deviants. This raise follows force theory for enhancing analytical functionalism Accordingly, such raising reflects the match between the forces of national prosperity and rejecting deviants. Forces brewed by national prosperity accentuate justice, lawfulness, and legal quality and lessen anomie, homicide, and theft (Bjornskov 2005; Rindermann 2008; Teymoori et al. 2016; van Wilsem 2004). Matching them are forces underlying deviance rejecting to uphold compliance, conformity, discipline, fairness, justice, morality, policing, security, and self-control and remove conflict, hostility, law violation, illegality, negativism, rebellion, and resistance (S. Henry 2009; Herman-Kinney 2003; Iacobucci and Frieh 2018; Kaplan et al. 2013; Vauclair and Fischer 2011; J. Williams 2011; Wright and DeLisi 2016).

National Globalization

National globalization elevated sociality regarding rejecting outsiders or xenophobia. According to force theory, as an enhancement of analytical functionalism, the elevation reflects the compatibility of forces between national globalization and the rejection of outsiders. Forces emitted by national globalization raise colonizing, competition, crime, exclusion, inequality, migration, stress, uncertainty, war, and cultural distancing and dampen solidarity (Arnett 2002; Brady et al. 2007; Kellner 2002; Munch 2012; Robertson 2001). Likewise, forces provoking xenophobia highlight classism, competition, conflict, crime, culturalism, deprivation, divisiveness, fear, frustration, stress, struggle, subordination, terrorism, threat, uncertainty avoidance, victimhood, victimization, and war and erode security (Banks and Valentino 2012; Blum 2008; Capdevila and Callaghan 2007; Davids 2011; de Figueiredo and Elins 2003; Elias and Feagin 2016; Feinberg et al. 2012; Husband and Alam 2011; Leong and Ward 2006; Marotta 2017; Meuleman et al. 2019; Ortona 2017; Rime et al. 2015; Savelkoul et al. 2011; Yi and Jung 2015). Notably, xenophobia represents avoiding uncertainty created by globalization.

National Government Effectiveness

National government effectiveness elevated sociality by providing power, utility, ideals, and norms to leverage analytical-functionalist mechanisms. Utility for sociality enhanced by government effectiveness has resided in justice experienced, living standards, social harmony experienced, satisfaction with democracy, and police and well-being generally (Bohnke 2008; Bratton and Mattes 2001; Tankebe 2009). Conversely, government effectiveness has diminished environmental problems as disutility against sociality (Wong and Wan 2011). Ideals for sociality raised by government effectiveness have prized generosity and institutional, political, and social trust (Grimes 2006; Guisan 2009; Heatherington and Globetti 2002; C. Wong et al. 2005). Conversely, government effectiveness has maintained the ideal against suicide to buttress sociality (Helliwell 2006). The ideal for suicide has impeded sociality by fomenting radicalism (Soliman et al. 2016). Norms for sociality strengthened by government effectiveness have spread prosperity and well-being (Guisan 2009; Rindermann 2018). Conversely, the norm for inequality has impaired sociality by provoking crime and violence (Ousey and Lee 2013; van Wilsem 2007).

Particularly, national government effectiveness boosted trust in others. Such boosting reflects the match of forces between national government and trust in others, based on force theory to enhance analytical functionalism. Forces delivered by national government effectiveness elevate harmony, justice, and social trust (Guisan 2009; R. Taylor et al. 2015; Wong and Shik 2011). Correspondingly, forces underpinning social trust generate bonding, cohesiveness, collaboration, confidence, cooperation, homogeneity, fairness, integration, justice, and reciprocity and resist conflict, diversity, and inequality (Buskens and Raub 2013; Li and He 2022; Mewes et al. 2021; Molm et al. 2007; Pretsch and Ehrhardt-Madapathi 2018; Rodrigo-Gonzalez et al. 2019; Ross and Jang 2000; ten Brinke and Keltner 2020; Vera-Toscano et al. 2013).

National Security

National security buttressed sociality by providing power, utility, ideals, and norms to leverage analytical-functionalist mechanisms. Power for sociality afforded by national security has derived from health and networking (Curley 2010; Ziersch et al. 2005). Utility for sociality given by national security has resided in well-being (Ziersch et al. 2005). Ideals for sociality cultivated by the security norm have highlighted cohesion, neighboring, and trust (Grannis 2009; Rochelle 2015). The norm for sociality maintained by national security has popularized quality (Olson et al. 2016).

Particularly, national security promoted confidence in institutions. According to force theory enhancing analytical functionalism, such promotion benefits from the congruence of forces between national security and confidence in institutions. Forces emanating from contextual security advance trust and dissolve fear and opposition (Barbarin and Richter 2001; Chiricos et al. 2000; Rochelle 2015). Likewise, forces underlying confidence in institutions breed authoritarianism, conservatism, empowerment, social capital, and trust (Bolger et al. 2020; Lowndes and Roberts 2013; Newton 2006; Pernia 2022; Suh et al. 2012). Authoritarianism embraces the forces of conformity, obedience, and submissiveness (Heller et al. 2022; Norris and Inglehart 2019; Pernia 2022). Similarly, conservatism displays or engenders the forces of allegiance, conformity, cooperation, loyalty, obedience, peace, respect, self-discipline, support, toleration, and trust and dismisses the forces of competition and transgression (Dutton and Rayner-Hilles 2022; Feinberg et al. 2019; Heilman and Kusev 2020; Kekes 1998; Lakoff 2009; Scruton 2014; Yoos 2007).

National Health

National health uplifted sociality by safeguarding power, utility, ideals, and norms to leverage analytical-functionalist mechanisms. Power enhanced by the norm for health has sprung from social capital (Portes and Vickstrom 2011). The norm raised by national health has popularized well-being (El-Ghannam 2002). Moreover, national health has stood on norms for prosperity, social capital, socioeconomic status, and trade to cultivate sociality (J. Jiang 2023; Bezo 2012; Rudra and Haggard 2005). Conversely, national health has maintained the norm against inequality and unemployment to secure sociality (J. Jiang 2023).

Particularly, national health facilitated sociality concerning the rejection of outsiders or xenophobia. This sustenance reflects the compatibility of forces between national health and xenophobia, considering force theory to enhance analytical functionalism. A force secured by national health develops social capital (Portes and Vickstrom 2011). Social capital manifests forces boosting belonging, bonding, cohesion, communitarianism, cooperation, homogeneity, homophily, nationalism, neighboring, and relatedness (Centola and Macy 2007; Chua et al. 2021; Coleman et al. 2022; Grootaert and van Bastelaer 2002; Harpham et al. 2002; Huxhold et al. 2022; Kirkby-Geddes et al. 2013; Rivera 2018; J. Son 2013; Wakefield and Poland 2005). Likewise, forces underpinning xenophobia accentuate assimilation, collectivism, communitarianism, conformity, cooperation, favoritism, groupism, homogeneity, ingroup identification, localism, nationalism, patriotism, and unity and discount conflict, diversity, mobility, pluralism, and variation (Amin 2012; Burchianti and Zapata-Barrero 2014; Elias and Feagin 2016; Hartmann et al. 2017; H. Kim et al. 2016; Macedo 2021; Jolly and DiGiusto 2014; Licata and Klein 2002; Marotta 2017; MuBotter 2024; Rindermann 2018; Vida and Reardon 2008; Wojcieszak and Garrett 2018; Zienkowski 2017).

National Life Satisfaction

National life satisfaction elevated sociality by affording norms to leverage analytical-functionalist mechanisms. Norms for sociality upheld by national satisfaction can popularize communitarianism, governance, and voting (Jackson and Miller 1995; Sciulli 2011; X. Zhu 2019). Conversely, national satisfaction can erode the norm for conflict to secure sociality (J. Turner 2013b).

National Democracy

National democracy eroded sociality by withdrawing ideals and norms for sociality through analytical-functionalist mechanisms. Ideals for sociality attenuated by national democracy have accentuated patriotism, social trust, and volunteering (Geys 2012; Kunovich 2009; Ruiter and De Graaf 2006). Norms against sociality enhanced by national democracy have popularized freedom (Moller and Skaaning 2013). Moreover, national democracy can evolve from norms for class conflict, diversity tolerance, individualism, and protesting (Beck et el. 1994; Hughes 2012; Moller and Skaaning 2013; Pourgerami 1991). In addition, national democracy stands on norms for competition, liberalism, and neoliberalism to impede sociality (Fishkin 2018; Moller and Skaaning 2013). National democracy also embraces norms for agonism, aggression, antagonism, appealing, argument, contesting, pluralism, polarization, self-interest, and selfishness to dampen sociality (Dryzek and Dunleavy 2009; Fairfield 2008; Minogue 2010; Moller and Skaaning 2013; Pappas 2019; Ringen 2007; Tracy and Hughes 2014; Yack 2012). Conversely, national democracy uses norms against Confucianism and conservatism to dampen sociality (Negri and Emery 2022; Shin 2012). National democracy also embraces norms against redistribution and unity to jeopardize sociality (Minogue 2010; Trainor 2008).

National Land

National land per capita obstructed sociality by withdrawing utility, ideals, and norms for sociality through analytical-functionalist mechanisms. Utility for sociality reduced by the national land share has resided in life satisfaction, neighborhood quality, and satisfaction (Oliver 2003; Whitham 2012). Ideals for sociality dampened by the national land share have prized civic engagement, collectivism, donation, neighboring, political participation, and prosocial behavior (Graddy and Wang 2009; Nai et al. 2018; Pattie et al. 2004; Swaroop and Morenoff 2006; Triandis 1995). Norms for sociality inhibited by the national land share have popularized economic growth and government spending (Obschonk et al. 2016; Pattie et al. 2004).

Particularly, the national land share diminished sociality regarding refuting misdeeds. This diminishment reflects the contradiction of forces between the land share and the misdeed refutation, based on force theory to enhance analytical functionalism. Forces given by the land share erode civicness, collectivism, donation, neighboring, and prosociality and breed suicide (Graddy and Wang 2009; Nai et al. 2018; O'Farrell et al. 2016; Swaroop and Morenoff 2006; Triandis 1995). These forces contradict those underlying refuting misdeeds that accept civilizing, communitarianism, morality, and prosocial socialization and resist antisociality, damage, escape, individualism, individualization, and risking (Agnew and Brezina 2010; Fitch et al. 2011; McLaughlin 2010; Merdian et al. 2017; Reiner 2016; Salisbury 2013; Sammons and Putwain 2019; Waiton 2008; Walsh 2014).

National Human Capital

National human capital reduced refuting unconventional sexuality. This reduction reflects the mismatch of forces between national human capital and the refutation, following force theory to enhance analytical functionalism. Forces incubated by national human capital raise aspiration and student status (Correll 2004; Hostetler et al. 2007). Student status evolves the force against childcare (Parrado 2005). On the contrary, forces underlying refutation against unconventional sexuality accept childcare or family obligation and resist sexual desire (Belliotti 1993; Jung 2016; Kirsch 2000).

National Income Inequality

National income inequality weakened sociality by withdrawing power, utility, ideals, and norms for sociality through analytical-functionalist mechanisms. Power for sociality weakened by income inequality has rested on health, social capital, and sympathy (Hitlin and Harkness 2018; Kim and Kawachi 2007; Portes and Vickstrom 2011). Moreover, income inequality has induced disability, illness, mortality, and poverty to eliminate power for sociality (A. Jones et al. 2015; Kawachi et al. 1997; Kim and Kawachi 2007). Utility for sociality reduced by income inequality has transpired in financial satisfaction (Winkelmann and Winkelmann 2010). Conversely, income inequality has bred disutility against sociality based on disadvantages, problems, and social exclusion experienced (Reardon and Bischoff 2011; Portes and Vickstrom 2011; Wilkinson and Pickett 2009). Ideals for sociality hampered by income inequality have supported social cohesion, social welfare, trust, volunteering, and voting (Gelissen 2002; Green et al. 2003; Lipford and Yandle 2009; Lister 2007; Oishi et al. 2011). Conversely, income inequality has diminished ideals against crime, education, and violence to impair sociality (Ousey and Lee 2013; Maurer 2011; van Wilsem 2007). Norms for sociality eroded by income inequality have popularized civic participation, fairness, justice, and trust (Eriksson et al. 2015; Oishi et al. 2011; Wilkinson and Pickett 2017; Uslaner 2002). Moreover, income inequality has risen with norms against education, employment, prosperity, and well-being to obstruct sociality (Inglehart 1997; Lobao and Hooks 2003; Sun 2011; Weakliem et al. 2005). Income inequality can also rise with norms against alliances, citizenship, coordination, social welfare, unionization, and universalism to hinder sociality (Edlund and Gronlund 2010; Guenther et al. 2016; Navarro 2002; Tomaskovic-Devey and Avent-Holt 2019). Conversely, norms against sociality heightened by income inequality have spread anomie, corruption, crime, depression, gambling, psychopathology, risk, theft, and vandalism (Hughes et al. 2015; Knack 2002; Teymoori et al. 2016; Uslaner 2008; Wilkinson and Pickett 2017; van Wilsem 2004). Moreover, income inequality has arisen from norms for dependency, despair, greed, immigration, minority status, prejudice, social exclusion, and unemployment to impede sociality (Alderson and

Nielsen 2002; Dorling 2010; C. Lin et al. 2015; Lobao and Hooks 2003; Nolan 1983). Income inequality can also grow with norms for capitalism, competition, differentiation, exploitation, individualization, neoliberalism, segmentation, social closure, and warfare to impair sociality (Baldus 2017; R. Brown 2017; Castells 2000; Guenther et al. 2016; Johnson and Johnson 2005; J. Turner 2010; Tomaskovic-Devey and Avent-Holt 2019).

Specifically, national income inequality diminished refutation against misdeeds. This diminishing reflects the contradiction of forces between national income inequality and the refutation, considering force theory to enhance analytical functionalism. Forces engendered by income inequality trigger corruption, crime, theft, vandalism, and violence and disrupt fairness and justice (Eriksson et al. 2015; Oishi et al. 2011; Uslaner 2008; Ousey and Lee 2013; van Wilsem 2007). Countering these forces are forces underlying refutation against misdeeds to establish punishment and prohibit antisociality, crime, externalizing behavior, homicide, and violence (Hoffmann 2023; Salisbury 2013; Sammons and Putwain 2019; Tanner-Smith et al. 2013).

National Economic Hardship

National economic hardship impaired sociality by withdrawing power, utility, ideals, and norms for sociality through analytical-functionalist mechanisms. Power for sociality reduced by national economic hardship has stemmed from civility, education, family income, family intactness, and wealth (L. Hao 1996; Owens and Walker 2018; Roscigno 1999). Conversely, national economic hardship has fostered dysfunction, illness, and social welfare dependency to reduce power to uphold sociality (Hirschl and Rank 1999; B. Johnson et al. 2006; A. Jones et al. 2015). Utility attenuated by national economic hardship has rested on neighborhood quality and satisfaction, relatedness, and security (Gaitan-Rossi and Shen 2018; Harris 2001; C. Ross et al. 2000). Ideals for sociality dismissed by national economic hardship have valorized civic engagement, community involvement, donation, and social trust (Abascal 2015; Broadbent and Papadopoulos 2011; Graddy and Wang 2009; Stoll 2001). Conversely, national economic hardship has fomented ideals for cynicism, suicide, theft, and violence to devalue sociality (Hagan et al. 2016; Krahe 2013; Piatkowska 2020). National income inequality has also impeded sociality by eroding social capital, support for redistribution and welfare, sympathy, trust, and volunteering (Busemeyer 2013; Hitlin and Harkness 2018; Lipford and Yandle 2009; Oishi et al. 2011; Portes and Vickstrom 2011).

Specifically, national income inequality dampened sociality regarding unfaith in religion. This dampening reflects the clash of forces between national income inequality and the unfaith, considering force theory to enrich analytical functionalism. Forces created by national income inequality uphold divinity and natural law (Diefenbach 2013). Contrariwise, forces underlying unfaith in religion resist divinity and natural law (Riordan 2008; Warburton 2005).

National Rejection of Deviants

National rejection of deviants reduced refutation against unconventional sexuality. This reduction reflects the clash of forces between national rejection of deviants and refutation against conventional sexuality. On the one hand, national rejection of deviants engenders the force of safety and diminishes the force of risk (Patterson and Keefe 2008). On the other hand, refutation against unconventional sex suggests the force of risk or unsafety in unconventional sex (Russell et al. 2020).

National Technology

National technology boosted unfaith in religion. This boosting reflects the match of forces between national technology and unfaith in religion, considering force theory to enrich analytical functionalism. Forces arising from national technology buttress emancipation, scientism, and self-expression (Welzel 2013; Welzel and Inglehart 2010; Y. Zhu 1995). Likewise, forces underpinning unfaith in religion highlight enlightenment, liberalism, rationality, scientification, self-enhancement, and subjectivity and resist strictness and traditionism (Cresswell 2018; Datler et al. 2013; Schlenker et al. 2012; von Stuckrad 2013; Wollschleger 2012).

However, national technology weakened refutation against misdeeds. This weakening reflects the mismatch of forces between national technology and refuting misdeeds, considering force theory to enrich analytical functionalism. Forces stemming from national technology champion risk and worsen sustainability (Roderick 2016; Welzel 2013). Contrariwise, forces underlying refutation against misdeeds accentuate survival and resist risk (de Castro-Rodrigues and Sacau 2015; Piquero et al. 2010).

National Bank Credit

National bank credit reduced the rejection of deviants. This reduction reflects the mismatch of forces between national bank credit and rejection of deviants, considering force theory to enrich analytical functionalism. Forces springing from national bank credit engender autonomy, creativity, freedom, individuality, and inequality (Godechot 2016; Haiven 2014). Contrariwise, forces underlying the rejection of deviants accept agreeableness, bonding, and consensus and resist independence, individualism, individualizing, and innovation (Iacobucci and Frieh 2018; Kaplan et al. 2013; Vauclair and Fischer 2011; J. Williams 2011; Wright and DeLisi 2016).

Meanwhile, national bank credit promoted unfaith in religion. This promotion reflects the match of forces between national bank credit and the unfaith, considering force theory to enrich analytical functionalism. Forces emanating from national bank credit propel autonomy, creativity, and possibility (Haiven 2014). Likewise, forces upholding unfaith in religion accept autonomy, diversity, individualism, and openness and resist conservatism, strictness, and traditionalism (Copen and Silverstein 2008; Grayling 2013; Land and Deane 1992; Pollack and Pickel 2007; Saucier and Skrzypinska 2006; Wollschleger 2012).

National Human Development

National human development reduced trust in other people. This reduction reflects the mismatch of forces between national human development and trust in others, considering force theory to enrich analytical functionalism. Forces arising from national human development breed corruption and freedom and weaken communitarianism and tradition (Davis and Robinson 2006; Nederveen Pieterse 2010; Quah 2003; Uslaner 2008). Contrariwise, forces underlying trust in others accept attachment, cohesiveness, collectivity, communitarianism, conservatism, cooperation, fairness, fraternity, justice, and morality and resist bribing, collusion, corruption, and liberty (Abascal 2015; Carter 2016; Halvorsen 2007; Herreros 2009; A. Hu 2013; Laroche et al. 2019; Olivera 2015; B. Six 2014; Uslaner 2008; Vera-Toscano et al. 2013; J. You 2012).

Meanwhile, national human development elevated unfaith in religion. This reduction elevation reflects the match of forces between national human development and unfaith in religion, considering force theory to enrich analytical functionalism. Forces arising from national human development display capability, capital, education, freedom, liberalization, pluralism, self-determination, self-direction, and wisdom and weaken tradition (Bond and Lun 2014; Hoekstra 2019; C. Johnson 2009; Nederveen Pieterse 2010; Quah 2003). Likewise, forces underlying unfaith in religion accept education, enlightenment, income, individualism, intelligence, liberalism, modernization, plurality, rationality and resist collectivism, communitarization, and traditionalism (De Graaf 2013; Grayling 2013; Immerzeel and van Tubergen 2013; Perlin 2011; Pollack and Pickel 2007; Requena and Stanek 2014; Rivera 2018; Saucier and Skrzypinska 2006; Schlenker et al. 2012; von Stuckrad 2013).

Irreligion

Irreligion dampened refutation against unconventional sexuality. This dampening reflects the clash of forces between irreligion and this refutation, considering force theory to enrich analytical functionalism. Forces brewed by irreligion buttress divorce and unconventional sex and lessen discipline, marriage, morality, normativity, parenthood, and traditionalism (Cochran et al. 2004; Ellison et al. 2013; Jost 2020;

Robert and Bukodi 2005; Saucier and Skrzypinska 2006; B. Turner 2009). Contrariwise, forces accepted by refutation against unconventional sexuality favor divorce and resist Catholicism, Christianity, marriage, morality, motherhood, normativity, parenthood, paternalism, procreation, religiousness, self-discipline, and traditionalism (Belliotti 1993; Bernasconi 2010; Jackson and Scott 2010; Jung 2016; Kirsch 2000; Malacrida and Boulton 2012; Primoratz 1999; Pruss 2013; Soble 2008).

Nonprofit Organizational Employment

Nonprofit organization employment particularly elevated unfaith in religion. This elevation reflects the match of forces between nonprofit organization employment and unfaith in religion, considering force theory to enrich analytical functionalism. Forces springing from nonprofit organization employment boost autonomy, empowerment, and flexibility (Islam and William 2012; Milligan and Fyfe 2005; Perotin 2001). Likewise, forces upholding unfaith in religion accept autonomy, enlightenment, intelligence, openness, and plurality and resist conservativeness and strictness (De Graaf 2013; Grayling 2013; Peifer 2010; Saucier and Skrzypinska 2006; Spilka et al. 2003; von Stuckrad 2013).

Independent Work

Independent work enhanced refuting misdeeds as sociality reflects the match of forces between independent work and this refutation, considering force theory to enhance analytical functionalism. Forces created by independent work secure citizenship, justice, safety, and solidarity as opposed to conflict (De Carlo et al. 2019; De Dreu and Nauta 2009; Man and Lam 2003; Parker et al. 2001; Younts and Mueller 2001). Meanwhile, forces underlying misdeed refutation establish agreeableness, agreement, attachment, civilizing, cohesion, community, consent, justice, protection, security, social capital, and social integration as opposed to competition, conflict, incivility, individualism, rebellion, risk (Jolley et al. 2019; Karstedt 2010; Kennedy et al. 1998; Messner et al. 2013; Ozer and Bertelsen 2019; Piquero et al. 2010; Reiner 2016; Tanner-Smith et al. 2013; Waiton 2008; Walsh 2014; Welch et al. 2008; Wright and DeLisi 2016).

Final Remarks

Social attitudes representing sociality showed the most pervasive differences between China and non-superpower countries. Similarly, the attitudes displayed the next most pervasive differences between the United States and non-superpower countries. Besides, the attitudes exhibited pervasive variations due to nonprofit organization employment, national population size, and national democracy. Notably, faith in religion manifested a decline with time. Furthermore, different social attitudes varied due to different national performances, including the national land share, technology, prosperity, income inequality, financialization, globalization, government effectiveness, human capital, human development, life satisfaction, economic hardship, security, and health.

National and temporal influences represent social changes, featuring denaturalization, globalization, individualization, industrialization, liberalization, rationalization, vitalization, and other ways of modernization (Harper and Leicht 2011; Morody and Giza-Poleszczuk 2018). Denaturalization, characterized by time and population size, elevated unfaith in religion, confidence in institutions, and refutation against unconventional sexuality. Globalization heightened the rejection of outsiders. Individualization, characterized by human capital, reduced refutation against unconventional sexuality. Industrialization, characterized by prosperity and technology, increased rejection of deviants and unfaith in religion but decreased refutation against misdeeds. Liberalization, characterized by democracy, diminished unfaith in religion, rejection of outsiders, and confidence in institutions. Rationalization, characterized by government effectiveness, increases trust in other people. Vitalization, characterized by human development, health, life satisfaction, and security as opposed to economic hardship, decreased trust in other people but increased unfaith in religion, confidence in institutions, and the rejection of outsiders.

As superpowers, China and the United States made pervasive differences in sociality, as indicated by the seven social attitudes. The differences stemmed from the combined differences in the superpower's bank credit, carbon dioxide emission, phone subscription, population size, and globalization. Specifically, the differences due to China sprang from the combined differences in irreligion, population size, and bank credit. China's differences furthermore reflect China's atypicality, distinctiveness, forcefulness, growth, power, and rise (Evans 2006; Han and Li 2024; Kachiga 2021; Yu and Chiu 2016; Zhang with Stening 2010). Meanwhile, the differences due to the United States reflected the combined differences in carbon dioxide emission, prosperity, government effectiveness, human capital, globalization, phone subscription, human development, bank credit, the rule of law, and liberty. These differences attest to American exceptionalism, impact, hyperpower, and massiveness (Chiozza 2023; Rollo 2023; Schroeder 2013). All the differences follow the premise of force theory that mass and acceleration or velocity, respectively based on size and rise, combine to produce influence (Mansfield and O'Sullivan 2011; Cheung 2013).

Sociality is ethical, considering its basis on the utility of national government effectiveness, health, life satisfaction, prosperity, and security as opposed to economic hardship. That is, sociality is a manifestation of national goods. Particularly, rejecting outsiders was a manifestation of national health and life satisfaction, and rejecting deviants was a manifestation of national prosperity. Refutation against unconventional sexuality was also a manifestation of national life satisfaction. Confidence in institutions was a manifestation of national security. Trust in others was a manifestation of national government effectiveness. Religious unfaith was a manifestation of low national economic hardship. Hence, according to deontological logic, sociality is good when its basis is sound (Killen 2018).

With time, sociality will rise, particularly involving refuting misdeeds and religion and rejecting outsiders. The increase in refuting misdeeds reflects civilization (M. Michael 2017; Rindermann 2018). The increase in religious unfaith registers secularization (Chakrabarti 2016). The increase in rejecting outsiders registers societalization, emphasizing homogeneity, membership, social cohesion, and socialization (Alexander and Adams 2023; Hayashi 2022; Kampen 2010; Semenova et al. 2020). Overall, the increase in sociality reflects communication growth (Tan 2003). Nevertheless, the rise in religious unfaith or secularization will be smaller in the United States. This smaller rise reflects the counterforces of multiculturalism, polarization, and Protestantism as a religion there (Boulianne et al. 2022; Cheng and Sikkink 2020; Hoyt and Goldin 2016). Multiculturalism means preserving heritage culture (Moghaddam 2008). Meanwhile, religion characterizes culture (Minkov 2011). Moreover, religion or its institutionalization necessarily retards secularization (Bompani and Brown 2015). Similarly, polarization prevents consensus in belief (Almogro 2023). Religion and secularization certainly build on belief (J. Turner et al. 2018).

Appendix

See Table 1.

Table 1 Means, standard deviation, and factor loadings on well-being

Correlate	Scoring	*M*	*SD*
Wave	5, 6	5.5	0.5
Population	million	834.8	530.3
Phone per capita	–	19.6	16.6
Land per capita	–	1.3	2.2
Technology per capita	–	175.5	293.1
Credit per capita	–	82.0	52.2
GDP	US$	7494.4	13,442.2
Gini	0–100	42.5	5.1
Globalization	–	58.2	9.9
Government effectiveness	–	0.1	0.6
Democracy	–	5.7	3.5
Liberty	–	40.1	34.4
Human development	–	0.7	0.1
Human capital	–	2.3	0.6
CO_2	–	4.7	4.7
Rule of law	–	43.8	10.0
Acquiescence	0–100	47.3	6.9
Female	0, 100	48.2	50.0

(continued)

C.-k. Cheung, *Social Attitudes in the Early 21st Century*,
https://doi.org/10.1007/978-981-96-9705-2

Table 1 (continued)

Correlate	Scoring	*M*	*SD*
Age	year	41.3	15.2
Education	0, 100	9.5	5.0
Irreligious	0, 100	36.6	48.2
Family income	0–100	37.7	23.7
Age squared	yeas^2	1.0	1.2
Married	0, 100	71.6	45.1
Cohabited	0, 100	4.5	20.7
Divorced	0, 100	2.3	15.0
Separated	0, 100	1.0	10.1
Widowed	0, 100	4.1	19.7
Kid	person	2.0	1.6
Mother immigrant	0, 100	7.0	25.5
Father immigrant	0, 100	6.7	25.0
Graduation age	year	18.8	10.6
Survey interest	0, 100	67.9	31.9
Living with parents	0, 100	36.0	48.0
Full-time employment	0, 100	25.3	43.5
Part-time employment	0, 100	10.1	30.1
Self-employment	0, 100	9.5	29.3
Retired	0, 100	12.5	33.1
Homemaking	0, 100	6.9	25.3
Student	0, 100	9.0	28.6
Unemployed	0, 100	6.5	24.6
Public employment	0, 100	25.3	43.5
Private business employment	0, 100	16.6	37.2
Nonprofit organization employment	0, 100	13.1	33.8
Intellectual work	0, 100	34.1	31.8
Creative work	0, 100	32.5	30.5
Independent work	0, 100	40.7	35.1
Supervision	0, 100	24.3	42.9
Earner status	0, 100	42.4	49.4
Earner employed	0, 100	86.4	34.3
Economic hardship	0–100	22.2	26.5
Neighborhood nuisance	0–100	24.3	24.6
Victimization	0–100	7.1	21.5

(continued)

Table 1 (continued)

Correlate	Scoring	*M*	*SD*
Security	0–100	73.6	22.5
Family saving	0–100	63.5	32.2
E-activity	0–100	23.9	38.0
Learning	0–100	48.1	30.6
Religious attendance	0–100	56.5	28.7
Risk aversion	0–100	67.3	40.3
Weapon carrying	0–100	11.0	31.3
Organizational participation	0–100	14.8	21.5
Appealing	0–100	14.1	26.6
Strike	0–100	9.2	28.9
Voting	0–100	86.4	21.1
Green demonstrating	0–100	7.1	25.7
Green donation	0–100	9.4	29.2
Health	0–100	62.3	29.1
Life satisfaction	0–100	63.5	25.6
Confidence in institutions	0–100	57.9	19.9
Justification for misdeeds	0–100	14.7	18.5
Justification for unconventional sexuality	0–100	23.7	27.3
Faith in religion	0–100	66.3	30.8
Acceptance of outsiders	0–100	21.4	31.1
Acceptance of deviants	0–100	57.9	31.5
Trust in others	0–100	50.2	18.6
China	0, 100	32.7	46.9
US	0, 100	7.5	26.3
China or US	0, 100	40.2	49.0

References

Abascal, M. 2015. "Love thy Neighbor: Ethnoracial Diversity and Trust Reexamined." *American Journal of Sociology* 121 (3): 622–782.

Abbey, Antonia, Rhiana Wegner, Jennifer Pierce, and Angela Jacques-Tiura. 2012. "Patterns of Sexual Aggression in a Community Sample of Young Men: Risk Factors Associated with Persistence, Desistance, and Initiation over a 1-Year Interval." *Psychology of Violence* 2 (1): 1–15.

Abbott, Pamela, Claire Wallace, and Roger Sapsford. 2011. "Surviving the Transformation: Social Quality in Central Asia and the Caucasus." *Journal of Happiness Studies* 12: 199–223.

Abegaz, Berhanu. 2013. "Political Parties in Business: Rent Seekers, Developmentalists, or Both?" *Journal of Development Studies* 49 (11): 1467–1483.

Abercrombie, Nicholas, Stephen Hill, and Bryan S. Turner. 1980. *The Dominant Ideology Thesis*. London: George Allen & Unwin.

Aberg, Yvonne. 2000. "Individual Social Action and Macro Level Dynamics: A Formal Theoretical Model." *Acta Sociologica* 43 (3): 193–205.

Abizadeh, Arash. 2010. "Citizenship, Immigration, and Boundaries." Pp.358–376 in *Ethics and World Politics*, edited by Duncan Bell. Oxford, UK: Oxford University Press.

Abouharb, M. Rodwan., and David Cingranelli. 2007. *Human Rights and Structural Adjustment*. Cambridge, UK: Cambridge University Press.

Abrutyn, Seth, and Jonathan H. Turner. 2011. "The Old Institutionalism Meets the New Institutionalism." *Sociological Perspectives* 54 (3): 283–306.

Abrutyna, Seth, and Anna S. Mueller. 2014. "Are Suicidal Behaviors Contagious in Adolescence? Using Longitudinal Data to Examine Suicide Suggestion." *American Sociological Review* 79 (2): 211–227.

Achilov, Dilshod. 2016. "Revisiting Political Islam: Explaining the Nexus between Political Islam and Contentious Politics in the Arab World." *Social Science Quarterly* 97 (2): 252–270.

Ackerman, Phillip L., and Stacey D. Wolman. 2007. "Determinants and Validity of Self-estimates of Abilities and Self-concept Measures." *Journal of Experimental Psychology: Applied* 13 (2): 57–78.

Adams, Matthew. 2007. *Self and Social Change*. London, CA: Sage.

Adamus, Magdalena, Eva Ballová Mikušková, Pavol Kačmár, Martin Guzi, Matuš Adamkovič, Maria Chayinska, and Jais Adam-Troian. 2024. "The Mediating Effect of Institutional Trust in the Relationship between Precarity and Conspiracy Beliefs: A Conceptual Replication of Adam-Troian et al. (2023)." *British Journal of Social Psychology* 63(3):1207–25.

Addad, Moshe. 1987. "Neuroticism, Extraversion and Meaning of Life: A Comparative Study of Criminals and Non-Criminals." *Personality & Individual Differences* 8 (6): 879–883.

C.-k. Cheung, *Social Attitudes in the Early 21st Century*,
https://doi.org/10.1007/978-981-96-9705-2

Adler, Emanuel, 2013. "Constructivism in International Relations: Sources, Contributions, and Debates." Pp. 112–144 in *Handbook of International Relations*, edited by Walter Carlsnaes, Thomas Risse and Beth A. Simmons. London, UK: SAGE.

Adloff, Frank. 2018. "Civil Society." Pp. 398–411 in *The SAGE Handbook of Political Sociology*, edited by William Outhwaite and Stephen Turner. London, UK: SAGE.

Adnanes, Marian. 2004. "Exit and/or Voice? Youth and Post-communist Citizenship in Bulgaria." *Political Psychology* 25 (5): 795–815.

Adongo, Raymond, Seongseop Kim, and Statia Elliot. 2019. "Give and Take: A Social Exchange Perspective on Festival Stakeholder Relations." *Annals of Tourism Research* 75: 42–57.

Adsera, Alicia. 2003. "Changing Fertility Rates in Developed Countries: The Impact of Labor Market Institutions." *Journal of Population Economics* 17: 17–43.

Ager, Alustair, and J. Ager. 2011. "Faith and the Discourse of Secular Humanitarianism." *Journal of Refugee Studies* 24 (3): 456–472.

Agnew, Robert S. 2007. "Strain Theory and Violent Behavior." Pp.519–528 in *The Cambridge Handbook of Violent Behavior and Aggression*, edited by Daniel J. Flannery, Alexander T. Vazsonyi and Irwin D. Waldman. Cambridge, UK: Cambridge University Press.

Agnew, Robert, and Timothy Brezina. 2010. "Strain Theories." Pp.96–113 in *The SAGE Handbook of Criminological Theory*, edited by Eugene McLaughlin and Tim Newburn. London, UK: SAGE.

Aguila, Cornelio, Alvaro Sicilia-Camacho, Antonio J. Rojas, Miguel A. Tejada, and Delgado-Noguera, and Michael Gard. 2008. "Postmodern Values and Leisure in Young Spanish University Students: An Exploratory Study." *Leisure Sciences* 30: 275–292.

Ahern, Melissa M., and Michael S. Hendryx. 2003. "Social Capital and Trust in Providers." *Social Science & Medicine* 57: 1195–1203.

Ahnquist, Johanna, Sarah P. Wamala, and Martin Lindstrom. 2012. "Social Determinants of Health: A Question of Social or Economic Capital? Interaction Effects of Socioeconomic Factors on Health Outcomes." *Social Science & Medicine* 74 (6): 930–939.

Aidnik, Martin. 2024. *The Public University as a Real Utopia: Towards a Renewal of Higher Education*. Cham, Switzerland: Springer.

Aiken, Lewis. 2002. *Attitudes and Related Psychosocial Constructs: Theories, Assessment, and Research*. Thousand Oaks, CA: Sage.

Aival-Naveh, Erez, Lily Rothschild-Yakar, and Jenny Kurman. 2019. "Keeping Culture in Mind: A Systematic Review and Initial Conceptualization of Mentalizing from a Cross? Cultural Perspective." *Clinical Psychology: Science & Practice* 26(4):12300. \117–116 Science and Practice 26(4):12300. \117–116.

Ajzen, Icek, and Martin Fishbein. 2014. "The Influence of Attitudes on Behavior." Pp. 173–221 in *The Handbook of Attitudes*, edited by Albarracin Dolores, T. Johnson Blair and P. Zanna Mark. Mahwah, NJ: Psychology.

Akaeda, Naoki. 2021. "Welfare States and the Health Impact of Social Capital: Focusing on the Crowding-out and Crowding-in Perspectives." *Social Indicators Research* 157 (3): 841–862.

Akiyama, Hiroko, and Toni Antonucci. 2002. "Gender Differences in Depressive Symptoms: Insights from a Life Span Perspective on Life Stages and Social Networks." *Advances in Medical Sociology* 8: 343–358.

Akman, Aynan. 2012. "Beyond the Objectivist Conception of Civil Society: Social Actors, Civility and Self-limitation." *Political Studies* 60: 321–340.

Alasuutari, Pertti. 2015. "The Discursive Side of New Institutionalism." *Cultural Sociology* 9 (2): 162–184.

Alderson, Arthur S., and Francois Nielsen. 2002. "Globalization and the Great U-turn: Income Inequality Trends in 16 OECD Countries." *American Journal of Sociology* 107 (5): 1244–1299.

Alderson, Arthur. 2004. "Explaining the Upswing in Direct Investment: A Test of Mainstream and Heterodox Theories of Globalization." *Social Forces* 83 (1): 81–122.

Aldridge, Stephen, and David Halpern. 2002. *Social Capital*. London: Performance & Innovation Unit.

Alesina, Alberto, and Eliana La Ferrara. 2002. "Who Trusts Others?" *Journal of Public Economics* 85 (2): 207–234.

Alessio, John C. 2011. *Social Problems and Inequality: Social Responsibility through Progressive Sociology*. Farnham, UK: Ashgate.

Alexander, Jeffrey C. 1997. "The Paradoxes of Civil Society." *International Sociology* 12 (2): 115–133.

Alexander, Jeffrey C., and Tracy Adams. 2023. "The Return of Antisemitism? Waves of Societalization and What Conditions Them." *American Journal of Cultural Sociology* 11: 251–268.

Algoe, Sara B., and Ruixue Zhaoyang. 2016. "Positive Psychology in Context: Effects of Expressing Gratitude in Ongoing Relationships Depend on Perceptions of Enactor Responsiveness." *Journal of Positive Psychology* 11 (4): 399–415.

Alharbi, Ahlam, and Mary Rucker. 2023. "Discursive Practices of the Performative Theory of Solidarity Discourse." *Language Sciences* 95: 101515.

Al-Kire, Rosemary, Michael Pasek, Jo-Ann Tsang, Joseph Leman, and Wade Rowatt. 2022. "Protecting America's Borders: Christian Nationalism, Threat, and Attitudes toward Immigrants in the United States." *Group Processes & Intergroup Relations* 25(2):354-78.

Al-krenawi, Alean, John R Graham, Fakir Al Gharaibeh. 2011. "A Comparison Study of Psychological, Family Function Marital and Life Satisfactions of Polygamous and Monogamous Women in Jordan." *Community Mental Health Journal* 47(5):594-602.

Allard, Scott, and Sheldon Danziger. 2000. "Welfare Magnets, Myth or Reality?" *Journal of Politics* 62 (2): 350–368.

Allen, Joseph P., Maryfrances R. Porter, F. Christy McFarland, and Penny Marsh. 2005. ' "The Two Faces of Adolescents' Success with Peers: Adolescent Popularity, Social Adaptation, and Deviant Behavior." *Child Development* 76 (3): 747–760.

Almakaeva, Anna, Christian Welzel, and Eduard Ponarin. 2018. "Human Empowerment and Trust in Strangers: The Multilevel Evidence." *Social Indicators Research* 139 (3): 923–962.

Alnsour, Jamal, and Julia Meaton. 2009. "Factors Affecting Compliance with Residential Standards in the City of Old Salt, Jordan." *Habitat International* 33: 301–309.

Alonso-Arbiol, Itziar, Nekane Balluerka, and Phillip R. Shaver. 2007. "A Spanish Version of the Experiences in Close Relationships (ECR) Adult Attachment Questionnaire." *Personal Relationships* 14: 45–63.

Alparone, Dario, Roberto Pozzetti, and Amelia Rizzo. 2024. "Sexuality in the Digital World: Treatment of a Case of Dating App Addiction." *Theory & Psychology* 34 (5): 630–645.

Altman, Andrew, and Christopher Heath Wellman. 2009. *A Liberal Theory of International Justice*. Oxford, UK: Oxford University Press.

Alumona, Ikenna Mike, and Stephen Nnaemeka Azom. 2018. "Politics of Identity and the Crisis of National Building in Africa." Pp. 291–306 in *The Palgrave Handbook of African Politics, Governance and Development*, edited by Samuel Ojo Oloruntoba and Toyin Falola. New York, NY: Palgrave.

Alvarez, R. Michael., and John Brehm. 2002. *Hard Choices, Easy Answers: Values, Information, and American Public Opinion*. Princeton, NJ: Princeton University Press.

Alvesson, Mats. 2002. *Postmodernism and Social Research*. Buckingham, UK: Open University Press.

Ambrey, Christopher L., and Christopher M. Fleming. 2014. "Valuing Ecosystem Diversity in South East Queensland: A Life Satisfaction Approach." *Social Indicators Research* 115: 45–65.

Ambrose, James. 2002. *Simplified Mechanics and Strength of Materials*. New York: John Wiley & Sons.

Amenta, Edwin. 2005. "State-centered and Political Institutional Theory: Retrospect and Prospect." Pp. 96–114 in *The Handbook of Political Sociology: States, Civil Societies, and Globalization*, edited by Thomas Janoski, Robert Alford, Alexander Hicks, and Mildred A. Schwartz. Cambridge, UK: Cambridge University Press.

Amin, Ash. 2012. *Land of Strangers*. Cambridge, UK: Polity.

Anciaes, Paulo Rui, Paul James Metcalfe, and Chris Heywood. 2017. "Social Impacts of Road Traffic: Perceptions and Priorities of Local Residents." *Impact Assessment & Project Appraisal* 35 (2): 172–183.

Andersen, Jorgen Goul. 1999. "Changing Labour Markets, New Social Divisions and Welfare State Support." Pp.13–33 in *The End of the Welfare State? Responses to State Retrenchment*, edited by Stefan Svallfors and Peter Taylor-Gooby. London: Routledge.

Anderson, C. Leigh., and Neil Nevitte. 2006. "Teach Your Children Well: Values of Thrift and Saving." *Journal of Economic Psychology* 27: 247–261.

Anderson, Mary R. 2010. "Community Psychology, Political Efficacy, and Trust." *Political Psychology* 31 (1): 59–84.

Anderson, RaeAnn E., Rachael L. Wandrey, Samuel C. Klossner, Shawn P. Cahill, and Douglas L. Delahanty. 2017. "Sexual Minority Status and Interpersonal Victimization in College Men." *Psychology of Sexual Orientation & Gender Diversity* 4 (1): 130–136.

Anderson-Butcher, Dawn, Angela Oliver Khairallah, and Janis Race-Bigelow. 2004. "Mutual Support Groups for Long-term Recipients of TANF." *Social Work* 49 (1): 131–140.

Andersson, Helle Wessel, Johan Hakon Bjorngaard, Silje Lill Kaspersen, Catharina E. A. WangIngunn, and Skre, and Thomas Dahl. 2010. "The Effects of Individual Factors and School Environment on Mental Health and Prejudiced Attitudes among Norwegian Adolescents." *Social Psychiatry & Psychiatric Epidemiology* 45 (5): 569–577.

Andreeva, Elena, Yuliya Myslyakova, Pavel Glukhikh, and Artem Ratner. 2017. "Economic and Social Impact of Modernization on Cultural Values." *Journal of International Studies* 10 (1): 193–208.

Andreouli, Eleni and Lia Figgou. 2019. "Critical Social Psychology of Politics." Pp. 148–165 in *The SAGE Handbook of Applied Social Psychology*, edited by Kieran C. O'Doherty and Darrin Hodgetts. London, UK: SAGE.

Andrews, Kenneth T., Kraig Beyerlein, and Tuneka Tucker Farnum. 2015. "The Legitimacy of Protest: Explaining White Southerners' Attitudes toward the Civil Rights Movement." *Social Forces* 94 (3): 1021–1044.

Angelis, Sophia, and Pamela Pensini. 2024. "Honesty-Humility Predicts Humanitarian Prosocial Behavior via Social Connectedness: A Parallel Mediation Examining Connectedness to Community, Nation, Humanity, and Nature." *Scandinavian Journal of Psychology* 64 (6): 810–818.

Angelusz, Robert, and Robert Tardos. 2001. "Change and Stability in Social Network Resources: The Case of Hungary under Transformation." Pp.297–323 in *Social Capital: Theory and Research*, edited by Nan Lin, Karen Cook, and Ronald S. Burt. New York: Aldine de Gruyter.

Anitha, Sundari, and Aisha K. Gill. 2018. "Making Politics Visible: Discourses on Gender and Race in the Problematisation of Sex-Selective Abortion." *Feminist Review* 120 (1): 1–19.

Anton, Charis E., and Carmen Lawrence. 2014. "Home is Where the Heart Is: The Effect of Place of Residence on Place Attachment and Community Participation." *Journal of Environmental Psychology* 40: 451–461.

Antonakis, John, Samuel Bendahan, Philippe Jacquart, and Rafael Lalive. 2010. "On Making Causal Claims: A Review and Recommendations." *Leadership Quarterly* 21: 1086–1120.

Antoni, Giacomo Degli, and Gianluca Grimalda. 2024. "Is Social Capital Bridging or Bonding? Evidence from a Field Experiment with Association Members." *Theory & Decision* 97 (1): 167–190.

Antonio, Robert J. 2000. "After Postmodernism: Reactionary Tribalism." *American Journal of Sociology* 106 (2): 40–87.

Apinunmahakul, Amornat, and Rose Anne Devlin. 2008. "Social Networks and Private Philanthropy." *Journal of Public Economics* 92: 309–328.

Aragno, Anna. 2014. "The Roots of Evil: A Psychoanalytic Inquiry." *Psychoanalytic Review* 101 (2): 249–288.

Arat, Gizem, and Narine N. Kerelian. 2019. "The Promotion of Socially Inclusive East Asian Society: The Hong Kong Case." *Journal of Human Rights & Social Work* 4 (4): 275–284.

Arce, José Manuel., and Rodríguez, and Michael James Winkelman. 2021. "Psychedelics, Sociality, and Human Evolution." *Frontiers in Psychology* 12: 729425.
Ariely, Gal, and Eric M. Uslaner. 2017. "Corruption, Fairness, and Inequality." *International Political Science Review* 38 (3): 349–362.
Arneson, Richard J. 2005. "Joel Feinberg and the Justification of Hard Paternalism." *Legal Theory* 11 (3): 259–284.
Arnett, Jeffrey Jensen. 2002. "The Psychology of Globalization." *American Psychologist* 57 (10): 774–783.
Aron, Arthur, Jodie L. Steele, Todd B. Kashdan, and M. A. X. Perez. 2006. "When Similars Do Not Attract: Tests of a Prediction from the Self-Expansion Model." *Personal Relationships* 13 (4): 387–396.
Arriaga, Ximena B., Rebecca J. Cobb, and Christine A. Daly. 2018. "Aggression and Violence in Romantic Relationships." Pp. 365–377 in *The Cambridge Handbook of Personal Relationships*, edited by Anita L. Vangelisti and Daniel Perlman. Cambridge, UK: Cambridge University Press.
Arseth, Annie K., Jane Kroger, Monica Martinussen, and Guro Bakken. 2009. "Intimacy Status, Attachment, Separation-Individuation Patterns, and Identity Status in Female University Students." *Journal of Social & Personal Relationships* 26 (5): 697–712.
Asendorpf, Jens B., Jaap J. A. Denissen, and Marcel A.G.. van Aken. 2008. "Inhibited and Aggressive Preschool Children at 23 Years of Age: Personality and Social Transitions into Adulthood." *Developmental Psychology* 44 (1): 997–1011.
Asendorpf, Jens B., Lars Penke, and Mitja D. Back. 2011. "From Dating to Mating and Relating: Predictors of Initial and Long-Term Outcomes of Speed-Dating in a Community Sample." *European Journal of Personality* 25 (1): 16–30.
Ashley, David. 1997. *History without a Subject: The Postmodern Condition.* Boulder, CO: Westview.
Ashworth, Andrew. 2006. *Principles of Criminal Law.* Oxford, UK: Oxford University Press
Ashworth, Peter D. 2013. The Gift Relationship. *Journal of Phenomenological Psychology* 44 (1): 1–36.
Aslani, Soroush, Jimena Ramirez-Marin, Zhaleh Semnani-Azad, Jeanne M. Brett, and Catherine Tinsley. 2013. "The Demise of the Rational Negotiator: Emotional Forces in Conflict and Negotiation." Pp. 249–282 in *Handbook of Research on Negotiation*, edited by Mara Olekalns and Wendi L. Adair. Cheltenham, UK: Elgar.
Aslanidis, Paris. 2018. "Populism as a Collective Action Master Frame for Transnational Mobilization." *Sociological Forum* 33 (2): 443–464.
Asongu, Simplice A. 2013. "How Has Mobile Phone Penetration Stimulated Financial Development in Africa?" *Journal of African Business* 14 (1): 7–18.
Assiter, Alison. 2003. *Revisiting Universalism.* Houndmills, UK: Palgrave.
Atkeson, Lonna Rae, and Cherie D. Maestas. 2012. *Catastrophic Politics: How Extraordinary Events Redefine Perceptions of Government.* New York: Cambridge University Press.
Atkins, Judi. 2008. "How Virtue-theoretic Arguments May Be Used in the Justification of Policy." *Politics* 28 (3): 129–137.
Atkinson, Giles, Andrew Healey, and Susana Mourato. 2005. "Valuing the Costs of Violent Crime: A Stated Preference Approach." *Oxford Economic Papers* 57 (4): 559–585.
Auerbach, Yehudith. 2009. "The Reconciliation Pyramid: A Narrative-based Framework for Analyzing Identity Conflicts." *Political Psychology* 30 (2): 291–318.
Avery, Eileen E., Joan M. Hermsen, and Danielle C. Kuhl. 2021. "Toward a Better Understanding of Perceptions of Neighborhood Social Cohesion in Rural and Urban Places." *Social Indicators Research* 157 (2): 523–541.
Axford, Barrie. 2013. *Theories of Globalization.* Cambridge, UK: Polity.
Ayalon, Hanna, Eliezer Ben-Rafael, and Abraham Yogev. 1993. *Community in Transition: Mobility, Integration, and Conflict.* Westport, CT: Greenwood.
Ayob, Abu H. 2020. "An Exploratory Study of Societal Values in Social Participation across Nations." *Social Science Journal* 57 (3): 310–325.

Aytac, Isik A., and Bruce H. Rankin. 2009. "Economic Crisis and Marital Problems in Turkey: Testing the Family Stress Model." *Journal of Marriage & Family* 71: 756–767.

Babrow, Austin S., and Katie M. Striley. 2015. "Problematic Integration Theory and Uncertainty Management Theory: Learning to Hear and Speak to Different Forms of Uncertainty." Pp.103–114 in *Engaging Theories in Interpersonal Communication: Multiple Perspectives*, edited by Dawn O. Braithwaite and Paul Schrodt. Thousand Oaks, CA: SAGE.

Bachkirova, Tatiana, and Elaine Cox. 2007. "A Cognitive-developmental Approach for Coach Development." Pp. 325–350 in *Handbook of Coaching Psychology: A Guide for Practitioners*, edited by Stephen Palmer and Alison Whybrow. Hove, UK: Routledge.

Backman, Olof, and Anders Nilsson. 2011. "Pathways to Social Exclusion: A Life-course Study." *European Sociological Review* 27 (1): 107–123.

Badea, Constantina, Kevin R. Binning, David K. Sherman, Mihaela Boza, and Anna Kende. 2021. "Conformity to Group Norms: How Group-Affirmation Shapes Collective Action." *Journal of Experimental Social Psychology* 95: 104153.

Badurdeen, Fathima Azmiya, Sahla Aroussi, and Michaelina Jakala. 2022. "Lived Realities and Local Meaning-Making in Defining Violent Extremism in Kenya: Implications for Preventing and Countering Violent Extremism in Policy and Practice." *Critical Studies on Terrorism* 16 (1): 1–22.

Bagherior, Reza, A. S. Bahaman, A. S. Asnarulkhadi, and A. Shamsudain. 2009. "A Social Exchange Approach to People's Participation in Watershed Management Programs in Iran." *European Journal of Scientific Research* 34 (3): 428–441.

Baik, Jiwoon. 2019. "One Belt One Road and the Geopolitics of Empire." *Inter-Asia Cultural Studies* 20 (3): 358–376.

Baildon, Mark, and Theresa Alviar-Martin. 2020. "Taming Cosmopolitanism: The Limits of National and Neoliberal Civic Education in Two Global Cities." *Asia Pacific Journal of Education* 40 (1): 98–111.

Bailey, Stephen J. 2004. *Strategic Public Finance*. Houndmills, UK: Palgrave.

Baker, Joseph O., and Buster G. Smith. 2009. "Growing up in Context: The Nones: Social Characteristics of the Religiously Unaffiliated." *Social Forces* 87 (3): 1251–1263.

Baldacci, Emanuele, Maria Teresa Guin-Siu, and Luiz de Mello. 2003. "More on the Effectiveness of Public Spending on Health Care and Education: A Covariance Structure Model." *Journal of International Development* 15: 709–725.

Baldner, Conrad, Daniela Di Santo, Alessandra Talamo, and Antonio Pierro. 2020. "Sympathy as Knowledge of the Other in Need: An Investigation into the Roles of Need for Closure and the Moral Foundations on Sympathy toward Immigrants." *Journal of Applied Social Psychology* 50 (4): 240–252.

Baldus, Bernd. 2017. *Origins of Inequality in Human Societies*. New York, NY: Routledge.

Baldwin, David A. 2013. "Power and International Relations." Pp. 273–297 in *Handbook of International Relations*, edited by Walter Carlsnaes, Thomas Risse and Beth A. Simmons. London, UK: SAGE.

Ball, Carlos A. 2003. *The Morality of Gay Rights: An Exploration in Political Philosophy*. New York: Routledge.

Ball, Michael. 2004. "Co-operation with the Community in Property-led Urban Regeneration." *Journal of Property Research* 21 (2): 119–142.

Ballard-Rosa, Cameron, Lucy Martin, and Kenneth Scheve. 2017. "The Structure of American Income Tax Policy Preferences." *Journal of Politics* 79 (1): 1–16.

Banks, Antoine J., and Nicholas A. Valentino. 2012. "Emotional Substrates of White Racial Attitudes." *American Journal of Political Science* 56 (2): 286–297.

Bannister, J. O. N., and Anthony O'Sullivan. 2013. "Civility, Community Cohesion and Antisocial Behaviour: Policy and Social Harmony." *Journal of Social Policy* 42 (1): 91–110.

Baofu, Peter. 2009. *The Future of Post-human Organization: A Preface to a New Theory of Communication, Decision-making and Leadership*. Newcastle, UK: Cambridge Scholars.

Baptista, N., José Carlos. Pinho, and Helena Alves. 2021. "Examining Social Capital and Online Social Support Links: A Study in Online Health Communities Facing Treatment Uncertainty." *International Review on Public & Nonprofit Marketing* 18 (1): 57–94.

Barabantseva, Elena. 2012. "Who Are Overseas Chinese Ethnic Minorities? China's Search for Transnational Ethnic Unity." *Modern China* 38: 78–109.

Barak, Adi. 2016. "Critical Consciousness in Critical Social Work: Learning from the Theatre of the Oppressed." *British Journal of Social Work* 46 (6): 1776–1792.

Barbarin, Oscar A., and Linda Richter. 2001. "Economic Status, Community Danger and Psychological Problems among South African Children." *Childhood* 8 (1): 115–133.

Barber, Jennifer S. 2004. "Community Social Context and Individualistic Attitudes toward Marriage." *Social Psychology Quarterly* 67 (3): 236–256.

Bardo, Michael T., Thomas Kelly, Donald R. Lynam, and Richard Milich. 2003. "Basic Science and Drug Abuse Prevention: Neuroscience, Learning, and Personality Perspectives." Pp.429–446 in *Handbook of Drug Abuse Prevention: Theory, Science, and Practice*, edited by Zili Sloboda and William J. Bukoski. New York: Kluwer Academic.

Barefoot, John C., Kimberly E. Maynard, Jean C. Beckham, Beverly H. Brummett, Karen Hooker, and Ilene C. Siegler. 1998. "Trust, Health, and Longevity." *Journal of Behavioral Medicine* 21 (6): 517–526.

Barkan, Steven E., and Steven F. Cohn. 2005. "Why Whites Favor Spending More Money to Fight Crime: The Role of Racial Prejudice." *Social Problems* 52 (2): 300–314.

Barker, David C., James D. Tinnick III. 2006. "Competing Visions of Parental Roles and Ideological Constraint." *American Political Science Review* 100 (2): 249–263.

Barkin, Shari, Shelley Kreiter, and Robert H. Du Rant. 2001. "Exposure to Violence and Intentions to Engage in Moralistic Violence during Early Adolescence." *Journal of Adolescence* 24: 777–789.

Barnawi, Fatima Hamza. 2017. "Prevalence and Risk Factors of Domestic Violence against Women Attending a Primary Care Center in Riyadh, Saudi Arabia." *Journal of Interpersonal Violence* 32 (8): 1171–1186.

Barr, Jeffrey A., Nambee G. Choi, Jun E. Mutchler, and Francis G. Caro. 2005. "Caregiving and Volunteering: A Private and Public Helping Behaviors Linked?" *Journal of Gerontology: Social Sciences* 60B (5): S247–S256.

Barr, Michael. 2012. "Nation Branding as Nation Building: China's Image Campaign." *East Asia* 29: 81–94.

Barr, Robert R. 2009. "Populists, Outsiders and Anti-Establishment Politics." *Party Politics* 15 (1): 29–48.

Barrett, Anne E. 1999. "Social Support and Life Satisfaction among the Never Married." *Research on Aging* 21 (1): 46–72.

Barry, Carolyn McNamara., and Allan Wigfield. 2002. "Social Perceptions of Friendship-making Ability and Perceptions of Friends" Deviant Behavior: Childhood to Adolescence." *Journal of Early Adolescence* 22 (2): 143–172.

Barry, Carolyn, Laura Padilla-Walker, and Larry Nelson Laura. 2012. "The Role of Mothers and Media on Emerging Adults" Religious Faith and Practices by Way of Internalization of Prosocial Values." *Journal of Adult Development* 19 (2): 66–78.

Barry, John Christopher. 2011. "Empire as a Gated Community: Politics of an American Strategic Metaphor." *Global Society* 25 (3): 287–309.

Barry, Monica, and Christine Hullett. 1998. *Social Exclusion and Social Work: Issues of Theory, Policy and Practice*. Dorset, UK: Russell House.

Bar-Tal, Daniel and Eran Halperin. 2013. "The Psychology of Intractable Conflicts: Eruption, Escalation, and Peacemaking." Pp.923–956 in *The Oxford Handbook of Political Psychology*, edited by Leone Huddy, David O. Sears and Jack S. Levy. New York: Oxford University Press.

Barthold, Charles, Stephen Dunne, and David Harvie. 2018. "Resisting Financialisation with Deleuze and Guattari: The Case of Occupy Wall Street." *Critical Perspectives on Accounting* 52: 4–16.

Basanez, Miguel. 2016. *A World of Three Cultures: Honor, Achievement and Joy*. New York: Oxford University Press.

Bask, Miia. 2005. "Welfare Problems and Social Exclusion among Immigrants in Sweden." *European Sociological Review* 21 (1): 73–89.

Batson, C. Daniel., and Tecia Moran. 1999. "Empathy-induced Altruism in a Prisoner's Dilemma." *European Journal of Social Psychology* 29: 909–924.

Batta, Anna. 2011. "Statism." Pp. 91–98 in *21st Century Political Science: A Reference Handbook*, edited by John T. Ishiyama and Marijke Breuning. Thousand Oaks, CA: SAGE.

Batto, Nathan F. 2019. "Cleavage Structure and the Demise of a Dominant Party: The Role of National Identity in the Fall of the KMT in Taiwan." *Asian Journal of Comparative* Politics 4(1):81-101.

Bauer, Isabelle, Carsten Wrosch, and Joelle Jobin. 2008. "I'm Better off Than Most Other People: The Role of Social Comparisons for Coping with Regret in Young Adulthood and Old Age." *Psychology & Aging* 23 (4): 800–811.

Bauman, Zygmunt. 2001. *The Individualized Society*. Cambridge, UK: Polity.

Bavetta, Sebastiano, Pietro Navarra, and Dario Maimone. 2014. *Freedom and the Pursuit of Happiness: An Economic and Political Perspective*. New York, NY: Cambridge University Press.

Beardsworth, Richard. 2011. *Cosmopolitanism and International Relations Theory*. Cambridge, UK: Polity.

Beardsworth, Richard. 2020, "Postmodernism Past, Present and Future." In *The SAGE Handbook of Political Science*, edited by Dirk Berg-Schlosser, Bertrand Badie and Leonardo Morlino. London, UK: SAGE.

Beauregard, Keth S., and David Dunning. 1998. "Turning up the Contrast: Self-enhancement Motives Prompt Egocentric Contrast Effects in Social Judgments." *Journal of Personality & Social Psychology* 74 (3): 606–621.

Bebber, Charles C. 1995. "Thematic Images Linking American Militancy Strikes of the 1980s and Rising U.S. Civil Violence." *Metaphor & Symbolic Activity* 10 (2): 139–154.

Becchetti, Leonardo, Elena Giachin Ricca, and Alessandra Pelloni. 2012. "The Relationship between Social Leisure and Life Satisfaction: Causality and Policy Implications." *Social Indicators Research* 108 (3): 453–490.

Beck, Ulrich, and Elisabeth Beck-Gernsheim. 2002. *Individualization: Institutionalized Individualism and Its Social and Political Consequences*. London: Sage.

Beck, Ulrich, Anthony Giddens, and Scott Lash. 1994. *Reflexive Modernization: Politics, Tradition and Aesthetics in the Modern Social Order*. Cambridge, UK: Polity.

Becker, Jan U., and Michel Clement. 2006. "Dynamics of Illegal Participation in Peer-to-peer Networks: Why Do People Illegally Share Media Files?" *Journal of Media Economics* 19 (1): 7–32.

Becker, Thomas E., Robert S. Billings, Daniel M. Eveleth, and Nicole W. Gilbert. 1997. "Validity of Scores on Three Attachment Style Scales: Exploratory and Confirmatory Evidence." *Educational & Psychological Measurement* 57 (3): 477–493.

Beckfield, Jason. 2004. "Does Income Inequality Harm Health: New Cross-national Evidence." *Journal of Health & Social Behavior* 45 (3): 231–248.

Bednall, Timothy C., Liliana L. Boveb, Ali Cheethamb, and Andrea L. Murray. 2013. "A Systematic Review and Meta-Analysis of Antecedents of Blood Donation Behavior and Intentions." *Social Science & Medicine* 96 (13): 86–94.

Beinc, Miehcel, Frederic Docquier, and Hillel Rapoport. 2001. "Brain Drain and Economic Growth: Theory and Evidence." *Journal of Development Economics* 64: 275–289.

Bekkers, Rene, Beate Volker, Martin van der Gaag, and Henk Flap. 2008. "Social Networks of Participants in Voluntary Associations." Pp.185–205 in *Social Capital: An International Research Program*, edited by Nan Lin and Bonnie H. Erickson. Oxford, UK: Oxford University Press.

Bekkers, Rene. 2005. "Participation in Voluntary Associations: Relations with Resources, Personality, and Political Values." *Political Psychology* 26 (3): 439–454.

Bekkers, Rene. 2008. "Straight from the Heart." *Advances in Medical Sociology* 10: 197–221.

Bekkers, Rene. 2010. "Who Gives What and When? A Scenario Study of Intentions to Give Time and Money." *Social Science Research* 39: 369–381.

Belanger, Eric, and Kees Aarts. 2006. "Explaining the Role of the LF: Issues, Discontent, and the 2002 Dutch Election." *Acta Politica* 41: 4–20.

Beldad, Ardion, Thea van der Geest, Menno de Jong, and Michael Steehouder. 2012. "A Cue or Two and I'll Trust You: Determinants of Trust in Government Organizations in Terms of Their Processing and Usage of Citizens' Personal Information Disclosed Online." *Government Information Quarterly* 29 (1): 41–49.

Bell, Daniel A. 1999. "Democracy with Chinese Characteristics: A Political Proposal for the Post-communist Era." *Philosophy East & West* 49 (4): 451–493.

Bellah, Robert N., Richard Madsen, William M. Sullivan, Ann Swidler, and Steven M. Tipton. 1991. *The Good Society*. New York: Vintage.

Bellani, Luna, and D'Ambrosio. Conchita. 2011. "Deprivation, Social Exclusion and Subjective Well-being." *Social Indicators Research* 104: 67–86.

Belle, Nicola, Paolo Belardinelli, Maria Cucciniello, and Greta Nasi. 2024. "Experimental Evidence on the Determinants of Citizens' Expectations toward Public Services." *Public Administration Review* 85 (1): 176–191.

Bellemare, Charles, and Sabine Kroger. 2007. "On Representative Social Capital." *European Economic Review* 51 (1): 183–202.

Belliotti, Raymond A. 1993. *Good Sex: Perspectives on Sexual Ethics*. Lawrence, KA: University Press of Kansas.

Bello, Valeria. 2016. "Inclusiveness as Construction of Open Identity: How Social Relationships Affect Attitudes Towards Immigrants in European Societies." *Social Indicators Research* 126 (1): 199–223.

Belzil, Christian and Jörgen Hansen. 2020. "The Evolution of the US Family Income–Schooling Relationship and Educational Selectivity." *Journal of Applied Econometrics* 35(7):841–59. \100–303.

Benassy-Quere, Agnes, Benoit Coeure, Pierre Jacquet, and Jean Pisani-Ferry. 2010. *Economic Policy: Theory and Practice*. New York: Oxford University Press.

Benda, Brent B. 2002. "A Test of Three Competing Theoretical Models of Delinquency Using Structural Equation Modeling." *Journal of Social Service Research* 29 (2): 55–91.

Bendek, Zoraida Mendiwelso. 2002. "Citizens of the Future: Beyond Normative Conditions through the Emergence of Desirable Collective Properties." *Journal of Business Ethics* 39 (1–2): 189–195.

Bender, Michael, and Athanasios Chasiotis. 2011. "Number of Siblings in Childhood Explains Cultural Variance in Autobiographical Memory in Cameroon, People's Republic of China, and Germany." *Journal of Cross-Cultural Psychology* 42 (6): 998–1017.

Bendixsen, Synnøve. 2018. "Differentiation of Rights in the Norwegian Welfare State: Hierarchies of Belonging and Humanitarian Exceptionalism." *Social Inclusion* 6 (3): 162–171.

Bengtson, Vern L., Robert A. Harootyan, Karl Kronebusch, Leora Lawton, Mark Schlesinger, Merril Silverstein, and Robert E. Vorek. 1994. *Intergenerational Linkages: Hidden Connections in American Society*. New York: Springer.

Bennardo, Giovanni, and Victor C. De Munck. 2014. *Cultural Models: Genesis, Methods, and Experiences*. New York: Oxford University Press.

Bennett, Jenna Karlsberg, Sarah O'Neill, Khushmand Rajendran, and Jeffrey M. Halperin. 2020. "Do Preschoolers' Neuropsychological Functioning and Hyperactivity/Inattention Predict Social Functioning Trajectories through Childhood?" *Journal of Pediatric Psychology* 45 (7): 793–802.

Benson, Michael L., and Sally S. Simpson. 2018. *White-collar Crime: An Opportunity Perspective*. New York: NY: Routledge.

Ben-Zur, Hasida. 2002. "Coping, Affect and Aging: The Roles of Mastery and Self-Esteem." *Personality & Individual Differences* 32 (2): 357–372.

Berard, T. J. 1999. "Michel Foucault, the History of Sexuality, and the Reformulation of Social Theory." *Journal for the Theory of Social Behaviour* 29 (3): 203–227.

Bergeman, C. S., and Pascal R. Deboeck. 2014. "Trait Stress Resistance and Dynamic Stress Dissipation on Health and Well-Being: The Reservoir Model." *Research in Human Development* 11 (2): 108–125.

Berger, John M. 2018. *Extremism*. Cambridge, MA: MIT.

Berger, Lawrence M. 2005. "Income, Family Characteristics, and Physical Violence toward Children." *Child Abuse & Neglect* 29 (2): 107–133.

Berger, Mark T. 2003. "Decolonisation, Modernisation and Nation-building: Political Development Theory and the Appeal of Communism in Southeast Asia, 1945–1975." *Journal of Southeast Asian Studies* 34 (3): 421–448.

Berger, Roni. 2015. *Stress, Trauma, and Posttraumatic Growth: Social Context, Environment, and Identities*. New York, NY: Routledge.

Berger-Schmitt, Reina. 2002. "Considering Social Cohesion in Quality of Life Assessments: Concept and Measurement." *Social Indicators Research* 58: 403–428.

Bernardo, Fatima, and Jose-Manuel. Palma-Oliveira. 2016. "Identification with the Neighborhood: Discrimination and Neighborhood Size." *Self & Identity* 15 (5): 579–598.

Bernardon, Stephanie, Kimberley A. Babb, Julie Hakim-Larson, and Marcia Gragg. 2011. "Loneliness, Attachment, and the Perception and Use of Social Support in University Students." *Canadian Journal of Behavioural Science* 43 (1): 40–51.

Bernauer, Thomas, and Vally Koubi. 2009. "Effects of Political Institutions on Air Quality." *Ecological Economics* 68 (5): 1355–1365.

Bernstein, Andrew. 2012. *Capitalist Solutions: A Philosophy of American Moral Dilemmas*. New Brunswick, NJ: Transaction.

Berry, Daniel R., Jonathan P. Hoerr, Selena Cesko, Amir Alayoubi, Kevin Carpio, Hannah Zirzow, Wesley Walters, Genny Scram, Katie Rodriguez, and Vanessa Beaver. 2020. "Does Mindfulness Training without Explicit Ethics-Based Instruction Promote Prosocial Behaviors? A Meta-Analysis." *Personality & Social Psychology Bulletin* 46 (8): 1247–1269.

Bersot, Heather Y., and Bruce A. Arrigo. 2015. "Responding to Sex Offenders." *Criminal Justice & Behavior* 42 (1): 32–44.

Besser-Jones, Lorraine. 2012. "The Role of Practical Reason in an Empirically Informed Moral Theory." *Ethical Theory & Moral Practice* 15 (2): 203–220.

Bessudnov, Alexey. 2016. "Ethnic Hierarchy and Public Attitudes Towards Immigrants in Russia." *European Sociological Review* 32 (5): 567–580.

Best, Samuel J., and Brian S. Krueger. 2010. "Government Monitoring and Political Participation in the United States: The Distinct Roles of Anger and Anxiety." *American Politics Research* 39 (1): 85–117.

Bettencourt, Fitzpatrick, E. Kathryn, Tammi Vacha-Haase, and Zinta S. Byrne. 2011. "Older and Younger Adults' Attitudes toward Feminism: The Influence of Religiosity, Political Orientation, Gender, Education, and Family." *Sex Roles* 64 (11–12): 863–874.

Beyerlein, Kraig, and David Sikkink. 2008. "Sorrow and Solidarity: Why Americans Volunteered for 9/11 Relief Effort." *Social Problems* 55 (2): 190–215.

Beynon-Jones, Siân. M. 2017. "Untroubling Abortion: A Discourse Analysis of Women's Accounts." *Feminism & Psychology* 27 (2): 225–242.

Bezo, Brent. 2012. "The Rights and Freedoms Gradient of Health: Evidence from a Cross-National Study." *Frontiers in Psychology* 3:441. \91–306, 100–355.

Bhochhibhoya, Shristi, Sarah B. Maness, Marshall Cheney, and Daniel Larson. 2021. "Risk Factors for Sexual Violence among College Students in Dating Relationships: An Ecological Approach." *Journal of Interpersonal Violence* 36 (15–16): 7722–7746.

Bian, Yanjie, Ronald Breiger, Deborah Davis, and Joseph Galashkiewicz. 2005. "Occupation, Class, and Social Networks in Urban China." *Social Forces* 83 (4): 1443–1468.

Bianchi, Andrea. 2016. *International Law Theories: An Inquiry into Different Ways of Thinking*. Oxford, UK: Oxford University Press.

Bickel, Robert. 2018. *Peter Berger on Modernization and Modernity: An Unvarnished Overview*. Abingdon, UK: Routledge.
Bierhoff, Hans-Werner. 2002. *Prosocial Behavior*. Hove, UK; Psychology.
Biersteker, Thomas J. 2013. "State, Sovereignty, and Territory." Pp. 245–272 in *Handbook of International Relations*, edited by Walter Carlsnaes, Thomas Risse and Beth A. Simmons. London, UK: SAGE.
Biggar, Nigel. 2020. *What's Wrong with Rights?* Oxford, UK: Oxford University Press.
Biggart, Nichole Woolsey, and Thomas D. Beanish. 2003. "The Economic Sociology of Conventions: Habit, Custom, Practice, and Routine in Market Order." *Annual Review of Sociology* 29: 443–464.
Biggs, Michael, and Steven Knauss. 2012. "Explaining Membership in the British National Party: A Multilevel Analysis of Contact and Threat." *European Sociological Review* 28 (5): 633–646.
Biggs, Simon, and Ariela Lowenstein. 2011. *Generational Intelligence: A Critical Approach to Age Relations*. Abingdon, UK: Routledge.
Billiet, Jaak, Bart Maddens, and Roeland Beerten. 2003. "National Identity and Attitude toward Foreigners in a Multinational State: A Replication." *Political Psychology* 24 (2): 241–257.
Bina, Florence, B. Paul, Y. Mbaya, and H. D. Dlakwa. 2020. "Effect of Insecurity on the Livelihood of Communities in Maiduguri Metropolis." *Journal of Public Administration* 2 (1): 31–36.
Birkett, Gemma. 2014. "Penal Reform Discourse for Women Offenders: Campaigners, Policy Strategies and Issue Reframing." *Crime, Media, Culture* 10 (2): 115–132.
Bish, Alison, and Susan Michie. 2010. "Demographic and Attitudinal Determinants of Protective Behaviors during Pandemic: A Review." *British Journal of Health Psychology* 15: 797–824.
Bishop, Brian J., Sheridan J. Coakes, and Pamela N. D'Rozario. 2002. "Sense of Community in Rural Communities: A Mixed Methodological Approach." Pp.271–290 in *Psychological Sense of Community: Research, Applications and Implications*, edited by Adrian T. Fisher, Christopher C. Sonn and Brian J. Bishop. New York: Kluwer Academic.
Bissell, David. 2010. "Passenger Mobilities: Affective Atmospheres and the Sociality of Public Transport." *Environment & Planning* 28 (2): 270–289.
Bix, Brian H. 2023. *Jurisprudence: Theory and Context*. London, UK: Reuters.
Bjarnegard, Elin, Karen Brounéus, and Erik Melander. 2019. "Violent Boyhoods, Masculine Honor Ideology, and Political Violence: Survey Findings from Thailand." *Journal of Interpersonal Violence* 36 (15–16): 7136–7160.
Bjornberg, Ulla, and Hans Ekbrand. 2008. "Financial and Practical Kin Support in Sweden: Normative Guidelines and Practice." *Journal of Comparative Family Studies* 39 (1): 73–95.
Bjornberg, Ulla, and Mia Latta. 2007. "The Roles of the Family and the Welfare State: The Relationship between Public and Private Financial Support in Sweden." *Current Sociology* 55 (3): 415–445.
Bjornskov, Christian, and Martin Paldam. 2012. "The Spirits of Capitalism and Socialism: A Cross-country Study of Ideology." *Public Choice* 150 (3): 469–498.
Bjornskov, Christian. 2005. "Does Political Ideology Affect Economic Growth?" *Public Choice* 123: 133–146.
Black, Richard, W. Neil Adger, Nigel W. Arnell, Stefan Dercon, Andrew Geddes, and David Thomas. 2011. "The Effect of Environmental Change on Human Migration." *Global Environmental Change* 21 (SUPPL. 1): S3–S11.
Blackwell, Brenda Sims, and Sarah Eschholz. 2002. "Sex Differences and Rational Choice: Traditional Tests and New Directions." Pp.109–135 in *Rational Choice and Criminal Behavior: Recent Research and Future Challenges*, edited by Alex R. Piquero and Stephen G. Tibbetts. New York: Routledge.
Blanc, Marie-Eve. 2005. "Social Construction of Male Homosexualities in Vietnam: Some Keys to Understanding Discrimination and Implications for HIV Prevention Strategy." *International Social Science Journal* 186: 661–673.

Blanchar, John C., and Scott Eidelman. 2013. "Perceived System Longevity Increases System Justification and The Legitimacy of Inequality." *European Journal of Social Psychology.* 43 (4): 238–245.

Blanchard, Tamar, Robert E. McGrath, and Eranda Jayawickreme. 2021. "Resilience in the Face of Interpersonal Loss: The Role of Character Strengths." *Applied Psychology: Health & Well-Being* 13 (4): 817–834.

Blanchette, Kelly, and Shelley L. Brown. 2006. *The Assessment and Treatment of Women Offenders: An Integrative Perspective.* Chichester, UK: Wiley.

Blank, Thomas, and Peter Schmidt. 2003. "National Identity in a United Germany: Nationalism or Patriotism? An Empirical Test with Representative Data." *Political Psychology* 24 (2): 289–312.

Blauza, Simon, Benedikt Heuckmann, Kerstin Kremer, and Alexander Georg Büssing. 2023. "Psychological Distance Towards COVID-19: Geographical and Hypothetical Distance Predict Attitudes and Mediate Knowledge." *Current Psychology* 42 (10): 8632–8643.

Bleidorn, Wiebke, Theo A. Klimstra, Jaap J. A. Denissen, Peter J. Rentfrow, Jeff Potter, and Samuel D. Gosling. 2013. "Personality Maturation around the World." *Psychological Science* 24 (12): 2530–2540.

Bloch, Katrina Rebecca, Tiffany Taylor, and Karen Martinez. 2020. "Playing the Race Card: White Injury, White Victimhood and the Paradox of Colour-Blind Ideology in Anti-Immigrant Discourse." *Ethnic & Racial Studies* 43 (7): 1130–1148.

Bloch, Katrina Rebecca. 2016. "It Is Just Sickening": Emotions and Discourse in an Anti-Immigrant Discussion Forum. *Sociological Focus* 49 (4): 257–270.

Blomberg, Helena, and Christian Kroll. 1999. "Who Wants to Preserve the Scandinavian Service State?" Pp.52–86 in The End of the Welfare State? Responses to State Retrenchment, edited by Stefan Svallfors and Peter Taylor-Gooby. London: Routledge.

Blum, Lawrence. 2008. "Ethnicity, Disunity, and Equality." Pp. 193–211 in *Contemporary Debates in Social Philosophy*, edited by Laurence Thomas. Malden, MA: Blackwell.

Bobo, Lawrence D., and Michael P. Massagli. 2001. "Stereotyping and Urban Inequality." Pp.89–102 in *Urban Inequality: Evidence from Four Cities*, edited by Alice O'Connor, Chris Tilly and Lawrence D. Bobo. New York: Russell Sage.

Bobo, Lawrence, and Vincent L. Hutchings. 1996. "Perceptions of Racial Group Competition: Extending Blumer's theory of Group Position to a Multiracial Social Context." *American Sociological Review* 61 (6): 951–972.

Bockler, Anne, Annika Rennert, and Tim Raettig. 2021. "Stranger, Lover, Friend? The Pain of Rejection Does Not Depend." *Social Psychology* 52 (3): 173–184.

Boer, Diana, and Ronald Fischer. 2013. "How and When Do Personal Values Guide Our Attitudes and Sociality? Explaining Cross-Cultural Variability in Attitude-Value Linkages." *Psychological Bulletin* 139 (5): 1113–1147.

Boeri, Tito, Gordon Hanson, and Barry McCormick. 2002. *Immigration Policy and the Welfare System.* Oxford, U: Oxford University Press.

Boert, Tito, Herbert Brucker, Frederic Pocquier, and Hilel Rapoport. 2012. *Brain Drain and Brain Gain: The Global Competition to Attract High-skilled Migrants.* Oxford, UK: Oxford University Press.

Boezeman, Edwin J., and Naomi Ellemers. 2008. "Volunteer Recruitment: The Role Of Organizational Support and Anticipated Respect in Non-Volunteers" Attraction to Charitable Volunteer Organizations." *Journal of Applied Psychology* 93 (5): 1013–1026.

Bogart, W. A. 2002. *Consequences: The Impact of Law and Its Complexity.* Toronto, Canada: University of Toronto Press.

Bohnke, Petra. 2008. "Does Society Matter? Life Satisfaction in the Enlarged Europe." *Social Indicators Research* 87: 189–210.

Bolet, Diane. 2023. "The Janus-Faced Nature of Radical Voting: Subjective Social Decline at the Roots of Radical Right and Radical Left Support." *Party Politics* 29 (3): 475–488.

Bolger, Daniel, Robert Thomson, and Elaine Howard Ecklund. 2020. "Determinants of Confidence in U.S. Institutions: Comparing Congress and Corporations." *Social Science Quarterly* 102 (1): 324–342.

Bolis, Ivan, Sandra N. Morioka, and Laerte I. Sznelwar. 2017. "Are We Making Decisions in a Sustainable Way? A Comprehensive Literature Review About Rationalities for Sustainable Development." *Journal of Cleaner Production* 145: 310–322.

Boman, John H., and Thomas J. Mowen. 2019. "Unpacking the Role of Conflict in Peer Relationships: Implications for Peer Deviance and Crime." *Deviant Behavior* 40 (7): 882–895.

Bompani, Barbara, and S. Terreni Brown. 2015. "A 'Religious Revolution'? Print Media, Sexuality, and Religious Discourse in Uganda." *Journal of Eastern African Studies* 9 (1): 110–126.

Bond, Michael Harris, and Virginia S.Y.. Kwan. 2000. "Decomposing a Sense of Superiority: The Differential Social Impact of Self-regard and Regard for Others." *Journal of Research in Personality* 34: 537–553.

Bond, Michael Harris, and Vivian Miu-Chi. Lun. 2014. "Citizen-making: The Role of National Goals for Socializing Children." *Social Science Research* 44: 75–85.

Bonini, Astra N. 2008. "Cross-national Variation in Individual Life Satisfaction: Effects of National Wealth, Human Development, and Environmental Conditions." *Social Indicators Research* 87: 223–236.

Booth, Jennifer, and John E. Martin. 1998. "Spiritual and Religious Factors on Substance Use, Dependence, and Recovery." Pp.175–200 in *Handbook of Religion and Mental Health*, edited by Harold G. Konenig. San Diego, CA: Academic.

Booth, John A. and Patricia Bayer Richard. 1998. "Civil Society and Political Context in Central America." *American Behavioral Scientist* 42(1):33–46. \57–349.

Borbath, Endre, and Theresa Gessler. 2020. "Different Worlds of Contention? Protest in Northwestern, Southern and Eastern Europe." *European Journal of Political Research* 59 (4): 910–935.

Borch, Christian. 2013. "Crowd Theory and the Management of Crowds: A Controversial Relationship." *Current Sociology* 61 (5–6): 584–601.

Bore, Miles, Don Munro, Ian Kerridge, and David Powis. 2005. "Not Moral Reasoning: A Libertarian-communitarian Dimension of Moral Orientation and Schwartz's Value Types." *Australian Journal of Psychology* 57 (1): 38–48.

Borjas, George. 1999. *Heaven's Door: Immigration Policy and the American Economy*. Princeton, NJ: Princeton University Press.

Bornschier, Volker, Mark Herkenrath, and Claudia Konig. 2005. "The Double Dividend of Expanding Education for Development." *International Sociology* 20 (4): 506–529.

Bornstein, Robert F. 2006. "The Complex Relationship between Dependency and Domestic Violence: Converging Psychological Factors and Social Forces." *American Psychologist* 62 (7): 709–711.

Boudon, Raymond. 2008. "How Can Axiological Feelings Be Explained?" *International Review of Sociology* 18 (3): 349–364.

Boulianne, Shelley, Chris Tenove, and Jordan Buffie. 2022. "Complicating the Resilience Model: A Four-Country Study about Misinformation." *Media & Communication* 10 (3): 169–182.

Bouwmeester, Onno. 2017. *The Social Construction of Rationality: Policy Debates and the Power of Good Reasons*. Abingdon, UK: Routledge.

Bowen, Natasha K., and Christopher J. Wretman. 2014. "Rural Neighborhoods and Child Aggression." *American Journal of Community Psychology* 54(3–4):304–315. \112–115.

Bowker, Matthew H. 2016. *Ideologies of Experience: Trauma, Failure, Deprivation, and the Abandonment of the Self*. New York, NY: Routledge.

Bowring, Finn. 2011. "Comparing Bauman and Arendt: Three Important Differences." *Sociology* 45 (1): 54–69.

Box, Richard C. 2008. *Making a Difference: Progressive Values in Public Administration*. Armonk, NY: Sharpe.

Boyd, Richard. 2006. "The Value of Civility?" *Urban Studies* 43 (5/6): 863–878.

Boyle, Gregory J., and Jeanne M. Joss-Reid. 2004. "Relationship of Humour to Health: A Psychometric Investigation." *British Journal of Health Psychology* 9 (1): 51–66.

Brady, David, and Kevin T. Leicht. 2008. "Party to Inequality: Right Party Power and Income Inequality in Affluent Western Democracies." *Research in Social Stratification & Mobility* 26: 77–106.

Brady, David, Jason Beckfield, and Wei Zhao. 2007. "The Consequences of Economic Globalization for Affluent Democracies." *Annual Review of Sociology* 33: 313–334.

Braithwaite, Valerie, and Eliza Ahmed. 2005. "A Threat to Tax Morale: The Case of Australian Higher Education Policy." *Journal of Economic Psychology* 26: 523–540.

Braithwaite, Valerie. 1998. "Communal and Exchange Trust Norms: Their Value Base and Relevance to Institutional Trust." Pp.46–74 in *Trust and Governance*, edited by Valerie Braithwaite and Margaret Levi. New York, NY: Russell Sage.

Bramley, Glen, and James Morgan. 2003. "Building Competitiveness and Cohesion: The Role of New Housebuilding in Central Scotland's Cities." *Housing Studies* 18 (4): 447–471.

Brand, Peter. 1999. "The Environment and Postmodern Spatial Consciousness: A Sociology of Urban Environmental Agendas." *Journal of Environmental Planning & Management* 42 (5): 631–648.

Brandt, Richard B. 1992. *Morality, Utilitarianism, and Rights*. Cambridge, UK: Cambridge University Press.

Brant, William Allen. 2019. *Beyond Legal Minds: Sex, Social Violence, Systems, Methods, Possibilities*. Leiden, Netherlands: Brill.

Branton, Regina, Valerie Martinez-Ebers, Tony E. Carey, Jr., and Tetsuya Matsubayashi. 2015. "Social Protest and Policy Attitudes: The Case of the 2006 Immigrant Rallies." *American Journal of Political Science* 59 (2): 390–402.

Bratton, Michael, and Robert Mattes. 2001. "Support for Democracy in Africa: Intrinsic or Instrumental?" *British Journal of Political Science* 31: 447–474.

Braun, Jerome. 2011. *To Break Our Chains: Social Cohesiveness and Modern Democracy*. Leiden, Netherlands: Brill.

Brawley, Mark R. 2003. *The Politics of Globalization: Gaining Perspective, Assessing Consequences*. Peterborough, Canada: Broadview.

Bray, Daniel. 2013. "Pragmatic Ethics and the Will to Believe in Cosmopolitanism." *International Theory* 5 (3): 446–476.

Brayne, Sarah. 2014. "Surveillance and System Avoidance: Criminal Justice Contact and Institutional Attachment." *American Sociological Review* 79 (3): 367–391.

Breakwell, Glynis M. 2007. *The Psychology of Risk*. Cambridge, UK: Cambridge University Press.

Brendgen, Mara, Frank Vitaro, and William M. Bukowski. 1998. "Affiliation with Delinquent Friends: Contributions of Parents, Self-esteem, Delinquent Behavior, and Rejection by Peers." *Journal of Early Adolescence* 18 (3): 244–265.

Brenig, Mattheus, and Till Proeger. 2018. "Putting a Price Tag on Security: Subjective Well-Being, and Willingness-to-Pay for Crime Reduction in Europe." *Journal of Happiness Studies* 19 (1): 145–166.

Brennan, Robert T., Rosalind Chart Barnett, and Karen C. Gareis. 2001. "When She Earns More than He Does: A Longitudinal Study of Dual-earner Couples." *Journal of Marriage & Family* 63: 168–182.

Brents, Barbara G. 2016. "Neoliberalism's Market Morality and Heteroflexibility: Protectionist and Free Market Discourses in Debates for Legal Prostitution." *Sexuality Research & Social Policy* 13 (4): 402–416.

Bretz, Shane, and Ron Sun. 2018. "Two Models of Moral Judgment." *Cognitive Science* 42: 4–37.

Brewer, Gayle, and Loren Abell. 2017. "Machiavellianism, Relationship Satisfaction, and Romantic Relationship Quality." *Europe's Journal of Psychology* 13 (3): 491–502.

Brewer, Marilynn B. 1996. "When contact Is Not Enough: Social Identity and Intergroup Cooperation." *International Journal of Intercultural Relations* 20 (3/4): 291–303.

Brewer, Paul R. 2003. "The Shifting Foundations of Public Opinion about Gay Rights." *Journal of Politics* 65 (4): 1208–1220.
Brezina, Timothy, and Alex R. Piquero. 2007. "Moral Beliefs, Isolation from Peers, and Abstention from Delinquency." *Deviant Behavior* 28 (5): 433–465.
Brezina, Timothy, and Robert Agnew. 2013. "General Strain and Urban Youth Violence." Pp. 143–159 in *The Oxford Handbook of Criminological Theory*, edited by Francis T. Cullen and Pamela Wilcox. New York: Oxford University Press.
Brigg, Morgan. 2018. "Humanitarian Symbolic Exchange: Extending Responsibility to Protect through Individual and Local Engagement." *Third World Quarterly* 39 (5): 838–853.
Briggs, Xavier, Joe T. de Souza, and Darden, and Angela Aidala. 1999. "In the Wake of Desegregation: Early Impacts of Scattered-site Public Housing on Neighborhoods in Yonkers New York." *Journal of the American Planning Association* 65 (1): 27–49.
Bright, Neil. 2018. *Rethinking Everything: Personal Growth through Transactional Analysis*. Lanham, MD: Rowman & Littlefield.
Brik, Tymofii, Andrew G. Livingstone, Maria Chayinska, and Evgeniya Bliznyuk. 2023. 'How Feeling Understood Predicts Trust and Willingness to Forgive in the Midst of Violent Intergroup Conflict: Longitudinal Evidence from Ukraine." *Social Psychological & Personality Science*.
Brines, Julie, and Kara Joyner. 1999. "The Ties that Bind: Principles of Cohesion on Cohabitation and Marriage." *American Sociological Review* 64: 333–355.
Brint, Steven. 2001. "Gemeinschaft Revisited: A Critique and Reconstruction of the Community Concept." *Sociological Theory* 19 (1): 1–23.
Brint, Steven. 2005. "Guide for the Perplexed: On Michael Burawoy's Public Sociology." *American Sociologist* 36 (3/4): 46–65.
Broadbent, Robyn, and Theo Papadopoulos. 2011. "Getting Wired@Collingwood: An ICT Project Underpinned by Action Research." *Community Development Journal* 47 (2): 248–265.
Brockmann, Hilke, Jan Delhey, Christian Welzel, and Hao Yuan. 2009. "The China Puzzle: Falling Happiness in a Rising Economy." *Journal of Happiness Studies* 10: 387–405.
Brody, David C., and Nicholas P. Lovrich. 2002. "Social Capital and Protecting the Rights of the Accused in the American States: An Investigation of the Dark Side of Social Capital." *Journal of Contemporary Criminal Justice* 18 (2): 115–131.
Brolis, Olivier, Marie Courtois, Ginette Herman, and Marthe Nyssens. 2018. "Do Social Enterprises Discriminate Less Than For-Profit Organizations? The Influence of Sector and Diversity Policies on Managers' Prejudice toward Immigrants." *Nonprofit & Voluntary Sector Quarterly* 47 (4): 745–766.
Bronk, Kendall Cotton, Patrick L. Hill, Daniel K. Lapsley, Tasneem L. Talib, and Holmes Finch. 2009. "Purpose, hope, and Life Satisfaction in Three Age Groups." *Journal of Positive Psychology* 4 (6): 500–510.
Broom, Alexander, K. R. David Sibbritt, Pamela Nilan Nayar, and Emma Kirby. 2013. "What Factors Predict Exposure to Caste, Political and Religious Violence in India? A Cross-Sectional Survey of 1000 Indian Men." *Asian Social Science* 9 (1): 1–8.
Brosius, Anna, E. J. van Elsas, and C. H. de Vreese. 2020. "Bad News, Declining Trust? Effects of Exposure to Economic News on Trust in the European Union." *International Journal of Public Opinion Research* 32 (2): 223–242.
Brown, Eleanor, and James M. Ferris. 2007. "Social Capital and Philanthropy: An Analysis of the Impact of Social Capital on Individual Giving and Volunteering." *Nonprofit & Voluntary Sector Quarterly* 36 (1): 85–99.
Brown, Graham, Barbara B. Brown, and Douglas D. Perkins. 2004. "New Housing as Neighborhood Revitalization: Place Attachment and Confidence among Residents." *Environment & Behavior* 36 (6): 749–775.
Brown, Jacob R., and Michael Zoorob. 2022. "Resisting Broken Windows." *Political Behavior* 44: 679–703.
Brown, Jason. 2019. *Anti-oppressive Counseling and Psychotherapy: Action for Personal and Social Change*. New York, NY: Routledge.

Brown, Jessica. 2016. "Social Support and Crime: A State-Level Analysis of Social Support Policies." *Journal of Sociology & Social Welfare* 43 (2): 135–156.
Brown, Kevin M., Russell Hoye, and Matthew Nicholson. 2014. "Generating Trust? Sport and Community Participation." *Journal of Sociology* 50 (4): 437–457.
Brown, Patrick. 2020. "Social Theories of Risk." Pp. 161–180 *Routledge Handbook of Social and Cultural Theory*, edited by Elliott, Anthony, London, UK: Routledge.
Brown, Randal D., and Daniel J. Weigel. 2018. "Exploring a Contextual Model of Sexual Self-Disclosure and Sexual Satisfaction." *Journal of Sex Research* 55 (2): 202–213.
Brown, Rebecca C. H. 2018. "Resisting Moralisation in Health Promotion." *Ethical Theory & Moral Practice* 21 (4): 997–1011.
Brown, Richard P. C., and John Connell. 2004. "The Migration of Doctors and Nurses from South Pacific Island Nations." *Social Science & Medicine* 58: 2193–2210.
Brown, Stephanie L., and R. Michael Brown. 2006. "Target Article: Selective Investment Theory: Recasting the Functional Significance of Close Relationships." *Psychological Inquiry* 17 (1): 1–29.
Browning, Christopher R., Tama Leventhal, and Jeanne Brooks-Gunn. 2005. "Sexual Initiation in Early Adolescence: The Nexus of Parental and Community Control." *American Sociological Review* 70 (5): 758–778.
Browning, Don S., and Terry D. Cooper. 2004. *Religious Thought and the Modern Psychologies*. Minneapolis, MN: Fortress.
Bruch, Sarah K., Myra Marx Ferree, and Joe Soss. 2010. "From Policy to Polity: Democracy, Paternalism, and the Incorporation of Disadvantaged Citizens." *American Sociological Review* 75 (2): 205–226.
Bruff, Ian. 2009. "The Totalisation of Human Social Practice: Open Marxists and Capitalist Social Relations, Foucauldians and Power Relations." *British Journal of Politics & International Relations* 11: 332–351.
Brugman, Daniel, Peter G. Heymans, Jan Boom, Andrei I. Podolskij, Olga Karabanova, and Olga Idobaeva. 2003. "Perception of Moral Atmosphere in School and Norm Transgressive Behaviour in Adolescents: An Intervention Study." *International Journal of Behavioral Development* 27 (4): 289–300.
Brundidge, Jennifer, and Ronald E. Rice. 2009. "Political Engagement Online: Do the Information Rich Get Richer and the Like-minded More Similar?" Pp. 144–156 in *Routledge Handbook of Internet Politics*, edited by Andrew Chadwick and Philip N. Howard. Abingdon, UK: Routledge.
Brynin, Malcolm, Alvaro Martinez Perez, and Simonetta Longhi. 2009. "How Close Are Couples?" Pp.93–108 in *Changing Relationships*, edited by Malcolm Brynin and John Ermisch. New York: Routledge.
Buchan, Nancy R., Rachel T.A.. Croson, and Robyn M. Dawes. 2002. "Swift Neighbors and Persistent Strangers: A Cross-cultural Investigation of Trust and Reciprocity in Social Exchange." *American Journal of Sociology* 108 (1): 168–206.
Buchanan, Kathryn E., and Anat Bardi. 2010. "Acts of Kindness and Acts of Novelty Affect Life Satisfaction." *Journal of Social Psychology* 150 (3): 235–237.
Buck, Nick. 2001. "Identifying Neighbourhood Effects on Social Exclusion." *Urban Studies* 38 (12): 2251–2275.
Buckley, F. H. 2009. *Fair Governance: Paternalism and Perfectionism*. New York: Oxford University Press.
Buechler, Steven M. 2011. *Understanding Social Movements: Theories from the Classical Era to the Present*. Boulder, CO: Paradigm.
Bukenya, Badru, and Frederick Golooba-Mutebi. 2020. "What Explains Sub-National Variation in Maternal Mortality Rates within Developing Countries? A Political Economy Explanation." *Social Science & Medicine* 256: 113066–113071.
Bukit, Mathew L. 2022. "Bangsamoro Separatism and Classical Counterinsurgency: Reconsidering Revolutionary War in the Southern Philippines." *Studies in Conflict & Terrorism* 47 (8): 911–939.

Bullock, John G. 2021. "Education and Attitudes toward Redistribution in the United States." *British Journal of Political Science* 51 (3): 1230–1250.

Bunringer, Gerhard, Hans-Ulrich. Wittchen, Katrin Gottlebe, Claudia Kufeld, and Thomas Goschke. 2008. "Why People Change? The Role of Cognitive-control Processes in the Onset and Cessation of Substance Abuse Disorders." *International Journal of Methods in Psychiatric Research* 17 (S1): S4–S15.

Burack, Cynthia. 2008. *Sin, Sex, and Democracy: Antigay Rhetoric and the Christian Right*. Albany, NY: State University of New York Press.

Burchianti, Flora, and Ricard Zapata-Barrero. 2014. "Is Catalonia Immune to Racism? An Analysis of Intolerant Political Discourses of Mainstream Party Representatives (2010–2011)." *Journal of Immigrant & Refugee Studies* 12 (4): 401–417.

Burgess, Adam. 2018. "Individualization Revisited: Global Family Developments, Uncertainty and Risk." *Journal of Risk Research* 21(1):83–95. \98–272.

Burgoon, Judee K., Laura K. Guerrero, and Kory Floyd. 2010. *Nonverbal Communication*. Columbus, MA: Allyn & Bacon.

Burke, Peter J., and Jan E. Stets. 1999. "Trust and Commitment through Self-verification." *Social Psychology Quarterly* 62 (4): 347–360.

Burt, S. Alexandra., Amber L. Pearson, Amanda Rzotkiewicz, Kelly L. Klump, and Jenae M. Neiderhiser. 2019. "It Really Does Take a Village: The Role of Neighbors in the Etiology of Nonaggressive Rule-Breaking Behavior." *Development & Psychopathology* 31 (2): 713–725.

Burton, Alexander L., Francis T. Cullen, Justin T. Pickett, Velmer S. Burton, and Angela J. Thielo. 2021. "Beyond the Eternal Criminal Record: Public Support for Expungement." *Criminology & Public Policy* 20 (1): 123–151.

Busemeyer, Marius R. 2013. "Education Funding and Individual Preferences for Redistribution." *European Sociological Review* 29 (6): 1122–1133.

Buskens, Vincent, and Werner Raub. 2013. "Rational Choice Research on Social Dilemmas: Embeddedness Effects on Trust." Pp. 113–150 in *The Handbook of Rational Choice Social Research*, edited by Rafael Wittek, Tom A. H. Snijders, and Victor Nee. Stanford, CA: Stanford University Press.

Bussey, Kay. 2020. "Development of Moral Disengagement: Learning to Make Wrong Right." Pp. 306–326 in *The Oxford Handbook of Moral Development: An Interdisciplinary Perspective*, edited by Lene Arnett Jensen. New York, NY: Oxford University Press.

Butler, Clark. 2008. *Human Rights Ethics: A Rational Approach*. West Lafayette, ID: Purdue University Press.

Butler, Judith. 2015. *Notes toward a Performative Theory of Assembly*. Cambridge, MA: Harvard.

Bystrov, Evgenia. 2012. "Religion, Demography and Attitudes toward Civil Marriage in Israel 1969–2009." *Current Sociology* 50 (6): 751–770.

Caballero-Dominguez, Carmen C., Jeimmy G. De Luque-Salcedo, and Adalberto Campo-Arias. 2021. "Social Capital and Psychological Distress During Colombian Coronavirus Disease Lockdown". *Journal of Community Psychology* 49(2), 691–702. Frank, Christine, Christopher G., Davis, and Frank J. Elgar. 2014. "Financial Strain, Social Capital, and Perceived Health During Economic Recession: A Longitudinal Survey in Rural Canada. *Anxiety, Stress, & Coping* 27 (4): 422–438.

Cacciatore, Michael A., Juan Meng, Bryan H. Reber, and Ben Boyd. 2018. "Globalization Effects or a Growing Cultural Divide? A Three-Year Comparative Analysis of Trust Predictors in the US and China." *Chinese Journal of Communication* 11 (1): 45–65.

Cacioppo, John T., and Louise C. Hawkley. 2009. "Loneliness." Pp. 227–240 in *Handbook of Individual Differences in Social Behavior*, edited by Mark R. Leary and Rick H. Hoyle. New York, NY: Guilford.

Cai, Tianji, Ruoyang Tang, Hongyu Wang, and Spencer De Li. 2022. "One Country Two Systems: A Comparative Study of National Identity between Hong Kong and Macau." *Chinese Sociological Review* 54 (2): 107–130.

Cairney, Paul. 2012. *Understanding Public Policy: Theories and Issues*. Houndmills, UK: Palgrave. (JF1525.P6C35) \80–350.

Cais, Jordi, Diego Torrente, and Catalina Bolancé. 2021. "The Effects of Economic Crisis on Trust: Paradoxes for Social Capital Theory." *Social Indicators Research* 153: 173–192.

Camara, Célia. F., Alejandra Sel, Carina C. J. M. de Klerk, and Paul H. P. Hanel. 2025. "Direct and Indirect Effects of Interpersonal Callousness on Aggression through Empathy and Moral Disengagement." *Personality & Individual Differences* 232: 112836.

Cameron, Gary. 2002. "Motivation to Join and Benefits from Participation in Parent Mutual Aid Organizations." *Child Welfare* 81 (1): 33–57.

Cameron, James E., Julie M. Duck, Deborah J. Terry, and Richard N. Lalonde. 2005. "Perceptions of Self and Group in the Context of a Threatened National Identity: A Field Study." *Group Processes & Intergroup Relations* 8 (1): 73–88.

Campagna, Desirée, Giulio Caperna, and Valentina Montalto. 2020. "Does Culture Make a Better Citizen? Exploring the Relationship between Cultural and Civic Participation in Italy." *Social Indicators Research* 149 (2): 657–686.

Campbell, Andrea Louise. 2003. "Participatory Reactions to Policy Threats: Senior Citizens and the Defense of Social Security and Medicare." *Political Behavior* 25 (1): 29–49.

Campbell, David E., and Christina Wolbrecht. 2020. "The Resistance as Role Model: Disillusionment and Protest among American Adolescents after 2016." *Political Behavior* 42 (4): 1143–1168.

Campbell, Heidi A., Katherine Arredondo, Katie Dundas, and Cody Wolf. 2018. "The Dissonance of "Civil" Religion in Religious-Political Memetic Discourse During the 2016 Presidential Elections." *Social Media + Society* 4(2):205630511878267. \1–1–342.

Campbell, Mary E., and Jennifer Eggerling-Boeck. 2006. "What about the Children? The Psychological and Social Well-being of Multiracial Adolescents." *Sociological Quarterly* 47: 147–173.

Campbell, Ross. 2011. "Socialist Values and Political Participation in Germany: A Barrier to 'Inner Unity'?" *West European Politics* 34 (2): 362–383.

Campbell, Tom. 2010. *Justice*. Houndmills, UK: Palgrave.

Campos-Castillo, Celeste, and Steven Hitlin. 2013. "Copresence: Revisiting a Building Block for Social Interaction Theories." *Sociological Theory* 31 (2): 168–192.

Canary, Danel J., Sandra G. Lakey, and Alan L. Sillars. 2013. "Managing Conflict in a Competent Manner: A Mindful Look at Events that Matter." Pp.263–289 in *The SAGE Handbook of Conflict Communication*, edited by John G. Oetzel and Stelle Ting-Toomey. Thousand Oaks, CA: SAGE.

Cano, Annmarie, and Dina Vivian. 2003. "Are Life Stressors Associated with Marital Violence?" *Journal of Family Psychology* 17 (3): 302–314.

Cao, Liqun, and Edward R. Maguire. 2013. "A Test of the Temperance Hypothesis: Class, Religiosity, and Tolerance of Prostitution." *Social Problems* 60 (2): 188–205.

Cao, Liqun, and Steven Stack. 2010. "Exploring Terra Incognita: Family Values and Prostitution Acceptance in China." *Journal of Criminal Justice* 38 (4): 531–537.

Cao, Liqun, Jihong Zhao, Ling Ren, and Ruohui Zhao. 2015. "Do In-Group and Out-Group Forms of Trust Matter in Predicting Confidence in the Order Institutions? A Study of Three Culturally Distinct Countries." *International Sociology* 30 (6): 674–693.

Cao, Liqun, Lanying Huang, and Ivan Sun. 2016. "From Authoritarian Policing to Democratic Policing: A Case Study of Taiwan." *Policing & Society* 26 (6): 642–658.

Capdevila, Rose, and Jane E.M.. Callaghan. 2007. "It's not Racist. It's Common Sense: A Critical Analysis of Political Discussion around Asylum and Immigration in the UK." *Journal of Community & Applied Social Psychology* 18: 1–16.

Caplan, Bryan. 2002. "Sociotropes, Systematic Bias, and Political Failure: Reflections on the Synergy of Americans and Economists on the Economy?" *Social Science Quarterly* 83 (2): 416–434.

Caplan, Leslie J., and Carmi Schooler. 2007. "Socioeconomic Status and Financial Coping Strategies: The Mediating Role of Perceived Control." *Social Psychology Quarterly* 70 (1): 43–58.

Caprara, Gian Vittorio and Michele Vecchione. 2013. "Personality Approaches to Political Behavior." Pp.23–58 in *The Oxford Handbook of Political Psychology*, edited by Leone Huddy, David O. Sears and Jack S. Levy. New York: Oxford University Press.

Caprara, Gian Vittorio, and Michele Vecchione. 2017. *Personalizing Politics and Realizing Democracy*. New York, NY: Oxford University Press.

Capraro, Valerio. 2024. "The Dual-Process Approach to Human Sociality: Meta-Analytic Evidence for a Theory of Internalized Heuristics for Self-Preservation." *Journal of Personality & Social Psychology* 126 (5): 719–757.

Caputo, Richard K. 2010. "Family Characteristics, Public Program Participation, & Civic Engagement." *Journal of Sociology & Social Welfare* 37 (2): 35–61.

Carbery, Julie, and Duane Buhrmester. 1998. "Friendship and Need Fulfillment during Three Phases of Young Adulthood." *Journal of Social & Personal Relationships* 15 (3): 393–409.

Carle, Adam C., Kurt J. Bauman, and Kathleen Short. 2009. "Assessing the Measurement and Structure of Material Hardship in the United States." *Social Indicators Research* 92: 35–51.

Carli, Linda L. 2013. "Gendered Communication and Social Influence." Pp.199–215 in *The SAGE Handbook of Gender and Psychology*, edited by Michelle K. Ryan and Myla R. Branscombe. London, UK: SAGE.

Carli, Linda L., and Alice E. Eagly. 2011. "Gender and Leadership." Pp. 103–117 in *The SAGE Handbook of Leadership*, edited by Alan Bryman, David Collinson, Keith Grint, Brad Jackson and Mary Uhl-Bien. London: SAGE.

Carlo, Gustoavo, George P. Knight, Camille D. Basilio, and Alexandra N. Davis. 2014. "Predicting Prosocial Tendencies among Mexican American Youth: The Intersection of Cultural Values, Social Cognitions, and Social Emotions." Pp. 242–257 in *Prosocial Development: A Multidimensional Approach,* edited by Laura M. Padilla-Walker and Gustavo Carlo. New York, NY: Oxford University Press.

Carlson, Per. 2004. "The European Health Divide: A Matter of Financial or Social Capital." *Social Science & Medicine* 59: 1985–1992.

Carlstrom, Charlotta. 2020. "God's Word Does Not Change as Trends Do" - Contemporary Discourses on Homosexuality in Swedish Christianity. *Theology & Sexuality* 26 (1): 28–44.

Carmeli, Abraham, Stephen Brammer, Emanuel Gomes, and Shlomo Y. Tarba. 2017. "An Organizational Ethic of Care and Employee Involvement in Sustainability-Related Behaviors: A Social Identity Perspective." *Journal of Organizational Behavior* 38 (9): 1380–1395.

Carollo, Luca, and Luca Solari. 2019. "Discourses of Professionalism in Front-Line Service Work: Insights from a Case Study in an Italian Bank." *Work, Employment & Society* 33 (5): 829–845.

Carpentier, Francesca R., and Dillman. 2017. "Priming Sexual and Romantic Representations in Two Media Environments: Sex Encourages and Romance Discourages Sexual Permissiveness … Sometimes." *Journal of Sex Research* 54 (6): 706–716.

Carpiano, Richard M. 2008. "Actual or Potential Neighborhood Resources and Access to Them: Testing Hypotheses of Social Capital for the Health of Female Caregivers." *Social Science & Medicine* 67: 568–582.

Carr, Deborah, and Michael A. Friedman. 2005. "Is Obesity Stigmatizing? Body weight, Perceived Discrimination and Psychological Well-being in the United States." *Journal of Health & Social Behavior* 46 (3): 244–259.

Carr, Patrick J. 2003. "The New Parochialism: The Implication of the Beltway Case for Arguments Concerning Informal Social Control." *American Journal of Sociology* 108(6):1249–1291.

Carrell, Michaell R., and Christina Heavrin. 2008. *Negotiating Essentials: Theory, Skills, and Practices*. Upper Saddle River, NJ: Pearson.

Carreras, Miguel. 2018. "Why No Gender Gap in Electoral Participation? A Civic Duty Explanation." *Electoral Studies* 52: 36–45.

Carrieri, Vincenzo. 2012. "Social Comparison and Subjective Well-being: Does the Health of Others Matter?" *Bulletin of Economic Research* 64 (1): 31–55.

Carson, Dena C. 2013. "Perceptions of Prosocial and Delinquent Peer Behavior and the Effect on Delinquent Attitudes: A Longitudinal Study." *Journal of Climate Justice* 41: 151–161.

Carter, Kameron M., Stacy L. Astrove, Brady M. Firth, Greg L. Stewart, and Samantha L. Solimeo. 2024. "Working at the Top of Their Capabilities: How Teamwork Support Attenuates Leader Role Conflict." *Group Dynamics* 28 (4): 292–308.

Carter, Michael J. 2016. "Microsociologies: Social Exchange, Trust, Justice, and Legitimacy." Pp. 369–386 in *Handbook of Contemporary Sociological Theory*, edited by Seth Abrutyn. Cham, Switzerland: Springer.

Carter, Niambi M., and Efren O. Perez. 2016. "Race and Nation: How Racial Hierarchy Shapes National Attachments." *Political Psychology* 37 (4): 497–513.

Carter, Travis M., and Scott E. Wolfe. 2021. "Explaining the Relationship between Neighborhood Disorder and Crime Fear: The Perceptual Role of Neighbors and the Police." *Journal of Criminal Justice* 77: 101867.

Caruana, Viv. 2014. "Re-thinking Global Citizenship in Higher Education: From Cosmopolitanism and International Mobility to Cosmopolitanisation, Resilience and Resilient Thinking." *Higher Education Quarterly* 68 (1): 85–104.

Cast, Alicia D. 2004. "Well-Being and The Transition to Parenthood: An Identity Theory Approach." *Sociological Perspectives* 47 (1): 55–78.

Cast, Alicia D., and Jan E. Stets. 2016. "The Self." Pp. 343–365 in *Handbook of Contemporary Sociological Theory*, edited by Seth Abrutyn. Cham, Switzerland: Springer.

Castelloe, Paul, and Dorothy N. Gamble. 2005. "Participatory Methods in Community Practice: Popular Education and Participating Rural Approach." Pp.261–275 in the *Handbook of Community Practice*, edited by Marie Weil. Thousand Oaks, CA: Sage.

Castells, Manuel. 2000. *End of Millennium*. Oxford, UK: Blackwell.

Castillo, Juan Carols. 2011. "Legitimacy of Inequality in Highly Unequal Context: Evidence from the Chilean Case." *Social Justice Research* 24: 314–340.

Castles, Francis G. 2000. "Putting the Economy First: Or Does Postmodernization Really Matter?" *Political Studies* 48 (1): 38–50.

Castro, Felice Gonzalez and Kate E. Murray. 2010. "Cultural Adaptation and Resilience: Controversies, Issues, and Emerging Models." Pp. 375–403 in *Handbook of Adult Resilience*, edited by John W. Reich, Alex J. Zautra and John Stuart Hall. New York, NY: Guilford.

Cattarello, Anne M. 2000. "Community-level Influences in Individuals?? Social Bonds, Peer Associations, and Delinquency: A Multilevel Analysis." *Justice Quarterly* 17 (1): 35–60.

Catterberg, Gabriela, and Alejandro Moreno. 2005. "The Individual Bases of Political Trust: Trends in New and Established Democracies." *International Journal of Public Opinion Research* 18 (1): 31–48.

Caulkins, D. Douglas. 2009. "Grid-group Analysis." Pp.57–72 in *Handbook of Social Capital: The Troika of Sociology, Political Science and Economics*, edited by Gert Tinggaard Svendsen and Gunnar Linad Haase Svendsen. Cheltenham, UK: Elgar.

Celso, B. G., D. J. Ebener, and E. J. Burkhead. 2003. "Humor Coping, Health Status, and Life Satisfaction among Older Adults Residing in Assisted Living Facilities." *Aging & Mental Health* 7 (6): 438–445.

Centola, Damon, and Michael Macy. 2007. "Complex Contagions and the Weakness of Long Ties." *American Journal of Sociology* 113 (3): 702–734.

Cerin, Ester, and Eva Leslie. 2008. "How Socio-economic Status Contributes to Participation in Leisure-time Physical Activity." *Social Science & Medicine* 66: 2596–2609.

Cerulo, Karen A., and Janet M. Ruane. 2014. "Apologies of the Rich and Famous: Cultural, Cognitive, and Social Explanations of Why We Care and Why We Forgive." *Social Psychology Quarterly* 77 (2): 123–149.

Ceva, Emanuela, and Federico Zuolo. 2013. "A Matter of Respect: On Majority-minority Relations in a Liberal Democracy." *Journal of Applied Psychology* 30 (3): 239–253.

Chahboun, Naima. 2024. "The Moral Benefits of Coercion: A Defense of Ideal Statism." *Politics, Philosophy & Economics* 23 (1): 47–66.

Chakrabarty, Debaj Yoti, Hajime Katayama, and Hanna Maslen. 2008. "Why Do the Rich Save More? A Theory and Australian Evidence." *Economic Record* 84: S32–S44.

Chalmers, Caitlin, Marilyn Anne Campbell, Barbara A. Spears, Des Butler, Donna Cross, Phillip Slee, and Sally Kift. 2016. "School Policies on Bullying and Cyberbullying: Perspectives across Three Australian States." *Educational Research* 58 (1): 91–109.

Chambers, Simone. 2002. "A Critical Theory of Civil Society." Pp.90–110 in *Alternative Conception of Civil Society*, edited by Simone Chambers and Will Kymlicka. Princeton, NJ: Princeton University Press.

Chan, David W. 2007. "Components of Leadership Giftedness and Multiple Intelligences among Chinese Gifted Students in Hong Kong." *Higher Ability Studies* 18 (2): 155–172.

Chan, Elaine. 2014. "Are Informal Connections a Functional Alternative to Associational Life in Enhancing Social Cohesion? Findings from Hong Kong." *Social Indicators Research* 119 (2): 803–821.

Chan, Kara, Sherrill Evans, Yu-Leung Ng, Marcus Yu-Lung Chiu, and Peter J. Huxley. 2014. "A Concept Mapping Study on Social Inclusion in Hong Kong." *Social Indicators Research* 119(1):121-37.

Chan, Raymond K.H.. 2012. "Competence Trust, Reflexivity and Risk Management in Hong Kong." *Asian Journal of Political Science* 20 (3): 267–283.

Chan, Siu Ming, Hung Wong, Tat Chor Au-Yeung, Xuan Huo, and Qin Gao. 2022. "Impacts of Poverty Stigma on Negative Affect among Welfare Recipients: Path Analysis on Mainland China and Hong Kong SAR." *Journal of Asian Public Policy* 15 (1): 145–164.

Chandler, Daniel. 2023. *Free and Equal: What Would a Fair Society Look Like?* Milton Keynes, UK: Lane.

Chaney, Paul. 2014. "Party Politicisation and the Formative Phase of Environmental Policy-Making in Multi-Level Systems: Electoral Discourse in UK Meso-Elections 1998–2011." *Political Studies* 62(2):252–72. \d12–4.2.

Chang, Cheng-Ping., Chih-Ting. Hsu, and I. Jun Chen. 2013. "The Relationship between the Playfulness Climate in the Classroom and Student Creativity." *Quality & Quantity* 47 (3): 1493–1510.

Chang, Han Il and Woo Chang Kang. 2018. "Why Do the Poor Oppose Income Redistribution? An Empirical Test on the Impacts of Nationalism and Fatalism." *Social Science Journal* 55(4):422-31.

Chang, Wen-Chun. 2009. "Social Capital and Subjective Happiness in Taiwan." *International Journal of Social Economics* 36(8):844-868.

Chanley, Virginia A., Thomas J. Rudolph, and Wendy M. Rahn. 2001. "Public Trust in Government in the Reagan Years and beyond." Pp.59–81 in *What Is It about Government that Americans Dislike?* edited by John R. Hibbing and Elizabeth Theiss-Morse. Cambridge, UK: Cambridge University Press.

Chappell, Neena L., and Michael J. Prince. 1997. "Reasons Why Canadian Seniors Volunteers." *Canadian Journal on Aging* 16 (2): 336–353.

Charles, Susan T., and Laura L. Carstensen. 2009. "Social and Emotional Aging." *Annual Review of Psychology* 61: 383–409.

Charles, Susan Turk, and Laura L. Carstensen. 2008. "Unpleasant Situations Elicit Different Emotional Responses in Younger and Older Adults." *Psychology and Aging* 23 (3): 495–504.

Chaskin, Robert J. 2001. "Building Community Capacity: A Definitional Framework and Case Studies from a Comprehensive Community Initiative." *Urban Affairs Review* 36 (3): 291–323.

Chaskin, Robert J., and Mark L. Joseph. 2010. "Building Community in Mixed-income Developments." *Urban Affairs Review* 45(3): 299–335.

Cheadle, Jacob E., and Philip Schwadel. 2012. "The Friendship Dynamics of Religion or the Religious Dynamics of Friendship? A Social Network Analysis of Adolescents Who Attend Small Schools." *Social Science Research* 41: 1198–1212.

Cheliotis, Leonidas K., and Suppho Xenukis. 2017. “The Moral Psychology of Penal Populism.” Pp. 176–190 in *The Routledge Handbook of Criminal Justice*, edited by Jonathan Jacobs and Jonathan Jackson, Abingdon, UK: Routledge.
Chen, Chih-Kai. 2008. “Causal Modeling of Knowledge-based Economy.” *Management Decision* 46 (3): 501–514.
Chen, Chuan-Yu, Carla L. Storr, and James C. Anthony. 2009. “Early-onset Drug Use and Risk for Drug Dependence Problems.” *Addictive Behaviors* 34(3):319-322.
Chen, Duan-Rung, Ly-Yun Chang, and Meng-Li Yang. 2008. “Gender-specific Responses to Social Determinants Associated with Self-perceived Health in Taiwan: A Multilevel Approach.” *Social Science & Medicine* 69:1630-1640.
Chen, Geoffrey C., and Charles Lees. 2018. “The New, Green Urbanization in China: Between Authoritarian Environmentalism and Decentralization.” *Chinese Political Science Review* 3 (2): 212–231.
Chen, Guo-hai, and Rod A. Martin. 2007. “A Comparison of Humor Styles, Coping Humor, and Mental Health between Chinese and Canadian University Students.” *Humor* 20 (3): 215–234.
Chen, Jie, and Yang Zhong. 1998. “Defining the Political System of Post-Deng China: Emerging Public Support for a Democratic Political System.” *Problems of Post-Communism* 45 (4): 30–42.
Chen, Jie. 2013. *A Middle Class without Democracy: Economic Growth and the Prospects for Democratization in China.* New York: Oxford University Press.
Chen, Juan. 2012a. “Seeking Help for Psychological Distress in Urban China.” *Journal of Community Psychology* 40 (3): 319–341.
Chen, Ni. 2012. “Branding National Image: The 2008 Beijing Summer Olympics, 2010 Shanghai World Expo, and 2010 Guangzhou Asian Games.” *Public Relations Review* 38:731-745.
Chen, Outong, Ranran Liu, and Xiaojing Zhao. 2025. “Impact of Army Morale on Suicidal Ideation: The Mediating Role of Grit and the Moderating Role of Social Support in a Chinese Navy Population.” *Military Psychology.*
Chen, Sheying. 1996. *Social Policy of the Economic State and Community Care in Chinese Culture: Aging, Family, Urban Change, and the Socialist Welfare Pluralism.* Aldershot, UK: Avebury.
Chen, Shu-Chen and Na-Ting Liu. 2019. “When and How Vicarious Abusive Supervision Leads to Bystanders” Supervisor-Directed Deviance.” *Personnel Review* 48(7):1734-55.
Chen, Sylvia Xiashua, and Winnie W.S.. Mak. 2008. “Seeking Professional Help: Etiology Beliefs about Mental Illness across Cultures.” *Journal of Counseling Psychology* 55 (4): 442–450.
Chen, Weixia, E. Xiaoyu Li, Scott Huebner, and Lili Tian. 2022. “Parent-Child Cohesion, Loneliness, and Prosocial Behavior: Longitudinal Relations in Children.” *Journal of Social & Personal Relationships* 39 (9): 2939–2963.
Chen, Xiangming, and Yuan Ren. 2016. “Modernity and Globalization: The Local and Global Sources of Individualistic and Materialistic Values in Shanghai.” *Globalizations* 13 (1): 16–31.
Chen, Xinguang, Peigang Wang, Rhiana Wegner, Jie Gong, Xiaoyi Fang, and Linda Kaljee. 2015. “Measuring Social Capital Investment: Scale Development and Examination of Links to Social Capital and Perceived Stress.” *Social Indicators Research* 120 (3): 669–687.
Chen, Xinxiang. 2011. “Tolerance and Economic Performance in American Metropolitan Areas: An Empirical Investigation.” *Sociological Forum* 26 (1): 71–97.
Chen, Xinyin, Lei Chang, Yunfeng He, and Hongyun Liu. 2005. “The Peer Group as a Context: Moderating Effects on Relations between Maternal Parenting and Social and School Adjustment in Chinese Children.” *Child Development* 76 (2): 417–434.
Chen, Xinyin. 2015. “Exploring the Implications of Social Change for Human Development: Perspectives, Issues and Future Directions.” *International Journal of Psychology* 50 (1): 56–59.
Chen, Zhenghui, and Gareth Davey. 2009. “Subjective Quality of Life in Zhuhai City, South China: A Public Survey Using the International Wellbeing Index.” *Social Indicators Research* 91: 243–258.
Cheng, Albert, and David Sikkink. 2020. “A Longitudinal Analysis of Volunteerism Activities for Individuals Educated in Public and Private Schools.” *Youth & Society* 52 (7): 1193–1219.

Cheng, Cecilia, Hsin-Yi Wang, Leif Sigerson, and Chor-Lam Chau. 2019. "Do the Socially Rich Get Richer? A Nuanced Perspective on Social Network Site Use and Online Social Capital Accrual." *Psychological Bulletin* 145(7):734-764.

Cheng, Cuiping, and Xiting Huang. 2017. "An Exploration of Courage in Chinese Individuals." *Journal of Positive Psychology* 12 (2): 141–150.

Cheng, Helen, John Bynner, Richard Wiggins, and Ingrid Schoon. 2012. "The Measurement and Evaluation of Social Attitudes in Two British Cohort Studies." *Social Indicators Research* 107 (2): 351–371.

Cheng, Joseph. 2016. "Business-Government Nexus: The Special Case of Hong Kong." *Asian Education & Development Studies* 5 (4): 454–467.

Cheng, Qiu, and Kinglun Ngok. 2020. "Welfare Attitudes Towards Anti-Poverty Policies in China: Economical Individualism, Social Collectivism and Institutional Differences." *Social Indicators Research* 150 (2): 679–694.

Cheng, Zhiming, and Russell Smyth. 2016. "Why Give It Away When You Need It Yourself? Understanding Public Support for Foreign Aid in China." *Journal of Development Studies* 52 (1): 53–71.

Chenoweth, Erica. 2021. *Civil Resistance: What Everyone Needs to Know*. New York, NY: Oxford University Press.

Cheung, Ada S., Olivia Ooi, Shalem Leemaqz, Pauline Cundill, Nicholas Silberstein, Ingrid Bretherton, Emily Thrower, Peter Locke, Mathis Grossmann, and Jeffrey D. Zajac. 2018. "Sociodemographic and Clinical Characteristics of Transgender Adults in Australia." *Transgender Health* 3 (1): 229–238.

Cheung, Cecilia Sin-Sze., and Eva M. Pomerantz. 2011. "Parents' Involvement in Children's Learning in the United States and China: Applications for Children's Academic and Emotional Adjustment." *Child Development* 82 (3): 332–350.

Cheung, Chau-kiu and Julian Chuk-ling Lai. 2020. "Public Priority for Allocating Kidney Transplants." Pp. 109–136 in *A Closer Look at Social Sustainability*, edited by Chau-kiu Cheung. New York: Nova.

Cheung, Chau-kiu, and Kwan-kwok Leung. 2011. "Neighborhood Homogeneity and Cohesion in Sustainable Community Development." *Habitat International* 35: 564–572.

Cheung, Chau-kiu, and Stephen Kum Ma. 2011. "Coupling Social Solidarity and Social Harmony in Hong Kong." *Social Indicators Research* 103 (3): 145–167.

Cheung, Chau-kiu. 1998. "Sophistication in Theorizing about Social Problems as a Condition for the Good Life." *Genetic, Social, General Psychology Monographs* 124 (3): 353–374.

Cheung, Chau-kiu. 2013. *Social Change and Psychosocial Responses: Social Force Theory Applied to Chinese Modernization and Postmodernization*. New York, NY: Nova.

Cheung, Chau-kiu. 2024. *Resilience Process and Its Personal and Social Bases*. Singapore: Springer.

Cheung, Karen Siu, and Lan, and Paul Siu Fai Yip. 2010. "Trends in Healthy Life Expectancy in Hong Kong SAR 1996–2008." *European Journal of Ageing* 7: 257–209.

Cheung, Nicole W.T.., and Yuet W. Cheung. 2006. "Is Hong Kong Experiencing Normalization of Adolescent Drug Use? Some Reflections on the Normalization Thesis." *Substance Use & Misuse* 41: 967–990.

Cheung, Yuet W., Susanne Y.P.. Choi, and Adam K.L.. Cheung. 2014. "Strain, Self-control, and Spousal Violence: A Study of Husband-to-wife Violence in Hong Kong." *Violence & Victims* 29 (2): 280–299.

Chhachhi, Amrita, and Linda Herrera. 2007. "Empire, Geopolitics and Development." *Development & Change* 38 (6): 1021–1040.

Chhotray, Vasudha and Gerry Stoker. 2009. *Governance Theory and Practice: A Cross-disciplining Approach*. Houndmills, UK: Palgrave.

Chi, Eunju, and Hyeok Yong Kwon. 2016. "The Trust-Eroding Effect of Perceived Inequality: Evidence from East Asian New Democracies." *Social Science Journal* 53 (3): 318–328.

Chi, Shang-xin, Shi-xi Su, and Ying Xu. 2021. "A Comparative Study from the Perspectives of Institutionalism and Culturalism of Patient Trust and Related Influencing Factors in the Chinese Mainland and Taiwan." *China* 19(4):188–209. \107–130.

Chiang, Shiao-Yun. 2010. "'Well, I'm a Lot of Things, but I'm Sure Not a Bigot': Positive Self-Presentation in Confrontational Discourse on Racism." *Discourse & Society* 21 (3): 273–294.

Child, Travers Barclay, and Elena Nikolova. 2020. "War and Social Attitudes." *Conflict Management & Peace Science* 37 (2): 152–171.

Chiozza, Giacomo. 2023. *Leverage and Cooperation in the U.S. World Order: The Shrewd Sheriff*. Cambridge, UK: Cambridge University Press.

Chiricos, Ted, Kathy Padgett, and Marc Gertz. 2000. "Fear, TV News, and the Reality of Crime." *Criminology* 38 (3): 755–785.

Cho, Seo-Young., Axel Dreher, and Eric Neumayer. 2013. "Does Legalized Prostitution Increase Human Trafficking?" *World Development* 41: 67–82.

Choi, Chonghyun, and Dongwook Kim. 2019. "The Determinants of Anti-Government Protests in Asia." *Journal of East Asian Studies* 19 (3): 315–338.

Choi, Susanne Y. P., and Roman David. 2012. "Lustration Systems and Trust: Evidence from Survey Experiments in the Czech Republic, Hungary, and Poland." *American Journal of Sociology* 117 (4): 1172–1201.

Choi, Wai Hong. 2004. *HKCSS Social Cohesion Indicators*. Hong Kong, China: Hong Kong Council of Social Service.

Chou, Kee-Lee. 2000. "Intimacy and Psychosocial Adjustment in Hong Kong Chinese Adolescents." *Journal of Genetic Psychology* 161 (2): 141–151.

Chouliaraki, Lilie.2013. *The Ironic Spectator: Solidarity in the Age of Post-Humanitarianism*. Cambridge, UK: Polity.

Chow, Chong Man, Duane Buhrmester, and Cin Cin Tan. 2014. "Interpersonal Coping Styles and Couple Relationship Quality: Similarity Versus Complementarity Hypotheses." *European Journal of Social Psychology* 44 (2): 175–186.

Christens, Brian D., Paul W. Speer, and N. Andrew Peterson. 2011. "Social Class as Moderator of the Relationship Between (Dis)Empowering Processes and Psychological Empowerment." *Journal of Community Psychology* 39 (2): 170–182.

Christians, Clifford G., Theodore L. Glasser, Denis McQuail, Kaarle Nordenstreng, and Robert A. White. 2009. *Normative Theories of the Media: Journalism in Democratic Societies*. Urbana, IL: University of Illinois Press.

Chu, Godwin C. 2001. "The Changing Concept of Zhong (Loyalty): Emerging New Chinese Political Culture." Pp.42–69 in *Chinese Political Culture, 1989–2000*, edited by Shiping Hua. Armonk, NY: Sharpe.

Chua, Lee-beng. 2002. *Psycho-Social Adaptation and the Meaning of Achievement for Chinese Immigrants*. New York: LFB.

Chua, Vincent, Gillian Koh, TanErn Ser, and Draw Shih. 2021. *Social Capital in Singapore: The Power of Network Diversity*. Singapore: Routledge.

Chui, Wing Hong, and Elliot W.Y.. Leung. 2014. "Youth in a Global World: Attitudes towards Globalization and Global Citizenship among University Students in Hong Kong." *Asia Pacific Journal of Education* 34 (1): 107–124.

Church, A. Timothy. 2010. "Measurement Issues in Cross-cultural Research." Pp. 151–175 in *The SAGE Handbook of Measurement*, edited by Geoffrey Walford, Eric Tucker, and Madhu Viswanathan. London, UK: SAGE.

Cichocka, Aleksandra, Marta Marchlewska, and Aleksandra Cislak. 2024. "Self-Worth and Politics: The Distinctive Roles of Self-Esteem and Narcissism." *Political Psychology* 45 (S1): 43–85.

Cisterna, Gustavo A., Andrés A. Acuña-Duarte, and César. A. Salazar. 2022. "Government Performance, Geophysical-Related Disasters, and Institutional Trust: A Comparison of Chilean and Haitian Responses after an Earthquake." *International Journal of Disaster Risk Reduction* 75: 102950.

Citrin, Jack, and Samantha Luks. 2001. "Political Trust Revisited: Deja Vu over Again?" Pp.9–27 in *What Is It about Government that Americans Dislike?* edited by John R. Hibbing and Elizabeth Theiss-Morse. Cambridge, UK: Cambridge University Press.

Ciziceno, Marco, and Giovanni A. Travaglino. 2019. "Perceived Corruption and Individuals' Life Satisfaction: The Mediating Role of Institutional Trust." *Social Indicators Research* 141 (2): 685–701.

Claassen, Ryan L., and Andrew Povtak. 2010. "The Christian Right Thesis: Explaining Longitudinal Change in Participation among Evangelical Christians." *Journal of Politics* 72 (1): 2–15.

Clark, Andrew E., Paul Frijters, and Michael A. Shields. 2008. "Relative Income Happiness and Utility: An Explanation for the Easterlin Paradox and Other Puzzles." *Journal of Economic Literature* 46 (1): 95–144.

Clark, Terry Nichols, and Ronald Inglehart. 1998. "The New Political Culture: Changing Dynamics of Support for the Welfare State and Other Policies in Postindustrial Societies." Pp.9–72 in *The New Political Culture*, edited by Terry Nichols Clark and Vincent Hoffmann-Martinot. Boulder, CO: Westview.

Clark, Terry Nichols. 2004. "A Political Theory of Consumption." *Research in Urban Policy* 19: 19–102.

Clegg, Stewart R. 2023. *Frameworks of Power*. London, UK: SAGE.

Clemence, Alain. 2001. "Social Positioning and Social Representations." Pp.83–95 in *Representations of the Social: Bridging Theoretical Traditions*, edited by Kay Deaux and Gina Philogene. Oxford, UK: Blackwell.

Clobert, Magali, Vassilis Saroglou, and Kwang-Kuo. Hwang. 2015. "Buddhist Concepts as Implicitly Reducing Prejudice and Increasing Prosociality." *Personality & Social Psychology Bulletin* 41 (4): 513–525.

Clubb, Gordon, and Ryan O'Connor. 2019. "Understanding the Effectiveness and Desirability of De-Radicalisation: How De-Radicalisation Is Framed in the Daily Mail." *British Journal of Politics & International Relations* 21 (2): 349–366.

Cobb-Clark, Deborah A., and Tue Gorgens. 2014. "Parents' Economic Support of Young-Adult Children: Do Socioeconomic Circumstances Matter?" *Journal of Population Economics* 27 (2): 447–471.

Cochran, John K., Mitchell B. Chamlin, Leonard Beeghley, and Melissa Fenwick. 2004. "Religion, Religiosity, and Nonmarital Sexual Conduct: An Application of Reference Group Theory." *Sociological Inquiry* 74 (1): 102–127.

Cochran, Susan D., and Vickie M. Mays. 2013. "Sexual Orientation and Mental Health." Pp.204–222 in *Handbook of Psychology and Sexual Orientation*, edited by Charlotte J. Patterson and Anthony R. D'Augelli. New York: Oxford University Press.

Cochrane, Allan. 2007. *Understanding Urban Policy: A Crucial Approach*. Malden, MA: Blackwell.

Cochrane, Tom. 2018. *The Emotional Mind: A Control Theory of Affective States*. Cambridge, UK: Cambridge University Press.

Coffe, Hilde, and Benny Geys. 2007. "Participation in Bridging and Bonding Associations and Civic Attitudes: Evidence from Flanders." *Voluntas: International Journal of Voluntary & Nonprofit Organizations* 18(4):385–406.

Coffe, Hilde, and Tanja van der Lippe. 2010. "Citizenship Norms in Eastern Europe." *Social Indicators Research* 96 (3): 479–496.

Cohen, Allan S., and David M. Bolt. 2005. "A Mixture Model Analysis of Differential Item Functioning." *Journal of Educational Measurement* 42 (2): 133–148.

Cohen, Andrew Jason. 2014. *Toleration*. Cambridge, UK: Polity.

Cohen, Bernard. 2019. "Police Enforcement of Street Prostitution as a Quality-of-Life Offense: New York City, United States, and Frankfurt Am Main, Germany." *Deviant Behavior* 40 (5): 526–543.

Cohen, Estee Shapiro, and Kim Fromme. 2002. "Differential Determinants of Young Adult Substance Use and High-risk Sexual Behavior." *Journal of Applied Social Psychology* 32 (6): 1124–1150.

Cohn, Ellen G., James Rotton, Amy G. Peterson, and Deborah B. Tarr. 2004. "Temperature, City Size, and the Southern Subculture of Violence: Support for Social Escape/Avoidance (Sea) Theory." *Journal of Applied Social Psychology* 34 (8): 1652–1674.

Cohrs, J. Christopher., Daniel J. Christie, Mathew P. White, and Chaitali Das. 2013. "Contributions of Positive Psychology to Peace: Toward Global Well-Being and Resilience." *American Psychologist* 68 (7): 590–600.

Cole, Wade M., Evan Schofer, and Kristopher Velasco. 2023. "Individual Empowerment, Institutional Confidence, and Vaccination Rates in Cross-National Perspective, 1995 to 2018." *American Sociological Review* 88 (3): 379–417.

Coleman, James S. 1988. "Social Capital in the Creation of Human Capital." *American Journal of Sociology* 94 (Supplement): S95–S120.

Coleman, Max E., Mohit K. Manchella, Adam R. Roth, Siyun Peng, and Brea L. Perry. 2022. "What Kinds of Social Networks Protect Older Adults' Health during a Pandemic? The Tradeoff between Preventing Infection and Promoting Mental Health." *Social Networks* 70: 393–402.

Collier, Andrew. 2001. *Christianity and Marxism: A Philosophical Contribution to Their Reconciliation.* London, UK: Routledge.

Collier, Michael W. 2002. "Explaining Corruption: An Institutional Choice Approach." *Crime, Law & Social Change* 38: 1–32.

Collier, Paul, and Anke Hoeffler. 2004. "Gre4ed and Grievance in Civil War." *Oxford Economic Papers* 56: 563–595.

Collins, Nancy L., and Brooke C. Feeney. 2004. "Working Models of Attachment Shape Perceptions of Social Support: Evidence from Experimental and Observational Studies." *Journal of Personality & Social Psychology* 87 (3): 363–383.

Collins, Nancy L., Maire B. Ford, and Brooke C. Feeney. 2011. "An Attachment-theory Perspective on Social Support in Close Relationships." Pp. 209–231 in *Handbook of Interpersonal Psychology Theory, Research, Assessment, and Therapeutic Interventions*, edited by Leonard M. Horowitz and Stephen Strack. Hoboken, NJ: Wiley.

Collins, Randall. 2001. "Civilizations as Zones of Prestige and Social Contact." *International Sociology* 16 (3): 421–437.

Collins, Randall. 2004. *Interaction Ritual Chains.* Princeton, NJ: Princeton University Press.
Dolinski, Dariusz. 2016. *Techniques of Social Influence: The Psychology of Gaining Compliance.* Hove, UK: Routledge.

Compton, Josh. 2013. "Inoculation Theory." Pp. 220–236 in *The SAGE Handbook of Persuasion*, edited by James Price Dillard and Lijing Shen. Thousand Oaks, CA: SAGE.

Comstock, Dana L., Tonya R. Hammer, Julie Strentzsch, Kristi Cannon, Jacqueline Parsons, and Gustavo Salazar Ii. 2008. "Relational-Cultural Theory: A Framework for Bridging Relational, Multicultural, and Social Justice Competencies." *Journal of Counseling & Development* 86 (3): 279–287.

Dias, Conde, Ana Rita, Carla Machado, and Miguel Gonçalves. 2012. "From 'Chastity as a Gift' to 'Doing It as a Sign of Love.'" *SAGE Open* 2 (4): 1–13.

Congdon, Peter. 2010. "A Multiple Indicator, Multiple Cause Method for Representing Social Capital with an Application to Psychological Distress." *Journal of Geographical Systems* 12 (1): 1–23.

Connolly, Willliam E. 2005. *Pluralism.* Durham, NC: Duke University Press.

Connors, Nicola A., Robert A. Bradley, Leanne Whiteside Mansell, Jeffrey Y. Liu, Tracy J. Roberts, Ken Burgadorf, and James M. Herrell. 2003. "Children of Mothers with Serious Substance Abuse Problems: An Accumulation of Risks." *American Journal of Drug & Alcohol Abuse* 29 (4): 743–758.

Conzo, Pierluigi, Arnstein Aassve, Giulia Fuochi, and Letizia Mencarini. 2017. "The Cultural Foundations of Happiness." *Journal of Economic Psychology* 62: 268–283.

Cooper, Cooper, Shane F. Blackman, and Kyle T. Keller. 2016. *The Science of Attitudes.* New York, NY: Routledge.

Cooper, Maisha, Alexander H. Updegrove, Shaun L. Gabbidon, George E. Higgins, and Hillary Potter. 2021. "Examining the Effects of Race/Ethnicity and Race Relations on Public Opinion about the Overrepresentation of Black People in U.S. Prisons." *Victims & Offenders* 16 (1): 1–19.

Copen, Casey E., and Merril Silverstein. 2008. "The Transmission of Religious Beliefs across Generations: Do Grandparents Matter?" *Journal of Comparative Family Studies* 39 (1): 59–71.

Corbin, Joanne N., and J. Camille Hall. 2019. "Resettlement Post Conflict: Risk and Protective Factors and Resilience among Women in Northern Uganda." *International Social Work* 62 (2): 918–932.

Corcoran, Katie E. 2013. "Divine Exchanges: Applying Social Exchange Theory to Religious Behavior." *Rationality & Society* 25 (3): 335–369.

Corcoran, Katie E., David Pettinicchio, and Jacob T.N.. Young. 2011. "The Context of Control: A Cross-national Investigation of the Link between Political Institutions Efficacy, and Collective Action." *British Journal of Social Psychology* 50: 575–605.

Cordes, Christian. 2006. "Darwinism in Economics: From Analogy to Continuity." *Journal of Evolutionary Economics* 16: 529–541.

Corlett, J. Angelo. 2006. *Responsibility and Punishment*. Dordrecht, Netherlands.

Cornelis, Ilse, Alain Van Hiel, Arne Roets, and Malgorzata Kossowska. 2009. "Age Differences in Conservatism: Evidence on the Mediating Effects of Personality and Cognitive Style." *Journal of Personality* 77: 51–87.

Cornwall, Benjamin. 2009. "Good Health and the Bridging of Structural Holes." *Social Networks* 31: 92–103.

Corr, Philip J., Shaun Hargreaves-Heap, Kei Tsutsui, Alexandra Russell, and Charles Seger. 2013. "Personality and Social Attitudes: Evidence for Positive-Approach Motivation." *Personality & Individual Differences* 55 (7): 846–851.

Corrigan, Michael W., Ann Higgins-D'Alessandro, and Philip Brown. 2013. "The Case of Adding Prosocial Education to Current Education Policy: Preparing Students for the Test of Life, Not Just a Life of Tests." *KEDI Journal of Educational Policy Special Issue* 2013: 37–50.

Corstange, Daniel, and Erin A. York. 2018. "Sectarian Framing in the Syrian Civil War." *American Journal of Political Science* 62 (2): 441–455.

Corvino, John. 2008. "Homosexuality, Harm, and Moral Principles." Pp. 79–93 in *Contemporary Debates in Social Philosophy*, edited by Laurence Thomas. Malden, MA: Blackwell.

Cosculluela, Victor. 1995. *The Ethics of Suicide*. New York, NY: Garland.

Cosic, Kreimir, Armano Srbljinovi, and Sinia Popovi. 2018. "Emotionally Based Strategic Communications in the Process of Societal Deradicalization." *International Journal of Strategic Communication* 12 (2): 196–214

Costa, Pedro J. C., Paulo A. S. Moreira, Sara Faria, and Joana Correia Lopes. 2023. "The Twenty Item Values Inventory (TwIVI) in Portuguese Adults: Factorial Structure, Internal Consistency, and Criterion-Related Validity." *Journal of Personality Assessment* 105 (1): 22–33.

Costello, Barbara J. 2013. "Hirschi's Criminology." Pp.131–142 in *The Oxford Handbook of Criminological Theory*, edited by Francis T. Cullen and Pamela Wilcox. New York: Oxford University Press.

Costello, Barbara J., and Paul R. Vowell. 1999. "Testing Control Theory and Differential Association: A Reanalysis of the Richmond Youth Project Data." *Criminology* 37 (4): 815–842.

Costello, Barbara J., and Trina L. Hope. 2016. *Peer Pressure, Peer Prevention: The Role of Friends in Crime and Conformity*. New York: Routledge.

Cote, James E. 2000. *Arrested Adulthood: The Changing Nature of Maturity and Identity*. New York: New York University Press.

Cotter, David A., JoAnn DeFiore, Joan M. Hermsen, Brenda Marsteller Kowalewsa, and Reeve Vanneman. 1998. "The Demand for Female Labor." *American Journal of Sociology* 103 (6): 1673–1712.

Cotter, David, Joan M. Hermsen, and Reeve Vanneman. 1999. "Systems of Gender, Race, and Class Inequality: Multilevel Analysis." *Social Forces* 78 (2): 433–460.

Cotterill, Stewart. 2017. *Performance Psychology: Theory and Practice*. Abingdon, UK: Routledge.
Cotterrell, Roger. 2018. *Sociological Jurisprudence: Juristic Thought and Social Inquiry*. Abingdon, UK: Routledge.
Cottrell, Catherine A., Steven L. Neuberg, and Norman P. Li. 2007. "What Do People Desire in Others? A Sociofunctional Perspective on the Importance of Different Valued Characteristics." *Journal of Personality & Social Psychology* 92(2):208-31.
Couldry, Nick and Andreas Hepp. 2017. *The Mediated Construction of Reality: Society, Culture, Mediatization*. Cambridge, UK: Polity.
Courtenay, Will H. 2000. "Constructions of Masculinity and Their Influence on Men??s Well-being: A Theory of Gender and Health." *Social Science & Medicine* 50: 1385–1401.
Cox, Amanda Barrett. 2016. "Mechanisms of Organizational Commitment: Adding Frames to Greedy Institution Theory." *Sociological Forum* 31 (3): 685–708.
Crafter, Sarah, Rachel Maunder, and Laura Soulsby. 2019. *Developmental Transitions: Exploring Stability and Change through the Lifespan*. Abingdon, UK: Routledge.
Craig, C. Samuel, and Susan P. Douglas. 2012. "Culture and Consumer Behavior: Contextual and Compositional Components." Pp.47–82 in *Handbook of Developments in Consumer Behavior*, edited by Victoria Wells and Gordon Foxall. Cheltenham, UK: Elgar.
Craig, Stephen C., Michael D. Martinez, James C. Kane, and Jason Gainous. 2005. "Core Values, Value Conflict and Citizens Ambivalence about Gay Rights." *Political Research Quarterly* 58 (1): 5–17.
Cramm, J. M., V. Moller, and A. P. Nieboer. 2012. "Individual- and Neighbourhood-level Indicators of Subjective Well-Being in a Small and Poor Eastern Cape Township: The Effect of Health, Social Capital, Marital Status, and Income." *Social Indicators Research* 105 (3): 581–593.
Crandall, Christian S., and Ryan K. Beasley. 2001. "A Perceptual Theory of Legitimacy: Politics, Prejudice, Social Institutions, and Moral Value." Pp.77–102 in *The Psychology of Legitimacy: Emerging Perspectives on Ideology, Justice, and Intergroup Relations*, edited by John T. Jost and Brenda Major. Cambridge, UK: Cambridge University Press.
Crane, M. F., B. J. Searle, M. Kangas, and Y. Nwiran. 2019. "How Resilience Is Strengthened by Exposure to Stressors: The Systematic Self-Reflection Model of Resilience Strengthening." *Anxiety, Stress, & Coping* 32 (1): 1–17.
Creed, Peter A., and Ruth-Eva. Gagliardi. 2015. "Career Compromise, Career Distress, and Perceptions of Employability: The Moderating Roles of Social Capital and Core Self-Evaluations." *Journal of Career Assessment* 23 (1): 20–34.
Cresswell, James. 2018. "Sociocultural Science of Religion and Natural Belief." Pp. 366–379 in *The Cambridge Handbook of Sociocultural Psychology*, edited by Alberto Rosa and Jaan Valsiner. Cambridge, UK: Cambridge University Press.
Crewe, Don and Ronnie Lippens. 2009. "Existentialism: Freedom, Being and Crime." Pp. 1–11 in *Existentialist Criminology*, edited by Ronnie Lippens and Don Crewe. Abingdon, UK: Routledge-Cavendish.
Crockett, Lisa J., Alexander Michael Wasserman, Kathleen Moritz Rudasill, Lesa Hoffman, and Irina Kalutskaya. 2018. "Temperamental Anger and Effortful Control, Teacher-Child Conflict, and Externalizing Behavior across the Elementary School Years." *Child Development* 89 (6): 2176–2195.
Cross, Patricia A., and Kim Matheson. 2006. "Understanding Sadomasochism: An Empirical Examination of Four Perspectives." *Journal of Homosexuality* 50 (2–3): 133–166.
Crossley, Nick, and Joseph Ibrahim. 2012. "Critical Mass, Social Networks and Collective Action: Exploring Student Political Worlds." *Sociology* 46 (4): 596–612.
Crowder, Kyle, Scott J. South, and Erick Chavez. 2006. "Wealth, Race, and Inter-neighborhood Migration." *American Sociological Review* 71: 72–94.
Crowe, Jonathan. 2009. *Legal Theory*. Pyrmont, Australia: Thomson Reuters.
Crowson, H. Michael. 2009. "Nationalism, Internationalism, and Perceived UN Irrelevance: Mediators of Relationships between Authoritarianism and Support for Military Aggression as Part of the War on Terror." *Journal of Applied Social Psychology* 39 (5): 1137–1162.

Croy, Gerry, Paul Gerrans, and Craig Speelman. 2010. "The Role and Relevance of Domain Knowledge, Perceptions of Planning Importance, and Risk Tolerance in Predicting Savings Intentions." *Journal of Economic Psychology* 31 (6): 860–871.

Cullen, Francis T., and Cheryl Lero Jonson. 2017. *Correctional Theory: Context and Consequences*. Thousand Oaks, CA: SAGE.

Cummins, Robert A. 1996. "The Domains of Life Satisfaction: An Attempt to Order Chaos." *Social Indicators Research* 38: 303–328.

Cummins, Robert A. 2016. "Happiness is the Right Metric to Measure Good Societal Functioning." *Society* 53(3):273–277.

Cummins, Robert A., Richard Eckersley, Julie Pallant, Jackie van Vugt, and Roseanne Misajon. 2003. "Developing a National Index of Subjective Wellbeing: The Australian Unity." *Social Indicators Research* 64: 159–190.

Curley, Alexandra M. 2010. "Relocating the Poor: Social Capital and Neighborhood Resources." *Journal of Urban Affairs* 32 (1): 79–103.

Currie, Janet, and Mark Stabile. 2009. "Mental Health in Childhood and Human Capital." Pp.115–148 in *The Problems of Disadvantaged Youth: An Economic Perspective*, edited by Jonathan Gruber. Chicago, IL: University of Chicago Press.

Curzer, Howard J. 2012. "An Aristotelian Account of Civility." Pp.80–98 in *Civility in Politics and Education*, edited by Deborah S. Mower and Wade L. Robison. New York: Routledge.

Cushing, Debra Flanders, and Evonne Miller. 2020. *Creating Great Place: Evidence-based Urban Design for Health and Wellbeing*. New York, NY: Routledge.

Cusick, Linda. 2002. "Youth Prostitution: A Literature Review." *Child Abuse Review* 11: 230–251.

Cutler, David M., and Adriana Lleras-Muney. 2008. "Education and Health: Evaluating Theories and Evidence." Pp.29–60 in *Making American Healthier: Social and Economic Policy as Health Policy*, edited by Robert F. Schoeni, James S. House, George A. Kaplan, and Harold Pollack. New York: Russell Sage.

Cutler, David M., Edward L. Glaeser, and Karen E. Norberg. 2001. "Explaining the Rise in Youth Suicide." Pp.219–269 in *Risky Behavior among Youth: An Economic Analysis*, edited by Jonathan Gruber. Chicago, IL: University of Chicago Press.

D'Ancona, Cea and Ma Angeles. 2018. "What Determines the Rejection of Immigrants through an Integrative Model?" *Social Science Research* 74:1-15.

d'Astous, Alain, and Dania Mouakhar-Klouz. 2022. "Self-Gift Giving and Satisfaction with Life: A Behavioural Tendency Perspective." *International Journal of Consumer Studies* 46 (1): 268–278.

D"raven, L. Lambert, and N. Pasha-Zaidi. 2016. "Using the PERMA Model in the United Arab Emirates." *Social Indicators Research* 125: 905–933.

Dabros, Matthew S., Suzanne L. Parker, and Mark W. Petersen. 2015. "Assessing the Stability of Trust in Government across Election Periods." *Social Science Quarterly* 96 (4): 996–1011.

Dahlberg, Stefan, Soren Holmberg, Bo Rothstein, Natalia Alvarado Pachon, and Richard Svensson. 2018. *The Quality of Government Basic Dataset* (Version Jan 18). University of Gothenburg: Quality of Government Institute, http://www.qog.pol.gu.se https://doi.org/10.18157/QoGBasJan18.

Dai, Yaoyao and Lu Wei Rose Luqiu. 2024. *Wolf Warrior Diplomacy and China's Ministry of Foreign Affairs: From Policy to Podium*. Lanham, MD: Lexington.

Dakka, Fadia. 2020. "Competition, Innovation and Diversity in Higher Education: Dominant Discourses, Paradoxes and Resistance." *British Journal of Sociology of Education* 41 (1): 80–94.

Dalbert, Claudia. 2001. *The Justice Motive as a Personal Resource: Dealing with Challenges and Critical Life Events*. New York, NY: Kluwer.

Dalla, Rochelle L. 2006. *Exposing the Pretty Woman Myth: A Qualitative Investigation of Street-level Prostituted Women*. Lanham, MD: Rowman & Littlefield.

Dambrun, Michaël, Donald M. Taylor, David A. McDonald, Jonathan Crush, and Alain Méot. 2006. "The Relative Deprivation-Gratification Continuum and the Attitudes of South Africans toward Immigrants: A Test of the V-Curve Hypothesis." *Journal of Personality & Social Psychology* 91 (6): 1032–1044.

Dandaneau, Steven P. 2001. *Taking It Big: Developing Sociological Consciousness in Postmodern Times*. Thousand Oaks, CA: Pine Forge.

Daneygier, Rafaela M., and Donald P. Green. 2010. "Hate Crime." Pp. 294–311 in *The SAGE Handbook of Prejudice, Stereotyping and Discrimination*, edited by John F. Dovidio, Miles Hewstone, Peter Glick and Victoria M. Esses. London, UK: SAGE.

Daniel, Ella, Anat Bardi, Ronald Fischer, Maya Benish-Weisman, and Julie A. Lee. 2022. "Changes in Personal Values in Pandemic Times." *Social Psychological & Personality Science* 13 (2): 572–582.

Dannreuther, Charlie, and Lew Perren. 2013. "Uncertain States: The Political Construction of the Small Firm, the Individualisation of Risk and the Financial Crisis." *Capital & Class* 37 (1): 37–64.

Darling, Carol Anderson, Lenore M. McWey, Stacy N. Howard, and Spencer B. Olmstead. 2007. "College Student Stress: The Influence of Interpersonal Relationships on Sense of Coherence." *Stress & Health* 23: 215–229.

Darwall, Stephen L. 2003. "Theories of Ethics." Pp.17–37 in *A Companion to Applied Ethics, edited by R.G. Frey and Christopher Heath Wellman*. Malden, MA: Blackwell.

Datler, Georg, Wolfgang Jagodzinski, and Peter Schmidt. 2013. "Two Theories on the Test Bench: Internal and External Validity of the Theories of Ronald Inglehart and Shalom Schwartz." *Social Science Research* 42: 906–925.

Davey, Gareth, and Ricardo Rato. 2011. "Subjective Wellbeing in China: A Review." *Journal of Happiness Studies* 13 (2): 333–346.

Davey, Gareth. 2012. "Happiness and Quality of Life in the People??s Republic of China." Pp.57–73 in *Happiness across Cultures*, edited by H. Selin and Gareth Davey. New York: Springer.

Davids, M. Fakhry. 2011. *Internal Racism: A Psychoanalytic Approach to Race and Difference.* Houndmills, UK: Palgrave.

Davies, Ian. 2009. "Latino Immigration and Social Change in the United States: Toward an Ethical Immigration Policy." *Journal of Business Ethics* 18: 377–391.

Davis, James A. 1985. *The Logic of Causal Order*. Beverly Hills, CA: Sage.

Davis, Nancy J., and Robert V. Robinson. 1999. "'Their Brothers' Keepers? Orthodox Religionists, Modernists, and Economic Justice in Europe." *American Journal of Sociology* 104 (6): 1631–1665.

Davis-Lipman, Angelina, Tom R. Tyler, and Susan M. Andersen. 2007. "Building Community One Relationship at a Time: Consequences for the Seeking and Acceptance of Help." *Social Justice Research* 20 (2): 187–206.

Dawkins, Casey J. 2006. "Are Social Networks the Ties that Bind Families to Neighborhoods." *Housing Studies* 21 (6): 867–881.

Dawson, Andrew. 2021. "The Achilles Heel of Democracy? A Macro Cross-National Assessment of the Correlates of State Legitimacy." *Social Science Research* 97: 102574.

Day, James. 2010. "Religion, Spirituality, and Positive Psychology in Adulthood: A Developmental View." *Journal of Adult Development* 17 (4): 215–229.

de Beer, Paul, and Ferry Kostere. 2009. *Sticking Together or Falling Apart? Solidarity in an Era of Individualization and Globalization.* Amsterdam, Netherlands: Amsterdam University Press.

de Bruyn, Eddy H., Maja Dekovic, and G. Wim Meijnen. 2003. "Parenting Goal Orientations, Classroom Behavior, and School Success in Early Adolescence." *Applied Developmental Psychology* 24: 393–412.

de C. R. Araujo, Magdalena Bobowik, Roosevelt Vilar, James H. Liu, Homero Gil de Zuñiga, Larissa Kus-Harbord, Nadezhda Lebedeva and Valdiney V. Gouveia. 2020. "Human Values and Ideological Beliefs as Predictors of Attitudes toward Immigrants across 20 Countries: The Country-Level Moderating Role of Threat." *European Journal of Social Psychology* 50 (3): 534–546.

De Carlo, Alessandro, Damiano Girardi, Alessandra Falco, Laura Dal Corso, and Annamaria Di Sipio. 2019. "When Does Work Interfere with Teachers? Private Life? An Application of the Job Demands-Resources Model." *Frontiers in Psychology* 10:1121.

de Castro-Rodrigues, Andreia, and Ana Sacau. 2015. "Judges' Perception on Causes of Criminality and Justifications for Crime." *European Journal of Probation* 7 (2): 124–142.

de Coster, Stacy. 2005. "Depression and Law Violation: Gendered Responses to Gendered Stresses." *Sociological Perspectives* 48 (2): 155–187.

de Courville Nicol, Valerie. 2011. *Social Economies of Fear and Desire: Emotional Regulation, Emotion Management, and Embodied Autonomy*. New York, NY: Palgrave.

De Deken, Johan Jeroen. 2002. "Christian Democracy, Social Democracy and the Paradoxes of Earnings-related Social Security." *International Journal of Social Welfare* 11:22–39. Andersson, Jenny. 2006. *Between Growth and Security: Swedish Social Democracy from a Strong Society to a Third Way*. Manchester, UK: Manchester University Press. Stefanski, Daniel and Łukasz Jach. 2022. "What Do People Think About Technological Enhancements of Human Beings? An Introductory Study Using the Technological Enhancements Questionnaire in the Context of Values, the Scientistic Worldview, and the Accepted Versions of Humanism." *Current Issues in Personality Psychology* 10(1):71–84.

De Dreu, Carsten K.W., and Aukje Nauta. 2009. "Self-interest and other-orientation in Organizational Behavior: Implications for Job Performance, Prosocial Behavior, and Personal Initiative." *Journal of Applied Psychology* 94(4):913-926.

de Figueiredo, Rui J. P., Jr., and Zachary Elins. 2003. "Are Patriots Bigots? An Inquiry into the Vices of Ingroup Pride." *American Journal of Political Science* 47 (1): 171–188.

de Graaf, Nan, Anthony Heath Dirk, and Ariana Need. 2001. "Declining Cleavages and Political Choices: The Interplay of Social and Political Factors in the Netherlands." *Electoral Studies* 20: 1–15.

De Graaf, Nan Dirk. 2013. "Secularization: Theoretical Controversies Generating Empirical Research." Pp. 322–354 in *The Handbook of Rational Choice Social Research*, edited by Rafael Wittek, Tom A. H. Snijders, and Victor Nee. Stanford, CA: Stanford University Press.

de Groot, Judith I.M.., and Linda Steg. 2009. "Morality and Prosocial Behavior: The Role of Awareness, Responsibility, and Norms in the Norm Activation Model." *Journal of Social Psychology* 149 (4): 425–449.

De Houwer, Jan, Bertram Gawronski, and Dermot Barnes-Holmes. 2013. "A Functional-Cognitive Framework for Attitude Research." *European Review of Social Psychology* 24(1):252-87.

de Jong, M. G., R. Pieters, and S. Stremersch. 2012. "Analysis of Sensitive Questions across Cultures: An Application of Multigroup Item Randomized Response Theory to Sexual Attitudes and Behavior." *Journal of Personality & Social Psychology* 103 (3): 543–564.

de Jonge, Jan. 2012. *Rethinking Rational Choice Theory: A Companion on Rational and Moral Action*. Houndmills, UK: Palgrave.

de la Ossa, Abigael, and Candelas. 2016. "Talk, Listen, Think: Discourses of Agency and Unintentional Violence in Consent Guidance for Gay, Bisexual and Trans Men." *Discourse & Society* 27 (4): 365–382.

de la Torre, Carlos. 2018. "Populism." Pp. 572–586 in *The SAGE Handbook of Political Sociology*, edited by William Outhwaite and Stephen Turner. London, UK: SAGE.

de Motte, Claire, and Mutale Gabriella. 2019. "How the Construction of Women in Discourse Explains Society's Challenge in Accepting That Females Commit Sexual Offences against Children." *Journal of Criminal Psychology* 9 (4): 155–165.

de Souza, Michel, Mauro Sayar Candido, and Ferreira, and Lízia de Figueiredo. 2023. "The Asymmetric Evolution of Economic Institutions: Evidence from Dynamic Panel Quantile Regression with IV and Fixed Effects." *Applied Economics Letters* 30 (11): 1531–1539.

De Vos, Jan. 2010. "Christopher Lasch's *The Culture of Narcissism*: The Failure of a Critique of Psychological Politics." *Theory & Psychology* 20(4):528-548.

De Vos, Jan. 2013. *Psychologization and the Subject of Late Modernity*. Houndmills, UK: Palgrave.

de Vries, Brian, and David Megathlin. 2009. "The Meaning of Friendship for Gay Men and Lesbians in the Second Half of Life." *Journal of GLBT Family Studies* 5 (1–2): 82–98.

de Vries, Jannes, and Paul M. de Graaf. 2008. "Is the Intergenerational Transmission of High Cultural Activities Biased by the Retrospective *Measurement* of Parental High Cultural Activities?" *Social Indicators Research.* 85 (2): 311–327.

Dean, Hartley. 2020. *Understanding* Human Need. Bristol, UK: Policy.

Dean, Mitchell. 2010. *Governmentality: Power and Rule in Modern Society.* Los Angeles, CA: SAGE.

Debus, Maike E., Charlotte Fritz, and Michel Philipp. 2019. "A Story of Gains and Losses: Intra-Individual Shifts in Job Characteristics and Well-Being When Transitioning to a Managerial Role." *Journal of Business & Psychology* 34 (5): 637–655.

Decuyper, Aron, Hanne Tack, Bénédicte. Vanblaere, Mathea Simons, and Ruben Vanderlinde. 2023. "Collaboration and Shared Responsibility in Team Teaching: A Large-Scale Survey Study." *Education Sciences* 13 (9): 896.

Deegan, Simone Jessica. 2021. "The Meaning of Murder: Family Members in the Lives of Juvenile Homicide Offenders." *British Journal of Criminology* 61 (1): 85–103.

Defoe, Ivy N., Judith Semon Dubas, Bernd Figner, and Marcel A. G. van Aken. 2015. "A Meta-Analysis on Age Differences in Risky Decision Making: Adolescents versus Children and Adults." *Psychological Bulletin* 141 (1): 48–84.

Degenne, Alain, Marie-Odile Lebeaux, and Yannick Lemel. 2004. "Does Social Capital Offset Social and Economic Inequalities?" Social Capital in Everyday Life." Pp.51–73 in *Creation and Returns of Social Capital: A New Research Program*, edited by Henk Flap and Beate Volker. London: Routledge.

Dekkers, Gijs J.M.. 2008. "Are You Unhappy? Then You Are Poor? Multi-dimensional Poverty in Belgium." *International Journal of Sociology & Social Policy* 28 (11/12): 502–545.

Bove, Del, Gian Vittorio Giannetta, Concetta Pastorelli Caprara, and Marinella Paciello. 2008. "Juvenile Firesetting in Italy: Relationship to Aggression, Psychopathology, Personality, Self-efficacy, and School Functioning." *European Child & Adolescence Psychiatry* 17: 235–244.

del Mar Bernad, Maria, Mateu Servera, Stephen P. Becker, and G. Leonard Burns. 2016. "Sluggish Cognitive Tempo and Adhd Inattention as Predictors of Externalizing, Internalizing, and Impairment Domains: A 2-Year Longitudinal Study." *Journal of Abnormal Child Psychology* 44 (4): 771–785.

Delanty, Gerard. 2009. *The Cosmopolitan Imagination: The Renewal of Critical Social Theory.* Cambridge, UK: Cambridge University Press.

Delbosc, Alexa, and Graham Currie. 2011. "Exploring the Relative Influences of Transport Disadvantage and Social Exclusion on Well-being." *Transport Policy* 18: 555–562.

DeLeon, Richard E., and Katherine C. Naff. 2004. "Identity Politics and Local Political Culture: Some Comparative Results from the Social Capital Benchmark Survey." *Urban Affairs Review* 39 (6): 689–719.

Delhey, Jan, Kenneth Newton, and Christian Welzel. 2011. "How General Is Trust in Most People? Solving the Radius of Trust Problem." *American Sociological Review* 76 (5): 786–807.

Delhey, Jan. 2010. "From Materialist to Post-materialist Happiness? National Affluence and Determinants of Life Satisfaction in Cross-national Perspective." *Social Indicators Research* 97: 65–84.

Deli, Gergely. 2020. *Just Living: Towards an Ethics-based Legal Theory.* Brussels, Belgium: Blue.

Deller, Steven, and Craig Maher. 2009. "Government, Effectiveness, Performance, and Local Property Values." *International Journal of Public Administration* 32 (13): 1182–1212.

Del-Teso-Craviotto, Marisol. 2009. "Racism and Xenophobia in Immigrants' Discourse: The Case of Argentines in Spain." *Discourse & Society* 20 (5): 571–592.

Delton, Andrew W., and Max M. Krasnow. 2017. "The Psychology of Deterrence Explains Why Group Membership Matters for Third-Party Punishment." *Evolution & Human Behavior* 38 (6): 734–743.

DeLue, Steven M., and Timothy M. Dale. 2009. *Political Thinking, Political Theory, and Civil Society.* New York: Pearson.

Demerath III, Nicholas J. 2002. "A Sinner among the Saints: Confessions of a Sociologist of Culture and Religion." *Sociological Forum* 17 (1): 1–19.
Demo, David H., and Cheryl Buehler. 2013. "Theoretical Approaches to Studying Divorce." Pp. 263–279 in *Handbook of Family Theories: A Content-based Approach*, edited by Mark A. Fine and Frank D. Fincham. New York: Routledge.
Dench, Geoff. 2006. "Putting Social Contribution back into Merit." *Political Quarterly* 77 (S1): 221–231.
Deng, Fang. 2011. *Unintended Outcomes of Social Movements: The 1989 Chinese Student Movement*. Abingdon, UK: Routledge.
Deng, Jun, and Craig A. Smith. 2018. "The Rise of New Confucianism and the Return of Spirituality to Politics in Mainland China." *China Information* 32 (2): 294–314.
Denisova, Irina, Markus Ellev, Timothy Frye, and Ekaterina Zhuravskaya. 2009. "Who Wants to Revise Privatization? The Complementarity of Market Skills and Institutions." *American Political Science Review* 103 (2): 284–304.
Dennison, Christopher R., and Raymond R. Swisher. 2019. "Postsecondary Education, Neighborhood Disadvantage, and Crime: An Examination of Life Course Relative Deprivation." *Crime & Delinquency* 65 (2): 215–238.
Denver, Megan, and Justin T. Pickett. 2022. "Race, Criminal Records, and Discrimination against Job Seekers: Examining Attitudinal Mechanisms." *Social Currents* 9 (3): 226–244.
Deptula, Daneen P., and Robert Cohen. 2004. "Aggressive, Rejected, and Delinquent Children and Adolescents: A Comparison for Their Friendships." *Aggression & Violent Behavior* 9: 75–104.
Deutsch, Morton. 2006. "A Framework for Thinking about Oppression and Its Change." *Social Justice Research* 19 (1): 7–41.
Devereux, Stephen. 2002. "Can Social Safety Nets Reduce Chronic Poverty?" *Development Policy Review* 20 (5): 657–675.
Devos, Thierry, Dario Spini, and Shalom H. Schwartz. 2002. "Conflicts among Human Values and Trust in Institutions." *British Journal of Social Psychology* 41: 481–494.
Dhal, Espen, Tone Flotten, and Thomas Lorentzen. 2008. "Poverty Dynamics and Social Exclusion: An Analysis of Norwegian Panel Data." *Journal of Social Policy* 37 (2): 231–249.
Di Domenico, Stefano I. and Marc A. Fournier. 2014. "Socioeconomic Status, Income Inequality, and Health Complaints: A Basic Psychological Needs Perspective." *Social Indicators Research* 119(3):1679-97.
Dickes, Paul, Marie Valentova, and Monique Borsenberger. 2010. "Construct Validation and Application of a Common Measure of Social Cohesion in 33 European Countries." *Social Indicators Research* 98: 451–473.
Dickson, Bruce J. 2001. "Cooptation and Corporatism in China: The Logic of Party Adaptation." *Political Science Quarterly* 115 (4): 517–540.
Diefenbach, Thomas. 2013. *Hierarchy and Organisation: Toward a General Theory of Hierarchical Social Systems*. New York, NY: Routledge.
Diesing, Paul. 1999. *Hegel's Dialectical Political Economy: A Contemporary Application*. Boulder, CO: Westview.
Dietz, Thomas, Linda Kalof, and Paul C Stern. 2002. "Gender Values, and Environmentalism." *Social Science Quarterly* 83 (1): 353–364.
Diez-Nicolas, Juan. 2002. "Two Contradictory Hypotheses on Globalization: Societal Convergence or Civilization Differentiation and Clash." *Comparative Sociology* 1 (3–4): 465–493.
DiGiuseppe, Raymond, Russell Leaf, Bernard Gorman, and Mitchell W. Robin. 2017. "The Development of a Measure of Irrational/Rational Beliefs." *Journal of Rational-Emotive & Cognitive-Behavior Therapy* 36 (1): 47–79.
Dijker, Anton J.M.., and Willem Koomen. 2007. *Stigmatization, Tolerance and Repair: An Integrative Psychological Analysis of Responses to Deviance*. New York: Cambridge University Press.
DiMaggio, Anthony Ross. 2015. "Class Sub-Conscious: Hegemony, False Consciousness, and the Development of Political and Economic Policy Attitudes." *Critical Sociology* 41 (3): 493–516.

DiMaggio, Paul, and Filiz Garip. 2011. "How Network Externalities Can Exacerbate Intergroup Inequality." *American Journal of Sociology* 116 (6): 1887–1933.
Dinesen, Peter Thisted, and Kim Mannemar Sonderskov. 2015. "Ethnic Diversity and Social Trust Evidence from the Micro-Context." *American Sociological Review* 80(3):550–573. \92–257.
Ding, Hao, Feng Xu, Jia-Ming Zhu, and Shenggang Li. 2021. "The Influence of Social Class on University Students" Prosocial Behavior Based on the Game Perspective." *Complexity* 2021:9951595.
Dinic, Bojana M., and Bojana Bodroza. 2021. "COVID-19 Protective Behaviors Are Forms of Prosocial and Unselfish Behaviors." *Frontiers in Psychology* 12: 647710.
Dioale, William, and Albert Seda. 2001. "Modernization as Changes in Cultural Complexity: New Cross-cultural Measurements." *Cross-Cultural Research* 35 (2): 129–153.
DiRenzo, Gordon J. 1990. "Socialization for Citizenship in Modern Democratic Society." Pp.25–46 in *Political Socialization, Citizenship, Education, and Democracy*, edited by Orit Ichilov. New York: Teachers College.
Dishion, Thomas J., and Kathryn Kavanagh. 2000. "A Multilevel Approach to Family-centered Prevention in Schools: Process and Outcome." *Addictive Behaviors* 25 (6): 899–911.
Dixon, John, and Shelley McKeown. 2021. "Negative Contact, Collective Action, and Social Change: Critical Reflections, Technological Advances, and New Directions." *Journal of Social Issues* 77 (1): 242–257.
Dixon, John, Kevin Dunheim, Colin G. Tredoux, Linda R. Tropp, Beverley Clack, Liberty Eaton, and Michael Quayle. 2010. "Challenging the Stubborn Core of Opposition to Equality: Racial Contact and Political Attitudes." *Political Psychology* 31 (6): 831–855.
Djupe, Paul A. 2018. "Religion and Politics." Pp. 958–972 in *The SAGE Handbook of Political Sociology*, edited by William Outhwaite and Stephen Turner. London, UK: SAGE.
Djupe, Paul A., and Andrew R. Lewis. 2015. "Solidarity and Discord of Pluralism: How the Social Context Affects Interest Group Learning and Belonging." *American Politics Research* 43 (3): 394–424.
Doane, Woody. 2017. "Humanist Sociology." Pp. 322–329 in *The Cambridge Handbook of Sociology, Vol. 2: Specialty and Interdisciplinary Studies*, edited by Kathleen Odell Korgen. New York, NY: Cambridge University Press.
Dobbin, Frank, Beth Simmons, and Geoffrey Garrett. 2007. "The Global Diffusion of Public Policies: Social Construction, Coercion, Competition, or Learning?" *Annual Review of Sociology* 33: 449–472.
Doerner, William G., and Steven P. Lab. 2012. *Victimology*. Burlington, MA: Anderson.
Doff, Wnda, and Reinout Kleinhans. 2011. "Residential Outcomes of Forced Relocation: Lifting a Corner of the Veil on Neighbourhood Selection." *Urban Studies* 48(4):661–680. \115–106.
Dolch, Norman A. 2003. "Role." Pp. 391–432 in *Handbook of Symbolic Interactionism*, edited by Larry T. Reynolds and Nancy J. Herman-Kinney. Lanham, MD: Rowman.
Domhoff, C. William. 2017. "The Class-dominance Theory of Power in the United States." Pp. 63–69 in *The Cambridge Handbook of Sociology*, Vol. 2: Specialty and Interdisciplinary Studies, edited by Kathleen Odell Korgen. New York, NY: Cambridge University Press.
Dominitz, Jeff, and Charles F. Manski. 1997. "Perceptions of Economic Insecurity: Evidence from the Survey of Economic Expectations." *Public Opinion Quarterly* 61: 261–287.
Donahue, Kelly L., Paul Lichtenstein, Niklas Langstrom, and Brian M. D'Onofrio. 2013. "Why Does Early Sexual Intercourse Predict Subsequent Maladjustment? Exploring Potential Familial Confounds." *Health Psychology* 32 (2): 180–189.
Donner, Michael R., Fabrício H. Chagas-Bastos, Richard W. Jeremiah, Simon M. Laham, and Naomi I. Eisenberger. 2024. "Pathogens or Promiscuity? Testing Two Accounts of the Relation between Disgust Sensitivity and Binding Moral Values." *Emotion* 24 (2): 465–478.
Dorff, Cassy. 2017. "Violence, Kinship Networks, and Political Resilience: Evidence from Mexico." *Journal of Peace Research* 54 (4): 558–573.
Dorling, Danny. 2010. "All in the Mind? Why Social Inequalities Persist." *Public Policy Research* 16 (4): 226–231.

Dotter, Daniel. 2004. *Creating Deviance: An Interactionist Approach*. Walnut Creek, CA: Altamira.
Douds, Kiara Wyndham. 2021. "The Diversity Contract: Constructing Racial Harmony in a Diverse American Suburb." *American Journal of Sociology* 126 (6): 1347–1388.
Dougherty, Lea R. 2006. "Children's Emotionality and Social Status: A Meta-analysis Review." *Social Development* 15 (3): 394–417.
Douglas, Emily M. 2006. "Familial Violence Socialization in Childhood and Later Life Approval of Corporal Punishment: A Cross-cultural Perspective." *American Journal of Orthopsychiatry* 76(10:23–30.
Douglass, Melanie D., Michael Stirrat, Monica A. Koehn, and Robert S. Vaughan. 2023. "The Relationship between the Dark Triad and Attitudes towards Feminism." *Personality & Individual Differences* 200: 111889.
Dovidio, John F., Jane Allyn Piliavin, David Al Schroeder, and Louis A. Penner. 2006. *The Social Psychology of Prosocial Behavior*. Mahwah, NJ: Lawrence Erlbaum.
Dowler, Elizabeth. 2002. "Food and Poverty in Britain: Rights and Responsibilities." *Social Policy & Administration* 36 (6): 698–717.
Downie, Michelle, Genevieve A. Mageau, and Richard Koestner. 2008. "What Makes for Pleasant Social Interaction? Motivational Dynamics of Interpersonal Relations." *Journal of Social Psychology* 148 (5): 523–534.
Draper, Thomas W., and Thomas B. Holman. 2005. "Locating the Big Five Personality Factors in the Relate Relationship Evaluation Measures." *Psychological Reports* 97 (3): 877–886.
Dreher, Axel, Noel Gaston, and Pim Martens. 2008. *Measuring Globalisation: Gauging Its Consequences*. New York: Springer.
Drollinger, Tanya. 2010. "A Theoretical Examination of Giving and Volunteering Utilizing Resource Exchange Theory." *Journal of Nonprofit & Public Sector Marketing* 22 (1): 55–66.
Dryzek, John S., and Patrick Dunleavy. 2009. *Theories of the Democratic State*. Houndmills, UK: Palgrave.
du Gay, Paul. 2012. "Leviathan Calling: Some Notes on Sociological Anti-Statism and Its Consequences." *Journal of Sociology* 48 (4): 397–409.
Duberstein, P. R., Y. Conwell, K. R. Conner, S. Eberly, J. S. Evinger, and E. D. Caine. 2004. "Poor Social Integration and Suicide: Fact or Artifact? A Case-control Study." *Psychological Medicine* 34: 1331–1337.
Dubois, Elizabeth, Sara Minaeian, Ariane Paquet-Labelle, and Simon Beaudry. 2020. "Who to Trust on Social Media: How Opinion Leaders and Seekers Avoid Disinformation and Echo Chambers." *Social Media + Society* 6(2):205630512091399.
Duffy, Ryan D., and Trisha L. Raque-Bogdan. 2010. "The Motivation to Serve Others: Exploring Relations to Career Development." *Journal of Career Assessment* 18 (3): 250–265.
Duhaime, Gerard, Edmund Searles, Peter J. Usher, Heather Myers, and Pierre Frechetti. 2004. "Social Cohesion and Living Conditions in the Canadian Arctic: From Theory to Measurement." *Social Indicators Research* 66: 295–317.
Dukes, Richard L., and Judith A. Stein. 2003. "Gender and Gang Membership: A Contrast of Rural and Urban Youth on Attitudes and Behavior." *Youth & Society* 34 (4): 415–440.
Dum, Christopher P., Kelly M. Socia, and Jason Rydberg. 2017. "Public Support for Emergency Shelter Housing Interventions Concerning Stigmatized Populations: Results from a Factorial Survey." *Criminology & Public Policy* 16 (3): 833–875.
Dunbar, Norah E., and Gordon Abra. 2021. "A Dyadic Power Theory Explanation of the Demand-Withdraw." *Personal Relationships* 28 (3): 586–606.
Duncan, Lauren E. 1999. "Motivation for Collective Action: Group Consciousness as Mediator of Personality, Life Experiences, and Women's Rights Activism." *Political Psychology* 20 (3): 611–635.
Duncan, Nick. 2017. *Positive Social Identity: The Quantitative Analysis of Ethics*. Abingdon, UK: Routledge.

Dunkel, Curtis S., Aaron W. Lukaszewski, and Kristine Chua. 2016. "The Relationships between Sex, Life History Strategy, and Adult Romantic Attachment Style." *Personality & Individual Differences* 98: 176–178.

Dunkle, Kristin L., Rachel K. Jewkes, Heather C. Brown, Glenda E. Gray, James A. McIntryre, and Sioban D. Harlow. 2004. "Transactional Sex among Women in Soweito, South Africa: Prevalence, Risk Factors and Association with HIV Infection." *Social Science & Medicine* 59: 1581–1592.

Dunn, Kevin M., James Forrest, Ian Burnley, and Amy McDonald. 2004. "Constructing Racism in Australia." *Australian Journal of Social Issues* 39 (4): 409–430.

Dunwoody, Philip T., and Friedrich Funke. 2016. "The Aggression-Submission-Conventionalism Scale: Testing a New Three Factor Measure of Authoritarianism." *Journal of Social & Political Psychology* 4 (2): 571–600.

Dutton, Edward and J. O. A. Rayner-Hilles. 2022. *The Past Is a Future Country: The Coming Conservative Demographic Revolution.* Exeter, UK: Imprint Academic.

Dutton, Edward, Guy Madison, and Richard Lynn. 2016. "Demographic, Economic, and Genetic Factors Related to National Differences in Ethnocentric Attitudes." *Personality & Individual Differences* 101: 137–143.

Duval-Diop, Dominique, Andrew Curtis, and Annie Clark. 2010. "Enhancing Equity with Public Participatory GIS in Hurricane Rebuilding: Faith-Based Organizations, Community Mapping, and Policy Advocacy." *Community Development* 41 (1): 32–49.

Dyck, Joshua J. 2012. "Racial Threat, Direct Legislation, and Social Trust." *Political Research Quarterly* 65 (3): 615–628.

Dyck, Joshua J., Edward L. Lascher, Jr. 2009. "Direct Democracy and Political Efficacy Reconsidered." *Political Behavior* 31: 401–427.

Dy-Liacco, Gabriel S., Ralph L. Piedmont, Nichole A. Murray-Swank, Thomas E. Rodgerson, and Martin F. Sherman. 2009. "Spirituality and Religiosity as Cross-Cultural Aspects of Human Experience." *Psychology of Religion & Spirituality* 1 (1): 35–52.

Eagly, Alice H., Amanda B. Diekman, Mary C. Johannesen-Schmidt, and Anne M. Koenig. 2004. "Gender Gaps in Sociopolitical Attitudes: A Social Psychological Analysis." *Journal of Personality & Social Psychology* 87 (6): 796–816.

Eakins, Danielle R., Elizabeth C. Neilson, Cynthia A. Stappenbeck, Hong V. Nguyen, Kelly Cue Davis, and William H. George. 2022. "Alcohol Intoxication and Sexual Risk Intentions: Exploring Cultural Factors among Heavy Drinking Women." *Addictive Behaviors* 131: 107314.

Earl, Jennifer, and Sarah A. Soule. 2001. "The Differential Protection of Minority Groups: The Inclusion of Sexual Orientation, Gender and Disability in State Hate Crime Laws, 1976–1995." *Research in Political Sociology* 9: 3–33.

Eastwood, Jonathan. 2015. "Can (and Should) We Construct an Evolutionary Psychological Theory of Institutions?" *Sociological Forum* 30 (1): 170–187.

Eatough, Virginia, Jonathan A. Smith, and Rachel Shaw. 2008. "Women, Anger, and Aggression: An Interpretative Phenomenological Analysis." *Journal of Interpersonal Violence* 23 (12): 1767–1799.

Eberl, Andreas. 2020. "The Effect of Informal Caregiving on Social Capital Investments." *Social Science Research* 85: 102319.

Economou, Marina, Elias Angelopoulos, Lily Evangelia Peppou, Kyriakos Souliotis, Chara Tzavara, Konstantinos Kontoangelos, Michael Madianos, and Costas Stefanis. 2016. "Enduring Financial Crisis in Greece: Prevalence and Correlates of Major Depression and Suicidality." *Social Psychiatry & Psychiatric Epidemiology* 51 (7): 1015–1024.

Edara, Inna Reddy. 2021. "Role of Social, Civic, and Governance Aspects in Life Satisfaction and Psychological Distress: Insights from Taiwan." *Current Psychology.* 41 (12): 8668–8677.

Edlund, Jonas, and Anne Gronlund. 2010. "Class Are Work Autonomy in 21 Countries: A question of Production Regime or Power Resource?" *Acta Sociologia* 53 (3): 213–228.

Edlund, Jonas. 2006. "Trust in the Capability of the Welfare State and General Welfare State Support: Sweden 1997–2002." *Acta Sociologica* 49 (4): 395–417.

Edney, Kingsley. 2012. "Soft Power and the Chinese Propaganda System." *Journal of Contemporary China* 21 (78): 899–914.
Edwards, Martin S. 2006. "Public Opinion Regarding Economic and Cultural Globalization: Evidence from a Cross-National Survey." *Review of International Political Economy* 13 (4): 587–608.
Edwards, Pearce, and Daniel Arnon. 2021. "Violence on Many Sides: Framing Effects on Protest and Support for Repression." *British Journal of Political Science* 51 (2): 488–506.
Edwards, Rosalind, and Val Gillies. 2004. "Support in Parenting: Values and Consensus Concerning Who to Turn to." *Journal of Social Policy* 33 (4): 627–647.
Edwards, Rosalind. 2004. "Present and Absent in Troubling Ways: Families and Social Capital Debates." *Sociological Review* 69: 1–21.
Edyvane, Derek. 2017. "The Passion for Civility." *Political Studies Review* 15 (3): 344–354.
Eger, Maureen A. 2010. "Even in Sweden: The Effect of Immigration on Support for Welfare State Spending." *European Sociological Review* 26 (2): 203–217.
Eggemeier, Matthew T. and Peter Joseph Fritz. 2020. *The Politics of Mercy: Catholic Life in an Era of Inequality, Racism, and Violence*. New York, NY: Crossroad.
Eggert, Nina, and Marco Giugni. 2015. "Does the Class Cleavage Still Matter? The Social Composition of Participants in Demonstrations Addressing Redistributive and Cultural Issues in Three Countries." *International Sociology* 30 (1): 21–38.
Ehrensuft, Miriam K., Patricia Cohen, Jocelyn Brown, Elizabeth Smailes, Henian Chen, and Jeffrey G. Johnson. 2003. "Intergenerational Transmission of Partner Violence: A 20-year Prospective Study." *Journal of Consulting & Clinical Psychology* 71 (4): 741–753.
Ehrke, Franziska, Gloria Grommisch, Emma Penelope Busch, and Magdalena C. Kaczmarek. 2023. "Populist Attitudes Predict Compliance-Related Attitudes and Behaviors During the Covid-19 Pandemic Via Trust in Institutions." *Social Psychology* 54 (1–2): 78–94.
Eibach, Richard P., Lisa K. Libby, and Joyce Ehrlinger. 2009. "Priming Family Values: How Being a Parent Affects Moral Evaluations of Harmless but Offensive Acts." *Journal of Experimental Social Psychology* 45 (5): 1160–1163.
Eibach, Richard P., Matthew O. Wilmot, and Lisa K. Libby. 2015. "The System-Justifying Function of Gratitude Norms." *Social & Personality Psychology Compass* 9 (7): 348–358.
Eikemo, Terje Andreas, Arne Matekaasa, and Kristen Ringdal. 2008. "Health and Happiness." Pp.48–64 in *Nordic Social Attitudes in a European Perspective*, edited by Heikki Ervasti, Torben Fridberg, Mikael Hjerm, and Kristen Ringdal. Cheltenham, UK: Edward Elgar.
Ein-Dor, Tsachi, and Gilad Hirschberger. 2012. "Sexual Healing." *Journal of Social & Personal Relationships* 29 (1): 126–139.
Eklund, Lisa, and Navtej Purewal. 2017. "The Bio-Politics of Population Control and Sex-Selective Abortion in China and India." *Feminism & Psychology* 27 (1): 34–55.
Elchardus, Mark, and Kobe De Keere. 2013. "Social Control and Institutional Trust: Reconsidering the Effect of Modernity on Social Malaise." *Social Science Journal* 50 (1): 101–111.
Elfenbein, Hillary Anger. 2013. "Individual Differences in Negotiation." Pp. 25–45 in *Handbook of Research on Negotiation*, edited by Mara Olekalns and Wendi L. Adair. Cheltenham, UK: Elgar.
Elfers, John, Patty Hlava, Farrah Sharpe, Sonia Arreguin, and Dawn Celeste McGregor. 2024. "Resilience and Loss: The Correlation of Grief and Gratitude." *International Journal of Applied Positive Psychology* 9 (1): 327–345.
El-Ghannam, Ashraf Ragab. 2002. "The Determinants of Social Well-Being, Economic Development, and Development Index in the Third World Countries." *Perspectives on Global Development & Technology* 1 (1): 51–69.
Elias, Sean, and Joe R. Feagin. 2016. *Racial Theories in Social Science: A Systemic Racism Critique*. New York, NY: Routledge.
Elliott, Anthony and Bryan S. Turner. 2012. *On Society*. Cambridge, UK: Polity.
Elliott, Anthony. 2003. *Critical Visions: New Directions in Social Theory*. Lanham, MD: Rowman & Littlefield.

Elliott, Anthony. 2022. *Making Sense of AI: Our Algorithmic World*. Cambridge, UK: Polity.

Elliott, Delbert S., and William Julius Wilson. 1996. "The Effects of Neighborhood Disadvantage on Adolescent Development." *Journal of Research in Crime & Delinquency* 33 (4): 389–416.

Ellis, Gary D., Patti A. Freeman, Tazim Jamal, and Jingxian Jiang. 2019. "A Theory of Structured Experience." *Annals of Leisure Research* 22 (1): 97–118.

Ellis, Ralph D., Norman Fischer, and James B. Sauer. 2006. *Foundations of Civic Engagement: Rethinking Social and Political Philosophy*. Lanham, MD: University Press of America.

Ellison, Christopher G., Jason D. Boardman, David R. Williams, and James S. Jackson. 2001. "Religious Involvement, Stress, and Mental Health: Findings from the 1995 Detroit Area Study." *Social Forces* 80 (1): 215–249.

Emer, Denise R., and Dennis L. Poepsel. 2021. "Under the Radar: Everyday Sadism Predicts Both Passive-Aggressive Harms and Beneficial Actions after Accounting for Prosocial Tendencies." *Personality & Individual Differences* 168: 110321.

Emery, Clifton R. and Shali Wu. 2020. "A Tale of Two Confucian Capitals: The Role of Friends and Secrecy in Beijing and Seoul." *Violence against Women* 26(5):458-81.

Emjaian, Brian, Sarah Beth Bell, Zachary Whitt, and C. Nathan De Wall. 2018. "Social-cognitive Processes in the Development of Antisocial and Violent Behavior." Pp. 259–277 in *The Cambridge Handbook of Violent Behavior and Aggression*, edited by Alexander T. Vazsonyi, David J. Flannery and Matt DeLisi. Cambridge, UK: Cambridge University Press.

Emler, Nicholas, and Elizabeth Frazer. 1999. "Politics: The Education Effect." *Oxford Review of Education* 25 (1/2): 251–273.

Engelstad, Fredrik. 2009. "Culture and Power." Pp. 210–238 in *The SAGE Handbook of Power*, edited by Stewart R. Clegg and Mark Haugaard. London, UK: SAGE.

Engle, Yuna, and Tim Kasser. 2005. "Why Do Adolescent Girls Idolize Male Celebrities?" *Journal of Adolescent Research* 20 (2): 263–283.

Epstein, William M. 1997. *Welfare in America: How Social Service Fails the Poor*. Madison, WI: University of Wisconsin Press.

Erhart, Ryan. 2016. "A Cross-National Examination of Prejudice toward Immigrants: The Role of Education and Political Ideology." *Journal of Aggression, Conflict & Peace Research* 8 (4): 279–289.

Erickson, Sarah J., and Sarah W. Feldstein. 2007. "Adolescent Humor and Its Relationship to Coping, Defense Strategies, Psychological Distress, and Well-being." *Child Psychology & Human Development* 37: 255–371.

Eriksson, Kimmo, Ali Kazemi, and Kjell Tornblom. 2015. "A New Look at Individual Differences in Perceptions of Unfairness: The Theory of Maximally Unfair Allocations in Multiparty Situations." *Social Justice Research* 28 (4): 401–414.

Erin, Calhoun, and Lisa V. Friel. 2001. "Adolescent Sexuality: Disentangling the Effects of Family Structure and Family Context." *Journal of Marriage & the Family* 63 (3): 669–681.

Erkkila, Tero. 2012. *Government Transparency: Impacts and Unintended Consequences*. Houndmills, UK: Palgrave.

Esaisason, Peter. 2014. "Nimbyism: A Reexamination of a Phenomenon." *Social Science Research* 48: 185–195.

Espelage, Dorothy L., Stanley Wasserman, and Mark Fleisher. 2007. "Social Networks and Violent Behavior." Pp.450–464 in *The Cambridge Handbook of Violent Behavior and Aggression*, edited by Daniel J. Flannery, Alexander T. Vazsonyi and Irwin D. Waldman. Cambridge, UK: Cambridge University Press.

Esposito, John L. 2002. *What Everyone Needs to Know about Islam*. New York: Oxford University Press.

Espvall, Majen, and Peter Dellgren. 2008. "Can We Count on Each Other? Reciprocity and Conflicts in Financial Support in Sweden." *International Journal of Social Welfare* 19: 84–94.

Esses, Victoria M., John F. Dovidio, Antoinette H. Semenya, and Lynne M. Jackson. 2005. "Attitudes toward Immigrants and Immigration: The Role of National and International Identity." Pp.317–337 in *The Social Psychology of Inclusion and Exclusion*, edited by Dominic Abrams, Michael A. Hogg and Jose M. Marque. New York: Psychology Press.

Etzioni, Amitai. 1996. "A Moderate Communitarian Proposal." *Political Theory* 24 (2): 155–171.

Evans, Paul. 2006. "Canada, Meet Global China." *International Journal* 61 (2): 283–297.

Evans, Paul. 2009. "Getting Global China Right." *Pacific Affairs* 82 (4): 677–686.

Evans, William N., Michael Hout, and Susan E. Mayer. 2004. "Assessing the Effect of Economic Inequality." Pp.933–968 in *Social Inequality*, edited by Kathryn M. Neckerman. New York: Russell Sage.

Evetts, Julia. 2013. "Professionalism: Value and Ideology." *Current Sociology*. 61(5–6):778–96. \d12–4.22.

Ewick, Patricia, and Susan Silbey. 2003. "Narrating Social Structure: Stories of Resistance to Legal Authority." *American Journal of Sociology* 108 (6): 1328–1372.

Fabrigar, Leandre R., Tara K. MacDonald, and Duane t. Wegener. 2014. "The Structure of Attitudes." Pp. 79–124 in *The Handbook of Attitudes*, edited by Albarracin Dolores, T. Johnson Blair and P. Zanna Mark. Mahwah, NJ: Psychology.

Fagot-Largeault, Anne. 2008. "The Fetus in Perspective: The Moral and Legal." Pp. 113–121 in *Contemporary Debates in Social Philosophy*, edited by Laurence Thomas. Malden, MA: Blackwell.

Fahey, James J. 2022. "Building Populist Discourse: An Analysis of Populist Communication in American Presidential Elections, 1896–2016." *Social Science Quarterly* 103 (4): 1268–1288.

Fahmy, Eldin. 2006. "Social Capital and Civic Action: A Study of Youth in the United Kingdom." *Young* 14 (2): 101–118.

Fairfield, Paul. 2008. *Why Democracy?* Albany, NY: State University of New York Press.

Falk, John H. 2018. *Born to Choose: Evolution, Self, and Well-being*. New York, NJ: Routledge.

Falkenberg, Andrcas W. 1998. "Quality of Life: Efficacy, Equity and Freedom in the United States and Scandinavia." *Journal of Socio-Economics* 27 (1): 1–27.

Fallman, Fredrik. 2010. "Useful Opium? Adapted Religion and Harmony in Contemporary China." *Journal of Contemporary China* 19 (67): 949–969.

Falomir-Pichastor, Juan Manuel, Armand Chatard, Leila Selimbegovic. Paul N'Dri Konan, and Gabriel Mugny. 2013. "Conformity and Counter-Conformity to Anti-Discrimination Norms: The Moderating Effect of Attitude toward Foreigners and Perceived In-Group Threat." *Journal of Applied Social* Psychology 43(Suppl.2):E206-E215.

Fan, Juan, Wenhui Liang, and Hanyi Zheng. 2022. "Government's Impression Management Strategies, Trust in Government and Social Cohesion: An Evidence from Songjiang University Town, China." *Frontiers in Psychology* 13: 951579.

Fang, Tongyi. 2003. *Spirit of Chinese Wisdom: From the Realm of Heaven-Human to the Border between Dao-Tactics*. Beijing, China: People.

Fanning, Bryan, Trutz Haase, and Neil O'Boyle. 2011. "Well-being, Cultural Capital and Social Inclusion: Immigrants in the Republic of Ireland." *International Migration & Integration* 12 (1): 1–24.

Fararo, Thomas J. 2001. *Social Action Systems: Foundation and Synthesis in Sociological Theory*. Westport, CT: Praeger.

Faricy, Christopher, and Christopher Ellis. 2014. "Public Attitudes toward Social Spending in the United States: The Differences between Direct Spending and Tax Expenditures." *Political Behavior* 36: 53–76.

Farla, Kristine. 2015. "Industrial Policy for Growth." *Journal of Industry, Competition & Trade* 15 (3): 257–282.

Farmer, Jane, Margaret Currie, Amanda Kenny, and Sarah-Anne. Munoz. 2015. "An Exploration of The Longer-Term Impacts of Community Participation in Rural Health Services Design." *Social Science & Medicine* 141: 64–71.

Farmer, Mark, Anne-Marie. McAlinden, and Shadd Maruna. 2016. "Sex Offending and Situational Motivation." *International Journal of Offender Therapy & Comparative Criminology* 60 (15): 1756–1775.

Farmer, Steven M., and Donald B. Fedor. 2001. "Changing the Focus on Volunteering: An Investigation of Volunteers Multiple Contributions to a Charitable Organization." *Journal of Management* 27: 191–211.

Farrell, Henry, and Abraham L. Newman. 2010. "Making Global Markets: Historical Institutionalism in International Political Economy." *Review of International Political Economy* 17 (4): 609–638.

Farrelly, Colin. 2007. *Justice, Democracy and Reasonable Agreement*. Houndmills, UK: Palgrave.

Farrington, David P. 2007. "Origins of Violent Behavior over the Life Span." Pp.19–48 in *The Cambridge Handbook of Violent Behavior and Aggression*, edited by Daniel J. Flannery, Alexander T. Vazsonyi and Irwin D. Waldman. Cambridge, UK: Cambridge University Press.

Farrington, David P. 2010. "Life-course and Developmental Theories in Criminology." Pp.259–270 in *The SAGE Handbook of Criminological Theory*, edited by Eugene McLaughlin and Tim Newburn. London, UK: SAGE.

Farrington, David P. 2018. "The Duration of Criminal Careers: How Many Offenders Do Not Desist up to Age 61?" *Journal of Developmental & Life Course Criminology* 5 (1): 4–21.

Farwell, Megan M., Micheal L. Shier, and Femida Handy. 2019. "Explaining Trust in Canadian Charities: The Influence of Public Perceptions of Accountability, Transparency, Familiarity and Institutional Trust." *VOLUNTAS: International Journal of Voluntary and Nonprofit Organizations* 30 (4): 768–782.

Fasel, Nicole, Oriane Sarrasin, Eva G. T. Green, and Eric Mayor. 2016. "Who Is to Blame? Official Discourse and Ethnic Diversity Attitudes during the 2011 Riots in England." *Political Psychology* 37 (5): 659–675.

Featherstone, Brid, and Kate Morris. 2012. "Feminist Ethics of Care." Pp.341–354 in *The SAGE Handbook of Social Work*, edited by Mel Gray, James Midgley and Stephen A. Webb. London, UK: SAGE.

Featherstone, Richard, and Mathieu Deflem. 2003. "Anomie and Strain: Context and Consequences of Merton's Two Theories." *Sociological Inquiry* 73 (4): 471–489.

Feeney, Brooke C., and Nancy L. Collins. 2001. "Predictors of Caregiving in Adult Intimate Relationships: An Attachment Theoretical Perspective." *Journal of Personality & Social Psychology* 80 (6): 972–994.

Feeney, Brooke C., and Nancy L. Collins. 2018. "Social Support in Close Relationships." Pp. 281–296 in *The Cambridge Handbook of Personal Relationships*, edited by Anita L. Vangelisti and Daniel Perlman. Cambridge, UK: Cambridge University Press.

Fehr, Beverley, and Ross Broughton. 2001. "Gender and Personality Differences in Conceptions of Love: An Interpersonal Theory Analysis." *Personal Relationships* 8 (2): 115–136.

Fein, Melvyn L. 2015. *Evolution versus Revolution: The Paradoxes of Social Change*. New Brunswick, NJ: Transaction.

Feinberg, Mark E., Louis D. Brown, and Marni L. Kan. 2012. "A Multi-Domain Self-Report Measure of Coparenting." *Parenting* 12 (1): 1–21.

Feinberg, Matthew, Elisabeth Wehling, Joanne M. Chung, Laura R. Saslow, and Ingrid Melvær Paulin. 2019. "Measuring Moral Politics: How Strict and Nurturant Family Values Explain Individual Differences in Conservatism, Liberalism, and the Political Middle." *Journal of Personality & Social Psychology* 118 (4): 777–804.

Feingold, Alan. 1994. "Gender Differences in Personality: A Meta-analysis." *Psychological Bulletin* 116 (3): 429–456.

Feinstein, Leon, and John Bynner. 2006. "Continuity and Discontinuity in Middle Childhood: Implications for Adult Outcomes in the UK 1970 Birth Cohort." Pp.327–349 in *Developmental Contexts in Middle Childhood: Bridges to Adolescence and Adulthood*, edited by Aletha C. Huston, and Marika N. Ripke. Cambridge, UK: Cambridge University Press.

Feldman, David B. 2006. "Can Suicide Be Ethical? A Utilitarian Perspective on the Appropriateness of Choosing to Die." *Death Studies* 30: 529–538.
Feldman, Yuval. 2018. *The Law of Good People: Challenging States. Ability to Regulate Human Behavior*. Cambridge, UK: Cambridge University Press.
Felson, Richard B., and Maureen C. Outlaw. 2007. "The Control Motive and Marital Violence." *Violence & Victims* 22 (4): 387–407.
Feltham-King, Tracey, and Catriona Macleod. 2016. "How Content Analysis May Complement and Extend the Insights of Discourse Analysis." *International Journal of Qualitative Methods* 15 (1): 1–9.
Fenwick, Tara. 2008. "Women Learning in Garment Work: Solidarity and Sociality." *Adult Education Quarterly* 58 (2): 110–128.
Fer, Seval. 2012. "Demographic Characteristics and Intellectual Styles." Pp.109–130 in *Handbook of Intellectual Styles: Preferences in Cognition, Learning, and Thinking*. New York: Springer.
Ferguson, Neil, and James W. McAuley. 2020. "Radicalization or Reaction: Understanding Engagement in Violent Extremism in Northern Ireland." *Political Psychology* 41 (2): 215–230.
Fernandes, April. 2018. "Red Lights and Handcuffs: The Effect of Arrests on the Fear of Crime." *Social Science Quarterly* 99 (4): 1390–1408.
Ferrara, Federico. 2022. *The Development of Political Institutions: Power, Legitimacy, Democracy*. Ann Arbor, MI: University of Michigan Press.
Ferretti, Fabio, Giacomo Gualtieri, Alessandra Masti, and Allison Uvelli. 2024. "Urban Safety and Psychological Distress During the Pandemic: The Results of a Longitudinal Study." *Frontiers in Psychology* 15: 1343585.
Ferssizidis, Patty, Leah M. Adams, Todd B. Kashdan, Christine Plummer, Anjali Mishra, and Joseph Ciarrochi. 2010. "Motivation for and Commitment to Social Values: The Roles of Age and Gender." *Motivation & Emotion* 34 (4): 354–362.
Ferwerda, Jeremy, and Nicholas L. Miller. 2014. "Political Devolution and Resistance to Foreign Rule: A Natural Experiment." *American Political Science Review* 108 (3): 642–660.
Fetvadjiev, Velichko H., and Jia He. 2019. "The Longitudinal Links of Personality Traits, Values, and Well-Being and Self-Esteem: A Five-Wave Study of a Nationally Representative Sample." *Journal of Personality & Social Psychology* 117 (2): 448–464.
Figueredo, Aurelio Jose, Emily Anne Patch, Marisol Perez-Ramos, and Gabriela Jacqueline Curz. 2018. "The Dark Violence Hybrid The Cross-cultural Validation of an Integrative Model." Pp. 65–80 *The Cambridge Handbook of Violent Behavior and Aggression*, edited by Alexander T. Vazsonyi, David J. Flannery and Matt DeLisi. Cambridge, UK: Cambridge University Press.
Filip, Agneessens, Hans Waege, and John Lievens. 2006. "Diversity in Social Support by Role Relations: A Typology." *Social Networks* 28: 427–441.
Fine, Gary Alan, and Lori Holyfield. 1996. "Secrecy, Trust, and Dangerous Leisure: Generating Group Cohesion on Voluntary Organizations." *Social Psychology Quarterly* 59 (1): 22–38.
Fine, Michael D. 2007. *A Caring Society? Care and the Dilemmas of Human Service in the Twenty-first Century*. Houndmills, UK: Palgrave.
Fingerman, Karen L., Yee To Ng, Shiyang Zhang, Katherine Britt, Gianna Colera, Kira S. Birditt, Susan T. Charles, and Deborah S. Carr. 2021. "Living Alone During Covid-19: Social Contact and Emotional Well-Being among Older Adults." *Journals of Gerontology* 76(3):e116-e21.
Fischer, Claude S., Michael Hout, Martin Sanchez Jankowski, Samuel R. Lucas, Ann Swindler, and Kim Voss. 1996. *Inequality by Design: Cracking the Bell Curve Myth*. Princeton, NJ: Princeton University Press.
Fischer, Peter, Tobias Greitemeyer, Suat Ilkay Omay, and Dieter Frey. 2007. "Mergers and Group Status: The Impact of High, Low and Equal Group Status on Identification and Satisfaction with a Company Merger, Experienced Controllability, Group Identity and Group Cohesion." *Journal of Community & Applied Social Psychology* 17 (3): 203–217.
Fisher, Robert J., and James E. Katz. 2000. "Social-desirability Bias and the Validity of Self-reported Values." *Psychology & Marketing* 17 (2): 105–120.

Fishkin, James. 2018. *Democracy When the People Are Thinking: Revitalizing Our Politics through Public Deliberation*. Oxford, UK: Oxford University Press.

Fitch, Brian D., Anthony H. Normore and David R. Werner. 2011. "Chapter 9 Theories of Criminal Justice: The Influence of Value Attributions on Correctional Education." *Advances in Educational Administration* 12:161–84.

Fives, Allyn. 2008. *Political and Philosophical Debates in Welfare*. Houndmills, UK: Palgrave.

Fjellvang, Tormod. 2011. "Socialization Values, Cultural-religious Zones and Modernization Theory." *European Sociological Review* 27 (2): 196–211.

Flanagan, Scott C., and Aie-Rie. Lee. 2000. "Value Change and Democratic Reform in Japan and Korea." *Comparative Political Studies* 33 (5): 626–659.

Flanagan, Scott C., and Aie-Rie. Lee. 2003. "The New Politics, Culture Wars, and the Authoritarian-libertarian Value Change in Advanced Industrial Democracies." *Comparative Political Studies* 36 (3): 235–270.

Flap, Henk, and Beate Volker. 2013. "Social Capital." Pp. 220–251 in *The Handbook of Rational Choice Social Research*, edited by Rafael Wittek, Tom A. H. Snijders, and Victor Nee. Stanford, CA: Stanford University Press.

Flavin, Patrick, and Michael J. Keane. 2011. "Life Satisfaction and Political Participation: Evidence from the United States." *Journal of Happiness Studies* 13 (1): 63–78.

Flett, Gordon L. 2018. *The Psychology of Mattering: Understanding the Human Need to Be Significant*. London, UK: Academic.

Fligstein, Neil, and Luke Dauter. 2007. "The Sociology of Markets." *Review of Sociology* 33: 105–128.

Florida, Richard. 2005. *Cities and the Creative Class*. New York: Routledge.

Flouri, Eirini, and Ann Buchanan. 2002. "The Protective Role of Parental Involvement in Adolescent Suicide." *Crisis* 23 (1): 17–22.

Flouri, Eirini. 2003. "Parental Socialization in Childhood and Offspring Materialist and Postmaterialist Values in Adult Life." *Journal of Applied Social Psychology* 33 (10): 2106–2122.

Follette, William C., Peter J. N. Linnerroth, and L. E. Ruckstuhl, Jr. 2001. "Positive Psychology: A Clinical Behavior Analytic Perspective." *Journal of Humanistic Psychology* 41(1):102–134. \87–244.

Fontana, David. 2003. *Psychology, Religion, and Spirituality*. Malden, MA; Blackwell. Harris, Kevin A., Desiree S. Howell, and Don W. Spurgeon. 2018. "Faith Concepts in Psychology: Three 30-Year Definitional Content Analyses." *Psychology of Religion & Spirituality* 10(1):1–29.

Forman, Tyrone A. 2001. "Social Determinants of White Youths" Racial Attitudes: Evidence from a National Survey." *Sociological Studies of Children and Youth* 8: 173–207.

Forsyth, James. 2003. *Psychological Theories of Religion*. Upper Saddle River, NJ: Prentice Hall.

Forsyth, Selina and Kaitlin P. Ward. 2022. "Media Use and Men's Approval of Intimate Partner Violence in Honduras." *Journal of Interpersonal Violence* 37(13–14):NP11541-NP56.

Foschi, Renato, and Marco Lauriola. 2014. "Does Sociability Predict Civic Involvement and Political Participation?" *Journal of Personality & Social Psychology* 106 (2): 339–357.

Foster, Dennis M., Alex Braithwaite, and David Sobek. 2013. "There Can Be No Compromise: Institutional Inclusiveness, Fractionalization and Domestic Terrorism." *British Journal of Political Science* 43 (3): 541–557.

Foster, Vivien, Susana Mourato, David Pearce, and Ece Ozdemiroglu. 2001. *The Price of Virtue: The Economic Value of the Charitable Sector*. Cheltenham, UK: Edward Elgar.

Foster-Fishman, Pennie G., Deborah A. Salem, Nichole E. Allen, and Kyle Fahrbach. 1999. "Ecological Factors Impacting Provider Attitudes towards Human Service Delivery Reform." *American Journal of Community Psychology* 27 (6): 785–816.

Fountain, Jane E. 2009. "Bureaucratic Reform and e-government in the United States: An Institutional Perspective." Pp. 99–113 in *Routledge Handbook of Internet Politics*, edited by Andrew Chadwick and Philip N. Howard. Abingdon, UK: Routledge.

Fowers, B. 2015. *The Evolution of Ethics: Human Sociality and the Emergence of Ethical Mindedness*. London, UK: Palgrave.

Fox, Bryanna H., Wesley G. Jennings, and David P. Farrington. 2015. "Bringing Psychopathy into Developmental and Life-Course Criminology Theories and Research." *Journal of Criminal Justice* 43 (4): 274–289.

Foy, Steven, Robert Freeland, Andrew Miles, Kimberly B. Rogers, and Lynn Smith-Lovin 2014. "Emotions and Affect as Source, Outcome and Resistance to Inequality." Pp. 295–324 in *Handbook of the Social Psychology of Inequality*, edited by, Jane D. McLeod, Edward J. Lawler, and Michael Schwalbe. Dordrecht, Netherland: Springer.

Fraley, R. Chris., Marie E. Heffernan, Amanda M. Vicary, and Claudia Chloe Brumbaugh. 2011. "The Experiences in Close Relationships-Relationship Structures Questionnaire: A Method for Assessing Attachment Orientations across Relationships." *Psychological Assessment* 23 (3): 615–625.

Francesconi, Marco, and Katrin Golsch. 2005. "The Process of Globalization and Transitions to Adulthood in Britain." Pp.249–276 in *Globalization, Uncertainty and Youth in Society*, edited by Hans-Peter Blossfeld, Erik Klijzing, Melinda Mills and Karin Kurz. London: Routledge.

Francois, Abel, and Raul Magni-Berton. 2013. "Individual Gendered Attitudes toward Immigrants. Empirical Evidence from French Surveys." *Social Science Journal* 50 (3): 321–330.

Frank, David John, and John W. Meyer. 2002. "The Profusion of Individual Roles and Identities in the Postwar Period." *Sociological Theory* 20 (1): 86–105.

Franklin, Leanne. 2012. *Gender.* Houndmills, UK: Palgrave.

Franks, Bradley, Adrian Bangerter, and Martin W. Bauer. 2013. "Conspiracy Theories as Quasi-Religious Mentality: An Integrated Account from Cognitive Science, Social Representations Theory, and Frame Theory." *Frontiers in Psychology* 4: 424.

Franzini, Luisa, Margaret Cauphy, William Spears, and Maria Eugenia Fernandez. Esquer. 2005. "Neighborhood Economic Conditions, Social Processes, and Self-rated Health in Low-income Neighborhoods in Texas: A Multilevel Latent Variables Model." *Social Science & Medicine* 61: 1135–1150.

Fraser, Ashley M., Laura M. Padilla-Walker, Sarah M. Coyne, Larry J. Nelson, and Laura A. Stockdale. 2012. "Associations between Violent Video Gaming, Empathic Concern, and Prosocial Behavior Toward Strangers, Friends, and Family Members." *Journal of Youth & Adolescence.* 41 (5): 636–649.

Fraser, Heather. 2005. "Four Different Approaches to Community Participation." *Community Development Journal* 40 (3): 286–300.

Frazer, Elizabeth. 1999. *The Problems of Communitarian Politics: Unity and Conflict*. Oxford, UK: Oxford University Pres.

Frederick, David A., Gaganjyot Sandhu, Patrick J. Morse, and Viren Swami. 2016. "Correlates of Appearance and Weight Satisfaction in a U.S. National Sample: Personality, Attachment Style, Television Viewing, Self-Esteem, and Life Satisfaction." *Body Image* 17: 191–203.

Fredman, Leah A., Brock Bastian, and William B. Swann. 2017. "God or Country? Fusion with Judaism Predicts Desire for Retaliation Following Palestinian Stabbing Intifada." *Social Psychological & Personality Science* 8 (8): 882–887.

Freeman, Daniel, Felicity Waite, Laina Rosebrock, Ariane Petit, Chiara Causier, Anna East, Lucy Jenner, Ashley-Louise Teale, Lydia Carr, Sophie Mulhall, Emily Bold, and Sinéad Lambe. 2022. "Coronavirus Conspiracy Beliefs, Mistrust, and Compliance with Government Guidelines in England." *Psychological Medicine*. 52(2):251–63.

Frei, Andreas, Kay W. Axhausen, and Timo Ohnmacht. 2009. "Mobilities and Social Network Geography: Size and Spatial Dispersion: The Zurich Case Study." Pp.99–120 in *Mobilities and Inequality*, edited by Timo Ohnmacht, Hanja Maksim, and Marfred Max Bergman. Farnham, UK: Ashgate.

Freitag, Markus, and Paul C. Bauer. 2016. "Personality Traits and the Propensity to Trust Friends and Strangers." *Social Science Journal* 53 (4): 467–476.

Freitag, Markus. 2003. "Social Capital in (Dis)similar Democracies: The Development of Generalized Trust in Japan and Switzerland." *Comparative Political Studies* 36 (8): 936–966.

French, Doran C., Nancy Eisenberg, Julie Vaughan, Urip Purwono, and Telie A. Suryanti. 2008. "Religious Involvement and the Social Competence and Adjustment of Indonesia Muslim Adolescents." *Developmental Psychology* 44 (2): 597–611.

Frerichs, Sabine, and Richard Munch. 2010. "Morality, Modernity, and World Society." Pp. 529–548 in *Handbook of the Sociology of Morality*, edited by Steven Hitlin and Stephen Vaisey. New York, NY: Springer.

Freund, Anat. 2005. "Work Attitudes of Social Workers across Three Sectors of Welfare Organization: Public, for-Profit, and Third Sector." *Journal of Social Service Research* 31 (3): 69–92.

Frey, Bruno S., Christine Benesch, and Alois Stutzer. 2007. "Does Watching TV Make Us Happy?" *Journal of Economic Psychology* 28: 283–313.

Frey, R. Scott., and Fengxiang Song. 1997. "Human Well-being in Chinese Cities." *Social Indicators Research* 42: 77–101.

Friborg, Oddgeir, Odin Hjemdal, Jan H. Rosenvinge, and Monica Martinussen. 2002. "A New Rating Scale for Adult Resilience: What Are the Central Protective Resources behind Healthy Adjustment?" *International Journal of Methods in Psychiatric Research* 12 (2): 65–76.

Fridberg, Torben and Olli Kangas. 2008a. "The Welfare State, Poverty and Social Exclusion." Pp.22–47 in *Nordic Social Attitudes in a European Perspective*, edited by Heikki Ervasti, Torben Fridberg, Mikael Hjerm, and Kristen Ringdal. Cheltenham, UK: Elgar.

Fridberg, Torben, and Olli Kangas. 2008b. "Social Capital." Pp.65–85 in *Nordic Social Attitudes in a European Perspective*, edited by Heikki Ervasti, Torben Fridberg, Mikael Hjerm, and Kristen Ringdal. Cheltenham, UK: Edward Elgar.

Friedkin, Noah. 2004. "Social Cohesion." *Annual Review of Sociology* 30: 409–425.

Friedman, Mark D. 2011. *Nozick's Libertarian Project: An Elaboration and Defense*. London: Continuum.

Friedman, Maurice. 1992. *Religion and Psychology: A Dialogical Approach*. New York: Paragon House.

Frohlich, Katherine L., Louise Potvin, Patrick Chabot, and Ellen Corin. 2002. "A Theoretical and Empirical Analysis of Context: Neighborhoods, Smoking and Youth." *Social Science & Medicine* 54: 1401–1417.

Frost, Natasha A., and Todd R. Clear. 2013. "Coercive Mobility." Pp.691–708 in *The Oxford Handbook of Criminological Theory*, edited by Francis T. Cullen and Pamela Wilcox. New York: Oxford University Press.

Frye, Victoria. 2007. "The Informal Social Control of Intimate Partner Violence against Women: Exploring Personal Attitudes and Perceived Neighborhood Social Cohesion." *Journal of Community Psychology* 35 (8): 1001–1018.

Fu, Xiwen. 2018. "The Contextual Effects of Political Trust on Happiness: Evidence from China." *Social Indicators Research* 139 (2): 491–516.

Fuchs, Christian. 2020. *Nationalism on the Internet: Critical Theory and Ideology in the Age of Social Media and Fake News*. New York, NY: Routledge.

Fuchs, Martin. 2015. "Processes of Religious Individualisation: Stocktaking and Issues for the Future." *Religion* 45 (3): 330–343.

Fujisawa, Yoshikazu, Tsuyashi Hamano, and Shogo Takegama. 2009. "Social Capital and Perceived Health in Japan: An Ecological and Multilevel Analysis." *Social Science & Medicine* 69: 500–505.

Fukuyama, Francis. 1992. *The End of History and the Last Man*. London: Penguin.

Fukuyama, Francis. 1995. *Trust: The Social Virtues and the Creation of Prosperity*. New York, NY: Free.

Fukuyama, Francis. 2001. "Social Capital, Civil Society, and Development." *Third World Quarterly* 22 (1): 7–20.

Fukuyama, Francis. 2018. *Identity: The Demand for Dignity and the Politics of Resentment*. New York, NY: Farrar, Straus & Giroux.

Fukuyama, Francis. 2018b. "Why National Identity Matters." *Journal of Democracy* 29 (4): 5–15.

Fuller, Steve. 2006. *The New Sociological Imagination*. London: Sage.
Fuller-Iglesias, Heather R., and Toni Antonucci. 2016. "Convoys of Social Support in Mexico: Examining Socio-Demographic Variation." *International Journal of Behavioral Development* 40 (4): 324–333.
Fung, Helene H., and Siu-Kei. Ng. 2006. "Age Differences in the Sixth Personality Factor: Age Differences in Interpersonal Relatedness among Canadians and Hong Kong Chinese." *Psychology & Aging* 21 (4): 810–814.
Funk, Carolyn L. 2001. "Process Performance: Public Reaction to Legislative Policy Debate." Pp.193–204 in *What Is It about Government that Americans Dislike?* edited by John R. Hibbing and Elizabeth Theiss-Morse. Cambridge, UK: Cambridge University Press.
Fyall, Rachel, and Beth Gazley. 2015. "Applying Social Role Theory to Gender and Volunteering in Professional Associations." *VOLUNTAS: International Journal of Voluntary and Nonprofit Organizations* 26 (1): 288–314.
Fyfe, R. 2005. "Making Space for Neo-communitarianism? The Third Sector, State and Civil Society in the UK." *Antipode* 536–557.
Gaertner, Samuel L., and John F. Dovidio. 2012. "The Common Ingroup Identity Model." Pp.439–457 in *Handbook of Theories of Social Psychology* (vol.2), edited by Paul A.M. Van Lange, Arie W. Kruglanski and E. Tory Higgins. London, CA: SAGE.
Gaffikin, Frank, and Mike Morriessey. 2011. "Community Cohesion and Social Inclusion: Unravelling a Complex Relationship." *Urban Studies* 48 (6): 1089–1118.
Gaines, N. Susan., and James C. Garand. 2010. "Morality, Equality, or Locality: Analyzing the Determinants of Same-sex Marriage." *Political Research Quarterly* 63 (3): 553–567.
Gaitan-Rossi, Pablo, and Ce Shen. 2018. "Fear of Crime in Mexico: The Impacts of Municipality Characteristics." *Social Indicators Research* 135(1):373-399.
Gallagher, Matthew W., and Shane J. Lopez. 2007. "Curiosity and Well-Being." *Journal of Positive Psychology* 2 (4): 236–248.
Galston, William A. 2005. *The Practice of Liberal Pluralism*. Cambridge, UK: Cambridge University Press.
Galupo, M. Paz., and Kirsten A. Gonzalez. 2013. "Friendship Values and Cross-Category Friendships: Understanding Adult Friendship Patterns across Gender, Sexual Orientation and Race." *Sex Roles* 68 (11–12): 779–790.
Galvin, Miranda A., Thomas A. Loughran, Sally S. Simpson, and Mark A. Cohen. 2018. "Victim Compensation Policy and White-Collar Crime." *Criminology & Public Policy* 17 (3): 553–594.
Gandjour, Afschin, and Karl Wilhelm Lauterbach. 2003. "Utilitarian Theories Reconsidered: Common Misconceptions, More Recent Developments, and Health Policy Implications." *Health Care Analysis* 11 (3): 229–244.
Gans, Chaim. 1992. *Philosophical Anarchism and Political Disobedience*. Cambridge, UK: Cambridge University Press.
Ganz, Aurora. 2023. "Emotions and Securitisation: A New Materialist Discourse Analysis." *European Journal of International Relations* 30 (2): 280–305.
Gao, Debu. 2018. *Values of China*. Beijing, China: Social Literature.
Gao, Huasheng, and Vanya Petrova. 2022. "Do Prostitution Laws Affect Rape Rates? Evidence from Europe." *Journal of Law & Economics* 65 (4): 753–789.
Gao, Yanjie, Hang Chen, Muhammad Zubair Tauni, Ibrahim Alnafrah, & Jiaqi Yu. 2024. "Unpacking the Impact of Financialization and Globalization on Environmental Degradation in BRICS Economies." *Resources Policy* 88: 104497.
Garb, Maja. 2015. "Public Trust in the Military: The Slovenian Armed Forces in a Comparative Analysis." *Current Sociology* 63 (3): 450–469.
Garcia, Enrique, and Juan Herrero. 2004. "Determinants of Social Integration in the Community: An Exploratory Analysis of Personal, Interpersonal, and Situational Variables." *Journal of Community & Applied Social Psychology* 14: 1–15.
Gardiner, Stephen M. 2009. "A Contract on Future Generations?" Pp.77–118 in *Intergenerational Justice*, edited by Axel Gosseries and Lukas H. Meyer. Oxford, UK: Oxford University Press.

Garland, Brett, Eric Wodahl, and Caryn Saxon. 2017. "What Influences Public Support of Transitional Housing Facilities for Offenders During Reentry?" *Criminal Justice Policy Review* 28 (1): 18–40.

Garnier, Helen E., and Judith A. Stein. 2002. "An 18-year Model of Family and Peer Effects on Adolescent Drug Use and Delinquency." *Journal of Youth & Adolescence* 31 (1): 45–56.

Garrett, Michael Tlanusta, Mark Parrish, Cyrus Williams, Lisa Grayshield, Tarrell Awe Agahe. Portman, Edil Torres Rivera, and Elizabeth Maynard. 2014. "Invited Commentary: Fostering Resilience among Native American Youth through Therapeutic Intervention." *Journal of Youth & Adolescence* 43 (3): 470–490.

Garrod, Joan and Mursha Jones. 2009. *Religion and Belief.* Houndmills, UK: Palgrave.

Garst, Barry A., Ryan J. Gagnon, Thomas Clanton, and Jay Woodward. 2021. "Cultivating Youth Affinity for College within the Context of Campus-Based Summer Camps." *Journal of Youth Development* 16 (5): 64–85.

Gattino, Silvia, Chiara Rollero, and Norma De Piccoli. 2015. "The Influence of Coping Strategies on Quality of Life from a Gender Perspective." *Applied Research in Quality of Life* 10 (4): 689–701.

Gault-Sherman, Martha. 2012. "It's a Two-Way Street: The Bidirectional Relationship between Parenting and Delinquency." *Journal of Youth & Adolescence* 41 (2): 121–145.

Gaus, Gerald F. 2003. *Contemporary Theories of Liberalism: Public Reason as a Post-Enlightenment Project*. London: Sage.

Gausel, Nicolay, Colin Wayne Leach, Vivian L. Vignoles, and Rupert Brown. 2012. "Defend or Repair? Explaining Responses to In-Group Moral Failure by Disentangling Feelings of Shame, Rejection, and Inferiority." *Journal of Personality & Social Psychology* 102 (5): 941–960.

Gay, David A., and John P. Lynxwiler. 2009. "The Impact of Race on Denominational Variations in Social Attitudes: The Issue and Its Dimensions." *Sociological Spectrum* 30 (1): 110–127.

Gazso, Amber. 2020. "Dueling Discourses, Power, and the Construction of the Recovering Addict: When Social Assistance Confronts Addiction in Toronto, Canada." *Critical Social Policy* 40 (1): 130–150.

Geboers, Ellen, Femke Geijsel, Wilfried Admiraal, and Geert ten Dam. 2013. "Review of The Effects of Citizenship Education." *Educational Research Review* 9: 158–173.

Gelade, Garry A. 1999. "Creativity in Conflict: The Personality of the Commercial Creative." *Journal of Genetic Psychology* 158 (1): 67–78.

Gelfand, Michele J., and Janetta Lun. 2013. "The Culture of the Situation: The Role of Situational Strength in Cultural Systems." *Asian Journal of Social Psychology* 16 (1): 34–38.

Gelissen, John. 2002. *Worlds of Welfare, Worlds of Consent? Public Opinion on the Welfare State.* Leiden, Netherlands: Brill.

Gelles, Richard J. 2007. "Family Violence." Pp.403–417 in *The Cambridge Handbook of Violent Behavior and Aggression*, edited by Daniel J. Flannery, Alexander T. Vazsonyi and Irwin D. Waldman. Cambridge, UK: Cambridge University Press.

Genevaz, Juliette. 2019. "Defense Education in Chinese Universities: Drilling Elite Youth." *Journal of Contemporary China* 28 (117): 453–467.

Georgas, Tames, Sophia Christakopoalou, Ype H. Poortinga, Alois Ahgleitner, Robin Goodwin, and Neophytos Charalambous. 1997. "The Relationship of Family Bonds to Family Structure and Function across Cultures." *Journal of Cross-Cultural Psychology* 28(3):303–320. \71–300.

Gerbasi, Alexandra, and Karen S. Cook. 2008. "The Effect off Perceived Trustworthiness on Affect in Negotiated and Reciprocal Exchange." Pp.141–165 in *Social Structure and Emotion*, edited by Jody Clay-Warner and Dawn T. Robinson. San Diego, CA: Academic.

Gerhards, Jürgen. 2010. "Non-Discrimination Towards Homosexuality: The European Union's Policy and Citizens' Attitudes Towards Homosexuality in 27 European Countries." *International Sociology* 25 (1): 5–28.

German, Miguelina, Nancy A. Gonzales, and Larry Dumka. 2009. "Familism Values as a Protective Factor for Mexican-origin Adolescents Exposed to Deviant Peers." *Journal of Early Adolescence* 29(1):16–42. \111–26.

Gershuny, Jonathan. 2000. *Changing Times: Work and Leisure in Postindustrial Society*. Oxford, UK: Oxford University Press.

Gerstein, Deon, et al. 1999. *Gambling Impact and Behavior Study*. Chicago, IL: National Opinion Research Center.

Geser, Hans. 1998. "Toward a One-dimensional Ideological Culture: Evidence from Swiss Local Parties." Pp.235–259 in *The New Political Culture*, edited by Terry Nichols Clark and Vincent Hoffmann-Martinot. Boulder, CO: Westview.

Gest, Scott D., Celene E. Domitrovich, and Janet A. Welsh. 2005. "Peer Academic Reputation in Elementary School: Association with Changes in Self-concept and Academic Skills." *Journal of Educational Psychology* 97 (3): 337–346.

Geys, Benny. 2012. "Association Membership and Generalized Trust: Are Connections between Associations Losing their Value?" *Journal of Civil Society* 8 (1): 1–15.

Gharaei, Nadya, Karen Phalet, and Fenella Fleischmann. 2018. "Contingent National Belonging: The Perceived Fit and Acceptance of Culturally Different Peers Predicts Minority Adolescents' Own Belonging." *Frontiers in Psychology* 9: 1975.

Ghimire, Ramesh. 2021. "Homeownership and Community Involvement: Results from the 2019 Metro Atlanta Speaks Survey." *Housing Policy Debate* 31 (6): 837–861.

Gibbs, John C. 2014. *Moral Development and Reality beyond the Theories of Kohlberg, Hoffman, and Haidt*. New York: Oxford University Press.

Gibson, James L. 2013. "Measuring Political Tolerance and General Support for Pro-Civil Liberties Policies." *Public Opinion Quarterly* 77 (S1): 45–68.

Gibson, James L., and Gregory A. Caldeira. 2003. "Defenders of Democracy? Legitimacy, Popular Acceptance and the South African Constitutional Court." *Journal of Politics* 65 (1): 1–30.

Giddens, Anthony. 1992. *The Transformation of Intimacy: Sexuality, Love and Eroticism in Modern Societies*. Cambridge, UK: Polity.

Gil de Zuniga, K., Matthew Barnidge Homero, and Andrés Scherman. 2017. "Social Media Social Capital, Offline Social Capital, and Citizenship: Exploring Asymmetrical Social Capital Effects." *Political Communication* 34 (1): 44–68.

Gil, Ana Isabel, and Jose Alberto Molina. 2007. "Human Development and Alcohol Abuse in Adolescence." *Applied Economics* 39: 1315–1323.

Gilberbloom, John I., John Po, and Markham. 1995. "The Impact of Homeownership on Political Beliefs." *Social Forces* 73 (4): 1589–1607.

Gilbert, Margaret. 2006. *A Theory of Political Obligation: Membership, Commitment, and the Bonds of Society*. Oxford, UK: Clarendon.

Gilens, Martin. 1999. *Why Americans Hate Welfare: Race, Media, and the Politics of Antipoverty Policy*. Chicago, IL: University of Chicago Press.

Gill, Anthony. 2004. "Weber in Latin America: Is Protestant Growth Enabling the Consolidation of Democratic Capitalism?" *Democratization* 11 (4): 42–65.

Gil-Lacruz, Marta, María I. Saz-Gil, and Ana I. Gil-Lacruz. 2019. "Benefits of Older Volunteering on Wellbeing: An International Comparison." *Frontiers in Psychology* 10: 2647.

Gillath, Omri, Gery C. Karantzas, and R. Chris Fraley. 2016. *Adult Attachment: A Concise Introduction to Theory and Research*. London: Academic.

Gillath, Omri, Phillip R. Shaver, Mario Mikulincer, Rachel E. Nitzberg, Ayelet Erez, and Marinus H. Van Ijzendoorn. 2005. "Attachment, Caregiving, and Volunteering: Placing Volunteerism in an Attachment-theoretical Framework." *Personal Relationships* 12 (4): 425–446.

Gilley, Bruce, and Heike Holbig. 2009. "The Debate on Party Legitimacy in China: A Mixed Quantitative Qualitative Analysis." *Journal of Contemporary China* 18 (59): 339–358.

Gilley, Bruce. 2009. *The Right to Rule: How States Win and Lose Legitimacy*. New York: Columbia University Press.

Gillham, Patrick F., Nathan C. Lindstedt, Bob Edwards, and Erik W. Johnson. 2019. "The Mobilizing Effects of Economic Threats and Resources on the Formation of Local Occupy Wall Street Protest Groups in 2011." *Sociological Perspectives* 62 (4): 433–454.

Brunie, Aurelie. 2009. "Meaningful Distinctions within a Concept: Relational, Collective, and Generalized Social Capital." *Social Science Research* 38: 251–265.

Gilson, Lucy. 2003. "Trust and the Development of Health Care as a Social Institution." *Social Science & Medicine* 56: 1453–1468.

Gino, Francesca, and Adam D. Galinsky. 2012. "Vicarious Dishonesty: When Psychological Closeness Creates Distance from One's Moral Compass." *Organizational Behavior & Human Decision Processes* 119 (1): 15–26.

Glaeser, Edward L., and Joshua D. Gottlieb. 2006. "Urban Resurgence and the Consumer City." *Urban Studies* 43 (8): 1275–1299.

Glaeser, Edward L., and Joshua D. Gottlieb. 2009. "The Wealth of Cities: Agglomeration Economies and Spatial Equilibrium in the United States." *Journal of Economic Literature* 47 (4): 983–1028.

Glaeser, Edward L., David L. Laibson, Jose A. Scheinkman, and Christine L. Soutter. 2000. "Measuring Trust." *Quarterly Journal of Economics* 115 (5): 811–846.

Glendinning, Anthony, Mark Nuttall, Leo Hendry, Marion Kleop, and Shila Wood. 2003. "Rural Communities and Well-being: A Good Place to Grow up?" *Sociological Review* 51 (1): 129–156.

Gnambs, Timo, and Bernad Batinic. 2012. "A Personality-Competence Model of Opinion Leadership." *Psychology & Marketing* 29 (8): 606–621.

Godechot, Olivier. 2016. "Financialization Is Marketization! A Study of the Respective Impacts of Various Dimensions of Financialization on the Increase in Global Inequality." *Sociological Science* 3 (22): 495–519.

Godoy, Richardo, Victoria Reyes-Garcia, Tomas Huanca, William R. Leonard, Ramona G. Olvera, Jonathan Bauchet, Zhao Ma, Jonathan St, Marisa Miodowski John, Oscar Zapata Rios, Vincent Vadez, and Craig Seyfried. 2007. "The Role of Community and Individuals in the Formation of Local Capital." *Human Ecology* 35: 709–721.

Goerres, Achim. 2007. "Why are Older People More Likely to Vote? The Impact of Ageing on Electoral Turnout in Europe." *British Journal of Politics & International Relations* 9 (1): 90–121.

Goetz, Stephan J., Mark D. Partridge, Dan S. Rickman, and Shibalee Majumdar. 2011. "Sharing the Gains of Local Economic Growth: Race-to-the-Top versus Race-to-the Bottom Economic Development." *Environment & Planning C: Government & Policy* 29: 428–456.

Goff, Brent G., and A. Wallace Goddard. 1999. "Terminal Care Values: Associated with Adolescent Problem Behaviors." *Adolescence* 34 (133): 47–60.

Goldstone, Jack A., and Bert Useem. 2012. "Putting Values and Institutions Back into the Theory of Strategic Action Fields." *Sociological Theory* 30 (1): 37–47.

Goodman, Sara Wallace. 2015. "Conceptualizing and Measuring Citizenship and Integration Policy." *Comparative Political Studies* 48 (14): 1905–1941.

Goodwin, Jeff. 2005. "Revolutions and Revolutionary Movements." Pp. 404–422 in *The Handbook of Political Sociology: States, Civil Societies, and Globalization*, edited by Thomas Janoski, Robert Alford, Alexander Hicks, and Mildred A. Schwartz. Cambridge, UK: Cambridge University Press.

Gordon, Ray. 2009. "Power and Legitimacy: From Weber to Contemporary Theory." Pp. 256–273 in *The SAGE Handbook of Power*, edited by Mark Haugaard and Stewart R. Clegg. London, UK: SAGE.

Gordon, Raymond. 2011. "Leadership and Power." Pp. 193–202 in *The SAGE Handbook of Leadership*, edited by Alan Bryman, David Collinson, Keith Grint, Brad Jackson and Mary Uhl-Bien. London: SAGE.

Gorsuch, Richard L. 1994. "Toward Motivational Theories of Intrinsic Religious Commitment." *Journal of the Scientific Study of Religion* 33 (4): 315–325.

Gotsbachner, Emo. 2001. "Xenophobic Normality: The Discriminatory Impact of Habitualized Discourse Dynamics." *Discourse & Society* 12 (6): 729–759.

Gottfredson, Michael R. 2018. "Self-control Theory and Criminal Violence." Pp. 301–323 in *The Cambridge Handbook of Violent Behavior and Aggression*, edited by Alexander T. Vazsonyi, David J. Flannery and Matt DeLisi. Cambridge, UK: Cambridge University Press.

Gottschalk, Marie. 2014. *Caught: The Prison State and the Lockdown of American Politics*. Princeton, NJ: Princeton University Press.

Gotzsche-Astrup, Oluf. 2020. "Pathways to Violence: Do Uncertainty and Dark World Perceptions Increase Intentions to Engage in Political Violence?" *Behavioral Sciences of Terrorism & Political Aggression* 13 (2): 142–159.

Goulding, Christina. 2000. "The Commodification of the Past, Postmodern Pastiche, and the Search for Authentic Experiences at Contemporary Heritage Attraction." *European Journal of Marketing* 34 (7): 835–853.

Gould-Williams, Julian, and Fiona Davies. 2005. "Using Social Exchange Theory to Predict the Effects of HRM Practice in Employee Outcomes: An Analysis of Public Sector Workers." *Public Management Review* 7 (1): 1–24.

Gowder, Paul. 2016. *The rule of law in the real world*. New York, NY: Cambridge University Press.

Graeff, Peter, and Gert Tinggaard Svendsen. 2013. "Trust and Corruption: The Influence of Positive and Negative Social Capital on the Economic Development in the European Union." *Quality & Quantity* 47 (5): 2829–2846.

Graham, Carol, and Stefano Pettinato. 2002. *Happiness and Hardship: Opportunity and Insecurity in New Market Economies*. Washington, DC: Brookings.

Graham, Carol, Soumya Chattopadhyay, and Mario Picon. 2010. "The Easterlin and Other Paradoxes: Why Both Sides of the Debate May be Correct." Pp.247–288 in *International Differences in Well-being*, edited by Ed Diener, John F. Helliwell and Daniel Kahneman. New York: Oxford University Press.

Grannis, Rick. 2009. *From the Ground up: Translating Geography into Community through Neighbor Networks*. Princeton, NJ: Princeton University Press.

Grant, Jill. 2006. *Planning the Good Community: New Urbanism in Theory and Practice*. London: Routledge.

Grant, Nickholas J., Gabriel J. Merrin, Matthew T. King, Dorothy L. Espelage, and Antonia Abbey. 2019. "Examining within-Person and between-Person Associations of Family Violence and Peer Deviance on Bullying Perpetration among Middle School Students." *Psychology of Violence* 9 (1): 18–27.

Granzin, Kent L., and Janeen E. Olsen. 1998. "Americans' Choice of Domestic over Foreign Products: A Matter of Helping Behavior?" *Journal of Business Research* 43: 39–54.

Granzin, Kent L., and Lois M. Haggard. 2000. "An Integrative Explanation for Quality of Life: Development and Test of a Structural Model." Pp.31–64 in *Advances in Quality of Life Theory and Research*, edited by Ed Diener and Don R. Rahtz. Dordrecht, Netherlands: Kluwer Academic.

Grasso, Maria T. 2014. "Age, Period and Cohort Analysis in A Comparative Context: Political Generations and Political Participation Repertoires in Western Europe." *Electoral Studies* 33: 63–76.

Grasso, Maria T., and Marco Giugni. 2016. "Protest Participation and Economic Crisis: The Conditioning Role of Political Opportunities." *European Journal of Political Research* 55: 663–680.

Grattan, Laura. 2016. *Populism's Power: Radical Grassroots Democracy in America*. New York: Oxford University Press.

Gravenkepper, Steve. 2007. "Building Community in Organizations: Principles of Engagement." *Consulting Psychology Journal* 59 (3): 203–208.

Gray, Emily, Maria Grasso, Stephen Farrall, Will Jennings, and Colin Hay. 2019. "Political Socialization, Worry about Crime and Antisocial Behaviour: An Analysis of Age, Period and Cohort Effects." *British Journal of Criminology* 59 (2): 435–460.

Gray, Mel. 2010. "Social Development and the Status Quo: Professionalization and Third Way Co-optation." *International Journal of Social Welfare* 19: 463–470.

Grayling, A. C. 2013. *The God Argument: The Case against Religion and for Humanism*. New York: Bloomsbury.

Graziano, William O., and Renee M. Tobin. 2009. "Agreeableness." Pp. 46–61 in *Handbook of Individual Differences in Social Behavior*, edited by Mark R. Leary and Rick H. Hoyle. New York, NY: Guilford.

Grcic, Joseph. 2000. *Ethics and Political Theory*. New York: Lanham.

Grealish, Annmarie, Sara Tai, Andrew Hunter, Richard Emsley, Trevor Murrells, and Anthony P. Morrison. 2017. "Does Empowerment Mediate the Effects of Psychological Factors on Mental Health, Well-Being, and Recovery in Young People?" *Psychology & Psychotherapy* 90 (3): 314–335.

Greco, Francesca, and Alessandro Polli. 2021. "Security Perception and People Well-Being." *Social Indicators Research* 153 (2): 741–758.

Green, Andy, and Jan Germen Janmaat. 2011. *Regimes of Social Cohesion: Societies and the Crisis of Globalization*. Houndmills, UK: Palgrave.

Green, Andy, John Preeton, and Ricardo Sabates. 2003. "Education, Equality and Social Cohesion: A Distributional Approach." *Compare* 33 (4): 453–470.

Greenberg, Jeff, and Jamie Arndt. 2012. "Terror Management Theory." Pp.398–415 in *Handbook of Theories of Social Psychology* (vol.1), edited by Paul A.M. Van Lange, Arie W. Kruglanski and E. Tory Higgins. Los Angeles, CA: SAGE.

Greenberg, Michael R. 1999. "Improving Neighborhood Quality: A Hierarchy of Needs." *Housing Policy Debate* 10 (3): 601–624.

Greene, Ida. 1991. *Soft Power Negotiation Skills*. San Diego, CA: PSI.

Greenwood, Ronni Michelle. 2008. "Intersectional Political Consciousness: Appreciation for Intra-group Differences and Solidarity in Diverse Groups." *Psychology of Women Quarterly* 32: 36–47.

Gregg, Benjamin. 2003a. *Coping in Politics with Indeterminate Norms: A Theory of Enlightened Localism*. Albany, NY: State University of New York Press.

Gregg, Benjamin. 2003b. *Coping in Politics with Indeterminate Norms*. Albany, NY: State University of New York Press.

Greslé-Favier, Claire. 2010. "The Legacy of Abstinence-Only Discourses and the Place of Pleasure in Us Discourses on Teenage Sexuality." *Sex Education* 10 (4): 413–422.

Griffin, Larry J., and Kenneth A. Bollen. 2009. "What Do These Memories Do? Civil Rights Remembrance and Racial Attitudes." *American Sociological Review* 74 (4): 594–614.

Griffiths, Mark, and Richard T.A.. Wood. 2000. "Risk Factors in Adolescence: The Case of Gambling, Videogame Playing, and the Internet." *Journal of Gambling Studies* 16 (2/3): 199–225.

Grijalva, Emily, Daniel A. Newman, M. Louis Tay, P. D. Brent Donnellan, Richard W. Harms, and Robins, and Taiyi Yan. 2015. "Gender Differences in Narcissism: A Meta-Analytic Review." *Psychological Bulletin* 141 (2): 261–310.

Grimes, Marcia. 2006. "Organizing Consent: The Role of Procedural Fairness in Political Trust and Compliance." *European Journal of Political Research* 45: 285–315.

Groot, Wim, and Henriette Maassen Van Den. Brink. 2003. "Sympathy and the Value of Health." *Social Indicators Research* 61: 97–120.

Groot, Wim, Henriette Maassen, and van den Brink, and Bernard van Praag. 2007. "The Compensating Income Variation of Social Capital." *Social Indicators Research* 82: 189–207.

Grootaert, Christiaan, and Thierry van Bastelaer. 2002. *Understanding and Measuring Social Capital: A Multidisciplinary Tool for Practitioners*. Washington, DC: World Bank.

Gross, Revital, and Shuli Brammli-Greenberg. 2004. "Evaluating the Effect of Regulatory Prohibitions against Risk Selection by Health Status on Supplemental Insurance Ownership in Israel." *Social Science & Medicine* 58: 1609–1622.

Grossi, Enzo, Angelo Compare, Cristina Lonardi, Renata Cerutti, Edward Callus, and Mauro Niero. 2013. "Gender-Related Effect of Cultural Participation in Psychological Well-Being: Indications from the Well-Being Project in the Municipality of Milan." *Social Indicators Research* 114 (2): 255–271.

Groves, Robert M., Eleanor Singer, and Amy Corning. 2000. "Leverage-saliency Theory of Survey Participation." *Public Opinion Quarterly* 64: 299–308.

Grzegorek, Jennifer L., Robert B. Slaney, Sarah Franze, and Kenneth G. Rice. 2004. "Self-Criticism, Dependency, Self-Esteem, and Grade Point Average Satisfaction among Clusters of Perfectionists and Nonperfectionists." *Journal of Counseling Psychology* 51 (2): 192–200.

Grzywacz, Joseph G., and David M. Almeida. 2008. "Stress and Binge Drinking: A Daily Process Examination of Stressor Pile-up and Socioeconomic Stress on Affect Regulation." *International Journal of Stress Management* 15 (4): 364–380.

Gu, Qing, and Michele Schweisfurth. 2015. "Transnational Connections, Competences and Identities: Experiences of Chinese International Students after Their Return Home." *British Educational Research Journal* 41 (6): 947–970.

Gu, Xiaorong. 2022. "Sacrifice and Indebtedness: The Intergenerational Contract in Chinese Rural Migrant Families." *Journal of Family Issues* 43 (2): 509–533.

Guan, Bin, Guoxian Bao, Qingchuan Liu, and Gary Raymond Raduziner. 2021. "Two-Way Risk Communication, Public Value Consensus, and Citizens' Policy Compliance Willingness about Covid-19: Multilevel Analysis Based on a Nudge View." *Administration & Society* 53 (7): 1106–1149.

Guan, Yanjun, Michael Harris Bond, Zheng Huang, Zhiyong Zhang, Hong Deng, Tian Hu, and Haiyan Gao. 2009. "Role of Personal Endorsement of Outgroup Members" Distinctive Values and Need for Cognitive Closure in Attitude towards the Outgroup." *Asian Journal of Social Psychology* 12:54-62.

Gubernskaya, Zoya. 2010. "Changing Attitudes Toward Marriage and Children in Six Countries." *Sociological Perspectives* 53 (2): 179–200.

Gudmundsdottir, Dora Gudrun. 2013. "The Impact of Economic Crisis on Happiness." *Social Indicators Research* 110 (3): 1083–1101.

Guenther, Katja M., Matthew C. Mahutga, and Panu Suppatkul. 2016. "Stratification." Pp. 229–245 in *Handbook of Contemporary Sociological Theory*, edited by Seth Abrutyn. Cham, Switzerland: Springer.

Guerin, Bernard. 2003. "Social Behaviors as Determined by Different Arrangements of Social Consequences: Diffusion of Responsibility Effects with Competition." *Journal of Social Psychology* 143 (3): 313–349.

Guerrero, Laura K. 2015. "Attachment Theory: A communication Perspective." Pp.321–334 in *Engaging Theories in Interpersonal Communication: Multiple Perspectives*, edited by Dawn O. Braithwaite and Paul Schrodt. Thousand Oaks, CA: SAGE.

Guillen, Laura, Lluis Coromina, and Willem E. Saris. 2011. "Measurement of Social Participation and Its Place in Social Capital Theory." *Social Indicators Research* 100 (2): 331–350.

Guimond, Serge, Armand Chatard, and Fabio Lorenzi-Cloldi. 2013. "The Social Psychology of Gender across Cultures." Pp.216–233 in *The SAGE Handbook of Gender and Psychology*, edited by Michelle K. Ryan and Myla R. Branscombe. London, UK: SAGE.

Guinjoan, Marc, and Guillem Rico. 2018. "How Perceptions of Inequality between Countries Diminish Trust in the European Union: Experimental and Observational Evidence." *Political Psychology* 39 (6): 1289–1303.

Guisan, M.-C. 2009. "Government Effectiveness, Education, Economic Development and Well-Being: Analysis of European Countries in Comparison with the United States and Canada, 2000–2007." *Applied Econometrics & International Development* 9 (1): 39–55.

Gundelach, Birte, and Anita Manatschal. 2017. "Ethnic Diversity, Social Trust and the Moderating Role of Subnational Integration Policy." *Political Studies* 65 (2): 413–431.

Gundert, Stefanie, and Christian Hohendanner. 2015. "Active Labour Market Policies and Social Integration in Germany: Do "One-Euro-Jobs" Improve Individuals' Sense of Social Integration?" *European Sociological Review* 31 (6): 780–797.

Guo, Baorong, and Jin Huang. 2005. "Marital and Sexual Satisfaction in Chinese Families: Exploring the Moderating Effects." *Journal of Sex & Marital Therapy* 31: 21–29.

Guo, Guang, Michael E. Roettger, and Tianji Cai. 2008. "The Integration of Genetic Propensities into Social-control Models of Delinquency and Violence among Male Youths." *American Sociological Review* 73: 543–568.

Guo, Yu, Hongzhe Xiang, and Yuhan Wang. 2023. "Understanding Self-Protective Behaviors During COVID-19 Pandemic: Integrating the Theory of Planned Behavior and O-S-O-R Model." *Current Psychology* 43(13):12071-12083.

Guo, Zhen, Ying Yang, Wenqi Li, Xiaonan Yao, and Yu Kou. 2023. "Longitudinal Relations among Honesty-Humility, Moral Disengagement, and Unethical Behavior in Adolescents: A between- and within-person Analysis." *Journal of Research in Personality* 106:104401.

Gurak, Douglas T., and Mary M. Kritz. 2000. "The Interstate Civilization of U.S. Immigrants: Individual and Contextual Determinants." *Social Forces* 78 (3): 1017–1039.

Gursimsek, Isik, and Melek Goregenli. 2005. "Humanistic Attitudes, Values, System Justification, and Control Beliefs in a Turkish Sample." *Social Behavior & Personality* 34 (7): 747–758.

Gustavsson, Gina. 2012. "Freedom in Mass Values: Egocentric, Humanistic, or Both? Using Isaiah Berlin to Understand a Contemporary Debate." *European Political Science Review* 4 (2): 241–262.

Gutmann, David. 1987. *Reclaimed Powers: Toward a New Psychology of Men and Women in Later Life*. New York: Basic.

Ha, Jung-Hwa, Hyunsook Yoon, Yeon Ok Lim, and Sun-Young Heo. 2016. "The Effect of Widowhood on Parent–Child Relationships in Korea: Do Parents' Filial Expectations and Geographic Proximity to Children Matter?" *Journal of Cross-Cultural Gerontology* 31(1):73-88.

Ha, Seong-Kyu. 2007. "Housing Regeneration and Building Sustainable Low-income Communities in Korea." *Habitat International* 31: 116–129.

Habibis, Daphne, Nicholas Hookway, and Anthea Vreugdenhil. 2016. "Kindness in Australia: An Empirical Critique of Moral Decline Sociology: Kindness in Australia." *British Journal of Sociology* 67 (3): 395–413.

Habibov, Nazim. 2014. "Individual and Country-Level Institutional Trust and Public Attitude to Welfare Expenditures in 24 Transitional Countries." *Journal of Sociology & Social Welfare* 41 (4): 23–48.

Hackel, Leor M., and Jamil Zaki. 2018. "Propagation of Economic Inequality through Reciprocity and Reputation." *Psychological Science* 29 (4): 604–613.

Hadden, Wilbur C., Gregory Pappas, and Abdul Qayyum Khan. 2003. "Social Stratification Development and Health in Pakistan: An Empirical Exploration of Relationships in Population-based National Health Examination Survey Data." *Social Science & Medicine* 57: 1863–1874.

Haddorff, David W. 2000. "Religion and the Market Opposition, Absorption, or Ambiguity." *Review of Social Economy* 58 (4): 483–503.

Hadjar, Andreas, and Robin Samuel. 2015. "Does Upward Social Mobility Increase Life Satisfaction? A Longitudinal Analysis Using British and Swiss Panel Data." *Research in Social Stratification & Mobility* 39: 48–58.

Hadlington, Lee, and Victoria Knight. 2022. "Public Acceptability of Prisoners" Access and Use of Digital Technologies in the UK." *Prison Journal* 102 (2): 237–255.

Hagan, John, Joshua Kaiser, and Anna Hanson. 2016. "The Theory of Legal Cynicism and Sunni Insurgent Violence in Post-Invasion Iraq." *American Sociological Review* 81 (2): 316–346.

Hagan, John, Susanne Rippl, Klaus Boehnke, and Hans Merkens. 1999. "The Interest in Evil: Hierarchic Self-interest and Right-wing Extremism among East and West German Youth." *Social Science Research* 28: 162–183.

Hagquist, Curt, and David Andrich. 2004. "Measuring Subjective Health among Adolescents in Sweden." *Social Indicators Research* 68: 201–220.

Hahn, Elizabeth A., David Cella, Rita K. Bode, and Rachel T. Hanrahan. 2010. "Measuring Social Well-Being in People with Chronic Illness." *Social Indicators Research* 96 (3): 381–401.

Haidt, Jonathan. 2012. *The Righteous Mind: Why Good People Are Divided by Politics and Religion.* New York: Pantheon.

Haiven, Max. 2014. *Cultures of Financialization: Fictitious Capital in Popular Culture and Everyday Life*. Houndmills, UK: Palgrave.

Hakhverdian, Armen, and Quinton Mayne. 2012. "Institutional Trust, Education, and Corruption: A Micro-Macro Interactive Approach." *Journal of Politics* 74 (3): 1739–1750.

Hald, Gert Martin and Neil N. Malamuth. 2915. "Experimental Effects of Exposure to Pornography: The Moderating Effect of Personality and Mediating Effect of Sexual Arousal." *Archives of Sexual Behavior* 44(1):99–109.

Hale, Carl S. 1999. "Eight Levels of Social Interest: Adult Development from an Adlerian Paradigm." *Adultspan Journal* 1 (2): 66–78.

Halevy, Nir, Eliran Halali, and Taya R. Cohen. 2019. "Brokering Orientations and Social Capital: Influencing Others' Relationships Shapes Status and Trust." *Journal of Personality & Social Psychology* 119 (2): 293–316.

Hall, Deborah L., David C. Matz, and Wendy Wood. 2010. "Why Don't We Practice What We Preach? A Meta-analytic Review of Religious Racism." *Personality & Social Psychology Review* 14 (1): 126–139.

Hall, John Stuart and Alex J. Zautra. 2010. "Indicators of Community Resilience: What Are They, Why Bother?" Pp. 350–371 in *Handbook of Adult Resilience*, edited by John W. Reich, Alex J. Zautra and John Stuart Hall. New York, NY: Guilford.

Hall, Richard A., and with Carolyn Brown Dennis, and Tere L. Chipman. 2000. *The Ethical Foundations of Criminal Justice*. Boca Raton, FL: CRC.

Hall, Steve. 2014. "The Socioeconomic Function of Evil." *Sociological Review* 62 (S2): 13–31.

Hall, Todd W., and Keith J. Edwards. 2002. "The Spiritual Assessment Inventory: A Theistic Model and Measurement for Assessing Spiritual Development." *Journal of the Scientific Study of Religion* 41 (2): 341–357.

Haller, Max, and Markus Hadler. 2006. "How Social Relations and Structures Can Produce Happiness and Unhappiness: An International Comparative Analysis." *Social Indicators Research* 75: 169–216.

Hallerod, Bjorn. 2006. "Sour Grapes: Relative Deprivation Adaptive Preferences and the Measurement of Poverty." *Journal of Social Policy* 35 (3): 371–390.

Hallsworth, Simon, and Tara Young. 2010. "Street Collectives and Group Delinquency: Social Disorganization, Subcultures and beyond." Pp.72–95 in *The SAGE Handbook of Criminological Theory*, edited by Eugene McLaughlin and Tim Newburn. London, UK: SAGE.

Halvorsen, Knut. 2007. "Legitimacy of Welfare States in Transitions from Homogeneity to Multiculturality: A Matter of Trust." Pp.239–259 in *Social Justice, Legitimacy and the Welfare State*, edited by Steffen Mau and Benjamin Veghte. Aldershot, UK: Ashgate.

Hameleers, Michael. 2019. "To Like Is to Support? The Effects and Mechanisms of Selective Exposure to Online Populist Communication on Voting Preferences." *International Journal of Communication* 13: 2417–2436.

Hamermesh, David S. 2019. *Spending Time: The Most Valuable Resource*. New York, NY: Oxford University Press.

Hammer, Raphaël, Eric D. Widmer, and Christian-Nils. Robert. 2009. "Subjective Proximity to Crime or Social Representations? Explaining Sentencing Attitudes in Switzerland." *Social Justice Research* 22 (4): 351–368.

Hample, Dale. 2018. *Interpersonal Arguing*. New York, NY: Lang.

Hampton, Keith N. 2010. "The Social Life of Wireless Urban Spaces: Internet Use, Social Networks, and the Public Realm." *Journal of Communication* 60 (4): 701–722.

Hampton, Keith N. 2016. "Why Is Helping Behavior Declining in the United States but Not in Canada? Ethnic Diversity, New Technologies, and Other Explanations: The Decline of Helping Behavior." *City & Community* 15 (4): 380–399.

Han, Enze, and Xiaojun Li. 2024. "Erosion of International Organizations' Legitimacy under Superpower Rivalry: Evidence on the International Court of Justice." *Canadian Journal of Political Science* 57 (1): 21–42.

Han, Ziqiang, Ivan Y. Sun, and Rong Hu. 2017. "Social Trust, Neighborhood Cohesion, and Public Trust in the Police in China." *Policing* 40(2):380-394.

Hanafi, Hasan. 2002. "Alternative Conceptions of Civil Society: A Reflective Islamic Approach." Pp.171–189 in *Alternative Conception of Civil Society*, edited by Simone Chambers and Will Kymlicka. Princeton, NJ: Princeton University Press.

Hand, Matthew M., Donna Thomas, Walter C. Buboltz, Eric D. Deemer, and Munkhsanaa Buyanjargal. 2013. "Facebook and Romantic Relationships: Intimacy and Couple Satisfaction Associated with Online Social Network Use." *Cyberpsychology, Behavior & Social Networking* 16 (1): 8–13.

Hannah, Frith, and Celia Kitzinger. 2001. "Reformulating Sexual Script Theory: Developing a Discursive Psychology of Sexual Negotiation." *Theory & Psychology* 11 (2): 209–232.

Hannah, Sean T., Patrick J. Sweeney, and Paul B. Lester. 2007. "Toward a Courageous Mindset: The Subjective Act and Experience of Courage." *Journal of Positive Psychology* 2 (2): 129–135.

Hansen, Thomas, Britt Slagsvold, and Reidun Ingebretsen. 2012. "The Strains and Gains of Caregiving: An Examination of the Effects of Providing Personal Care to a Parent on a Range of Indicators of Psychological Well-Being." *Social Indicators Research* 114 (2): 323–343.

Hansen-Nord, Nete, Sloth Mette Skar, Finn Kjaerulf, Juan Almendarez, Sergio Bohr, Oscar Sosa, Julio Castro, Anne-Marie Nybo. Andersen, and Jens Modvig. 2014. "Social Capital and Violence in Poor Urban Areas of Honduras." *Aggression & Violent Behavior* 19 (6): 643–648.

Hanson, Rochelle F., Genelle K. Sawyer, Angela M. Begle, and Prace S. Hubel. 2010. "The Impact of Crime Victimization on Quality of Life." *Journal of Traumatic Stress* 23 (2): 189–197.

Hao, Lingxin. 1996. "Family Structure, Private Transfers, and the Economic Well-being of Families with Children." *Social Forces* 75 (1): 269–292.

Harambam, Jaron, and Stef Aupers. 2015. "Contesting Epistemic Authority: Conspiracy Theories on the Boundaries of Science." *Public Understanding of Science* 24 (4): 466–480.

Harman, Chris. 2009. *Zombie Capitalism: Global Crisis and the Relevance of Marx*. Chicago, IL: Haymarket.

Harper, Charles L., and Kevin T. Leicht. 2011. *Exploring Social Change: America and the World*. Boston, MA: Prentice Hall.

Harpham, Trudy, Emma Grant, and Elizabeth Thomas. 2002. "Measuring Social Capital within Health Surveys: Key Issues." *Health Policy & Planning* 17 (1): 106–111.

Harrington, Austin. 2004. *Art and Social Theory: Sociological Arguments in Aesthetics*. Cambridge, UK: Polity.

Harrington, Maureen, and Simone Fullagar. 2013. "Challenges for Active Living Provision in an Era of Healthism." *Journal of Policy Research in Tourism, Leisure & Events* 5 (2): 139–157.

Harris, David R. 2001. "Why Are Whites and Blacks Averse to Black Neighbors?" *Social Science Research* 30: 100–116.

Hartmann, Douglas, Paul R. Croll, Ryan Larson, Joseph Gerteis, and Alex Manning. 2017. "Colorblindness as Identity: Key Determinants, Relations to Ideology, and Implications for Attitudes about Race and Policy." *Sociological Perspectives* 60 (5): 866–888.

Harvey, David. 2016. *The Ways of the World*. New York, NY: Oxford University Press.

Harvey, John H., and Amy Wenzel. 2006. "Theoretical Perspectives in the Study of Close Relationships." Pp.35–49 in *The Cambridge Handbook of Personal Relationships*, edited by Anita L. Vangelisti and Daniel Perlman. New York: Cambridge University Press.

Harvie, Peter, and Tonoy Manzis. 2011. "Interpreting Multi-agency Partnership: Ideology, Discourse and Domestic Violence." *Social & Legal Studies* 26 (1): 79–85.

Harzing, Anne-Wil. 2006. "Response Styles in Cross-national Survey Research: A 26-country Study." *International Journal of Cross Cultural Management* 6 (2): 243–266.

Haslam, S. Alexander, Stephen D. Reicher, and Michael J. Platow. 2011. *The New Psychology of Leadership, Identity, Influence, and Power*. Hove, UK: Psychology.

Hassan, Riaz. 1995. *Suicide Explained: The Australian Experience*. Victoria, Australia: Melbourne University Press.

Hassan, Riaz. 2000. "Faithlines: Institutional Configurations and Trust in Religious Institutions in Muslim Societies." *Comparative Sociology* 41 (2): 202–223.

Hatch, Stephani L. 2007. "Economic Stressors, Social Integration, and Drug Use among Women in an Inner-city Community." *Journal of Drug Issues* 37: 257–280.

Hathaway, Andrew D. 2003. "Cannabis Effects and Dependency Concerns in Long-term Frequent Users: A Missing Piece of the Public Health Puzzle." *Addiction Research & Theory* 11 (6): 441–458.

Hattery, Angela, and Earl Smith. 2012. *The Social Dynamics of Family Violence*. Boulder, CO: Westview.

Haugaard, Mark. 2003. "Reflections on Seven Ways of Creating Power." *European Journal of Social Theory* 6 (1): 87–113.

Haugaard, Mark. 2020. *The Four Dimensions of Power: Understanding Domination, Empowerment and Democracy*. Manchester, UK: Manchester University Press.

Haugaard, Mark. 2021. "The Four Dimensions of Power: Conflict and Democracy." *Journal of Political Power* 14 (1): 153–175.

Havinga, Tetty. 2002. "The Effects and Limits of Anti-discrimination Law in the Netherlands." *International Journal of the Sociology of Law* 30: 75–90.

Hawdon, James, Colin Bernatzky, and Matthew Costello. 2019. "Cyber-Routines, Political Attitudes, and Exposure to Violence-Advocating Online Extremism." *Social Forces* 98 (1): 329–354.

Hawdon, James, John Ryan, and Catherine Mobley. 2000. "An Evaluation of Community Antiviolence Programs: Implications of Some Preliminary Findings." *Research in Community Sociology* 10: 165–187.

Hawley, Patricia H. 2014. "Evolution, Prosocial Behavior, and Altruism: A Roadmap for Understanding Where the Proximate Meets the Ultimate." Pp. 3–69 in *Prosocial Development: A Multidimensional Approach*, edited by Laura M. Padilla-Walker and Gustavo Carlo. New York, NY: Oxford University Press.

Hayashi, Mahito. 2022. "Theorizing Regulzation-in-City for Homeless People's Subaltern Strategy and Informality: Societalization, Metabolism, and Classes with(out) Housing." *Critical Sociology* 48 (2): 323–339.

Hayes, Diane, and Catherine E. Ross. 1986. "Body and Mind: The Effect of Exercise, Overweight, and Physical Health on Psychological Well-being." *Journal of Health & Social Behavior* 27: 387–400.

Hayo, Bernd. 2004. "Public Support for Creating a Market Economy in Eastern Europe." *Journal of Comparative Economics* 32: 720–744.

Hays, R. Allen., and Alexandra M. Kogl. 2007. "Neighborhood Attachment, Social Capital Building, and Political Participation: A Case Study of Low- and Moderate-income Residents of Waterloo, Iowa." *Journal of Urban Affairs* 29 (2): 181–205.

Hayslip, Bert, Jr., Persephanie Silverthorn, R. Jerald Shori, and Craig E. Henderson. 2000. "Determinants of Custodial Grandparents" Perceptions of Problem Behavior in Their Grandchildren." Pp.255–268 in *Grandparents Raising Grandchildren: Theoretical, Empirical, and Clinical Perspectives*, edited by Bert Hayslip, Jr., and Robin Goldberg-Glen. New York: Springer.

He, Alex Jingwei, and Liang Ma. 2021. "Citizen Participation, Perceived Public Service Performance, and Trust in Government: Evidence from Health Policy Reforms in Hong Kong." *Public Performance & Management Review* 44 (3): 471–493.

He, Cai, and Xiaoping Wu. 2006. "Social Changes and Occupational Gender Inequality." *Chinese Sociology & Anthropology* 38(4):37-53.

He, Jia, Dave Bartram, Ilke Inceoglu, and Fons J. R. van de Vijver. 2014. "Response Styles and Personality Traits: A Multilevel Analysis." *Journal of Cross-Cultural Psychology* 45 (7): 1028–1045.

He, Zili, and Chuanghi Wang. 2024. "Understanding the Unique Characteristics and Essential Requirements of Chinese Modernization." *International Critical Thought* 14 (1): 1–17.

Headey, Bruce. 2008. "Life Goals Matter to Happiness: A Revision of Set-point Theory." *Social Indicators Research* 86: 213–231.

Headey, Bruce. 2010. "The Set Point Theory of Well-being Has Serious Flaws: On the Eve of a Scientific Revolution?" *Social Indicators Research* 97: 7–21.

Heaphy, Brian. 2007. *Late Modernity and Societal Change: Reconstructing Social and Personal Life*. Abingdon, UK: Routledge.

Heatherington, Marc J., and Suzanne Globetti. 2002. "Political Trust and Racial Policy Preferences." *American Journal of Political Science* 46 (2): 253–295.

Heckscher, Charles. 2015. *Trust in a Complex World: Enriching Community*. Oxford, UK: Oxford University Press.

Heffernan, Troy, Mark Morrison, Parikshit Basu, and Arthur Sweeney. 2010. "Cultural Differences, Learning Styles and Transnational Education." *Journal of Higher Education Policy & Management* 32 (1): 27–39.

Hegtvedt, Karen A., and Heather L. Scheuerman. 2010. "The Justice/Morality Link." Pp. 331–360 in *Handbook of the Sociology of Morality*, edited by Steven Hitlin and Stephen Vaisey. New York, NY: Springer.

Heidemeier, Heike, and Ursula M. Staudinger. 2012. "Self-evaluation Process in Life Satisfaction: Uncovering Measurement Non-equivalence and Age-related differences." *Social Indicators Research* 105: 39–61.

Heilman, Renata M., and Petko Kusev. 2020. "Personal Values Associated with Prosocial Decisions." *Behavioral Sciences* 10 (4): 77.

Heinemann, Friedrich. 2008. "Is the Welfare State Self-destructive? A Study of Government Benefit Morale." *Kyklos* 61 (2): 237–257.

Heinze, Eric A., and Brandy J. Jolliff. 2011. "Idealism and Liberalism." Pp. 319–326 in *21st Century Political Science: A Reference Handbook*, edited by John T. Ishiyama and Marijke Breuning. Thousand Oaks, CA: SAGE.

Heitmeyer, Wilhelm and Reimund Anhut. 2008. "Disintegration, Recognition, and Violence: A Theoretical Perspective." *New Directions for Youth Development* 119:25–37. \90–295.

Held, David. 2010. *Cosmopolitanism: Ideals and Realities*. Cambridge, UK: Polity. Herrmann, Therese. 2023. "Cosmopolitanism, Global Justice and Refugees: Minimal Moral Conditions for EU Refugee Policy." Pp. 172–199 in *Cosmopolitan Norms and European Values: Ethical Perspectives on Europe's Refugee Policy*, edited by Marie Gobel and Andreas Niederberger. Milton, UK: Taylor & Francis.

Held, Virginia. 2008. *How Terrorism is Wrong: Morality and Political Violence*. New York: Oxford University Press.

Helliwell, John F. 2006. "Well-being, Social Capital, and Public Policy." *Economic Journal* 116: C34–C45.

Helliwell, John F., and Robert D. Putnam. 2005. "The Social Context of Well-being." Pp.435–459 in *The Science of Well-being*, edited by Felica A. Huppert, Nick Baylis and Barry Keverne. Oxford, UK: Oxford University Press.

Helliwell, John F., Chris Burrington-Leigh, Anthony Harris, and Haifang Huang. 2010. "International Evidence on the Social Context of Well-being." Pp.291–327 in *International Differences in Well-being*, edited by Ed Diener, John F. Helliwell and Daniel Kahneman. New York: Oxford University Press. (HN25.I58) \90–89.

Hellwig, Timothy T. 2001. "Interdependence, Government Constraints, and Economic Voting." *Journal of Politics* 63 (4): 1141–1162.

Helly, Denise. 2003. "Social Cohesion and Cultural Plurality." *Canadian Journal of Sociology* 28 (1): 19–42.

Henderson, Shannon D., and Stan H. Hodges. 2007. "Music, Song, and the Creation of Community and Community Spirit by Gay Subculture." *Sociological Spectrum* 27: 57–80.

Hendricks, Carmen Ortiz, and Glynn Rudich. 2000. "A Community Building Perspective in Social Work Education." *Journal of Community Practice* 8 (3): 21–36.

Hendriksen, Pauline A., Pantea Kiani, Johan Garssen, Gillian Bruce, and Joris C. Verster 2021. "Living Alone or Together During Lockdown: Association with Mood, Immune Fitness and Experiencing Covid-19 Symptoms." *Psychology Research & Behavior Management* 14: 1947–1957.

Hendry, Leo B. and Marion Kloep. 2012. *Adolescence and Adulthood: Transitions and Transformations*. Houndmills, UK: Palgrave.

Hener, Timo, Helmut Rainer, and Thomas Siedler. 2016. "Political Socialization in Flux? Linking Family Non-Intactness During Childhood to Adult Civic Engagement." *Journal of the Royal Statistical Society* 179 (3): 633–656.

Hennessy, Michael, Michael X. Delli, Michael B. Carpini, Kenneth Winneg Blank, and Kathleen Hall Jamieson. 2015. "Using Psychological Theory to Predict Voting Intentions." *Journal of Community Psychology* 43 (4): 466–483.

Henry, Julie D., William von Hippel, and Kate Baynes. 2009. "Social Inappropriateness, Executive Control, and Aging." *Psychology & Aging* 24 (1): 239–244.

Henry, Stuart. 2009. *Social Deviance*. Cambridge, UK: Polity.

Hepper, Erica G., Tim Wildschut, Constantine Sedikides, Sara Robertson, and Clay D. Routledge. 2020. "Time Capsule: Nostalgia Shields Psychological Wellbeing from Limited Time Horizons." *Emotion* 21 (3): 644–664.

Herd, Pamela, James S. House, and Robert F. Schoeni. 2008. "Income Support Policies and Health among the Elderly." Pp. 97–121 in *Making American Healthier: Social and Economic Policy as Health Policy*, edited by Robert F. Schoeni, James S. House, George A. Kaplan, and Harold Pollack. New York: Russell Sage.

Herian, Mitchel N., Louis Tay, Joseph A. Hamm, and Ed Diener. 2014. "Social Capital, Ideology, and Health in the United States." *Social Science & Medicine* 105:30–37.

Herman-Kinney, Nancy J. 2003. "Deviance." Pp. 695–720 in *Handbook of Symbolic Interactionism*, edited by Larry T. Reynolds and Nancy J. Herman-Kinney. Lanham, MD: Rowman.

Hernandez, Bernardo, Ana M. Martin, Cristina Ruiz, and M. del Carmen Hidalgo. 2010. "The Role of Place Identity and Place Attachment in Breaking Environmental Protection Laws." *Journal of Environmental Psychology* 30 (2): 281–288.

Herr, Ranjoo Seodu. 2012. "Confucian Family for a Feminist Future." *Asian Philosophy* 22 (4): 327–346.

Herrmann, Richard K., Pierangelo Isernia, and Paslo Segatti. 2009. "Attachment to the Nation and International Relations: Dimensions of Identity and Their Relationship to War and Peace." *Political Psychology* 30 (5): 721–754.

Herzog, Sergio. 2005. "The Relationship between Economic Hardship and Crime: The Case of Israel and the Palestinians." *Sociological Perspectives* 48 (2): 189–211.

Heshmati, Saeideh and Zita Oravecz. 2022. "I Feel Loved When Other People Feel Loved: Cultural Congruence in Beliefs on Love Is Related to Well-Being." *Journal of Social & Personal Relationships* 39(2):347–71. \94–273.

Heung, Amy Liu, and Mei, and David Zweig. 2011. "Hong Kong??s Contribution to Mainland China's Property Sector." *Asian Survey* 51 (4): 739–768.

Hewstone, Miles, Ed Cairns, Alberto Voci, Stefania Paolini, Frances McLernon, Richard J. Crisp, Ulrike Niens, and Jean Craig. 2005. "Intergroup Contact in a Divided Society: Challenging Segregation in Northern Ireland." Pp.265–292 in *The Social Psychology of Inclusion and Exclusion*, edited by Dominic Abrams, Michael A. Hogg and Jose M. Marque. New York: Psychology Press.

Hicks, Sarah, and Sarah Brown. 2013. "Perceptions of Risk: A Review of the Effects of Individual and Community-Level Variables on Perceptions of Risk." *International Review of Victimology* 19 (3): 249–267.

Hickson, Kevin. 2013. "The Localist Turn in British Politics and Its Critics." *Policy Studies* 34 (4): 408–421.

Hilbig, Benjamin E., Ingo Zettler, Felix Leist, and Timo Heydasch. 2013. "It Takes Two: Honesty-Humility and Agreeableness Differentially Predict Active versus Reactive Cooperation." *Personality & Individual Differences* 54 (5): 598–603.

Hill, Charles T. 2019. *Intimate Relationships across Cultures: A Comparative Study*. Cambridge, UK: Cambridge University Press.

Hill, Taylor G., Sean P. Mackinnon, and Bryan Smale. 2023. "Relative Importance of Individual and Community Predictors of Wellbeing." *International Journal of Community Well-Being* 6 (3): 279–299.

Hindman, Elizabeth Blanks. 2009. "Protecting Childhood: Rights, Social Goals and the First Amendment in the Context of the Child Online Protection Act." *Communication Law & Policy* 15 (1): 1–23.

Hinds, Lyn. 2007. "Building Police—Youth Relationships: The Importance of Procedural Justice." *Youth Justice* 7 (3): 195–209.

Hirono, Miwa. 2013. "Three Legacies of Humanitarianism in China." *Disasters* 37 (S2): S202–S220.

Hirschl, Thomas, and Mark R. Rank. 1999. "Community Effect on Welfare Participation." *Sociological Forum* 14 (1): 155–174.

Hitlin, Steven, and Sarah K. Harkness. 2018. *Unequal Foundations: Inequality, Morality, and Emotions across Cultures*. New York, NY: Oxford University Press.

Hitlin, Steven, and Kevin Pinkston. 2013. "Values, Attitudes, and Ideologies: Explicit and Implicit Constructs Shaping Perception and Action." Pp. 319–339 in *Handbook of Social Psychology*, edited by John Delamater and Amanda Ward. Dordrecht, Netherlands: Springer.

Hitlin, Steven. 2006. "Parental Influences on Children's Values and Aspirations: Bridging Two Theories of Social Class and Socialization." *Sociological Perspectives* 49 (1): 25–46.

Hjelm, Titus. 2014. "Religion, Discourse and Power: A Contribution towards a Critical Sociology of Religion." *Critical Sociology* 40 (6): 855–872.

Hjemdal, Odin, Antonio Roazzi, B. B. Maria da Graça, and Dias, and Oddgeir Friborg. 2015. "The Cross-Cultural Validity of the Resilience Scale for Adults: A Comparison between Norway and Brazil." *BMC Psychology* 3 (1): 18.

Hjerm, L. Berg. 2010. "National Identity and Political Trust." *Perspectives on European Politics & Society* 11 (4): 390–407.

Hjortskov, Morten. 2019. "Citizen Expectations and Satisfaction over Time: Findings from a Large Sample Panel Survey of Public School Parents in Denmark." *American Review of Public Administration* 49 (3): 353–371.

Ho, David Y.F., Albert W.L.. Chau, Chi-yue Chiu, and S. Q. Peng. 2003. "Ideological Orientation and Political Transition in Hong Kong: Confidence in the Future." *Political Psychology* 24 (2): 403–413.

Ho, David Yau-fai, Si-qing Peng, and Chi-yue Chiu. 2006. *Social Way and Human Consciousness*. Hong Kong, China: Joint.

Ho, Wing Chung, and Lin Li. 2022. "The Time-Space Tactics of Chinese Buddhist and Taoist Believers under State-Religion Tension." *China Information* 36 (2): 241–261.

Hoare, Carol Hren. 2002. *Erikson on Development in Adulthood: New Insights from the Unpublished Papers*. New York: Oxford University Press.

Hobbs, Valerie. 2020. "The Discourse of Divorce in Conservative Christian Sermons." *Critical Discourse Studies* 17 (2): 193–210.

Hobfoll, Steven E., and Jeremiah A. Schumm. 2002. "Conservation of Resources Theory: Application to Public Health Promotion." Pp.285–312 in *Emerging Theories in Health Promotion Practice and Research Strategies for Improving Public Health*, edited by Ralph J. DiClemente, Richard A. Crosby, and Michelle C. Kegler. San Francisco, CA: Jossey-Bass.

Hobolt, Sara Binzer, and Robert Klemmensen. 2005. "Welfare to Vote: The Effect of Government Spending on Turnout." Paper prepared for presentation at the *Comparative Study of Electoral Systems*, August 30–31, 2005, Washington, DC, United States.

Hobson, Barbara. 2005. "Feminist Theorizing and Feminisms in Political Sociology." Pp. 135–152 in *The Handbook of Political Sociology: States, Civil Societies, and Globalization*, edited by Thomas Janoski, Robert Alford, Alexander Hicks, and Mildred A. Schwartz. Cambridge, UK: Cambridge University Press.

Hocksmann, Hynn. 2004. *On Philosophy in China*. Toronto, Canada: Thomson.

Hoekstra, Erin. 2021. "Not a Free Version of a Broken System: Medical Humanitarianism and Immigrant Health Justice in the United States." *Social Science & Medicine* 285: 114287.

Hoffman, Lily M. 2003. "The Marketing of Diversity in the Inner City: Tourism and Regulation in Harlem." *International Journal of Urban & Regional Research* 27 (2): 286–299.

Hoffman, Lisa. 2006. "Autonomous Choices and Patriotic Professionalism: On Governmentability in Late-socialist China." *Economy & Society* 35 (4): 550–570.

Hoffmann, John P. 2023. "Family Structure, Unstructured Socializing, and Delinquent Behavior." *Journal of Criminal Justice* 87: 102086.

Hoffmann, John P., and Lanced. Erickson, And Karen R. Spence. 2013. "Modeling the Association between Academic Achievement and Delinquency: An Application of Interactional Theory." *Criminology* 51 (3): 629–659.

Holbig, Heike. 2011. "International Dimensions of Legitimacy: Reflections on Western Theories and the Chinese Experience." *Journal of Chinese Political Science* 16 (2): 161–181.

Holbrook, Allyson L., Melanie C. Green, and Jon A. Krosnick. 2003. "Telephone versus Face-to-face Interviewing of National Probability Samples with Long Questionnaires: Comparisons of Respondent Satisficing and Social Desirability Response Bias." *Public Opinion Quarterly* 67: 79–125.

Holdo, Markus. 2022. "How Can We Trust a Political Leader? Ethics, Institutions, and Relational Theory? Institutions and Relational Theory." *International Political Science Review* 43 (3): 236–239.

Holland, Janet, Tracey Reynolds, and Susie Weller. 2007. "Transitions, Networks and Communities: The Significance of Social Capital in the Lives of Children and Young People." *Journal of Youth Studies* 10 (1): 97–116.

Holliday, Adrian. 2011. *Intercultural Communication and Ideology*. London, UK: SAGE. Smith, Michael. 2000. "Moral Religion." Pp.15–37 in *The Blackwell Guide to Ethical Theory*, edited by Hugh LaFollette. Malden, MA: Blackwell.

Holliday, Ian, and Waikeung Tam. 2001. "Social Capital in Hong Kong." *East Asia: An International Quarterly* 19 (1/2): 144–170.

Holliman, Andrew, Daniel Waldeck, Bethany Jay, Summayah Murphy, Emily Atkinson, Rebecca J. Collie, and Andrew Martin. 2021. "Adaptability and Social Support: Examining Links with Psychological Wellbeing among UK Students and Non-students." *Frontiers in Psychology* 12: 636520.

Hollinger, Franz. 2017. "Value Orientations and Social Attitudes in the Holistic Milieu: Value Orientations and Social Attitudes." *British Journal of Sociology* 68 (2): 293–313.

Holloway, Evan D., Johanna B. Folk, Catalina Ordorica, and Marina Tolou-Shams. 2022. "Peer, Substance Use, and Race-Related Factors Associated with Recidivism among First-Time Justice-Involved Youth." *Law & Human Behavior* 46 (2): 140–153.

Holowchak, M., and Andrew. 2008. *The Stoics: A Guide for the Perplexed*. London: Continuum.

Holzel, Lars, Martin Harter, Christina Reese, and Levente Kriston. 2011. "Risk Factors for Chronic Depression: A Systematic Review." *Journal of Affective Disorders* 129(1–3):1–13. \116–362.

Hombrados-Mendieta, Maria Isabel, Luis Gomez-Jacinto, Juan Manuel Dominguez-Fuentes, and Patricia Garcia-Leiva. 2013. "Sense of Community and Satisfaction with Life among Immigrants and the Native Population." *Journal of Community Psychology* 41 (5): 601–614.

Hong, Jun Sung, Dong Ha Kim, and Alex R. Piquero. 2017. "Assessing the Links between Punitive Parenting, Peer Deviance, Social Isolation and Bullying Perpetration and Victimization in South Korean Adolescents." *Child Abuse & Neglect* 73:63-70.

Hong, Jun Sung, Michael J. Kral, Dorothy L. Espelage, and Paula Allen-Meares. 2012. "The Social Ecology of Adolescent-Initiated Parent Abuse: A Review of the Literature." *Child Psychiatry & Human Development* 43 (3): 431–454.

Honohan, Iseult. 2002. *Civic Republicanism*. London: Routledge.

Hood, Christopher. 1991. "Stabilization and Cutbacks: A Catastrophe for Government Growth Theory?" *Journal of Theoretical Politics* 3 (1): 37–63.

Hooghe, Marc, and Anna Kern. 2015. "Party Membership and Closeness and the Development of Trust in Political Institutions: An Analysis of the European Social Survey, 2002¨C2010." *Party Politics* 21 (6): 944–956.

Hooghe, Marc, Ruth Dassonneville, and Sofie Marien. 2015. "The Impact of Education on the Development of Political Trust: Results from a Five-Year Panel Study among Late Adolescents and Young Adults in Belgium." *Political Studies* 63 (1): 123–141.

Hooghe, Marc. 2003. "Participation in Voluntary Associations and Value Indicators: The Effect of Current and Previous Participation Experiences." *Nonprofit & Voluntary Sector Quarterly* 32 (1): 47–69.

Hookway, Nicholas. 2017. "Zygmunt Bauman's Moral Saint." *Acta Sociologica.* 60 (4): 358–367.

Hookway, Nicholas. 2019. *Everyday Moralities: Doing It Ourselves in an Age of Uncertainty*. Abingdon, UK: Routledge.

Hopcroft, Rosemary L. 2016. *Evolution and Gender: Why It Matters for Contemporary Life*. New York: Routledge.

Horell, Harold D. 2014. "On Learning to See the World Religiously: Moral Awareness, Faith, and Public Moral Discourse." *Religious Education* 109 (4): 424–439.

Horn, Stacey S. 2013. "Attitudes about Sexual Orientation." Pp. 239–251 in *Handbook of Psychology and Sexual Orientation*, edited by Charlotte J. Patterson and Anthony R. D'Augelli. New York, NY: Oxford University Press.

Hornsey, Matthew J., and Jolanda Jetten. 2004. "The Individual within the Group: Balancing the Need to Belong with the Need to Be Different." *Personality & Social Psychology Review* 8 (3): 248–264.

Horowitz, Jonathan. 2018. "Relative Education and the Advantage of a College Degree." *American Sociological Review* 83 (4): 771–801.

Hou, Jack W. 2011. "Economic Reform of China: Cause and Effects." *Social Science Journal* 48 (3): 419–434.

Hou, Weiqin, Yingchun Zhang, Mingli Huang. 2003. *Conflict and Integration*. Beijing: China: Chinese People.

Hough, Mike. 2012. "Researching Trust in the Police and Trust in Justice: A UK Perspective." *Policing & Society* 22 (3): 332–345.

Hounkpatin, Osafo, Alex M. Hilda, Christopher J. Wood, and Boyce, and Graham Dunn. 2015. "An Existential-Humanistic View of Personality Change: Co-Occurring Changes with Psychological Well-Being in a 10-Year Cohort Study." *Social Indicators Research* 121 (2): 455–470.

Houser, Daniel, and Erte Xiao. 2015. "House Money Effects on Trust and Reciprocity." *Public Choice* 163 (1/2): 187–199.

Houtman, Disk. 2000. "The Working Class and the Welfare State Support for Economic Redistribution, tolerance for Nonconformity and the Conditionality of Solidarity with the Unemployed." *Netherlands' Journal of Social Sciences* 36 (1): 37–55.

Hovermann, Andreas, and Steven F. Messner. 2019. "Institutional Imbalance, Marketized Mentality, and the Justification of Instrumental Offenses: A Cross-National Application of Institutional Anomie Theory." *Justice Quarterly* 38 (3): 406–432.

Howard, Matt C., and Kent K. Alipour. 2014. "Does the Courage Measure Really Measure Courage? A Theoretical and Empirical Evaluation." *Journal of Positive Psychology* 9 (5): 449–459.

Howell, Jude. 2012. "Civil Society, Corporatism and Capitalism in China." *Journal of Comparative Asian Development* 11 (2): 271–297.

Hoyt, Crystal L., and Aleah Goldin. 2016. "Political Ideology and American Intergroup Discrimination: A Patriotism Perspective." *Journal of Social Psychology* 156 (4): 369–381.

Hraba, Joseph, Rehan Mullick, Frederick Lorenz, and Jiri Vecernik. 2001. "'Age and Czechs' Attitudes toward the Postcommunist Economic Reforms." *Sociological Quarterly* 42 (3): 421–435.

Hsee, Christopher K., George F. Loewenstein, Sally Blount, and Max H. Bazerman. 1999. "Preference Reversals between Joint and Separate Evaluations of Options: A Review and Theoretical Analysis." *Psychological Bulletin* 125 (5): 576–590.

Hsiao, Yangji. 2004. *Shaping Modern Citizens: Study of the Development and Cultivation of Senior Secondary Student Citizenship*. Taipei, Taiwan: Weber Culture.

Hsieh, Chang-Ming. 2002. "Trends in Financial Satisfaction: Does Poverty Make a Difference?" *International Journal of Aging & Human Development* 54 (1): 15–30.

Hsu, Han-Yu, Li-Li Huang and Kwang-Kuo Hwang. 2019. "Liberal–Conservative Dimension of Moral Concerns Underlying Political Faction Formation in Taiwan." *Asian Journal of Social Psychology* 22(3):301-15.

Hu, Anning. 2013. "Generalized Trust among Christians in Urban China: Analysis Based on Propensity Score Matching." *Current Sociology* 61 (7): 1021–1039.

Hu, Jieren, Yue Tu, and Tong Wu. 2018. "Selective Intervention in Dispute Resolution: Local Government and Community Governance in China." *Journal of Contemporary China* 27(111):423-39.

Hu, Yang. 2016. "Sex Ideologies in China: Examining Interprovince Differences." *Journal of Sex Research* 53 (9): 1118–1130.

Hu, Yiliang. 2005. *Guanxi Community*. Beijing, China: People.

Huang, Qing. 2018. "Public Trust in Local Governments and Environmental Risks in China: The Effects of Media Use, Perceived Dread, and Perceived Inequality." *Chinese Journal of Communication* 11 (1): 88–104.

Huang, Xian, and Qin Gao. 2018. "Does Social Insurance Enrollment Improve Citizen Assessment of Local Government Performance? Evidence from China." *Social Science Research* 70: 28–40.

Huber, Max A., Louis D. Brown, Rosalie N. Metze, Martin Stam, Tine Van Regenmortel, and Tineke N. Abma. 2022. "Exploring Empowerment of Participants and Peer Workers in a Self-Managed Homeless Shelter." *Journal of Social Work* 22 (1): 26–45.

Huber, Saskia, Sebastian Sattler, and Mehlkop Guido. 2023. "Mechanisms of Perceived Social Norms: The Mediating and Moderating Role of Morality and Outcome Expectations on Prescription Drug Misuse in the Working Population." *Deviant Behavior* 44 (3): 359–380.

Huberman, Jennifer. 2022. *The Spirit of Digital Capitalism*. Cambridge, UK: Polity.

Hudders, Liselot, and Mario Pandelaere. 2012. "The Silver Lining of Materialism: The Impact of Luxury Consumption on Substance Well-being." *Journal of Happiness Studies* 13: 411–437.

Huddy, Leonie, Alessandro Del Ponte, and Caitlin Davies. 2021. "Nationalism, Patriotism, and Support for the European Union." *Political Psychology* 42 (6): 995–1017.

Huddy, Leonie, and Stanley Feldman. 2011. "Americans Respond Politically to 9/11: Understanding the Impact of the Terrorist Attacks and Their Aftermath." *American Psychologist* 66 (6): 455–467.

Huddy, Leonie. 2013. "From Group Identity to Political Cohesion and Commitment." Pp.737–773 in *The Oxford Handbook of Political Psychology*, edited by Leone Huddy, David O. Sears and Jack S. Levy. New York: Oxford University Press.

Hudson, Alexandra. 2023. *The Soul of Civility: Timeless Principles to Heal Society and Ourselves*. New York, NY: St. Martin's Press.

Hudson, Christopher G. 2000. "From Social Darwinism to Self-organization: Implications for Social Change Theory." *Social Service Review* 74 (4): 533–559.

Huemer, Michael. 2013. *The Problem of Political Authority: An Examination of the Right to Coerce and the Duty to Obey*. Houndmills, UK: Palgrave.

Huesmann, L. Rowell, and Lucyna Kirwil. 2007. "Why Observing Violence Increases the Risk of Violent Behavior by the Observer." Pp.545–570 in *The Cambridge Handbook of Violent Behavior and Aggression*, edited by Daniel J. Flannery, Alexander T. Vazsonyi and Irwin D. Waldman. Cambridge, UK: Cambridge University Press.

Huesmann, L. Rowell, Eric F. Dubgos, Leonard D. Eron, and Paul Boxer. 2006. "Middle Childhood Family-contextual and Personal Factors as Predictors of Adult Outcomes." Pp.62–86 in *Developmental Contexts in Middle Childhood: Bridges to Adolescence and Adulthood*, edited by Aletha C. Huston and Marika N. Ripke. Cambridge, UK: Cambridge University Press.

Huesmann, L. Rowell. 2018. "The Contagion of Violence." Pp.527–556 in *The Cambridge Handbook of Violent Behavior and Aggression*, edited by Alexander T. Vazsonyi, David J. Flannery and Matt DeLisi. Cambridge, UK: Cambridge University Press.

Hughes, Chelsea M., Brandon J. Griffin, and Everett L. Worthington. 2017. "A Measure of Social Behavior in Team-Based, Multiplayer Online Games: The Sociality in Multiplayer Online Games (SMOG) Scale." *Computers in Human Behavior* 69: 386–395.

Hughes, Chris. 2012. *Liberal Democracy or the End of History: Fukuyama and Postmodern Challenges*. Abington, UK: Routledge.

Hughes, Diane. 2001. "Cultural and Contextual Correlates of Obligation to Family and Community among Urban Black and Latino Adults." Pp.179–224 in *Caring and Doing for Others: Social Responsibility in the Domain of Family, Work, and Community*, edited by Alice S. Rossi. Chicago, IL: University of Chicago Press.

Hughes, John R. 2006. "A General Review of Recent Reports on Homosexuality and Lesbianism." *Sexuality & Disability* 24: 195–205.

Hughes, Lorine A., Lonnie M. Schaible, and Benjamin R. Gibbs. 2015. "Economic Dominance, the American Dream, and Homicide: A Cross-National Test of Institutional Anomie Theory." *Sociological Inquiry* 85 (1): 100–128.

Hui, Chin Ming, Daniel C. Molden, and Eli J. Finkel. 2013. "Loving Freedom: Concerns with Promotion or Prevention and the Role of Autonomy in Relationship Well-Being." *Journal of Personality & Social Psychology* 105 (1): 61–85.

Hui, Victoria Ka-ying, Michael Harris Bond, and Timmy Sze Wing Ng. 2007. "General Beliefs about the World as Defensive Mechanisms against Death Anxiety." *Omega* 54(3):199-214.

Huiras, Jessica, Christopher Uggen, and Barbara McMorris. 2000. "Career Jobs, Survival Jobs, and Employee Deviance: A Social Investment Model of Workplace Misconduct." *Sociological Quarterly* 41 (2): 245–263.

Hulse, Kath, and Wendy Stone. 2007. "Social Cohesion, Social Capital and Social Exclusion: A Cross-cultural Comparison." *Policy Studies* 28 (2): 109–126.

Hunt, Diana. 1989. *Economic Theories of Development: An Analysis of Competing Paradigms*. New York: Harvester Wheatsheaf.

Hunt, Nicholas C., Govind S. Iyer, and Peggy Jimenez. 2019. "Election Outcome and Tax Compliance: The Role of Political Party Affiliation, Affect Balance, and Trust in Government." *Applied Psychology* 68 (2): 341–372.

Hunter, Bronwyn A., Leonard A. Jason, and Christopher B. Keys. 2013. "Factors of Empowerment for Women in Recovery from Substance Use." *American Journal of Community Psychology* 51 (1–2): 91–102.

Hunter, Lance Y. 2016. "Terrorism, Civil Liberties, and Political Rights: A Cross-National Analysis." *Studies in Conflict & Terrorism* 39 (2): 165–193.

Huntington, Samuel P. 2004. *Who Are We? The Challenges to America's National Identity*. New York, NY: Simon & Schuster.

Husband, Charles, and Yunis Alam. 2011. *Social Cohesion and Counter-terrorism: A Policy Contradiction?* Bristol, UK: Policy.

Huta, Veronika. 2014. "Eudaimonia." Pp.201–213 in *the Oxford Handbook of Happiness*, edited by Susan A. David, Ilona Boniwell and Amanda Conley Ayers. Oxford, UK: Oxford University Press. (BF575.H27O95) \83–115.

Hutcherson, Donald T. 2012. "Crime Pays." *Prison Journal* 92 (3): 315–335.

Hutchings, Kimberly. 2010. "Feminism." Pp.164–180 in *Ethics and World Politics*, edited by Duncan Bell. Oxford, UK: Oxford University Press.

Huxhold, Oliver, Katherine L. Fiori, and Tim Windsor. 2022. "Rethinking Social Relationships in Adulthood: The Differential Investment of Resources Model." *Personality & Social Psychology Review* 26 (1): 57–82.

Huxhold, Oliver, Martina Miche, and Benjamin Schuz. 2014. "Benefits of Having Friends in Older Ages: Differential Effects of Informal Social Activities on Well-Being in Middle-Aged and Older Adults." *Journals of Gerontology. Series B, Psychological Sciences & Social Sciences* 69(3):366–375.

Huyck, Margaret Hellie, and David Leo Gutmann. 2006. "Men and Their Wives: Why Are Some Married Men Vulnerable at Midlife?" Pp.27–50 in *Men in Relationships: A New Look from a Life Course Perspective*, edited by Victoria Hilkevitch Bedford, and Barbara Formaniak Turner. New York: Springer.

Hwang, Kwang-Kuo., and Jeffrey Chang. 2009. "Self-Cultivation: Culturally Sensitive Psychotherapies in Confucian Societies." *Counseling Psychologist* 37 (7): 1010–1032.

Hwang, Woosang, Jeung Hyun Kim, Maria T. Brown, and Merril Silverstein. 2022. "Are Filial Eldercare Norms Related to Intergenerational Solidarity with Older Parents? A Typological Developmental Approach." *Journal of Family Psychology* 36 (4): 585–596.

Hybels, C. F., D. G. Blazer, and B. H. Kaplan. 2000. "Social and Personal Resources and the Prevalence of Phobic Disorder in a Community Population." *Psychological Medicine* 30: 705–716.

Hyggen, Christer. 2006. "Risks and Resources: Social Capital among Social Assistance Recipients in Norway." *Social Policy & Administration* 40 (5): 493–508.

Iacobucci, Alaina C., and Emma C. Frieh. 2018. "(In)dependence and Addictions: Governmentality across Public and Private Treatment Discourses." *Theoretical Criminology* 22 (1): 83–98.

Igarashi, Akira. 2021. "Threats and Norms: Multicultural Policies and Natives' Attitudes towards Immigrants." *Sociological Quarterly* 63 (3): 426–448.

Igarashi, Hiroki, and Hiro Saito. 2014. "Cosmopolitanism as Cultural Capital: Exploring the Intersection of Globalization, Education and Stratification." *Cultural Sociology* 8(3):222–239. \86–310.

Iida, Takeshi, and Tetsuya Matsubayashi. 2010. "Constitutions and Public Support for Welfare Policies." *Social Science Quarterly* 91 (1): 42–62.

Ikeda, Kenichi, and Sean E. Richey. 2005. "Japanese Network Capital: The Impact of Social Networks and Japanese Political Participation." *Political Behavior* 27 (3): 239–260.

Ikels, Charlotte. 1989. "Becoming a Human Being in Theory and Practice: Chinese Views of Human Development." Pp.109–134 in *Age Structuring in Comparative Perspective*, edited by David I. Kertzer and K. Warner Schaie. Hillsdale, NJ: Lawrence Erlbaum Associates.

Immerzeel, Tim, and Frank van Tubergen. 2013. "Religion as Reassurance? Testing the Insecurity Theory in 26 European Countries." *European Sociological Review* 29 (2): 359–372.

Inglehart, Ronald F. 2010. "Faith and Freedom: Traditional and Modern Ways to Happiness." Pp.351–397 in *International Differences in Well-being*, edited by Ed Diener, John F. Helliwell and Daniel Kahneman. New York: Oxford University Press.

Inglehart, Ronald, and Christian Welzel. 2005. *Modernization, Cultural Change, and Democracy: The Human Development Sequence*. New York: Cambridge University Press.

Inglehart, Ronald, and Wayne E. Baker. 2000. "Modernization, Cultural Change, and the Persistence of Traditional Values." *American Sociological Review* 65: 1–51.

Inglehart, Ronald. 1997. *Modernization and Postmodernization: Cultural, Economic, and Political Change in 43 Societies*. Princeton, NJ: Princeton University Press.

Inglehart, Ronald. 1999. "Postmodernization Erodes Respect for Authority, but Increases Support for Democracy." Pp.236–256 in *Critical Citizens: Global Support for Democratic Government*, edited by Pippa Norris. Oxford, UK: Oxford University Press.

Inglehart, Ronald. 2003. "Modernization and Volunteering." Pp.55–70 in *The Values of Volunteering: Cross-cultural Perspectives*, edited by Paul Dekker and Loek Halman. New York: Kluwer.

Inglehart, Ronald. 2018. *Cultural Evolution: People's Motivations Are Changing and Reshaping the World*. Cambridge, UK: Cambridge University Press.

Inglis, Fred. 2004. *Culture*. Cambridge, UK: Polity.

Ingram, Jason R., and Sameer Hinduja. 2008. "Neutralizing Music Piracy? An Empirical Examination." *Deviant Behavior* 29: 334–366.

Inoguchi, Takashi. 2017. "Social Capital in Ten Asian Societies." Pp. 13–27 in *Trust with Asian Characteristics*, edited by Takashi Inoguchi and Yasuharu Tokuda. Singapore: Sprinter.

Ip, Po-Keung. 2014. "Harmony as Happiness? Social Harmony in Two Chinese Societies." *Social Indicators Research* 117(3):719-41.

Irwin, Michael D. 2016. "The Concept of Community as Theoretical Ground: Contention and Compatibility across Levels of Analysis and Standpoints of Social Processes." Pp. 247–268 in *Handbook of Contemporary Sociological Theory*, edited by Seth Abrutyn. Cham, Switzerland: Springer.

Isaacowitz, Derek M., George E. Vaillant, and Martin E.P.. Seligman. 2003. "Strengths and Satisfaction across the Adult Lifespan." *International Journal of Aging & Human Development* 57 (2): 181–201.

Isham, Jonathan, Jane Kolodinsky, and Garrett Kimberly. 2006. "The Effects of Volunteering for Nonprofit Organizations on Social Capital Formation: Evidence from a Statewide Survey." *Nonprofit & Voluntary Sector Quarterly* 35 (3): 367–383.

Ishii, Kenichi. 2009. "Nationalistic Sentiments of Chinese Consumers: The Effects and Determinants of Animosity and Consumer Ethnocentrism." *Journal of International Consumer Marketing* 21: 299–308.

Ishii, Tatsunori, and Katsumi Watanabe. 2023. "Do Empathetic People Have Strong Religious Beliefs? Survey Studies with Large Japanese Samples." *International Journal for the Psychology of Religion* 33 (1): 1–18.

Ishio, Yoshito. 2010. "Social Bases of American Patriotism: Examining Effects of Dominant Social Statuses and Socialization." *Current Sociology* 38 (1): 67–93.

Islam, Jonathan, Jane Kolodinsky, and Garrett Kimberly. 2006. "The Effects of Volunteering for Nonprofit Organizations on Social Capital Formation: Evidence from a Statewide Survey." *Nonproft & Voluntary Sector Quarterly* 35 (3): 367–383.

Izquierdo, Honorio Martin, and Almudena Moreno Minguez. 2003. "Sociological Theory of education in the Dialectical Perspective." Pp. 21–41 in *The International Assessment of New Research and Theory*, edited by Carlos Alberto Torres and Ari Antikainen. Lanham, MD: Rowman.

Jackman, Danielle M., and David MacPhee. 2017. "Self-Esteem and Future Orientation Predict Adolescents? Risk Engagement." *Journal of Early Adolescence* 37 (3): 339–366.

Jackson, Linda A., John E. Hunter, and Carolyn H. Hodge. 1993. "Physical Attractiveness and Intellectual Competence: A Meta-analytic Review." *Social Psychology Quarterly* 58 (2): 108–127.

Jackson, Robert W., and Ross A. Miller. 1995. "Voter Turnout in the Industrial Democracies during the 1980s." *Comparative Political Studies* 27 (4): 467–492.

Jackson, Stevi and Sue Scott. 2010. *Theorizing Sexuality*. New York: NY: Open University Press.

Jackson, Todd, Hong Chen, Cheng Guo, and Xiao Gao. 2006. "Stories We Love by: Conceptions of Love among Couples from the People's Republic of China and the United States." *Journal of Cross-Cultural Psychology* 37 (4): 446–464.

Jackson, William A. 2019. *Markets: Perspectives from Economic and Social Theory*. Abingdon, UK: Routledge.

Jacobs, David, and Jason T. Carmichael. 2002. "Subordination and Violence against State Control Agents: Testing Political Explanations for Lethal Assaults against the Police." *Social Forces* 80 (4): 1223–1251.

Jacobs, David, and Jason T. Carmichael. 2004. "Ideology, Social Threat, and the Death Sentence: Capital Sentences across Time and Space." *Social Forces* 83 (1): 249–278.

Jacques, Jeffrey M. 1998. "Changing Marital and Family Patterns: A Test of the Post-Modern Perspective." *Sociological Perspectives* 41 (2): 381–413.

Jagers, Jan, and Stefaan Walgrave. 2007. "Populism as Political Communication Style: An Empirical Study of Political Parties" Discourse in Belgium." *European Journal of Political Research* 46 (3): 319–345.

Jagger, Alison M. 2000. "Feminist Ethics." Pp.348–374 in *The Blackwell Guide to Ethical Theory*, edited by Hugh LaFollette. Malden, MA: Blackwell.

Jakobsson, Niklas, and Andreas Kotsadam. 2011. "Gender Equity and Prostitution: An Investigation of Attitudes in Norway and Sweden." *Feminist Economics* 17 (1): 31–58.

James, Jeffrey. 2010. "Penetration and Growth Rates of Mobile Phones in Developing Countries: An Analytical Classification." *Social Indicators Research* 99 (1): 135–145.

Jang, Jongick, Tae-Hwan. Kim, Hoon Hong, Chung Sik Yoo, and Jonghyun Park. 2018. "Statistical Estimation of the Causal Effect of Social Economy on Subjective Well-Being." *VOLUNTAS: International Journal of Voluntary and Nonprofit Organizations* 29 (3): 511–525.

Jang, Sung Joon. 1999. "Age-varying Effects of Family, School and Peers on Delinquency: A Multilevel Modeling Test of Interactional Theory." *Criminology* 37 (3): 643–685.

Janmaat, Jan Germen and Nathalie Mons. 2023. "Tracking and Political Engagement: An Investigation of the Mechanisms Driving the Effect of Educational Tracking on Voting Intentions among Upper Secondary Students in France." *Research Papers in Education*.

Janmaat, Jan Germen. 2011. "Social Cohesion as a Real-life Phenomenon: Assessing the Explanatory Power of the Universalist and Particularist Perspectives." *Social Indicators Research* 100: 61–83.

Jarvinen, Markus, and Minna Branders. 2020. "Contracts as Trust Builders." *Journal of Trust Research* 10 (1): 46–65.

Jasso, Guillermina. 2002. "Seven Secrets of Doing Theory." Pp.317–342 in *New Directions in Contemporary Sociological Theory*, edited by Joseph Berger and Morris Zelditch, Jr. Lanham, MD: Rowman & Littlefield.

Jau, Jasmin, and David Hodgson. 2018. "How Interaction with Animals Can Benefit Mental Health: A Phenomenological Study." *Social Work in Mental Health* 16 (1): 20–33.

Javakhishvili, Nino, and Gvantsa Jibladze. 2018. "Analysis of Anti-Domestic Violence Policy Implementation in Georgia Using Contextual Interaction Theory (CIT)." *Journal of Social Policy* 47 (2): 317–334.

Jaworsky, Bernadette Nadya. 2014. "Terrorists at the Gates? Unauthorized Migrants and Discourses of Danger." *Migration Letters* 8 (1): 43–54.

Jayaratne, Toby Epstein, Oscar Ybarra, Jane P. Sheldon, Tony N. Brown, Merle Feldbaum, Carla A. Pfeffer, and Elizabeth M. Petty. 2006. White Americans" Genetic Lay Theories of Race Differences and Sexual Orientation: Their Relationship with Prejudice toward Blacks, and Gay Men and Lesbians. *Group Process & Intergroup Relations* 9 (1): 77–94.

Jaye, Chrystal, Jessica Young, Richard Egan, Rebecca Llewellyn, Wayne Cunningham, and Peter Radue. 2018. "The Healthy Lifestyle in Longevity Narratives." *Social Theory & Health* 16 (4): 361–378.

Jeffreys, Elaine. 2012. *Prostitution Scandals in China: Policing, Media and Society*. Abington, UK: Routledge.

Jeffries, Vincent. 2000. "Virtue and Marital Conflict: A Theoretical Formulation and Research Agenda." *Sociological Perspectives* 43 (2): 231–246.

Jenkins, J. Craig., and Michael Wallace. 1996. "The Generalized Action Potential of Protest Movements: The New Class, Social Trends, and Political Exclusion Explanations." *Sociological Forum* 11 (2): 183–207.

Jenkins, J. Craig, and William Form. 2005. "Social Movements and Social Change." Pp. 331–349 in *The Handbook of Political Sociology: States, Civil Societies, and Globalization*, edited by Thomas Janoski, Robert Alford, Alexander Hicks, and Mildred A. Schwartz. Cambridge, UK: Cambridge University Press.

Jenkins-Smith, Hank C., and Kerry G. Herron. 2009. "Rock and a Hard Place: Public Willingness to Trade Civil Rights and Liberties for Greater Security." *Politics & Policy* 37 (5): 1095–1129.

Jennings, Freddie J., and Frank M. Russell. 2019. "Civility, Credibility, and Health Information: The Impact of Uncivil Comments and Source Credibility on Attitudes About Vaccines." *Public Understanding of Science* 28 (4): 417–432.

Jensen, Gary F. 2007. "Social Learning and Violent Behavior." Pp.636–646 in *The Cambridge Handbook of Violent Behavior and Aggression*, edited by Daniel J. Flannery, Alexander T. Vazsonyi and Irwin D. Waldman. Cambridge, UK: Cambridge University Press.

Jensen, Tina Gudrun, Kristina Weibel, and Kathrine Vitus. 2017. "'There Is No Racism Here': Public Discourses on Racism, Immigrants and Integration in Denmark." *Patterns of Prejudice* 51 (1): 51–68.

Jensen, Tina Gudrun, Kristina Weibel, and Kathrine Vitus. 2017. "'There Is No Racism Here': Public Discourses on Racism, Immigrants and Integration in Denmark." *Patterns of Prejudice* 51 (1): 51–68.

Jeong, Jisu, and Seunghui Han. 2020. "Trust in Police as an Influencing Factor on Trust in Government: 2sls Analysis Using Perception of Safety." *Policing* 43 (4): 541–558.

Jessop, Bob. 2016. *The State: Past, Present, Future.* Cambridge, UK: Polity.

Jia, Qifan, Jie Zhou, and Mingquan Huang. 2020. "Life Satisfaction Predicts Perceived Social Justice: The Lower Your Life Satisfaction, the Less Just You Perceive Society to Be." *Frontiers in Psychology* 11: 540835.

Jiang, Junfeng. 2023. "Heterogeneous Influence of Socioeconomic Inequality on Population Health: A Cross-National Study." *Social Indicators Research* 169 (3): 1109–1124.

Jiang, Shiqing, Ming Lu, and Hiroshi Sato. 2011. "Identity, Inequality, and Happiness: Evidence from Urban China." *World Development* 40(6):1190–1200.

Jiang, Zhengcheng. 2012. *Xuanzi's Saying So.* Beijing, China: Overseas Chinese.

Jin, Guantao, and Qingfeng Liu. 1993. *The Transformation of Chinese Society: The Fate of Its Ultrastable Structure in Modern Times.* Hong Kong: Chinese University of Hong Kong. (HN737.C456) \63–359.

Jin, Yinghuai. 2003. *Interpretation of the Theory of Socialism with Chinese Characteristics.* Xian, China: Xian Communication University.

John, Karen. 2001. "Measuring Children's Social Functioning." *Child Psychology & Psychiatry Review* 6 (4): 181–188.

Johnson, Blair T., Gregory R. Maio, and Aaron Smith-McLallen. 2014. "Communication and Attitude Change, Causes, Processes, and Effects." Pp. 617–669 in *The Handbook of Attitudes*, edited by Albarracin Dolores, T. Johnson Blair and P. Zanna Mark. Mahwah, NJ: Psychology.

Johnson, Branden. 2004. "Varying Risk Comparison Elements: Effects of Public Reactions." *Risk Analysis* 24 (1): 103–114.

Johnson, Bruce D., Flutura Bardhi, Stephen J. Sifaneck, and Eloise Dunlap. 2006. "Marijuana Argot as Subculture Threads." *British Journal of Criminology* 46: 46–77.

Johnson, Craig. 2009. *Arresting Development: The Power of Knowledge for Social Change.* Abingdon, UK: Routledge.

Johnson, David W., and Roger T. Johnson. 2005. "New Developments in Social Interdependence Theory." *Genetic, Social, & General Psychology Monographs* 131 (4): 285–358.

Johnson, Katherine E. 2015. *Sexuality: A Psychosocial Manifesto.* Cambridge, UK: Polity.

Johnson, Tim, Mikhail G. Myagkov, and John M. Orbell. 2013. "Distinctive Preferences toward Risk in the Substantive Domain of Sociality." *Political Psychology* 34 (1): 1–22.

Johnston, Nicolas, and Srinjoy Bose. 2020. "Violence, Power and Meaning: The Moral Logic of Terrorism." *Global Policy* 11 (3): 315–325.

Jolley, Daniel, Karen M. Douglas, Ana C. Leite, and Tanya Schrader. 2019. "Belief in Conspiracy Theories and Intentions to Engage in Everyday Crime." *British Journal of Social Psychology* 58 (3): 534–549.

Jolliffe, Darrick, and David P. Farrington. 2010. "Individual Differences and Offending." Pp.40–55 in *The SAGE Handbook of Criminological Theory*, edited by Eugene McLaughlin and Tim Newburn. London, UK: SAGE.

Jolly, Seth K., and Gerald M. DiGiusto. 2014. "Xenophobia and Immigrant Contact: French Public Attitudes toward Immigration." *Social Science Journal* 51 (3): 464–473.

Jones, Antwan, Gregory D. Squires, and Cynthia Ronzio. 2015. "Foreclosure Is Not an Equal Opportunity Stressor: How Inequality Fuels the Adverse Health Implications of the Nation's Financial Crisis." *Journal of Urban Affairs* 37 (5): 505–529.

Jones, Daniel N., and Delroy L. Paulhus. 2009. "Machiavellianism." Pp. 93–108 in *Handbook of Individual Differences in Social Behavior*, edited by Mark R. Leary and Rick H. Hoyle. New York, NY: Guilford.

Jones, David W. 2016. *Disordered Personalities and Crime: An Analysis of the History of Moral Insanity*. Abingdon, UK: Routledge.

Jones, James Holland, and Brodie Ferguson. 2009. "Demographic and Social Predictors of Intimate Partner Violence in Colombia." *Human Nature: An Interdisciplinary Biosocial Perspective* 20 (2): 184–203.

Jones, Lindsey, and Marco d'Errico. 2019. "Whose Resilience Matters? Like-for-Like Comparison of Objective and Subjective Evaluations of Resilience." *World Development* 124: 104632.

Jones, Rachel K., and April Brayfield. 1997. "Life's Greatest Joy? European Attitudes toward the Centrality of Children." *Social Forces* 75 (4): 1239–1270.

Jones, Russell, Derek Heim, Simon Hunter, and Anne Ellaway. 2014. "The Relative Influence of Neighbourhood Incivilities, Cognitive Social Capital, Club Membership and Individual Characteristics on Positive Mental Health." *Health & Place* 28: 187–193.

Jones, Stanton L., and Mark A. Yarhouse. 2000. *Homosexuality: The Use of Scientific Research in the Church's Moral Debate*. Downers Grove, IL: InterVarsity.

Jonsson, Sofia, and Niklas Jakobsson. 2017. "Is Buying Sex Morally Wrong? Comparing Attitudes Toward Prostitution Using Individual-Level Data Across Eight Western European Countries." *Women's Studies International Forum* 61: 58–69.

Jorgensen, Bradley S., Robert D. Jamieson, and John F. Martin. 2010. "Income, Sense of Community and Subjective Well-being: Combining Economic and Psychological Variables." *Journal of Economic Psychology* 31: 612–643.

Joseph, Jonathan. 2006. *Marxism and Social Theory*. Houndmills, UK: Palgrave.

Joseph, Lauren J., and Pamela Black. 2012. "Who's the Man? Fragile Masculinities, Consumer Masculinities, and the Profile of Sex Work Client." *Men & Masculinities* 15 (5): 486–506

Joslyn, Mark R., and Donald P. Haider-Markel. 2002. "Framing Effects on Personal Opinion and Perception of Public Opinion: The Cases of Physician-Assisted Suicide and Social Security." *Social Science Quarterly* 83 (3): 690–706.

Jost, John T. 2020. *A Theory of System Justification*. Cambridge, MA: Harvard University Press.

Jost, John T., Brett W. Pelham, Oliver Sheldon, and Billian Ni Sullivan. 2003. "Social Inequality and the Reduction of Ideological Dissonance on Behalf of the System: Evidence of the Enhanced System Justification among the Disadvantaged." *European Journal of Social Psychology* 33:13-36.

Jou, Willy. 2011. "How Do Citizens in East Asian Democracies Understand Left and Right?" *Japanese Journal of Political Science* 12 (1): 33–55.

Juhl, Jacob, Tim Wildschut, Constantine Sedikides, Tara Diebel, Wing-Yee. Cheung, and Ad. J. J. M. Vingerhoets. 2019. "Nostalgia Proneness and Empathy: Generality, Underlying Mechanism, and Implications for Prosocial Behavior." *Journal of Personality* 88 (3): 485–500.

Jukes, Matthew C. H., Stephanie S. Zuilkowski, and Elena L. Grigorenko. 2018. "Do Schooling and Urban Residence Develop Cognitive Skills at the Expense of Social Responsibility? A Study of Adolescents in the Gambia, West Africa." *Journal of Cross-Cultural Psychology* 49 (1): 82–98.

Jung, Jinkyung J., and Eunsun E. Kwon. 2011. "Trust Development in Volunteering: An Exploratory Study of Social Trust and Volunteer Activities in Korea." *International Review of Public Administration* 16 (1): 157–179.

Jung, Joo-young. 2016. "Are You an Opinion Giver, Seeker, or Both? Re-Examining Political Opinion Leadership in the New Communication Environment." *International Journal of Communication* 10: 4439–4459.

Jupille, Joseph Henri, and James A. Caporaso. 2022. *Theories of Institutions*. Cambridge, UK: Cambridge University Press.

Kabashima, Ikuo, Jonathan Marshall, Takayoshi Ukekami, and Dae-Song. Hyun. 2000. "Casual Cynics or Disillusioned Democrats? Political Alienation in Japan." *Political Psychology* 21 (4): 779–804.

Kaczmarek, Lukasz D., and Dariusz Drążkowski. 2014. "MMORPG Escapism Predicts Decreased Well-Being: Examination of Gaming Time, Game Realism Beliefs, and Online Social Support for Offline Problems." *Cyberpsychology, Behavior & Social Networking* 17 (5): 298–302.

Kadianaki, Irini, Eleni Andreouli, and Mario Carretero. 2018. "Using National History to Construct the Boundaries of Citizenship: An Analysis of Greek Citizens' Discourse About Immigrants' Rights." *Qualitative Psychology* 5 (1): 172–187.

Kagotani, Koji. 2015. "National Security Environments, Patriotism, and Japanese Public Opinion." *Japanese Journal of Political Science* 16 (1): 96–113.

Kahne, Joseph, Bernadette Chi, and Ellen Middaugh. 2006. "Building Social Capital for Civic and Political Engagement: The Potential of High-school Civics Courses." *Canadian Journal of Education* 29 (2): 387–409.

Kahneman, Daniel, David A. Schkade, Calude Fishler, Alan B. Krueger, and Amy Krilla. 2010. "The Structure of Well-being in Two Cities: Life Satisfaction and Experience and Happiness in Columbus, Ohio and Rennes, France." Pp.16–33 in *International Differences in Well-being*, edited by Ed Diener, John F. Helliwell and Daniel Kahneman. New York: Oxford University Press.

Kaiser, Florian G., and Katarzyna Byrka. 2015. "The Campbell Paradigm as a Conceptual Alternative to the Expectation of Hypocrisy in Contemporary Attitude Research." *Journal of Social Psychology* 155 (1): 12–29.

Kalish, Yuval. 2008. "Bridging in Social Networks: Who Are the People on Structural Holes and Why Are They There?" *Asian Journal of Social Psychology* 11: 53–66.

Kallhoff, Angela. 2011. *Why Democracy Needs Public Goods*. Lanham, MD: Lexington.

Kalu, Kalu N. 2019. *A Functional Theory of Government, Law, and Institutions*. Lanham, MD: Lexington Books.

Kampen, Jarl K. 2010. "On the (in)Consistency of Citizen and Municipal Level Indicators of Social Capital and Local Government Performance." *Social Indicators Research* 97 (2): 213–228.

Kanan, James W., and Matthew V. Pruitt. 2002. "Modeling Fear of Crime and Perceived Victimization Risk: The (In)significance of Neighborhood Integration." *Sociological Inquiry* 72 (4): 527–548.

Kang, Xiaoguang. 2005. *Benevolent Rule: Third Way of Chinese Political Development*. Singapore: Global.

Kaplan, Howard B., and Xiaoru Liu. 2000. "Social Movements as Collective Coping with Spoiled Personal Identities: Intimation from a Panel Study of Changes in the Life Course Between Adolescence and Adulthood." Pp.215–238 in *Self, Identity, and Social Movements*, edited by Sheldon Stryker, Timothy J. Owens, and Robert W. White. Minneapolis, MN: University of Minnesota Press.

Kaplan, Howard B., Feodor A. Gostjev, and Robert J. Johnson. 2013. "Social Psychological Perspectives on Deviance." Pp. 563–594 in *Handbook of Social Psychology*, edited by John Delamater and Amanda Ward. Dordrecht, Netherlands: Springer.

Kapur, Kanika. 1998. "The Impact of Health on Job Mobility: A Measure of Job Lock." *Industrial and Labor Relations Review* 51 (2): 282–298.

Karekla, Maria, and Georgia Panayiotou. 2011. "Coping and Experiential Avoidance: Unique or Overlapping Constructs?" *Journal of Behavior Therapy & Experimental Psychiatry* 42 (2): 163–170.

Karger, Howard, James Midgley, Peter A. Kindle, and C. Brene Brown. 2007. *Controversial Issues in Social Policy*. Boston, MA: Pearson.

Karremans, Johan C., Melanie P. J. Schellekens, and Gesa Kappen. 2017. "Bridging the Sciences of Mindfulness and Romantic Relationships: A Theoretical Model and Research Agenda." *Personality & Social Psychology Review* 21 (1): 29–49.
Karstedt, Susanne, and Stephen Farrall. 2006. "The Moral Economy of Everyday Crime." *British Journal of Criminology* 46: 1011–1036.
Karstedt, Susanne. 2010. "New Institutionalism in Criminology: Approaches, Theories and Themes." Pp.337–359 in *The SAGE Handbook of Criminological Theory*, edited by Eugene McLaughlin and Tim Newburn. London, UK: SAGE.
Karuppannan, Sadasivam, and Alpana Sivam. 2011. "Social Sustainability and Neighborhood Deisgn: An Investigation of Residents? Satisfaction in Delhi." *Local Environment* 16 (9): 849–880.
Kas, Judith, Joyce Delnoij, Rense Corten, and Paolo Parigi. 2022. "Trust Spillovers in the Sharing Economy: Does International Airbnb Experience Foster Cross-National Trust?" *Journal of Consumer Behaviour* 21 (3): 509–522.
Kasser, Tim. 2016. "Materialistic Values and Goals." *Annual Review Psychology* 67: 489–514.
Katz-Gerro, Tally, and Yossi Shavit. 1998. "The Stratification of Leisure and Taste: Classes and Lifestyles in Israel." *European Sociological Review* 14 (4): 369–386.
Kaufmann, Eric, Anne Goujon, and Vegard Skirbekk. 2012. "The End of Secularization in Europe? A Socio-demographic Perspective." *Sociology of Religion* 73 (1): 69–91.
Kaufman-Parks, Angela M., Alfred Demaris, Peggy C. Giordano, Wendy D. Manning, and Monica A. Longmore. 2017. "Parents and Partners: Moderating and Mediating Influences on Intimate Partner Violence across Adolescence and Young Adulthood." *Journal of Social & Personal Relationships* 34 (8): 1295–1323.
Kaukinen, Catherine. 2004. "Status Compatibility, Physical Violence, and Emotional Abuse in Intimate Relationships." *Journal of Marriage & Family* 66: 452–471.
Kaurin, Pauline Shanks. 2020. *On Obedience: Contrasting Philosophies for the Military, Citizenry and Community.* Annapolis, MD: Naval.
Kawachi, Ichiro, Bruce P. Kennedy, Kimberly Lochner, and Deborah Prothrow-Stith. 1997. "Social Capital, Income Inequality, and Mortality." *American Journal of Public Health* 87(9):1491–1498. \71–217.
Kay, Aaron C., Danielle Gaucher, Jamie L. Napier, Mitchell J. Callan, and Kristin Laurin. 2008. "God and the Government: Testing a Compensatory Control Mechanism for the Support of External Systems." *Journal of Personality & Social Psychology* 95 (1): 18–35.
Kayabol, Nazlı Büşra., and Akçabozan, and Zeynep Hatipoğlu Sümer. 2022. "How to Maintain a Marriage: Maintenance Behaviors, Equity, and Appreciation in Understanding Marital Satisfaction+." *Current Psychology* 41 (9): 5781–5794.
Kayser, Daniela Niesta, Tobias Greitemeyer, Peter Fischer, and Dieter Frey. 2010. "Why Mood Affects Help Giving, but not Moral Courage: Comparing Two Types of Prosocial Behaviour." *European Journal of Social Psychology* 40: 1136–1157.
Kazarian, Shane S., and Rod A. Martin. 2006. "Humor Styles, Culture-related Personality, Well-being, and Family Adjustment among Armenians in Lebanon." *Humor* 19 (4): 405–423.
Kearns, Ade, and Elise Whitley. 2015. "Getting there? The Effects of Functional Factors, Time and Place on the Social Integration of Migrants." *Journal of Ethnic & Migration Studies* 41 (13): 2105–2129.
Keeting, Caroline F. 2016. "The Life and Times of Nonverbal Communication Theory and Research: Past, Present, Future." Pp. 17–42 in *APA Handbook of Nonverbal Communication*, edited by David Matsumoto, Hyisung C. Hwang and Mark G. Frank. Washington, DC: American Psychological Association.
Kegley, Charles W. and Gregory A. Raymond. 2021. *Great Powers and World Order: Patterns and Prospects.* Thousand Oaks, CA; SAGE.
Keightley, Michelle L., Gordon Winocur, Hana Burianova, Donaya Hongwanishkul, and Cheryl L. Grady. 2006. "Age Effects on Social Cognition: Faces Tell a Different Story" *Psychology & Aging* 21 (3): 558–572.

Keijsers, Loes, Rolf Loeber, Susan Branje, and Wim Meeus. 2011. "Bidirectional Links and Concurrent Development of Parent-child Relationships and Boys' Offending Behavior." *Journal of Abnormal Psychology* 120 (4): 878–889.

Keillor, Bruce, Deborah Owens, and Charles Pettijohn. 2001. "A Cross-cultural Cross-national Study of Influencing Factors and Socially Desirable Response Biases." *International Journal of Market Research* 43 (1): 63–84.

Kekes, John. 1997. *Against Liberalism.* Ithaca, NY: Cornell University Press.

Kekes, John. 2006. *The Enlargement of Life: Moral Imagination at Work.* Ithaca, NY: Cornell University Press.

Kelley, Douglas L., Vincent R. Waldron, and Dayna N. Kloeber. 2019. *A Communicative Approach to Conflict, Forgiveness, and Reconciliation: Reimagining Our Relationships.* New York, NY: Routledge.

Kelley, Jonathan, and Nan Dirk De Graaf. 1997. "National Context, Parental Socialization and Religious Belief: Results from 15 Nations." *American Sociological Review* 62:639-659.

Kelly, Brendan D. 2012. "Contemplative Traditions and Meditation." Pp. 307–325 in *The Oxford Handbook of Psychology and Spirituality*, edited by Lisa J. Miller. New York, NY: Oxford University Press.

Kelly, Diann Cameron. 2009. "In Preparation for Adulthood: Exploring Civic Participation and Social Trust among Young Minorities." *Youth & Society* 40 (4): 526–540.

Kelly, Eric Damian, and Barbara Becker. 2000. *Community Planning: An Introduction to the Comprehensive Plan.* Washington, DC: Island.

Kelly, Megan M., Bryann B. DeBeer, Elizabeth Chamberlin, Tracy Claudio, J. Brooke Duarte, Irene Harris, Meaghan A. Kennedy, Steven Shirk, and Erin D. Reilly. 2022. The Effects of Loneliness and Psychological Flexibility on Veterans" Substance Use and Physical and Mental Health Functioning During the Covid-19 Pandemic. *Journal of Contextual Behavioral Science* 26: 217–226.

Kelly, Orla. 2020. "The Silver Bullet? Assessing the Role of Education for Sustainability." *Social Forces* 99 (1): 178–204.

Kemmis, Stephen, and Robin McTaggart. 2005. "Participatory Action Research." Pp.559–603 in *The Sage Handbook of Qualitative Research* (3rd ed.), edited by Norman K. Denzin and Yvonne S. Lincoln. Thousand Oaks, CA: Sage.

Kende, Judit, Charis Psaltis, Julia Reiter, Kyriaki Fousiani, Huseyin Cakal, and Eva Green. 2022. Past and Present Intergroup Contact and Conflict among Inhabitants of Former Mixed Villages of Cyprus: The Role of Individual and Collective Experiences in Predicting Attitudes and Trust. *Political Psychology* 43 (4): 751–768.

Kendler, Kenneth S., Charles O. Gardner, and Carol A. Prescott. 2006. "Toward a Comprehensive Developmental Model for Major Depression in Men." *American Journal of Psychiatry* 163 (1): 115–124.

Kennedy, Bruce D., Ichiro Kawachi, and Elizabeth Brainerd. 1998. "The Role of Social Capital in the Russia Mortality Crisis." *World Development* 26 (11): 2029–2043.

Kennedy, Paul. 2010. *Local Lives and Global Transformations towards World Society.* Houndmills, UK: Palgrave.

Kent, Martha and Mary C. Davis. 2010. "The Emergence of Capacity-building Programs and Models of Resilience." Pp. 427–449 in *Handbook of Adult Resilience*, edited by John W. Reich, Alex J. Zautra and John Stuart Hall. New York, NY: Guilford.

Kentmen, Cigdem. 2010. "Bases of Support for the EU's Common Foreign and Security Policy: Gender, Attitudes toward Economic Integration, and Attachment to Europe." *International Political Science Review* 31 (3): 285–299.

Kernis, Michael H., and Brian M. Goldman. 2006. "A Multicomponent Conceptualization of Authenticity: Theory and Research." *Advances in Experimental Social Psychology* 38: 283–357.

Kerrissey, Jasmine, and Evan Schofer. 2013. "Civic and Political Participation: Union Membership and Political Participation in the United States." *Social Forces* 91 (3): 895–928.

Kertzer, Joshua D., Kathleen E. Powers, Brian C. Rathbun, and Ravi Iyer. 2014. "Moral Support: How Moral Values Shape Foreign Policy Attitudes." *Journal of Politics* 76 (3): 825–840.

Kesebir, Pelin, and Selin Kesebir. 2012. "The Cultural Salience of Moral Character and Virtue Declined in Twentieth Century America." *Journal of Positive Psychology* 7 (6): 471–480.

Kessler, Ronald C., Kristin D. Mickelson, Ellen E. Walters, Shenyang Zhao, and Lana Hamilton. 2004. "Age and Depression in the MIDUS Survey." Pp.227–251 in *How Healthy Are We: A National Study of Well-being at Midlife*, edited by Orville Gilbert Brim, Carol D. Ryff and Ronald C. Kessler. Chicago, IL: University of Chicago Press.

Ketelaars, Pauline, Stefaan Walgrave, and Ruud Wouters. 2017. "Protesters on Message? Explaining Demonstrators" Differential Degrees of Frame Alignment." *Social Movement Studies* 16 (3): 340–354.

Kettrey, Heather Hensman. 2016. "What's Gender Got to Do with It? Sexual Double Standards and Power in Heterosexual College Hookups." *Journal of Sex Research* 53 (7): 754–765.

Keyes, Corey L.M.. 2002. "Social Civility in the United States." *Sociological Inquiry* 72 (3): 393–408.

Keyes, Corey L.M., and Adam D. Shapiro. 2004. "Social Well-being in the United States: A Descriptive Epidemiology." Pp.350–372 in *How Healthy Are We: A National Study of Well-being at Midlife*, edited by Orville Gilbert Brim, Carol D. Ryff and Ronald C. Kessler. Chicago, IL: University of Chicago Press.

Khamis, Vivian. 2006. "Family Environment and Parenting as Predictors of Attention-deficient and Hyperactivity among Palestinian Children." *Journal of Social Service Research* 32 (4): 99–116.

Khatchadourian, Haig. 1999. *Community and Communitarianism*. New York: Peter Lang.

Khomyakov, Maxim. 2020. "Russia: Colonial, Anticolonial, Postcolonial Empire?" *Social Science Information* 59 (2): 225–263.

KhosraviNik, Majid. 2010. "The Representation of Refugees, Asylum Seekers and Immigrants in British Newspapers." *Journal of Language & Politics* 9 (1): 1–28.

Kick, Edward L., and Laura A. McKinney. 2014. "Global Context, National Interdependencies, and the Ecological Footprint." *Sociological Perspectives* 57 (2): 256–279.

Kilburn, Johnn C., Jr., and Michael O. Maume. 2000. "The Paradox of Neighborhood Association Existence and Membership." *Research in Community Sociology* 10:327–344. Peng, Yusheng. 2004. "Kinship Networks and Entrepreneurs in China's Transitional Economy. *American Journal of Sociology* 109 (5): 1045–1074.

Kilian, Britta, Manfred Hofer, and Claudia Kuhnle. 2013. "Conflicts between On-Task and Off-Task Behaviors in the Classroom: The Influences of Parental Monitoring, Peer Value Orientations, Students' Goals, and Their Value Orientations." *Social Psychology of Education* 16 (1): 77–94.

Killen, Melanie. 2018. "The Origins of Morality: Social Equality, Fairness, and Justice." *Philosophical Psychology* 31 (5): 767–803.

Kilminster, Richard. 2008. "Narcissism or Informalization? Christopher Lasch, Norbert Elias and Social Diagnosis." *Theory, Culture & Society* 25 (3): 131–151.

Kim, Andrew Enungi. 2004. "The Social Perils of the Korean Financial Crisis." *Journal of Contemporary Asia* 34 (2): 221–337.

Kim, Daniel, and Ichiro Kawachi. 2007. "U.S. State-Level Social Capital and Health-Related Quality of Life: Multilevel Evidence of Main, Mediating, and Modifying Effects." *Annals of Epidemiology* 17 (4): 258–269.

Kim, Heejung S., David K. Sherman, and John A. Updegraff. 2016. "Fear of Ebola." *Psychological Science* 27 (7): 935–944.

Kim, Myunghee, and Mychal Voorhees. 2011. "Government Effectiveness and Institutional Trust in Japan, South Korea, and China." *Asian Politics & Policy* 3 (3): 413–432.

Kim, Sookyung. 2012. "Racism in the Global Era: Analysis of Korean Media Discourse around Migrants, 1990–2009." *Discourse & Society* 23 (6): 657–678.

Kim, Sungmoon. 2019. "The Political Economy of Confucian Harmony: A Xunzian Vision." *American Journal of Economics & Sociology* 78 (2): 493–521.

Kim, Uichol, Geir Helgesen, and Byung Man Ahn. 2002. "Democracy, Trust, and Political Efficacy: Comparative Analysis of Danish and Korean Political Culture." *Applied Psychology* 51 (2): 318–353.

Kim, Yeung Yun. 2013. "The Identity Factor in Intercultural Conflict." Pp. 639–660 in *The SAGE Handbook of Conflict Communication*, edited by John G. Oetzel and Stelle Ting-Toomey. Thousand Oaks, CA: SAGE.

Kim, Young-Il, and W. Bradford Wilcox. 2013. "Bonding Alone: Familism, Religion, and Secular Civic Participation." *Social Science Research* 42(1):31-45.

Kinchy, Abby et al. 2008. "Against Free Markets, against Science? Regulating the Socio-economic Effects of Biotechnology." *Rural Sociology* 73(2):147-179.

King, Rosalind Berkowitz. 2005. "The Case of American Women: Globalization and the Transition to Adulthood in an Individualistic Regime." Pp.305–325 in *Globalization, Uncertainty and Youth in Society*, edited by Hans-Peter Blossfeld, Erik Klijzing, Melinda Mills and Karin Kurz. London: Routledge.

Kingston, Beverly, David Huizinga, and Delbert Elliott. 2009. "A Test of Social Disorganization Theory in High-risk Urban Neighborhoods." *Youth & Society* 41 (1): 53–79.

Kipnis, Andrew. 2002. "Practices of Guanxi: Production and Practices of Guanxi." Pp.21–36 in *Social Connection in China: Institutions, Culture, and the Changing Nature of Guanxi*, edited by Thomas Gold, Doug Guthrie, and David Wank. Cambridge, UK: Cambridge.

Kirchler, Erich, and Boris Maciejovsky. 2001. "Tax Compliance within the Context of Gain and Loss Situations, Expected and Current Asset Position, and Profession." *Journal of Economic Psychology* 22: 173–194.

Kirk, David S., and Andrew V. Papachristos. 2011. "Cultural Mechanisms and the Persistence of Neighborhood Violence." *American Journal of Sociology* 116 (4): 1190–1233.

Kirkby-Geddes, Emma, Nigel King, and Alison Bravington. 2013. "Social Capital and Community Group Participation: Examining Bridging and Bonding in the Context of a Healthy Living Centre in the UK." *Journal of Community & Applied Social Psychology* 23 (4): 271–285.

Kirkpatrick, Daniel. 2020. *Political Expression and Conflict Transformation in Divided Societies: Criminalising Politics and Politicising Crime*. Abingdon, UK: Routledge.

Kirmanoglu, Hasan, and Cem Baslevent. 2014. "Life Satisfaction of Ethnic Minority Members: An Examination of Interactions with Immigration, Discrimination, and Citizenship." *Social Indicators Research* 116: 173–184.

Kirsch, Max H. 2000. *Queer Theory and Social Change*. London: Routledge.

Kiser, Edgar, and Erin Powers. 2013. "Rational Choice Approach to State-making." Pp. 443–470 in *The Handbook of Rational Choice Social Research*, edited by Rafael Wittek, Tom A. H. Snijders, and Victor Nee. Stanford, CA: Stanford University Press.

Kisliuk, Sarah, and Kristina S. Weißmüller. 2023. "Social Capital as a Resource for Prosocial Donation Behavior? Quantitative Evidence on the Dark Side of Strategic Networking." *Social Sciences & Humanities Open* 8 (1): 100573.

Kitayama, Shinsbu, and Anzel Rose Markus. 2000. "The Pursuit of Happiness and the Realization of Sympathy: Cultural Patterns of Self, Social Relations, and Well-being." Pp.113–161 in *Culture and Subjective Well-being*, edited by Ed Diener and Eunkook M. Suh. Cambridge, MA: MIT.

Kitchen, Peter, and Allison Williams. 2010. "Quality of Life and Perceptions of Crime, Saskatoon, Canada." *Social Indicators Research* 95:33–61. \103–10.

Kitts, James. 2003. "Egocentric Bias on Information Management? Selective Disclosure and the Social Roots of Norm Misperception." *Social Psychology Quarterly* 66 (3): 222–237.

Kitzinger, Celia, and Sue Wilkinson. 1995. "Transitions from Heterosexuality to Lesbianism: The Discursive Production of Lesbian Identities." *Developmental Psychology* 31 (1): 95–104.

Kivisto, Peter and Thomas Faist. 2010. *Beyond a Border: The Causes and Consequences of Contemporary Immigration*. Thousand Oaks, CA: Pine Forge.

Kjell, O. N. E., D. Daukantaitė, K. Hefferon, and S. Sikström. 2016. "The Harmony in Life Scale Complements the Satisfaction with Life Scale: Expanding the Conceptualization of the Cognitive Component of Subjective Well-Being." *Social Indicators Research* 126 (2): 893–919.

Klandermans, Bert, and Jacquelien van Stekelenburg. 2013. "Social Movements and the Dynamics of Collective Action." Pp.774–811 in *The Oxford Handbook of Political Psychology*, edited by Leone Huddy, David O. Sears and Jack S. Levy. New York: Oxford University Press.

Klein, Carlo. 2013. "Social Capital or Social Cohesion: What Matters for Subjective Well-Being?" *Social Indicators Research* 110 (3): 891–911.

Kleiner, Tuuli-Marja. 2018. "Public Opinion Polarisation and Protest Behaviour." *European Journal of Political Research* 57 (4): 941–962.

Kleinhans, Reinout, Hugo Priemus, and Godfried Engbersen. 2007. "Understanding Social Capital in Recently Restructured Urban Neighborhoods: Two Case Studies in Rotterdam." *Urban Studies* 44 (5/6): 1069–1091.

Kleinhans, Reinout. 2009. "Does Social Capital Affect Residents' Propensity to Move from Restructured Neighborhoods?" *Housing Studies* 24 (5): 629–651.

Kloos, Noortje, J. W. J. R. Judith Austin, and van't Klooster, Constance Drossaert, and Ernst Bohlmeijer. 2022. "Appreciating the Good Things in Life during the Covid-19 Pandemic: A Randomized Controlled Trial and Evaluation of a Gratitude App." *Journal of Happiness Studies* 23 (8): 4001–4025.

Klucarova, Sona, and Xie He. 2021. "Status Consumption and Charitable Donations: The Power of Empowerment." *Psychology & Marketing* 39: 1116–1128.

Kluegel, James R., and Masaru Miyano. 1995. "Justice Beliefs and Support for the Welfare State in Advanced Capitalism." Pp.81–105 in *Social Justice and Political Change: Public Opinion in Capitalist and Post-communist States*, edited by James R. Kluegel, David S. Mason, and Bernd Wegener. New York: Aldine de Gruyer.

Klussman, Kristine, Austin Lee Nichols, and Julia Langer. 2020. "The Role of Self-Connection in the Relationship between Mindfulness and Meaning: A Longitudinal Examination." *Applied Psychology: Health & Well-Being* 12 (3): 636–659.

Klyukanov, Igor E. 2021. *Principles of Intercultural Communication*. New York, NY: Routledge.

Knab, Jean, Irv Garfinkel, and Sara McLanahan. 2008. "The Effects of Welfare and Child Support Policies on Maternal Health and Well-being." Pp.281–303 in *Making American Healthier: Social and Economic Policy as Health Policy*, edited by Robert F. Schoeni, James S. House, George A. Kaplan, and Harold Pollack. New York: Russell Sage.

Knack, Stephen. 2002. "Social Capital, Growth, and Poverty: A Survey of Cross-country Evidence." Pp.42–84 in *The Role of Social Capital in Development: An Empirical Assessment*, edited by Christiaan Grootaert and Thierry van Bastelaer. Cambridge, UK: Cambridge University Press.

Knight, Kyle W., and Eugene A. Rosa. 2011. "The Environmental Efficiency of Well-Being: A Cross-National Analysis." *Social Science Research* 40 (3): 931–949.

Kobayashi, Emiko, and Harold R. Kerbo. 2012. "Differences in Perceived Levels of Informal Punishments for Noncompliance and Rewards for Compliance: A Comparison of Japanese and American Workers." *Deviant Behavior* 33: 40–57.

Kochak, Sana. 2022. "Women, Morality and Law: Prostitution in Kashmir." *South Asian Review* 43 (1–2): 74–93.

Koegl, Christopher J., and David M. Day. 2019. "The Monetary Costs of Crime for a Sample of Offenders in Ontario." *Canadian Journal of Criminology & Criminal Justice* 61 (3): 21–44.

Koehler, Daniel, and Verena Fiebig. 2019. "Knowing What to Do: Academic and Practitioner Understanding of How to Counter Violent Radicalization." *Perspectives on Terrorism* 13 (3): 44–62.

Koerner, Ascan. 2018. "Relationship Typologies." Pp. 65–76 in *The Cambridge Handbook of Personal Relationships*, edited by Anita L. Vangelisti and Daniel Perlman. Cambridge, UK: Cambridge University Press.

Kolers, Avery. 2016. *A Moral Theory of Solidarity*. Oxford, UK: Oxford University Press.

Kolker, Emily S. 2004. "Framing as a Cultural Resource in Health Social Movements: Funding Activism and the Breast Cancer Movement in the U.S. 1990–1993." *Sociology of Health & Illness* 26 (6): 820–844.

Komotar, Maruša Hauptman. 2020. "Discourses on Quality and Quality Assurance in Higher Education from the Perspective of Global University Rankings." *Quality Assurance in Education* 28 (1): 78–88.

Konarska, Joanna. 2005. "Sources of Social Activity of People with Visual and Motor Impairments." *Social Behavior & Personality* 33 (8): 751–766.

Kong, Dejun Tony. 2013. "Intercultural Experience as an Impediment of Trust: Examining the Impact of Intercultural Experience and Social Trust Culture on Institutional Trust in Government." *Social Indicators Research* 113 (3): 847–858.

Kong, Feng, Xu Wang, Jingjing Zhao. 2014. "Dispositional Mindfulness and Life Satisfaction: The Role of Core Self-evaluations." *Personality & Individual Differences* 56:165-169.

Koning, Lukas, and Eric van Dijk. 2013. "Motivational Cognition in Negotiation." Pp. 46–74 in *Handbook of Research on Negotiation*, edited by Mara Olekalns and Wendi L. Adair. Cheltenham, UK: Elgar.

Kono, Shintaro, and Eiji Ito. 2021. "Effects of Leisure Constraints and Negotiation on Activity Enjoyment: A Forgotten Part of the Leisure Constraints Theory." *Annals of Leisure Research* 26 (5): 647–666.

Konty, Mark. 2007. "'When in Doubt, Tell the Truth': Pragmatism and the Sociology of Deviance." *Deviant Behavior* 28 (2): 153–170.

Koomen, Wilem, and Joop van der Pligt. 2016. *The Psychology of Radicalization and Terrorism.* Abingdon, UK: Routledge.

Koppel, Stephen, and Mark R. Fondacaro. 2017. "The Retributism Heuristic." Pp. 191–202 in *The Routledge Handbook of Criminal Justice*, edited by Jonathan Jacobs and Jonathan Jackson, Abingdon, UK: Routledge.

Kornienko, Olga, Thomas J. Dishion, and Thao Ha. 2018. "Peer Network Dynamics and the Amplification of Antisocial to Violent Behavior among Young Adolescents in Public Middle Schools." *Journal of Emotional & Behavioral Disorders* 26 (1): 21–30.

Koromeckyj-Cox, Tanya, Amy Mehraban Pienta, and Tyson H. Brown. 2007. "Women of the 1950s and the Normative Life Course: The Implications of Childlessness, Fertility timing, and Marital Status for Psychological Well-being in Late Midlife." *International Journal of Aging & Human Development* 64 (4): 299–330.

Korostelina, Karyna. 2008. "Concepts of National Identity and the Readiness for Conflict Behaviour." *National Identities* 10 (2): 207–223.

Koster, Ferry. 2013. "Sociality in Diverse Societies: A Regional Analysis across European Countries." *Social Indicators Research* 111 (2): 579–601.

Koumenta, Maria. 2015. "Public Service Motivation and Organizational Citizenship." *Public Money & Management* 35 (5): 341–348.

Koven, Steven G. 2015. *Public Sector Ethics: Theory and Applications.* Boca Raton, FL: CRC.

Kozuch, Barbara, and Zbyslaw Dobrowolski. 2014. *Creating Public Trust: An Organisational Perspective.* Frankfurt, Germany: Peter Lang.

Kraaykamp, Gerbert, and Koen van Eijck. 2005. "Personality, Media Preferences, and Cultural Participation." *Personality & Individual Differences* 38 (7): 1675–1688.

Kraft, Kenneth L., and Anusom Singhapakdi. 1991. "The Role of Ethics and Social Responsibility in Achieving Organizational Effectiveness: Students versus Managers." *Journal of Business Ethics* 10 (9): 679–686.

Krahe, Barbara. 2013. *The Social Psychology of Aggression.* Hove, UK: Psychology.

Kral, Michael J. 2019. *The Idea of Suicide: Contagion, Imitation, and Cultural Diffusion.* New York, NY: Routledge.

Kramer, Betty J., and James David Lambert. 1999. "Caregiving as a Life Course Transition among Older Husbands: A Prospective Study." *The Gerontologist* 39 (6): 658–667.

Kramer, Roderick M. 1999. "Trust and Distrust in Organizations: Emerging Perspectives, Enduring Questions." *Annual Review of Psychology* 50: 569–598.

Kriesi, Hanspeter. 1993. *Political Mobilization and Social Change: The Dutch Case in Comparative Perspective.* Aldershot, UK: Avebury.

Kroenig, Matthew, Melissa McAdam, and Steven Weber. 2010. "Taking Soft Power Seriously." *Comparative Strategy* 29 (5): 412–431.

Kroneberg, Clemens, and Andreas Wimmer. 2012. "Struggling over the Boundaries of Belonging: A Formal Model of National Building, Ethnic Closure, and Populism." *American Journal of Sociology* 118 (1): 176–230.

Kruglanski, Arie W., and Wolfgang Stroebe. 2014. "The Influence of Beliefs and Goals on Attitudes: Issues of Structure, Function, and Dynamics." Pp. 323–368 in *The Handbook of Attitudes*, edited by Albarracin Dolores, T. Johnson Blair and P. Zanna Mark. Mahwah, NJ: Psychology.

Kruglanski, Arie W., Katarzyna Jasko, Marina Chernikova, Michelle Dugas, and David Webber. 2017. "To the Fringe and Back: Violent Extremism and the Psychology of Deviance." *American Psychologist* 72 (3): 217–230.

Krulichova, Eva. 2019. "The Relationship between Fear of Crime and Risk Perception across Europe." *Criminology & Criminal Justice* 19 (2): 197–214.

Krumrei-Mancuso, Elizabeth J. 2017. "Intellectual Humility and Prosocial Values: Direct and Mediated Effects." *Journal of Positive Psychology* 12 (1): 13–28.

Krupp, Daniel Brian, Lindsay A. Sewall, Martin L. Lalumière, Craig Sheriff, and Grant T. Harris. 2012. "Nepotistic Patterns of Violent Psychopathy: Evidence for Adaptation?" *Frontiers in Psychology* 3: 305.

Kruse, Keven M. 2015. *One Nation under God: How Corporate America Invented Christian America.* New York, NY: Basic.

Krys, Kuba, Yukiko Uchida, Shigehiro Oishi, and Ed Diener. 2019. "Open Society Fosters Satisfaction: Explanation to Why Individualism Associates with Country Level Measures of Satisfaction." *Journal of Positive Psychology* 14(6):768–78.

Krzyzanowski, Michał. 2020. "Discursive Shifts and the Normalisation of Racism: Imaginaries of Immigration, Moral Panics and the Discourse of Contemporary Right-Wing Populism." *Social Semiotics* 30 (4): 503–527.

Kuiper, Nicholas A., and Sorrel Nicholl. 2004. "Thoughts of Feeling Better? Sense of Humor and Physical Health." *Humor* 17 (1/2): 37–66.

Kukreja, Sunil, and James D. Miley. 1989. "Government Repression: A Test of the Conflict, World-System Position, and Modernization Hypotheses." *International Journal of Contemporary Sociology* 26 (3–4): 147–157.

Kulik, Liat. 2002. "The Impact of Social Background on Gender-role Ideology: Parents' versus Children's Attitudes." *Journal of Family Issues* 23 (1): 53–73.

Kullgen, John. 1995. *Autonomy and Intervention: Parentalism in the Caring Life.* New York: Oxford University Press.

Kumlin, Staffan, Miroslav Nemčok, and Arno Van Hootegem. 2025. "Welfare State Evaluations, Normative Expectations, and Political Trust: Longitudinal Evidence from Germany and Norway." *Public Management Review.*

Kung, Winnie W. 2003. "'Chinese Americans' Help Seeking for Emotional Distress." *Social Service Review* 77: 110–134.

Kunovich, Robert M. 2009. "The Sources and Consequences of National Identification." *American Sociological Review* 74: 573–593.

Kunovich, Robert M., and Randy Hudson. 1999. "Civil War, Social Integration and Mental Health in Croatia." *Journal of Health & Social Behavior* 40: 323–343.

Kunovich, Robert M., and Randy. Hodson. 1999. "Conflict, Religious Identity, and Ethnic Intolerance in Croatia." *Social Forces* 78 (2): 643–669.

Kunst, Jonas R., Talieh Sadeghi, Hajra Tahir, David Sam, and Lotte Thomsen. 2016. "The Vicious Circle of Religious Prejudice: Islamophobia Makes the Acculturation Attitudes of Majority and Minority Members Clash." *European Journal of Social Psychology* 46 (2): 249–259.

Kuper, Niclas, Lara Kroencke, Gabriella M. Harari, and Jaap J. A. Denissen. 2023 Who Benefits from Which Activity? On the Relations between Personality Traits, Leisure Activities, and Well-Being". *Journal of Personality & Social Psychology* 125(1), 141–72. Fields, Scott A., and John R. McNamara. 2003. "The Prevention of Child and Adolescent Violence: A Review. *Aggression & Violent Behavior* 8: 61–91.

Kuperus, Tracy, and Richard Asante. 2021. "Christianity, Citizenship, and Political Engagement among Ghanaian Youth." *African Studies Quarterly* 20 (2): 37–61.

Kuppens, Toon, Russell Spears, Antony S. R. Manstead, Bram Spruyt, and Matthew J. Easterbrook. 2018. "Educationism and the Irony of Meritocracy: Negative Attitudes of Higher Educated People Towards the Less Educated." *Journal of Experimental Social Psychology* 76: 429–447.

Kurz, Tim, and Ngaire Donaghue. 2013. "Gender and Discourse." Pp.61–77 in *The SAGE Handbook of Gender Psychology*, edited by Michelle K. Ryan and Nyla R. Branscombe. London: SAGE.

Kutlaca, Maja, Martijn van Zomeren, and Kai Epstude. 2020. "Friends or Foes? How Activists and Nonactivists Perceive and Evaluate Each Other." *PLoS ONE* 15 (4): e0230918.

Kwak, Dae-Hoon., Chaudia E. San, and Miguel, and Diana L. Carreon. 2010. "Political Legitimacy and Public Confidence in Police: An Analysis of Attitudes toward Mexican Police." *Policing* 35 (1): 124–146.

Kwan, Alex Yui-huen, and Beatrice Kwai-king Law. 1994. "Attitudes of Student/Pupil Nurses toward the Aged in Hong Kong: Implications for Nursing Education." *Hong Kong Journal of Gerontology* 8 (1): 43–51.

Kwan, Letty Y.-Y., and Chi-yue Chiu. 2018. "Cultural Diversity, Fractionalization and Economic Complexity: Effects on Innovation Performance and Human Development." Pp. 105–121 in *Handbook of Culture and Creativity: Basic Processes and Applied Innovations*. New York, NY: Oxford University Press.

Kwok, Sylvia Y. C. L., Leveda Cheng, Bonnie W. Y. Chow, and Chloe C. Y. Ling. 2015. "The Spillover Effect of Parenting on Marital Satisfaction Among Chinese Mothers." *Journal of Child and Family Studies* 24 (3): 772–783.

Kyriacou, Andreas P. 2020. *Inequality and Governance*. Abingdon, UK: Routledge.

La Grange, Adrienne, and Ngai Ming Yip. 2001. "Social Belonging, Social Capital and the Promotion of Home Ownership: A Case Study of Hong Kong." *Housing Studies* 16 (3): 291–310.

La Grange, Adrienne. 2011. "Neighbourhood and Class: A Study of Three Neighbourhoods in Hong Kong." *Urban Studies* 48 (6): 1181–1200.

Labonne, Julien, and Robert S. Chase. 2011. "Do Community-driven Development Projects Enhance Social Capital? Evidence from the Philippines." *Journal of Development Economics* 96: 348–358.

Labrecque, Lauren I. 2014. "Fostering Consumer-Brand Relationships in Social Media Environments: The Role of Parasocial Interaction." *Journal of Interactive Marketing* 28 (2): 134–148.

Ladouceur, Robert, Normand Boudreault, Christian Jacques, and Frank Vitaro. 1999. "Pathological Gambling and Related Problems among Adolescents." *Journal of Child & Adolescent Substance Abuse* 8 (4): 55–68.

Lagerwey, John. 2010. *China: A Religious State*. Hong Kong, China: University of Hong Kong Press.

Lahey, Benjamin B., and Irwin D. Waldman. 2007. "Personality Dispositions and the Development of Violence and Conduct Problems." Pp.260–287 in *The Cambridge Handbook of Violent Behavior and Aggression*, edited by Daniel J. Flannery, Alexander T. Vazsonyi and Irwin D. Waldman. Cambridge, UK: Cambridge University Press.

Lahusen, Christian. 2021. *The Political Attitudes of Divided European Citizens: Public Opinion and Social Inequalities in Comparative and Relational Perspective*. Abingdon, UK: Routledge.

Lai, Julian, and Julia Tao. 2006. "Perception of Environmental Risks among the Chinese People." *International Journal of Environmental, Cultural, Economic & Social Sustainability* 1 (5): 125–158.

Lakoff, George. 2002. *Moral Politics: How Liberals and Conservatives Think*. Chicago, IL: University of Chicago Press.

Lakoff, George. 2006. *Thinking Points: Communicating Our American Values and Vision*. New York, NY: Farrar, Straus & Giroux.

Lakoff, George. 2009. *The Political Mind: A Cognitive Scientist's Guide to Your Brain and Its Politics*. New York, NY: Penguin.

Lambert, Nathaniel M., Steven M. Graham, Frank D. Fincham, and Tyler F. Stillman 2009. "A Changed Perspective: How Gratitude Can Affect Sense of Coherence through Positive Reframing." *Journal of Positive Psychology* 4 (6): 461–470.

Lambie, John A. 2008. "On the Irrationality of Emotion and the Rationality of Awareness." *Consciousness & Cognition* 17 (3): 946–971.

LaMothe, Ryan. 2012. "State-Corporate Capitalism, Political Polarization, and a Culture of Unquiet Desperation: A Pastoral Analysis and Responses." *Pastoral Psychology* 61 (1): 15–29.

Lancee, Bram, and Sergi Pardos-Prado. 2013. "Group Conflict Theory in a Longitudinal Perspective: Analyzing the Dynamic Side of Ethnic Competition." *International Migration Review* 47 (1): 106–131.

Lancee, Bram, and Jaap Dronkers. 2011. "Ethnic, Religious and Economic Diversity in Dutch Neighbourhoods: Explaining Quality of Contact with Neighbours, Trust in the Neighbourhood and Inter-Ethnic Trust." *Journal of Ethnic & Migration Studies* 37 (4): 597–618.

Land, Kenneth C., and Glenn Deane. 1992. "On the Large-sample Estimation of Regression Models with Spatial-or-network Effects Terms: A Two-stage Least Squares Approach." *Sociological Methodology* 22: 221–248.

Land, Kenneth C., Patricia L. McCall, and Daniel S. Nagin. 1996. "A Comparison of Poisson, Negative Binomial, and Semiparametric Mixed Poisson Regression Models with Empirical Applications to Criminal Careers Data." *Sociological Methods & Research* 24 (4): 387–442.

Landsberger, Stefan R. 2009. "Harmony, Olympic Manners and Morals: Chinese Television and the New Propaganda of Public Service Advertising." *European Journal of East Asian Studies* 8 (2): 331–355.

Lane, Dylan, and Danielle Sulikowski. 2017. "Bleeding-Heart Conservatives and Hard-Headed Liberals: The Dual Processes of Moral Judgements." *Personality & Individual Differences* 115: 30–34.

Lane, Robert E. 1991. *The Market Experience*. Cambridge, UK: Cambridge University Press.

Lange, Jens, Liz Redford, and Jan Crusius. 2019. "A Status-Seeking Account of Psychological Entitlement." *Personality & Social Psychology Bulletin* 45 (7): 1113–1128.

Lange, Matthew, and Andrew Dawson. 2009. "Dividing and Ruling the World? A Statistical Test of the Effects of Colonisation on Postcolonial Civil Violence." *Social Forces* 88 (2): 785–818.

Langenderfer, Jeff, and Terence A. Shimp. 2001. "Consumer Vulnerability to Scams, Swindles, and Fraud: A New Theory of Visceral Influences on Persuasion." *Psychology & Marketing* 18 (7): 763–783.

Langman, Lauren. 2005. "From Virtual Public Spheres to Global Justice: A Critical Theory of Internetworked Social Movements." *Sociological Theory* 23 (1): 42–74.

Lapan, Richard T., Norman C. Gysbers, and Gregory F. Petroski. 2001. "Helping Seventh Graders Be Safe and Successful: A Statewide Study of the Impact of Comprehensive Guidance and Counseling Programs." *Journal of Counseling & Development* 79: 320–330.

Laroche, Hervé, Véronique. Steyer, and Christelle Théron. 2019. "How Could You Be So Gullible? Scams and Over-Trust in Organizations." *Journal of Business Ethics* 160 (3): 641–656.

Larsen, Christian Albrekt. 2013. *The Rise and Fall of Social Cohesion: The Construction and Deconstruction of Social Trust in the US, UK, Sweden, and Denmark*. Oxford, UK: Oxford University Press.

Larsen, Knud S. 2018. *Adaptation and Well-Being: Meeting the Challenges of Life*. Abingdon, UK: Routledge.

Larsen, Sean. 2015. "Natural Law and the 'Sin Against Nature.'" *Journal of Religious Ethics* 43 (4): 629–673.

Larson, Reed W. 2000. "Toward a Psychology of Positive Youth Development." *American Psychologist* 55 (1): 170–183.

Larson, Reed W., Kathrin C. Walker, and Gina McGovern. 2020. "Youth Programs as Contexts for Development of Ethical Judgment and Action." Pp. 552–559 in *The Oxford Handbook of Moral*

Development: An Interdisciplinary Perspective, edited by Lene Arnett Jensen. New York, NY: Oxford University Press.
Laruffa, Francesco. 2020. "What is a Capability-enhancing Social Policy? Individual Autonomy, Democratic Citizenship and the Insufficiency of the Employment-focused Paradigm." *Journal of Human Development & Capabilities* 21 (1): 1–16.
Lasch, Christopher. 1984. *The Minimal Self: Psychic Survival in Troubled Times*. New York, NY: Norton.
Lassey, Marie L., William R. Lassey, and Martin J. Jinks. 1997. *Health Care Systems around the World: Characteristics, Issues, Reforms*. Upper Saddle River, NJ: Prentice Hall.
Lau, Anna L.D.., Iris Chi, Robert A. Cummins, Tatia M.C.. Lee, and Kee-L. Chou, and Lawrence W.M. Chung. 2008. "The SARS (Severe Acute Respiratory Syndrome) Pandemic in Hong Kong: Effects on the Subjective Wellbeing of Elderly and Younger People." *Ageing & Mental Health* 12 (6): 746–760.
Lau, Maggie, and Wanxin Li. 2011. "The Extent of Family and School Social Capital Promoting Positive Subjective Well-being among Primary School children in Shenzhen, China." *Children & Youth Services Review* 33: 1573–1582.
Lau, Patrick S.Y.., Man Tak Yuen, and Raymond M.C.. Chan. 2005. "Do Demographic Characteristics Make a Difference to Burnout among Hong Kong Secondary School Teachers?" *Social Indicators Research* 71: 491–516.
Lauder, William, Kerry Mummery, and Siobhan Sharkey. 2006. "Social Capital, Age and Religiosity in People Who Are Lonely." *Journal of Clinical Nursing* 15 (3): 334–340.
Launay, Jacques, and Robin I. M. Dunbar. 2015. "Does Implied Community Size Predict Likeability of a Similar Stranger?" *Evolution & Human Behavior* 36 (1): 32–37.
Laurence, James. 2011. "The Effect of Ethnic Diversity and Community Disadvantage on Social Cohesion: A Multi-level Analysis of Social Capital and Interethnic Relations in UK Communities." *European Sociological Review* 27 (1): 70–89.
Lauriola, Marco, Renato Foschi, and Luca Marchegiani. 2015. "Integrating Values and Cognitive Style in a Model of Right-Wing Radicalism." *Personality & Individual Differences* 75: 147–153.
Lavis, John N., and Gregory L. Stoddart. 2003. "Social Cohesion and Health." Pp.121–149 in *Economic Implications of Social Cohesion*, edited by Lars Osberg. Toronto, Canada: University of Toronto Press.
Lavrijsen, Jeroen, and Ides Nicaise. 2017. "Returns on Vocational Education over the Life Cycle: Between Immediate Labour Market Preparation and Lifelong Employability." *International Review of Education* 63 (2): 257–280.
Lavy, Shiri, Mario Mikulincer, and Phillip R. Shaver. 2010. "Autonomy's Proximity Imbalance: An Attachment Theory Perspective on Intrusiveness in Romantic Relationships." *Personality & Individual Differences* 48: 552–556.
Law, Kam-yee. 2009. "The Portrayal of Chinese Top Party-state Leaders in the American Mainstream News Media, 1978–2008: Thirty Years of Reform Have Not Changed Chinese Yet?" *China Report* 45 (1): 35–51.
Lawler, Edward J. 2002. "Micro Social Order." *Social Psychology Quarterly* 65 (1): 4–17.
Lawler, Edward J., and Shane R. Thye. 2006. "Social Exchange Theory of Emotions." Pp. 295–320 in *Handbook of the Sociology of Emotions*, edited by Jan E. Stets and Jonathan H. Turner. Boston, MA: Springer.
Lawler, Edward J., Shane R. Thye, and Jeongkoo Yoon. 2009. *Social Commitments in a Depersonalized World*. New York: Russell Sage.
Lawler, Edward J., Shane R. Thye, and Jeongkoo Yoon. 2016. "The Problem of Social Order in Nested Group Structures." Pp. 149–166 in *Handbook of Contemporary Sociological Theory*, edited by Seth Abrutyn. Cham, Switzerland: Springer.
Lawrence, Rich L., and Steven E. Daniels. 1997. "Procedural Justice and Public Involvement in Natural Resource Decision Making." *Society & Natural Resources* 10 (6): 577–589.
Lawton, M. Powell., Miriam S. Moss, Laraine Winter, and Christine Hoffman. 2002. "Motivation in Later Life: Personal Projects and Well-being." *Psychology & Aging* 17 (4): 539–547.

Layous, Kristin, S. Katherine Nelson, Eva Oberle, Kimberly A. Schonert-Reichl, Sonja Lyubomirsky, and Frank Krueger. 2012. "Kindness Counts: Prompting Prosocial Behavior in Preadolescents Boosts Peer Acceptance and Well-Being." *PLoS ONE* 7 (12): e51380.

Le Monkhouse, Lien, Bradley R. Barnes, and Thi Song Hanh Pham. 2013. "Measuring Confucian Values among East Asian Consumers: A Four Country Study." *Asia Pacific Business Review* 19(3):320-36.

Leask, Marita. 2013. "From Bad Women to Mad Women: A Genealogical Analysis of Abortion Discourses in Aotearoa New Zealand." *New Zealand Sociology* 28 (2): 104–118.

Ledbetter, Andrew M., Heather M. Stassen-Ferrara, and Megan M. Dowd. 2013. "Comparing Equity and Self-Expansion Theory Approaches to Relational Maintenance." *Personal Relationships* 20 (1): 38–51.

Lee, Chien-chiang, and Chun-ping Chang. 2006. "Social Security Expenditure and GDP in OECD Countries: A Conintegrated Panel Analysis." *International Economic Journal* 20 (3): 303–320.

Lee, Ching Kwan, and Yonzhong Zhang. 2013. "The Power of Instability: Unraveling the Mirco-foundations of Bargained Authoritarianism in China." *American Journal of Sociology* 118 (6): 1475–1508.

Lee, Dan, Kap-Young. Jeong, and Sean Chae. 2011. "Measuring Social Capital in East Asia and Other World Regions: Index of Social Capital for 72 Countries." *Global Economic Review* 40 (4): 385–407.

Lee, Ellie. 2017. "Constructing Abortion as a Social Problem: 'Sex Selection' and the British Abortion Debate." *Feminism & Psychology* 27 (1): 15–33.

Lee, Francis L. F. 2022. "Pandemic Control and Public Evaluation of Government Performance in Hong Kong." *Chinese Journal of Communication* 15 (2): 284–302.

Lee, Francis L. F. 2022. "Pandemic Control and Public Evaluation of Government Performance in Hong Kong." *Chinese Journal of Communication* 15 (2): 284–302.

Lee, Francis L. F., and Joseph Man Chan. 2016. "Digital Media Activities and Mode of Participation in a Protest Campaign: A Study of the Umbrella Movement, Information." *Communication & Society* 19 (1): 4–22.

Lee, Francis L.F.. 2012. "Does Discussion with Disagreement Discourage All Topics of Political Participation? Survey Evidence from Hong Kong." *Communication Research* 39 (4): 543–562.

Lee, Francis L.F.., and Joseph M. Chan. 2011. *Media, Social Mobilization, and Mass Protests in Post-colonial Hong Kong*. Abingdon, UK: Routledge.

Lee, Jae Kook, and Renita Coleman. 2014. "Testing Generational, Life Cycle, and Period Effects of Age on Agenda Setting." *Mass Communication & Society* 17 (1): 3–25.

Lee, Kibeom, and Michael C. Ashton. 2012. "Getting Mad and Getting Even: Agreeableness and Honesty-Humility as Predictors of Revenge Intentions." *Personality & Individual Differences* 52 (5): 596–600.

Lee, Kin Cheung, Alice Oh, Qianru Zhao, Fang-Yi Wu, Shiyun Chen, Thomas Diaz, and Chez Kuang Ong. 2017. "Repentance in Chinese Buddhism: Implications for Mental Health Professionals." *Journal of Spirituality in Mental Health* 19 (3):210–26.

Lee, Yejin, Juliette L. Ratchford, Mason S. Ming, Rosemary L. Al-Kire, Perry L. Glanzer, Kevin D. Dougherty, and Sarah A. Schnitker. 2023. "A Person-Centered Approach to the Dark Triad Traits and Religiousness: Examining Differences in Intellectual Humility, Prosociality, and Mental Health in U.S. College Students." *Psychology of Religion & Spirituality* 16 (1): 93–103.

Lee-Baggley, Dayna, Anita DeLongis, Paul Voorhoeave, and Esther Greenglass. 2004. "Coping with the Threat of Severe Acute Respiratory Syndrome: Role of Threat Appraisals and Coping Responses in Health Behaviors." *Asian Journal of Social Psychology* 7: 9–12.

Lee-Treweek, Geraldine. 2002. "Trust in Complementary Medicine: The Case of Cranial Osteopathy." *Sociological Review* 50: 50–68.

Leflot, Geertje, Pol A. C. van Lier, Karine Verschueren, Patrick Onghena, and Hilde Colpin. 2011. "Transactional Associations among Teacher Support, Peer Social Preference, and Child Externalizing Behavior: A Four-wave Longitudinal Study." *Journal of Clinical Child & Adolescent Psychology* 40 (1): 87–99.

Lehmann, Curtis S., and Richard L. Gorsuch. 2017. "The Relevance of Religiousness and Reasoned Action for Adolescent Moral and Immoral Behavioral Intentions." *Psychology of Religion & Spirituality* 9 (S1): S49–S59.

Lehmann, Robert J. B., Alexander F. Schmidt, and Sara Jahnke. 2021. "Stigmatization of Paraphilias and Psychological Conditions Linked to Sexual Offending." *Journal of Sex Research* 58 (4): 438–447.

Lelli, Sara. 2008. "Operationalizing Sen's Capability Approach: The Influence of the Selected Technique." Pp.310–361 in *The Capability Approach: Concepts, Measures and Applications*, edited by Flavio Comim, Mozaffar Qizilbash and Sabina Alinre. Cambridge, UK: Cambridge University Press.

Lemay, Edward P., Arie W. Kruglanski, Erica Molinario, Maximilian Agostini, Jocelyn J. Bélanger, Ben Gützkow, Jannis Kreienkamp, Anne Margit Reitsema, Michelle R. vanDellen, PsyCorona Collaboration, and N. Pontus Leander. 2023. "The Role of Values in Coping with Health and Economic Threats of COVID-19." *Journal of Social Psychology* 163 (6): 755–772.

Lemay, Edward P., Jr., Margaret S. Clark, and Brooke C. Feeney. 2007. "Proportion of Responsiveness to Needs and the Construction of Satisfying Communal Relationships." *Journal of Personality & Social Psychology* 92(5):834–853. \103–312.

Lemon, M. C. 2003. *Philosophy of History: A Guide for Students*. London, UK: Routledge.

Lennartsson, Carin. 2010. "Need and Support: Determinants of Intra-familial Financial Transfers in Sweden." *International Journal of Social Welfare* 20: 66–74.

Lenz, A. Stephen. 2016. "Relational-Cultural Theory: Fostering the Growth of a Paradigm through Empirical Research." *Journal of Counseling & Development* 94 (4): 415–428.

Lenzi, Michela, Jill Sharkey, Alessio Vieno, Ashley Mayworm, Danielle Dougherty, and Karen Nylund-Gibson. 2015. "Adolescent Gang Involvement: The Role of Individual, Family, Peer, and School Factors in a Multilevel Perspective." *Aggressive Behavior* 41 (4): 386–397.

Leong, Chan-Hoong. 2008. "A Multilevel Research Framework for the Analyses of Attitudes toward Immigrants." *International Journal of Intercultural Relations* 32 (2): 115–129.

Lepkowski, James M., and Mick P. Couper. 2002. "Nonresponse in the Second Wave of Longitudinal Household Surveys." Pp.259–272 in *Survey Nonresponse*, edited by Robert M. Groves, Don A. Dillman, John L. Eltinge and Roderick J.A. Little. New York: John Wiley.

Letki, Natalia. 2006. "Investigating the Roots of Civic Morality: Trust, Social Capital, and Institutional Performance." *Political Behavior* 28: 305–325.

Letki, Natalia. 2008. "Does Diversity Erode Social Cohesion? Social Capital and Race in British Neighborhoods." *Political Studies* 56 (1): 99–126.

Leu, Chao-Hsien. Ke-Mei Chen, and Hsiu-Hui Chen. 2016. "A Multidimensional Approach to Child Poverty in Taiwan." *Children & Youth Services Review* 66:35-44.

Leung, Carson Kai-Sang., Syed K. Tanbeer, and Juan J. Cameron. 2014. "Interactive Discovery of Influential Friends from Social Networks." *Social Network Analysis & Mining* 4 (1): 154.

Leung, Chan-Hoong., and Colleen Ward. 2006. "Cultural Values in Attitudes toward Immigrants and Multiculturalism: The Case of the Eurobarometer Survey on Racism and Xenophobia." *International Journal of Intercultural Relations* 30: 799–810.

Leung, Joe C.B.., and Richard C. Nann. 1995. *Authority and Benevolence: Social Welfare in China*. Hong Kong: Chinese University Press.

Lever, Joaquina Palomar, Nuria Lanzagorta Pinol, and Jorge Hernandez Uralde. 2005. "Poverty, Psychological Resources and Subjective Well-being." *Social Indicators Research* 73: 375–408.

Levesque, Gabriel, and Maude Benoit. 2020. "Legalize or Prohibit It? Quebec's Exceptionalism on Cannabis Regulation and the Framing of Evidence in Policymaking." *American Review of Canadian Studies* 50 (3): 371–385.

Levi, Margaret, and Laura Strker. 2000. "Political Trust and Trustworthiness." *Annual Review of Political Science* 3: 475–507.

Levin, Jeffrey S., and Linda M. Chatters. 1998. "Research on Religion and Mental Health: An Overview on Empirical Findings and Theoretical Issues." Pp.33–50 in *Handbook of Religion and Mental Health*, edited by Harold G. Konenig. San Diego, CA: Academic.

Levitt, Mary J., and Ayse Cici-Gokaltun. 2011. "Close Relationships across the Life Span." Pp.457–486 in *Handbook of Life-Development*, edited by Karen L. Fingerman, Cynthia A. Berg, Jacque Smith and Toni C. Antonucci. New York: Springer.

Levitt, Steven D., and Lance Lochner. 2001. "The Determinants of Juvenile Crime." Pp.327–373 in *Risky Behavior among Youth: An Economic Analysis*, edited by Jonathan Gruber. Chicago, IL: University of Chicago Press.

Lewicki, Roy J., and Beth Polin. 2013. "Trust and Negotiation." Pp. 161–190 in *Handbook of Research on Negotiation*, edited by Mara Olekalns and Wendi L. Adair. Cheltenham, UK: Elgar.

Lewin-Epstein, Noah, Amit Kaplan, and Asaf Levanon. 2003. "Distributive Justice and Attitudes toward the Welfare State." *Social Justice Research* 16 (1): 1–27.

Lewis, Penney. 2001. "Rights Discourse and Assisted Suicide." *American Journal of Law & Medicine* 27 (1): 45–99.

Li, Bingqin, and Guy Mayraz. 2017. "Infrastructure Spending in China Increases Trust in Local Government." *Social Indicators Research* 132 (1): 341–356.

Li, Chunkai, Song Wang, Yajun Zhao, Feng Kong, and Jingguang Li. 2017. "The Freedom to Pursue Happiness: Belief in Free Will Predicts Life Satisfaction and Positive Affect among Chinese Adolescents." *Frontiers in Psychology* 7: 02027.

Li, Gu, Will W. L. Sham, and Wang Ivy Wong. 2023. "Are Romantic Orientation and Sexual Orientation Different? Comparisons Using Explicit and Implicit Measurements." *Current Psychology* 42(28):24288-24301.

Li, H. 2021. *The Relationship between Regime Type and Civic Education, Governance and Citizenship in Asia.* Singapore: Springer.

Li, Han Z., Zhi Zhang, Gira Bhatt, and Young-Ok Yum. 2006. "Rethinking Culture and Self-Construal: China as a Middle Land." *Journal of Social Psychology* 146(5):591-610.

Li, Hui, Ting Gong, and Hanyu Xiao. 2016. "The Perception of Anti-corruption Efficacy in China: An Empirical Analysis." *Social Indicators Research* 125 (3): 885–903.

Li, Ji. 2003. "Strategic Human Resource Management and MNEs' Performance in China." *International* Journal of *Human Resource Management* 14(2):157-173.

Li, Jin, Yu Sun, Mei Li, Hui"e Li, Wei Fan, and Yiping Zhong. 2020. "Social Distance Modulates Prosocial Behaviors in the Gain and Loss Contexts: An Event-Related Potential (ERP) Study." *International Journal of Psychophysiology* 150:83-91.

Li, Jingpeng, and Dingguo Song. 1992. "Political Consciousness and Political Behavior of Contemporary China's Youth. Beijing, China: China's People Public Order University. Filho, Mario Gloria, and João Gabriel Modesto. 2019. Morality, Activism and Radicalism in the Brazilian Left and the Brazilian Right." *Trends in Psychology* 27 (3): 763–777.

Li, Mengfan. 2023a. "The Adjustment of Social Trust and Internet Use on Cognitive Bias in Social Status: Perspective of Performance Perception." *Asian Journal of Social Psychology* 26 (2): 270–286.

Li, Mianguan, and Robert Walker. 2018. "Targeting Social Assistance: Dibao and Institutional Alienation in Rural China." *Social Policy & Administration* 52 (3): 771–789.

Li, Na and Mang He. 2022. "Social Security Satisfaction and People's Subjective Wellbeing in China: The Serial Mediation Effect of Social Fairness and Social Trust." *Frontiers in Psychology* 13:855530.

Li, Qiong, and Marilynn B. Brewer. 2004. "What Does It Mean to Be an American? Patriotism, Nationalism and American Identity after 9/11." *Political Psychology* 25 (5): 727–739.

Li, Shi. 2014. "How to Make a Grateful Child? Reflection on Gratitude Campaigns in China in Recent Years." *SAGE Open* 4 (4): 215824401455901.

Li, Shuxian, Xinyuan Fu, Mengyuan Zhang, Ruoran Fu, Mei Zhang, and Yu Kou. 2024. "Effect of Economic Inequality on Generosity: A Social Norm Perspective." *International Journal of Psychology* 59(6):801-811.

Li, Xiaoqing. 2023b. "Mobile Social Networking Sites for Emotional Support: Moderating Effect of Gender." *Current Psychology* 42 (10): 7998–8009.

Li, Yunqing, and Kenneth F. Ferraro. 2006. "Volunteering in Middle and Later Life: Is Health a Benefit, Barrier or Both?" *Social Forces* 85 (1): 497–518.

Li, Yu-sheng, and Ying-chih Chung. 2008. "Neighborhood Effects on an Individual's Health Using Neighborhood Measurements Developed by Factor Analysis and Cluster Analysis." *Journal of Urban Health* 86 (1):5-18.

Liang, Yan. 2010. "China and the Global Financial Crisis: Assessing the Impacts and Policy Responses." *China & World Economy* 18 (3): 56–72.

Licata, Laurent, and Olivier Klein. 2002. "Does European Citizenship Breed Xenophobia? European Identification as a Predictor of Intolerance towards Immigrants." *Journal of Community & Applied Social Psychology* 12: 323–337.

Lichterman, Paul. 2012. "Religion in Public Action." *Sociological Theory* 30 (1): 15–36.

Liebler, Carolyn A., and Gary D. Sandefur. 2002. "Gender Differences in the Exchange of Social Support with Friends, Neighbors, and Coworkers at Midlife." *Social Science Research* 31: 364–391.

Like, Taya Z. 2011. "Urban Inequality and Racial Differences in Risk for Violent Victimization." *Crime & Delinquency* 57 (3): 432–457.

Lilly, J. Robert, Francis T. Cullen, and Richard A. Ball. 2011. *Criminological Theory: Context and Consequences*. Los Angeles, CA: SAGE.

Lim, Chaeyoon, and Robert D. Putnam. 2010. "Religion, Social Networks, and Life Satisfaction." *American Sociological Review* 75 (6): 914–933.

Lim, Joseph Y., and Manuel F. Montes. 2000. "The Structure of Employment and Structural Adjustment in the Philippines." *Journal of Development Studies* 36 (4): 149–181.

Lim, Lena L. 2009. "The Influences of Harmony Motives and Implicit Beliefs on Conflict Styles of the Collectivist." *International Journal of Psychology* 44 (6): 401–409.

Lin, Chun-Hung A., Suchandra Lahiri, and Ching-Po Hsu. 2015. "Population Aging and Regional Income Inequality in Taiwan: A Spatial Dimension." *Social Indicators Research* 122(3):757-777.

Lin, Cunguang. 2003. *Formation of Confucian China: Evolution of Early Confucianism and Chinese Political Culture*. Jinan, China: Qi Lu Book.

Lin, Delia. 2017. *Civilising Citizens in Post-Mao China: Understanding the Rhetoric of Suzhi*. Abington, UK: Routledge.

Lin, Ka, Yun Xu, Tianhai Huang, and Jiahua Zhang. 2013. "Social Exclusion and Its Cause in East Asian Societies: Evidence from SQSQ Survey Data." *Social Indicators Research* 112(3):641-660.

Lin, Shen. 2018. "We Work Like Ants…We Avoid Being Troublemakers: An Exploratory Inquiry on Resilience of Chinese Street Vendors in the Urban Village." *International Journal of Sociology & Social Policy* 38 (11/12): 1024–1040.

Lin, Yi-Ying, Dena Phillips Swanson, and Ronald David Rogge. 2021. "The Three Teachings of East Asia (TTEA) Inventory: Developing and Validating a Measure of the Interrelated Ideologies of Confucianism, Buddhism, and Taoism." *Frontiers in Psychology* 12: 626122.

Lindblad, Mark R., Kim R. Manturuk, and Roberto G. Quercia. 2013. "Sense of Community and Informal Social Control among Lower Income Households: The Role of Homeownership and Collective Efficacy in Reducing Subjective Neighborhood Crime and Disorder." *American Journal of Community Psychology* 51 (1–2): 123–139.

Lindstrom, Martin, and Maria Rosvall. 2015. "Life Course Perspectives on Economic Stress and Generalized Trust in Other People." *Social Science Journal* 53 (1): 7–13.

Lineres, L. Oriann. 2004. "Social Connection to Neighbors, Multiple Victimization, and Current Health among Women Residing in High Crime Neighborhoods." *Journal of Family Violence* 19 (6): 355–366.

Lingiadi, Vittorio, and Paloa Capozzi. 2004. "Psychoanalytic Attitudes towards Homosexuality: An Empirical Research." *International Journal of Psychoanalysis* 85: 137–158.

Linquiti, Peter D. 2023. *Rebooting Policy Analysis: Strengthening the Foundation, Expanding the Scope*.Thousand Oaks, CA: SAGE.

Lipford, Jody W., and Bruce Yandle. 2009. "The Determinants of Purposeful Voluntarism." *Journal of Socio-Economics* 38 (1): 72–79.
Lippa, Richard A. 2005. *Gender, Nature, and Nurture*, 2nd ed. Mahwah, NJ: Lawrence Erlbaum.
Lista, Peter, and Fabio Rojas. 2018. "Institutions." Pp. 312–329 in *The SAGE Handbook of Political Sociology*, edited by William Outhwaite and Stephen Turner. London, UK: SAGE.
Litman, Jordan A., Oliver C. Robinson, and James D. Demetre. 2017. "Intrapersonal Curiosity: Inquisitiveness about the Inner Self." *Self & Identity* 16 (2): 231–250.
Littlejohn, Stephen W., Karen A. Foss, and John G. Oetzel. 2017. *Theories of Human Communication.* Long Grove, IL: Waveland.
Liu, Aichun, Shichao Wang, Renjie Li, Yulei Chen, Zhaojun Chen, and Jianpeng Guo. 2025 "The Impact of Perception of School Moral Atmosphere on College Students' Moral Sensitivity." *Ethics & Behavior*.
Liu, Bingsheng, Yu Zhai, Yan Li, Ling Li, Guobin Wu, and Si Chen. 2023. "Effects of Social Influence on Relationships among Citizens' Expectation Confirmation, Satisfaction and Acceptance under Different Urban Renewal Compensation Modes." *Public Performance & Management Review* 46 (6): 1413–1441.
Liu, Fengbo, Ning Li, and Yue Xi. 2024. "Impacts of Family Functioning on Social Avoidance and Distress among People with Disabilities: A Moderated Mediating Model." *Current Psychology* 43 (24): 21072–21082.
Liu, James H. and Felicia Pratto 2018. "Colonization, Decolonization, and Power Ruptures and Cultural Junctures out of Dominance." Pp. 261–280 in *The Oxford Handbook of Social Psychology*, edited by Phillp L. Hammack. New York, NY: Oxford University Press.
Liu, James, Rebekah Goldstein Hawes, Dennis Hilton, Li-li Huang, Cecilia Gastardo-Conaco, Emma Dresler Hawke, Florence Pittolo, Ying-ying Hong, Colleen Ward, Sheela Abraham, Yoshihisa Kashima, Emiko Kashima, Megumi M. Ohashi, Masaki Yuki, and Yukako Hidaka. 2005. "Social Representation of Events and People in World History across 12 Cultures." *Journal of Cross-Cultural Psychology* 36 (2):1–21.
Liu, Jindian, Ning Neil Yu, Mingwang Cheng, and Chunyan Wu. 2023. "Internet Use and Better-Informed Divorce in China." *Behavioral Sciences* 13(2):177.
Liu, Mingtang, and Kellee S. Tsai. 2021. "Structural Power, Hegemony, and State Capitalism: Limits to China's Global Economic Power." *Politics & Society* 49 (2): 235–267.
Liu, Xianchen, and Jenn Yun Tein. 2005. "Life Events, Psychopathology, and Suicide Behavior in Chinese Adolescents." *Journal of Affective Disorders* 86: 195–203.
Liu, Zhangming. 2008. "Pondering Harmonious Development. Beijing, China: People. Lalander, Rickard and Maija Merimaa. 2018. The Discursive Paradox of Environmental Conflict: Between Ecologism and Economism in Ecuador." *Forum for Development Studies* 45 (3): 485–511.
Liu, Zhengjia, and Dan Berkowitz. 2014. "Where is our Steve Jobs? A Case Study of Consumerism and Neo-Liberal Media in China." *Journalism* 15 (8): 1006–1022.
Livingstone, Andrew G., Summer L. Bedford, Aya Afyouni, Ngoc Vu, Ioanna Kapantai, Damilola Makanju, Maria Chayinska, Roberto González, Pía Carozzi, Camila Contreras, Sarosha Byrne, Jennifer Guy, Lara King, Clarissa H. C. Lo, Harriet Pearson, and Calandra Tapp. 2023. "You Get Us, So You Like Us: Feeling Understood by an Outgroup Predicts More Positive Intergroup Relations Via Perceived Positive Regard." *Journal of Personality & Social Psychology* 126(2):262-281.
Lizardo, Omar. 2006. "How Cultural Tastes Shape Personal Networks." *American Sociological Review* 71 (5): 778–807.
Lizardo, Omar. 2016. "Cultural Theory." Pp. 99–120 in *Handbook of Contemporary Sociological Theory*, edited by Seth Abrutyn. Cham, Switzerland: Springer.
Lloyd, Christopher E. M., Brittney S. Mengistu, and Graham Reid. 2022. "His Main Problem Was Not Being in a Relationship with God": Perceptions of Depression, Help-Seeking, and Treatment in Evangelical Christianity. *Frontiers in Psychology* 13: 831534.
Lo, Ming-cheung Miriam., and Christopher P. Bettinger. 2009. "Civic Solidarity in Hong Kong and Taiwan." *China Quarterly* 197: 183–203.

Lo, Sonny Shiu-Hing. 2021. *The Dynamics of Peaceful and Violent Protests in Hong Kong: The Anti-Extradition Movement*, Singapore: Palgrave.

Loader, Ian, and Neil Walker. 2007. *Civilizing Security*. Cambridge, UK: Cambridge University Press.

Lobao, Linda, and Gregory Hooks. 2003. "Public Employment, Welfare Transfers, and Economic Well-Being across Local Populations: Does a Lean and Mean Government Benefit the Masses?" *Social Forces* 82 (2): 519–556.

Lobao, Linda, Lazarus Adua, and Gregory Hooks. 2014. "Privatization, Business Attraction and Social Services across the United States: Local Government's Use of Market-oriented, Neoliberal Policies in the Post-2000 Period." *Social Problems* 61 (4): 644–672.

Lochner, Kimberly, Ichiro Kawachi, Robert T. Brennan, and Stephen L. Burka. 2003. "Social Capital and Neighborhood Mortality Rates in Chicago." *Social Science & Medicine* 36: 1797–1805.

Lodewijkx, Hein F.M.., Gaby L.E.. "Kersten, and Martijn van Zomeren. 2008. Dual Pathways to Engage in Silent Marches against Violence: Moral Outrage, Moral Cleansing and Modes of Identification." *Journal of Community & Applied Social Psychology* 8: 153–167.

Loewy, Erich H. 1993. *Freedom and Community: The Ethics of Interdependence*. Albany, NY: State University of New York Press.

Lofors, Jonas, and Kristina Sundquist. 2007. "Law-linking Social Capital as a Predictor of Mental Disorders: A Cohort Study of 4.5 Million Swedes." *Social Science & Medicine* 64: 21–34.

Loftus, Jeni. 2001. "America??s Liberalization in Attitudes toward Homosexuality, 1973–1998." *American Sociological Review* 66: 762–782.

Logan, Jill M., and Rebecca J. Cobb. 2013. "Trajectories of Relationship Satisfaction: Independent Contributions of Capitalization and Support Perceptions." *Personal Relationships* 20 (2): 277–293.

Loh, Christine, and Kee Foong. 2005. *Hong Kong as a World City: Assessing Its Attractiveness to Global Talent*. Hong Kong: Civic Exchange.

Loh, Dylan. 2017. "Defending China's National Image and Defensive Soft Power: The Case of Hong Kong's Umbrella Revolution." *Journal of Chinese Political Science* 22 (1): 117–134.

Lohman, Margaret C. 2006. "Factors Influencing Teachers' Engagement in Informal Learning Activities." *Journal of Workplace Learning* 18(3):141–56. \93–301.

Long, D. Adam., and Douglas D. Perkins. 2007. "Community Social and Place Predictors of Sense of Community: A Multilevel and Longitudinal Analysis." *Journal of Community Psychology* 35 (5): 563–581.

Loo, Jeff Hai-chi. 2020. "The Myth of Hong Kong Nationalism." *Asian Education & Development Studies* 9 (4): 535–545.

Lopez-Concepcion, Arelys, Ana Gil-Lacruz, Isabel Saz-Gil, and Víctor. Bazán-Monasterio. 2023. "Social Well-Being for a Sustainable Future: The Influence of Trust in Big Business and Banks on Perceptions of Technological Development from a Life Satisfaction Perspective in Latin America." *Sustainability* 15 (1): 628.

Lopez-Sanders, Laura, and Hana E. Brown. 2020. "Political Mobilisation and Public Discourse in New Immigrant Destinations: News Media Characterisations of Immigrants During the 2006 Immigration Marches." *Journal of Ethnic & Migration Studies* 46 (4): 820–838.

Louis, Vincent V., and Shanyang Zhao. 2002. "Effects of Family Structure, Family SES, and Adulthood Experience on Life Satisfaction." *Journal of Family Issues* 23 (8): 986–1005.

Louis, Winnifred R., Morgana Lizzio-Wilson, Mikaela Cibich, Craig McGarty, Emma F. Thomas, Catherine E. Amiot, Nathan Weber, Joshua Rhee, Grace Davies, Timothy Rach, Syasya Goh, Zoe McMaster, Orla Muldoon, Naoimh Howe, and Fathali Moghaddam. 2022. "Failure Leads Protest Movements to Support More Radical Tactics." *Social Psychological & Personality Science* 13 (3): 675–687.

Low, Sabina, and Joann Wu Shortt. 2017. "Family, Peer, and Pubertal Determinants of Dating Involvement among Adolescents." *Journal of Research on Adolescence* 27(1):78-87.

Lowe, Seana S. 2001. "The Art of Community Transformation." *Education & Urban Society* 33 (4): 457–471.

Lowndes, Vivien, and Mark Roberts. 2013. *Why Institutions Matter: The New Institutionalism in Political Science*. Houndmills, UK: Palgrave.
Lowrey-Kinberg, Belen, Hillary Mellinger, and Erin M. Kearns. 2020. "How Social Dominance Orientation Shapes Perceptions of Police." *Policing* 43 (4): 607–624.
Lu, Hong, Lening Zhang, and Terance D. Mieche. 2002. "Interdependency, Communitarianism and Reintegrative Shaming in China." *Social Science Journal* 39: 189–201.
Lu, Jie. 2014. "A Cognitive Anatomy of Political Trust and Respective Bases: Evidence from a Two-City Survey in China." *Political Psychology* 35 (4): 477–494.
Lu, Luo, and Shu-fang Kao. 2002. "Traditional and Modern Characteristics across the Generations: Similarities and Discrepancies." *Journal of Social Psychology* 142 (1): 45–59.
Lu, Peiqi, Jeewon Oh, Katelin E. Leahy, and William J. Chopik. 2021. "Friendship Importance around the World: Links to Cultural Factors, Health, and Well-Being." *Frontiers in Psychology* 11:570839.
Lu, Yao, and Donald J. Treiman. 2008. "The Effect of Sibship Size on Educational Attainment in China: Period Variations." *American Sociological Review* 73 (5): 813–834.
Lubbers, Mareel, Marcel Coenders, and Peer Scheepers. 2006. "Objections to Asylum Seeker Centres: Individual and Contextual Determinants of Resistance to Small and Large Centres in the Netherlands." *European Sociological Review* 32 (3): 243–257.
Lubell, Mark. 2003. "Collaborative Institutions, Belief-systems, and Perceived Policy Effectiveness." *Political Research Quarterly* 56 (3): 309–323.
Lubis, Syahid Izharuddin, and Agnes Sianipar. 2022. "How Religious Tolerance Can Emerge among Religious People: An Investigation on the Roles of Intellectual Humility, Cognitive Flexibility, and Trait Aggressiveness." *Asian Journal of Social Psychology* 25 (2): 276–287.
Lucas, Brian J., and Nour S. Kteily. 2018. "(Anti-)Egalitarianism Differentially Predicts Empathy for Members of Advantaged Versus Disadvantaged Groups." *Journal of Personality & Social Psychology* 114 (5): 665–692.
Lucas, Brian J., and Robert W. Livingston. 2014. "Feeling Socially Connected Increases Utilitarian Choices in Moral Dilemmas." *Journal of Experimental Social Psychology* 53: 1–4.
Lucas, Todd, Ludmila Zhdanova, Craig A. Wendorf, and Sheldon Alexander. 2013. "Procedural and Distributive Justice Beliefs for Self and Others: Multilevel Associations with Life Satisfaction and Self-Rated Health." *Journal of Happiness Studies* 14 (4): 1325–1341.
Luhmann, Maike, Richard E. Lucas, Michael Eid, and Ed Diener. 2013. "The Prospective Effect of Life Satisfaction on Life Events." *Social Psychological & Personality Science* 4(1):39–45.
Luk, Pattie Yuk, and Yee Fong. 2001. "Comparing Contexts for Developing Personal and Social Education in Hong Kong." *Comparative Education* 37 (1): 65–87.
Lundasen, Susanne Wallman, and Dag Wollebaek. 2013. "Diversity and Community Trust in Swedish Local Communities." *Journal of Elections, Public Opinion & Parties* 23 (3): 299–321.
Lupton, Deborah. 2013. *Risk*. Milton Park, UK: Routledge.
Luria, Gil, Ram A. Cnaan, and Amnon Boehm. 2019. "National Culture of Indulgence as Predictor of Prosocial Behavior: Governmental Effectiveness as Boundary Condition." *VOLUNTAS: International Journal of Voluntary and Nonprofit Organizations* 30 (5): 1164–1175.
Luthar, Timothy C. 2009. *Hegel's Critique of Modernity: Reconciling Individual Freedom and the Community*. Lanham, MD: Lexington.
Ly, Bora, and John Kwame Boateng. 2021. "China Quest for Global Governance Overhaul." *Cogent Social Sciences* 7 (1): 1932031.
Ly, Bora, and Richard Meissner. 2020. "China and Global Governance: Leadership through Bri." *Cogent Social Sciences* 6 (1): 1801371.
Lyng, Stephen, Rick Matthews, and William J. Miller. 2009. "Existentialism Edgework and the Contingent Body: Exploring the Criminalized Implications of Ultimate fighting." Pp. 94–126 in *Existentialist Criminology*, edited by Ronnie Lippens and Don Crewe. Abingdon, UK: Routledge-Cavendish.
Lynxwiler, John, and David Gay. 2000. "Moral Boundaries and Deviant Music: Public Attitudes toward Heavy Metal and Rap." *Deviant Behavior* 21 (1): 63–85.

Lytkina, Ekaterina and Tim Reeskens. 2025. "Rally around the Government or a Populist Response? How Concerns About Covid-19 and Emotional Responses Relate to Institutional Trust and Support for Right-Wing Populism." *American Behavioral Scientist.*

Lyubomirsky, Sonja, Chris Tkach, and M. Robin DiMatteo. 2006. "What Are the Differences between Happiness and Self-esteem?" *Social Indicators Research* 78:363–404. \d09–12.2.

Ma, Hing Keung, Ping Chung Cheung, and Daniel T.L.. Shek. 2007. "The Relation of Prosocial Orientation to Peer Interactions, Family Social Environment and Personality of Chinese Adolescents." *International Journal of Behavioral Development* 31 (1): 12–18.

Ma, Joyce L.C.., Timothy K.Y.. Wong, Yuk King Lau, and Shuk Han Pun. 2009. "Perceived Family Functioning and Family Resources of Hong Kong Families: Implications for Social Work Practice." *Journal of Family Social Work* 12: 244–263.

Ma, Mac Zewei. 2021. Testing the Parasite-Stress Theory of Sociality Based on the Circular Model of Human Values: A Multilevel Analysis Approach. *Personality & Individual Differences* 168: 110277.

Maass, Anne, Mara Carinu, and Silvia Galdi. 2013. "Sexual Harassment: Motivations and Consequences." Pp.341–388 in *The SAGE Handbook of Gender and Psychology*, edited by Michelle K. Ryan and Myla R. Branscombe. London, UK: SAGE.

Macedo, Stephen. 2021. "Populism, Localism and Democratic Citizenship." *Philosophy & Social Criticism* 47 (4): 447–476.

MacGregor, Casimir, Alan Petersen, and Christine Parker. 2021. "Promoting a Healthier, Younger You: The Media Marketing of Anti-Ageing Superfoods." *Journal of Consumer Culture* 21 (2): 164–179.

Macias, Thomas. 2015. "Risks, Trust, and Sacrifice: Social Structural Motivators for Environmental Change." *Social Science Quarterly* 96 (5): 1264–1276.

Mackinnon, Sean P. 2012. "Perceived Social Support and Academic Achievement: Cross-Lagged Panel and Bivariate Growth Curve Analyses." *Journal of Youth and Adolescence* 41 (4): 474–485.

Macmillan, Ross, and Arturo Baiocchi. 2010. "Conceptualizing the Dynamics of Lives and Historical Times: Life Course Phenomena, Institutional Dynamics and Sociohistorical Change." Pp.73–97 in *Social Change and Human Development: Concept and Results*, edited by Rainer K. Silbereisen. Los Angeles, CA: SAGE.

Madsen, Richard. 2002. "Confucian Conceptions of Civil Society." Pp.190–204 in *Alternative Conception of Civil Society*, edited by Simone Chambers and Will Kymlicka. Princeton, NJ: Princeton University Press.

Magdol, Lynn, and Diane R. Bessel. 2003. "Social Capital, Social Currency, and Portable Assets: The Impacts of Residential Mobility on Exchanges of Social Support." *Personal Relationships* 10: 149–169.

Magee, Marc Porter. 2008. "Civic Participation and Social Capital: A Social Network Analysis in Two American Counties." Pp.308–327 in *Social Capital: An International Research Program*, edited by Nan Lin and Bonnie H. Erickson. Oxford, UK: Oxford University Press.

Magnani, Elisabetta, and Rong Zhu. 2018. "Does Kindness Lead to Happiness? Voluntary Activities and Subjective Well-Being." *Journal of Behavioral & Experimental Economics* 77: 20–28.

Mahfud, Yara, Constantina Badea, Maykel Verkuyten, and Kate Reynolds. 2018. "Multiculturalism and Attitudes toward Immigrants: The Impact of Perceived Cultural Distance." *Journal of Cross-Cultural Psychology* 49 (6): 945–958.

Mahmud, Rifat. 2021. "What Explains Citizen Trust in Public Institutions? Quality of Government, Performance, Social Capital, or Demography." *Asia Pacific Journal of Public Administration* 43 (2): 106–124.

Mahoney, Dennis J. 2004. *Politics and Progress: The Emergence of American Political Science.* Lanham, MD: Lexington.

Mahoney, James. 2021. *The Logic of Social Science.* Princeton, NJ: Princeton University Press.

Mair, Christine A., Feinian Chen, Guangya Liu, and Jonathan R. Brauer. 2016. "Who in the World Cares? Gender Gaps in Attitudes toward Support for Older Adults in 20 Nations." *Social Forces* 95 (1): 411–438.

Major, Brenda, Mark Appelbaum, Linda Beckman, Mary Ann Dutton, Nancy Felipe Russo, and Carolyn West. 2009. “Abortion and Mental Health: Evaluating the Evidence.” *American Psychologist* 64 (9): 863–890.

Makarios, Matthew D., and Tara L. Sams. 2013. “Social Support and Crime.” Pp.160–185 in *The Oxford Handbook of Criminological Theory*, edited by Francis T. Cullen and Pamela Wilcox. New York: Oxford University Press.

Makhanova, Anastasia, and Melissa A. Shepherd. 2020. “Behavioral Immune System Linked to Responses to the Threat of Covid-19.” *Personality & Individual Differences* 167: 110221.

Malahy, Lori W., Michelle A. Rubinlicht, and Cheryl R. Kaiser. 2009. “Justifying Inequality: A Cross-temporal Investigation of U.S. Income Disparities and Just-world Beliefs from 1973 and 2006.” *Social Justice Research* 22: 369–383.

Malesevic, Siniša. 2022. *Why Humans Fight: The Social Dynamics of Close-Range Violence*. Cambridge, UK: Cambridge University Press.

Malizia, Emil, Edward Feser, Henry Renski, and Joshua Drucker. 2021. *Understanding Local Economic Development*. Abingdon, UK: Routledge.

Malka, Ariel, and Christopher J. Soto. 2011. “The Conflicting Influences of Religiosity on Attitude toward Torture.” *Personality & Social Psychology Bulletin* 37 (8): 1091–1103.

Mallinas, Stephanie R., Jarret T. Crawford, and Jeremy A. Frimer. 2020. “Subcomponents of Right-Wing Authoritarianism Differentially Predict Attitudes toward Obeying Authorities.” *Social Psychological & Personality Science* 11 (1): 134–143.

Malone, David M. and Rohinton P. Medhora. 2020. “Multilateralism.” In *The SAGE Handbook of Political Science*, edited by Dirk Berg-Schlosser, Bertrand Badie and Leonardo Morlino. London, UK: SAGE.

Maloutas, Thomas, and Maro Pantelidou Malouta. 2004. “The Glass Menagerie of Urban Governance and Social Cohesion: Concepts and Stakes / Concepts as Stakes.” *International Journal of Urban & Regional Research* 28 (2): 449–465.

Maltseva, Kateryna. 2016. “Prosocial Morality in Individual and Collective Cognition.” *Journal of Cognition & Culture* 16 (1–2): 1–36.

Man, Derek C., and Simon S.K.. Lam. 2003. “The Effects of Job Complexity and Autonomy on Cohesiveness in Collectivistic and Individualistic Work Groups: A Cross-cultural Analysis.” *Journal of Organizational Behavior* 24 (8): 979–994.

Manassis, Katharina. 2017. *Developing Empathy: A Biopsychosocial Approach to Understanding Compassion for Therapists and Parents*. New York, NY: Routledge.

Mancini, Anthony D., Gabriele Prati, and George A. Bonanno. 2011. “Do Shattered Worldviews Lead to Complicated Grief? Prospective and Longitudinal Analyses.” *Journal of Social & Clinical Psychology* 30 (2): 184–215.

Mancini, Christina, Justin T. Pickett, Kristen M. Budd, Stephanie Bontrager, and Dominique Roe-Sepowitz. 2020. “Examining Policy Preferences for Prostitution Regulation among American Males: The Influence of Contextual Beliefs.” *Criminal Justice Review* 45 (4): 413–429.

Mangum, Maruice. 2012. “Explaining African-American Political Trust: Examining Psychological Involvement, Policy Satisfaction, and Reference Group Effect.” *International Social Science Review* 87 (1&2): 3–18.

Mangum, Maruice. 2019. “Revisiting Economic Threat and Cultural Concerns: Public Opinion toward Immigration and Non-Citizens by Race.” *Social Science Research* 83: 102309.

Mannan, Md. 2007. “Student Attrition and Academic and Social Integration: Application of Tinto 's Model at the University of Papua New Guinea.” *Higher Education* 53(2):147-165.

Manning, Matthew, Christopher L. Ambrey, Christopher M. Fleming, and Shane D. Johnson. 2018. “The Impact of Field Court Attendance Notices on Property Crime in New South Wales, Australia.” *Journal of Quantitative Criminology* 34 (4): 971–998.

Manning, Matthew, Christopher M. Fleming, and Christopher L. Ambrey. 2016. “Life Satisfaction and Individual Willingness to Pay for Crime Reduction.” *Regional Studies* 50 (12): 2024–2039.

Mannion, Greg. 2003. "Children??s Participation in School Grounds Developments: Creating a Place for Education that Promotes Children??s Social Inclusion." *International Journal of Inclusive Education* 7 (2): 175–192.

Manturuk, Kim, Mark Lindblad, and Roberto Quercia. 2010. "Friends and Neighbors: Homeownership and Social Capital among Low- to Moderate-Income Families." *Journal of Urban Affairs* 32 (4): 471–488.

Mantzvavinos, C. 2011. "Institutions." Pp.399–412 in *The SAGE Handbook of the Philosophy of Social Sciences*, edited by Ian C. Jarvie and Jesus Zamora-Bonilla. London, UK: SAGE.

March, Evita. 2019. "Psychopathy, Sadism, Empathy, and the Motivation to Cause Harm: New Evidence Confirms Malevolent Nature of the Internet Troll." *Personality & Individual Differences* 141: 133–137.

Marcum, Christopher Steven. 2013. "Age Differences in Daily Social Activities." *Research on Aging* 35 (5): 612–640.

Mare, Robert D. 1996. "Demography and the Evolution of Educational Inequality." Pp.117–151 in *Social Differentiation and Social Inequality*, edited by James N. Barron, David B., Grusky, and Donald J. Treiman. Boulder, CO: Westview.

Marien, Sofie, and Marc Hooghe. 2011. "Does Political Trust Matter? An Empirical Investigation into The Relation Between Political Trust and Support for Law Compliance." *European Journal of Political Research* 50 (2): 267–291.

Marien, Sofie. 2011. "The Effect of Electoral Outcomes on Political Trust: A Multi-level Analysis of 23 Countries." *Electoral Studies* 30: 712–726.

Marien, Sofie. 2017. "Assessing the Role of Television, the Family, and the School in the Development of Political Trust in Adolescence." *Social Science Quarterly* 98 (3): 818–835.

Marini, Margaret Mooney, and Burton Singer. 1988. "Causality in the Social Sciences." Pp.347–409 in *Sociological Methodology 1988*, Vol.18, edited by Clifford C. Clogg. Washington, DC: American Sociological Association.

Markey, Patrick M., and Charlotte N. Markey. 2007. "The Interpersonal Meaning of Sexual Promiscuity." *Journal of Research in Personality* 41 (6): 1199–1212.

Markiewicz, Dorothy, Anna Beth Doyle, and Mara Brendgen. 2001. "The Quality of Adolescents' Friendships: Associations with Mothers' Interpersonal Relationships, Attachments to Parents and Friends, and Prosocial Behaviors." *Journal of Adolescence* 24 (4): 429–445.

Markowitz, Fred E. 2001. "Attitudes and Family Violence: Linking Intergenerational and Cultural Theories." *Journal of Family Violence* 16 (2): 205–218.

Markowski, Radoslaw. 2006. "Political Accountability and Institutional Design in New Democracies." *International Journal of Sociology* 36 (2): 45–75.

Marks, Nadine F. 1996. "Flying Solo at Midlife: Gender, Marital Status and Psychological Well-being." *Journal of Marriage and the Family* 58: 917–932.

Markus, Gregory B. 2001. "American Individualism Reconsidered." Pp.401–432 in *Citizens and Politics: Perspectives from Political Psychology*, edited by James H. Kukinski. Cambridge, UK: Cambridge University Press.

Marotta, Vince. 2017. *Theories of the Stranger: Debates on Cosmopolitanism, Identity and Cross-cultural Encounters*. Abington, UK: Routledge.

Marozzi, Marco. 2015. "Measuring Trust in European Public Institutions." *Social Indicators Research* 123 (3): 879–895.

Marres, Noortje. 2017. *Digital Sociology: The Reinvention of Social Research*. Cambridge, UK: Polity.

Marschall, Melissa J., and Dietlind Stolle. 2004. "Race and the City: Neighborhood Context and Development of Generalized Trust." *Political Behavior* 26 (2): 125–153.

Marsh, Dylan R., and Bryan J. Dik. 2021. "Beyond-the-Self Callings: The Role of a Transcendent Summons for Undergraduates and Working Adults." *Journal of Career Assessment* 29 (4): 570–588.

Marsh, Kerry L. and Harry M. Wallace. 2014. "The Influence of Beliefs and goals on Attitudes: Issues of Structure, Function, and Dynamics." Pp. 369–395 in *The Handbook of Attitudes*, edited by Albarracin Dolores, T. Johnson Blair and P. Zanna Mark. Mahwah, NJ: Psychology.
Marsh, Timothy, and Jac Brown. 2011. "Homonegativity and Its Relationship to Religiosity, Nationalism and Attachment Style." *Journal of Religion & Health* 50 (3): 575–591.
Martela, Frank, and Richard M. Ryan. 2016. "The Benefits of Benevolence: Basic Psychological Needs, Beneficence, and the Enhancement of Well-Being." *Journal of Personality* 84 (6): 750–764.
Martin, Christopher. 2020. "Educational Justice and the Value of Knowledge." *Journal of Philosophy of Education* 54 (1): 164–182.
Martin, Jeffrey T. 2014. "The Confucian Ethic and the Spirit of East Asian Police: A Comparative Study in the Ideology of Democratic Policing." *Crime, Law, & Social Change* 61 (4): 461–490.
Martin, Rod A. 2007. *The Psychology of Humor: An Integrative Approach*. Burlington, MA: Elsevier.
Martinelli, Alberto. 2005. *Global Modernization: Rethinking the Project of Modernity*. London: SAGE.
Martinez, Teresa A., and Steve L. McMullin. 2004. "Factors Affecting Decisions to Volunteer in Nongovernmental Organizations." *Environment & Behavior* 36 (1): 112–126.
Marzana, Daniela, Elena Marta, and Maura Pozzi. 2012. "Social Action in Young Adults: Voluntary and Political Engagement." *Journal of Adolescence* 35 (3): 497–507.
Mason, Andrew. 2012. *Living Together as Equals: The Demands of Citizenship*. Oxford, UK: Oxford University Press.
Masters, Roger D. 2001. "cognitive Neuroscience, Emotion, and Leadership." Pp. 68–102 in *Citizens and Politics: Perspectives from Political Psychology*, edited by James H. Kuklinski. Cambridge, UK: Cambridge University Press.
Masterson, Suzanne S. 2001. "A Trickle-Down Model of Organizational Justice: Relating Employees' and Customers' Perceptions of and Reactions to Fairness." *Journal of Applied Psychology* 86 (4): 594–604.
Masui, Keita. 2023. "Interactional Effects of Adverse Childhood Experiences, Psychopathy, and Everyday Sadism on Internet Trolling." *Personality & Individual Differences* 214: 112327.
Mata, Fernando, and Ravi Pendakur. 2014. "Social Capital, Diversity and Giving or Receiving Help among Neighbours." *Social Indicators Research* 118 (1): 329–347.
Mathis, Arlesia, Ronica Rooks, and Daniel Kruger. 2016. "Improving the Neighborhood Environment for Urban Older Adults: Social Context and Self-Rated Health." *International Journal of Environmental Research and Public Health* 13 (3): 1–13.
Matthewman, Steve. 2011. *Technology and Social Theory*. Houndmills, Palgrave.
Matthews, Christopher R., and Alex Channon. 2016. "It's Only Sport: The Symbolic Neutralization of Violence." *Symbolic Interaction* 39 (4): 557–576.
Matts, Jacqueline S., Wizdom Powell Hammond, Nyusha Grayman, Meredith Bonacci-William. Brennan, Sheri-Ann. Cowie, Lina Ladyzhenskaya, and Sara So. 2009. "The Social Production of Altruism: Motivations for Caring Action in a Low-income Urban Community." *American Journal of Community Psychology* 43: 71–84.
Matusov, Eugene. 2024. "Community Versus Society: The Normative Vision of Sociality in Joint Self-Education." *Culture & Psychology* 30 (1): 3–29.
Mau, Steffen. 2005. "Democratic Demand for a Social Europe? Preferences of the European Citizenry." *International Journal of Social Welfare* 14: 76–85.
Maule, Linda S., and Robert K. Goidel. 2003. "Adultery, Drugs, and Sex: An Experimental Investigation of Individual Reactions to Unethical Behavior by Public Officials." *Social Science Journal* 40: 65–78.
Maume, Michael O., and Matthew R. Lee. 2003. "Social Institutions and Violence: A Sub-national Test of Institutional Anomie Theory." *Criminology* 41 (4): 1137–1172.
Maurer, Markus. 2011. "Education and Social Integration: Comprehensive Schooling in Europe." *European Educational Research Journal* 10 (1): 160–167.

May, David C. 1999. "Tolerance of Nonconformity and Its Effect on Attitudes toward the Legalization of Prostitution: A Multivariate Analysis." *Deviant Behavior* 20 (4): 335–358.

May, Simon. 2011. *Love: A History*. New Haven, CT: Yale University Press.

Mayda, Anna Maria, and Dani Rodrik. 2005. "Why Are Some People (and Countries) More Protectionist Than Others?" *European Economic Review* 49: 1393–1430.

Mayer, Adam. 2017. "Social Capital, Economic Hardship, and Health: A Test of the Buffering Hypothesis in Transition and Nontransition Countries." *Sociological Spectrum* 37 (2): 111–126.

Mazziotta, Agostino, Amélie. Mummendey, and Stephen C. Wright. 2011. "Vicarious Intergroup Contact Effects." *Group Processes & Intergroup Relations* 14 (2): 255–274.

McAllister, Ian. 1999. "The Economic Performance of Government." Pp.188–203 in *Critical Citizens: Global Support for Democratic Government*, edited by Pippa Norris. Oxford, UK: Oxford University Press.

McCabe, Brian J. 2012. "Homeownership and Social Trust in Neighbors." *City & Community* 11 (4): 389–408.

McCabe, Brian J. 2014. "Are Homeowners Better Citizens? Homeownership and Community Participation in the United States." *Social Forces* 91 (3): 929–954.

McCaffoee, Kevin. 2016. "Sociology in the Study of Morality." Pp. 435–456 in *Handbook of Contemporary Sociological Theory*, edited by Seth Abrutyn. Cham, Switzerland: Springer.

McCarthy, Gerard, and Barbara Maughan. 2010. "Negative Childhood Experiences and Adult Love Relationships: The Role of Internal Working Models of Attachment." *Attachment & Human Development* 12 (5): 445–461.

McCauley, Clark, and Sophia Moskalenko. 2017. "Understanding Political Radicalization: The Two-Pyramids Model." *American Psychologist* 72 (3): 205–216.

McClurg, Scott D. 2006. "The Electoral Resources of Political Talk: Examining Disagreement and Expertise Effects in Social Networks on Political Participation." *American Journal of Political Science* 50 (3): 737–754.

McCrae, Robert R. 2009. "Personality Profiles of Cultures: Patterns of Ethos." *European Journal of Personality* 23: 205–227.

McCright, Aaron M., and Riley E. Dunlap. 2008. "The Nature and Social Bases of Progressive Social Movement Ideology: Examining Public Opinion toward Social Movements." *Sociological Quarterly* 49 (4): 825–848.

McCright, Aaron M., and Terry Nichols Clark. 2006. "The Political Opportunity Structure of the Environmental Movement in U.S. Communities." *Research in Urban Policy* 10: 199–240.

McDevitt, Michael. 2018. "Political Socialization and Child Development." Pp. 797–811 in *The SAGE Handbook of Political Sociology*, edited by William Outhwaite and Stephen Turner. London, UK: SAGE.

McDonell, James R., Natallia Sianko, Jill D. McLeigh, and William Spaulding. 2021. "Neighborhood, Neighborliness, and Family and Child Well-Being." *American Journal of Orthopsychiatry* 91 (3): 310–321.

McDowell, Michael and Nathan Robert Brown. 2009. *World Religions: At Your Fingertips*. New York, NY: Alpha.

McGhee, Derek. 2003. "Moving to Our Common Ground: A Critical Examination of Community Cohesion Discourse in Twenty-First Century Britain." *Sociological Review* 51 (3): 376–404.

McGraw, Kathleen M. 2001. "Political Accounts and Attribution Processes." Pp.160–197 in *Citizens and Politics: Perspectives from Political Psychology*, edited by James H. Kuklinski. Cambridge, UK: Cambridge University Press.

McGraw, Kathleen M., Milton Lodge, and Jeffrey M. Jones. 2002. "The Pandering Politician of Suspicious Minds." *Journal of Politics* 14 (2): 362–383.

McKnight, D. Harrison, and Norman L. Chervany. 2006. "Reflection on an Initial Trust-building Model." Pp. 29–51 in *Handbook of Trust Research*, edited by Reinhard Bachmann and Akbar Zaheer. Cheltenham, UK: Elgar.

McLaughlin, Eugene. 2010. "Critical Criminology." Pp.153–174 in *The SAGE Handbook of Criminological Theory*, edited by Eugene McLaughlin and Tim Newburn. London, UK: SAGE.

McLeod, Branden A., Jasmine Gilmore, Laura G. Daughtery, Joseph T. Jones, Jr. 2018. "A Nonprofit Organization's Approach to Cognize Community Responses to Historic and Perpetuated Structural Racism in Baltimore City." *Journal of Public & Nonprofit Affairs* 4 (2): 223–240.

McLevey, John, and Ryan Deschamps. 2018. "Public Policy Formation and Implementation." Pp. 924–942 in *The SAGE Handbook of Political Sociology*, edited by William Outhwaite and Stephen Turner. London, UK: SAGE.

McMullin, Julie Ann, and John Cairney. 2004. "Self-esteem and the Intersection of Age, Class, and Gender." *Journal of Aging Studies* 18 (1): 75–90.

McNamara, Luke, Julia Quilter, Russell Hogg, Arlie Loughnan, Heather Douglas, David Brown, and Lindsay Farmer. 2021. "Understanding Processes of Criminalisation: Insights from an Australian Study of Criminal Law-Making." *Criminology & Criminal Justice* 21 (3): 387–407.

McNeeley, Susan, and Yue Yuan. 2017. "A Multilevel Examination of the Code of the Street?s Relationship with Fear of Crime." *Crime & Delinquency* 63 (9): 1146–1167.

McVeigh, Rory, and Maria-Elena D. Diaz. 2009. "Voting to Ban Same-sex Marriage: Interest, Values, and Communities." *American Sociological Review* 74 (6): 891–915.

McVeigh, Rory, Daniel J. Myers, and David Sikkink. 2004. "Corn, Klansmen, and Coolidge: Structure and Framing in Social Movements." *Social Forces* 83 (2): 653–690.

Meadows, Chris M. 2014. *A Psychological Perspective on Joy and Emotional Fulfillment*. New York: NY: Routledge.

Mededovic, Janko, and Uroš Kovacevic. 2021. "Sadism as a Key Dark Trait in the Link between Football Fandom and Criminal Attitudes." *Journal of Individual Differences* 42 (1): 9–18.

Medvedovski, Dmitri, and Kirk Allison. 2017. "Paternal Religious Affiliation and Practice in Lithuania: Spiritual Goods or Secular Utilities?" *International Journal of Social Economics* 44 (12): 1758–1777.

Meier, Kenneth J. 1994. *The Politics of Sin: Drugs, Alcohol, and Public Policy*. Armonk, NJ: Sharpe.

Melzer, Silvia Maja. 2011. "Does Migration Make You Happy? The Influence of Migration on Subjective Well-being." *Journal of Social Research & Policy* 2 (2): 73–92.

Menahem, Gila. 2001. "Urban Civic World: A Conceptual and Empirical Exploration." *Local Government Studies* 27 (1): 37–60.

Menard, Scott, and Barbara J. Mose. 1984. "A Structuralist Critique of the IQ-Delinquency Hypotheses: Theory and Evidence." *American Journal of Sociology* 89: 1347–1378.

Meng, Fanhua. 2011. *Phenomena of Chinese Culture in the Turn of the 21st Century*. Singapore: Silkroad.

Meng, Tianguang, and He Chen. 2014. "A Multilevel Analysis of Social Capital and Self-Rated Health: Evidence from China." *Health & Place* 27:38-44.

Menon, Anand. 2011. "Power, Institutions and the CSDP: The Promise of Institutionalist Theory." *Journal of Common Market Studies* 49 (1): 83–100.

Merdian, Hannah, Danielle Kettleborough, Kieran McCartan, and Derek E. Perkins. 2017. "Strength-Based Approaches to Online Child Sexual Abuse: Using Self-Management Strategies to Enhance Desistance Behaviour in Users of Child Sexual Exploitation Material." *Journal of Criminal Psychology* 7 (3): 182–191.

Mesch, Gustavo S. 1996. "The Effect of Environmental Concerns and Governmental Incentives on Organized Action in Local Areas." *Urban Affairs Review* 31 (3): 346–366.

Mesch, Gustavo S. 2009. "Social Bonds and Internet Pornographic Exposure among Adolescents." *Journal of Adolescence* 32: 601–618.

Mesch, Gustavo S., and Orit Manor. 1998. "Social Ties, Environmental Perception, and Local Attachment." *Environment & Behavior* 30 (4): 504–519.

Mesoudi, Alex. 2011. *Cultural Evolution: How Darwinian Theory Can Explain Human Culture and Synthesize the Social Sciences*. Chicago, IL: University of Chicago Press. Minkov, Michael. 2011. *Cultural Differences in a Globally World*. Bingley, UK: Emerald. Rose, David C. 2019. *Why Culture Matter Most*. New York, NY: Oxford University Press.

Messner, Steven F., Helmut Thome, and Richard Rosenfeld. 2008. "Institutions, Anomie, and Violent Crime: Clarifying and Elaborating Institutional-anomie Theory." *International Journal of Conflict & Violence* 2 (2): 163–181.

Messner, Steven F., Richard Rosenfeld, and Susanna Karstedt. 2013. "Social Institutions and Crime." Pp.405–423 in *The Oxford Handbook of Criminological Theory*, edited by Francis T. Cullen and Pamela Wilcox. New York: Oxford University Press.

Meszaros, Istvan. 2015. *The Necessity of Social Control*. New York: NY: Monthly Review.

Meuleman, Bart, Koen Abts, Koen Slootmaeckers, and Cecil Meeusen. 2019. "Differentiated Threat and the Genesis of Prejudice: Group-Specific Antecedents of Homonegativity, Islamophobia, Anti-Semitism, and Anti-Immigrant Attitudes." *Social Problems* 66 (2): 222–244.

Mewes, Jan, Malcolm Fairbrother, Giuseppe Nicola Giordano, Cary Wu, and Rima Wilkes. 2021. "Experiences Matter: A Longitudinal Study of Individual-Level Sources of Declining Social Trust in the United States." *Social Science Research* 95:102537.

Meyer, Gerhard, and Michael A. Stadler. 1999. "Criminal Behavior Associated with Pathological Gambling." *Journal of Gambling Studies* 15 (1): 29–43.

Michael, John, Luke McEllin, and Annalena Felber. 2020. "Prosocial Effects of Coordination – What, How and Why?" *Acta Psychologica* 207: 103083.

Michael, Mike. 2017. *Actor-network Theory: Trials, Trails, and Translations*. London, UK: SAGE.

Michaeli, Yossi, Daniel J. Dickson, Maor Kalfon Hakhmigari, Miri Scharf, and Shmuel Shulman. 2022. "Change in Self-Criticism across Emerging Adulthood and Psychological Well-Being at Age 35: The Mediating Role of Reflectivity." *Emerging Adulthood* 10 (2): 323–334.

Michalos, Alex C., and Bruno D. Zumbo. 2001. "Ethnicity, Modern Prejudice and the Quality of Life." *Social Indicators Research* 53: 189–222.

Michalos, Alex C., Harvey V. Thommasen, Rua Read, Nancy Anderson, and Bruno D. Zumbo. 2005. "Determinants of Health and the Quality of Life in the Bella Coola Valley." *Social Indicators Research* 72: 1–50.

Michalski, Joseph H. 2005. "Explaining Intimate Partner Violence: The Sociological Limitation of Victimization Studies." *Sociological Forum* 20 (4): 623–640.

Michel, Lacie M. 2007. "Personal Responsibility and Volunteering after a Natural Disaster: The Case of Hurricane Katrina." *Sociological Spectrum* 27: 633–652.

Midgley, James, and Michelle Livermore. 2005. "Development Theory and Community Practice." Pp.153–168 in the *Handbook of Community Practice*, edited by Marie Weil. Thousand Oaks, CA: Sage.

Mihailidis, Paul, and Benjamin Thevenin. 2013. "Media Literacy as a Core Competency for Engaged Citizenship in Participatory Democracy." *American Behavioral Scientist* 57 (11): 1611–1622.

Mihailov, Emilian. 2023. "Measuring Impartial Beneficence: A Kantian Perspective on the Oxford Utilitarianism Scale." *Review of Philosophy & Psychology* 14 (3): 989–1004.

Mikulincer, Mario, and Phillip R. Shaver. 2018. "Attachment Theory as a Framework for Studying Relationship Dynamics and Functioning." Pp. 175–185 in *The Cambridge Handbook of Personal Relationships*, edited by Anita L. Vangelisti and Daniel Perlman. Cambridge, UK: Cambridge University Press.

Miles-Johnson, Toby, and Yurong Wang. 2018. "Hidden Identities": Perceptions of Sexual Identity in Beijing. *British Journal of Sociology* 69 (2): 323–351.

Milgram, Roberta M., and Eunsook Hong. 1994. "Creative Thinking and Creative Performance in Adolescents as Predictors of Creative Attainments in Adults: A Follow-up Study after 18 Years." Pp.212–228 in *Beyond Terman: Contemporary Longitudinal Studies of Giftedness and Talent*, edited by Rena F. Subotnik, and Karen D. Arnold. Norwood, NJ: Ablex.

Millar, Jeff. 2013. "An Interdiscursive Analysis of Language and Immigrant Integration Policy Discourse in Canada." *Critical Discourse Studies* 10 (1): 18–31.

Miller, Alan S. 1995. "A Rational Choice Model of Religious Behavior in Japan." *Journal for the Scientific Study of Religion* 34 (2): 234–244.

Miller, Alistair. 2022. "The Existential Turn in Philosophy of Education. In Defence of Liberal Autonomy." *Journal of Philosophy of Education* 56 (2): 356–370.

Miller, David, and Richard Dagger. 2003. "Utilitarianism and beyond: Contemporary Analytical Political Theory." Pp.446–469 in *The Cambridge History of Twentieth-century Political Thought*, edited by Terence Ball and Richard Bellamy. Cambridge, UK: Cambridge University Press.

Miller, Seumas. 2010. *The Moral Foundations of Social Institutions: A Philosophy Study*. New York: Cambridge University Press.

Miller, Susan M. 2015. "Public Support for Sale Government Spending and Public Approval of Federal Agency Performance." *American Politics Research* 44 (3): 523–547.

Milligan, Christine, and Nicholas R. Fyfe. 2005. "Preserving Space for Volunteers: Exploring the Links between Voluntary Welfare Organizations, Volunteering and Citizenship." *Urban Studies* 42 (3): 417–433.

Mills, Melinda, and Kadri Taht. 2010. "Nonstandard Work Schedules and Partnership Quality: Quantitative and Qualitative Findings." *Journal of Marriage & the Family* 72 (4): 860–875.

Milner, Helen V. 2020. "Globalization." In *The SAGE Handbook of Political Science*, edited by Dirk Berg-Schlosser, Bertrand Badie and Leonardo Morlino. London, UK: SAGE.

Milner, Henry. 2002. *Civic Literacy: How Informed Citizens Make Democracy Work*. Hanover, NH: University Press of New England.

Milner, Judith, and Steve Myers. 2007. *Working with Violence: Policies and Practices in Risk Assessment and Management*. Houndmills, UK: Palgave.

Milstein, Brian. 2021. "Security and Democratic Equality." *Contemporary Political Theory* 20 (4): 836–857.

Mingo, Isabella, and Maria Paola Faggiano. 2020. "Trust in Institutions between Objective and Subjective Determinants: A Multilevel Analysis in European Countries." *Social Indicators Research* 151 (3): 815–839.

Minogue, Kenneth. 2010. *The Servile Mind: How Democracy Erodes the Moral Life*. New York: Encounter.

Mirivel, Julien C. 2014. *The Art of Positive Communication: Theory and Practice*. New York, NY: Lang.

Mirowsky, John, and Catherine E. Ross. 2001. "Age and Effect of Economic Hardship on Depression." *Journal of Health & Social Behavior* 42: 132–150.

Mishler, William, and John P. Willerton. 2003. "The Dynamics of Presidential Popularity in Post-communist Russia: Cultural Imperative versus Neo-institutional Choice?" *Journal of Politics* 65 (1): 111–141.

Mishler, William, and Richard Rose. 1997. "Trust, Distrust and Skepticism: Popular Evaluation of Civil and Political Institutions in Post-communist Societies." *Journal of Politics* 59 (2): 418–451.

Mistry, Roshmitas, and Edward D. Lowe. 2006. "What Earnings and Income Buy: The Basics Plus a Little Extra: Implications for Family and Child Well-being." Pp.173–205 in *Making It Work: Low-wage Employment, Family Life, and Child Development*, edited by Hirskazu Yoshikawa, Thomas S. Weisner, and Edward D. Lowe. New York: Russell Sage.

Mitchell, Neil J. 2005. "Calculating and Believing: Ideological Norms in the Cradle of Utility Maximization." *Social Justice Research* 18 (3): 243–256.

Mitrut, Andreea, and Francois-Charles. Wolff. 2011. "Do Private and Public Transfers Received Affect Life Satisfaction: Evidence from Romania." *Journal of Economic Psychology* 32: 969–979.

Mitts, Tamar. 2019. "From Isolation to Radicalization: Anti-Muslim Hostility and Support for ISIS in the West." *American Political Science Review* 113 (1): 173–194.

Miyata, Kakuko, Kenichi Ikeda, and Tetsuro Kobayashi. 2008. "The Internet, Social Capital, Civic Engagement, and Gender in Japan." Pp.206–233 in *Social Capital: An International Research Program*, edited by Nan Lin and Bonnie H. Erickson. Oxford, UK: Oxford University Press.

Moeller, Hans-Georg. 2004. *Daoism Explained: From the Dream of the Butterfly to the Fishnet Allegory*. Chicago, IL: Open Court.

Moeller, Scott J., Jennifer Crocker, and Brad J. Bushman. 2009. "Creating Hostility and Conflict: Effects of Entitlement and Self-Image Goals." *Journal of Experimental Social Psychology* 45 (2): 448–452.

Moghaddam, Fathali M. 2008. *Multiculturalism and Intergroup Relations: Psychological Implications for Democracy in Global Context*. Washington, DC: American Psychological Association.

Molana, Hanieh H., and Richard E. Adams. 2019. "Evaluating Sense of Community in the Residential Environment from the Perspectives of Symbolic Interactionism and Architectural Design." *Journal of Community Psychology* 47 (7): 1591–1602.

Mole, Richard. 2011. "Nationality and Sexuality: Homophobic Discourse and the 'National Threat' in Contemporary Latvia." *Nations & Nationalism* 17 (3): 540–560.

Molina, Oscar, and Martin Rhodes. 2002. "Corporatism: The Past, Present, and Future of a Concept." *Annual Review of Political Science* 5: 305–331.

Molitor, Fred, Melissa Rossi, Lisa Branton, and Julie Field. 2011. "Increasing Social Capital and Personal Efficacy through Small-Scale Community Events." *Journal of Community Psychology* 39 (6): 749–754.

Moller, Jorgen, and Svend-Erik. Skaaning. 2013. *Democracy and Democratization in Comparative Perspective: Conceptions, Conjunctures, Causes, and Consequences*. Abingdon, UK: Routledge.

Moller, Stephanie, and Huiping Li. 2009. "Segregation in Organizations: Parties, Unions, Policies and Occupational Sex Segregation in the United States." *Social Forces* 87 (3): 1529–1560.

Moller, Valerie. 2005. "Resilient or Resigned? Criminal Victimisation and Quality of Life in South Africa." *Social Indicators Research* 72: 263–317.

Mollon, Phil. 2005. "The Inherent Shame of Sexuality." *British Journal of Psychotherapy* 22 (2): 167–178.

Molm, Linda D. 1997. *Coercive Power in Social Exchange*. Cambridge, UK: Cambridge University Press.

Molm, Linda D. 2008. "The Structure of Reciprocity and Integrative Bonds: The Role of Emotions." Pp.167–192 in *Social Structure and Emotion*, edited by Jody Clay-Warner and Dawn T. Robinson. San Diego, CA: Academic.

Molm, Linda D., David A. Schaefer, and Jessica L. Collett. 2007. "The Value of Reciprocity." *Social Psychology Quarterly* 70 (2): 199–217.

Molm, Linda D., Nobuyuki Takahashi, and Gretchen Peterson. 2003. "In the Eye of the Beholder: Procedural Justice in Social Exchange." *American Sociological Review* 68 (1): 128–152.

Mols, Frank, and Jolanda Jetten. 2017. *The Wealth Paradox: Economic Prosperity and the Hardening of Attitudes*. Cambridge, UK: Cambridge University Press.

Momonoki, Yoshie S., and Hidetoki Ishii. 2023. "Modeling the Direct and Indirect Relationships between Cognitive Style, Daily Life Stress and Mental Distress." *Journal of Affective Disorders Reports* 13: 100594.

Montgomery, Diane, Pamela A. Hodges, and Judith S. Kuafman. 2004. "An Exploratory Study of the Relationship between Mood States and Creativity Self-perceptions." *Creativity Research Journal* 16 (2&3): 341–344.

Moore, Alfred. 2017a. *Critical Elitism: Deliberation, Democracy and the Problem of Expertise*. Cambridge, UK: Cambridge University Press.

Moore, Dahlia, and Salem Aweiss. 2003. "Outcome Expectations in Prolonged Conflicts: Perceptions of Sense of Control and Relative Deprivation." *Sociological Inquiry* 73 (2): 190–211.

Moore, Kathleen A. 2017. "Mindfulness at Work." Pp.453–467 in *Research Handbook on Work and Well-being*, edited by Ronald J. Burke and Kathryn M. Page. Cheltenham, UK: Elgar.

Moore, Margaret. 2001. *The Ethics of Nationalism*. Oxford, UK: Oxford University Press.

Moore, Margaret. 2010. "Defending Community: Nationalism, Patriotism, and Culture." Pp.130–145 in *Ethics and World Politics*, edited by Duncan Bell. Oxford, UK: Oxford University Press.

Moore, Margaret. 2015. *A Political Theory of Territory*. Oxford, UK: Oxford University Press.

Moran, James B., Nicholas Kerry, Jin X. Goh, and Damian R. Murray. 2021. "Parasites and Promiscuity: Acute Disease Salience Leads to More Restricted Sexual Attitudes." *Journal of Social & Personal Relationships* 38 (11): 3333–3349.

Moreira, Pollyana De Lucena, Jolio Rique Neto, Jos-Manuel Sabucedo, and Cleonice Pereira Dos Santos Camino. 2018. "Moral Judgment, Political Ideology and Collective Action." *Scandinavian Journal of Psychology* 59(6):610-620.

Morenoff, Jeffrey D., and Robert J. Sampson. 1997. "Violent Crime and the Spatial Dynamics of Neighborhood Transition: Chicago, 1970–1990." *Social Forces* 76 (1): 31–64.

Morgan, Gareth. 1997. *Images of Organization*, 2nd ed. Thousand Oaks, CA: Sage.

Morgan, Jessica, and Oliver Robinson. 2013. "Intrinsic Aspirations and Personal Meaning across Adulthood: Conceptual Interrelations and Age/Sex Differences." *Developmental Psychology* 49 (5): 999–1010.

Morgan, Seiriol. 2021. "Entitlement, Domination and Violence: A Philosophical Model of a Deviant Sense of Justification, and Its Implications for Understanding Human Rights Abuses." *International Journal of Human Rights* 25 (9): 1543–1573.

Morody, Mioslawa, and Anna Giza-Poleszczuk. 2018. *Transformation of Social Bonds: The Outline of the Theory of Social Change*. Berlin, Germany: Lang.

Morokoff, Patricia J., Colleen A. Redding, Lisa L. Harlow, Sookhyun Cho, Joseph S. Rossi, Kathryn S. Meier, Kenneth H. Mayer, Beryl Koblin, and Pamela Brown-Peterside. 2009. "Associations of Sexual Victimization, Depression, and Sexual Assertiveness with Unprotected Sex: A Test of the Multifaceted Model of HIV Risk across Gender." *Journal of Applied Biobehavioral Research* 14 (1): 30–54.

Moroni, Stefano. 2010. "An Evolutionary Theory of Institutions and a Dynamic Approach to Reform." *Planning Theory* 9 (4): 275–297.

Morris, Stephen D., and Joseph L. Klesner. 2010. "Corruption and Trust: Theoretical Considerations and Evidence from Mexico." *Comparative Political Studies* 43 (10): 1258–1285.

Morrison, Brenda. 2006. "School Bullying and Restorative Justice toward a Theoretical Understanding of the Role of Respect, Pride, and Shame." *Journal of Social Issues* 62 (2): 371–392.

Morrison, Keith. 2005. "Structuration Theory, Habitus, and Complexity Theory: Elective Affinities or Old Wine in New Bottles?" *British Journal of Sociology of Education* 26 (3): 311–326.

Morselli, Davide, and Stefano Passini. 2018. "Exclusive and Inclusive Protest in Europe: Investigating Values, Support for Democracy, and Life Conditions." *Journal of Community & Applied Social Psychology* 28 (3): 123–141.

Moschis, George P., and Fon Sim Ong. 2011. "Religiosity and Consumer Behavior of Older Adults: A Study of Subcultural Influences in Malaysia." *Journal of Consumer Behavior* 10: 8–17.

Mosher, Michael A. 2002. "Are Civil Societies the Transmission Belts of Ethical Tradition?" Pp.207–230 in *Alternative Conception of Civil Society*, edited by Simone Chambers and Will Kymlicka. Princeton, NJ: Princeton University Press.

Moskalenko, Sphia, Clark McCauley, and Paul Rozin. 2007. "Group Identification under Conditions of Threat: College Students" Attachment to Country, Family, Ethnicity, Religion, and University before and after September 11, 2001." *Political Psychology* 27 (1): 77–97.

Moss, Jeremy. 2014. *Reassessing Egalitarianism*. Houndmills, UK: Palgrave.

Moticjunaite, Akvile, and Zhanna Kravchenko. 2008. "Family Policy, Employment and Gender-role Attitudes: A Comparative Analysis of Russia and Sweden." *Journal of European Social Policy* 18 (1): 38–49.

Motschenbacher, Heiko. 2013. "Now Everybody Can Wear a Skirt: Linguistic Constructions of Non-Heteronormativity at Eurovision Song Contest Press Conferences." *Discourse & Society* 24 (5): 590–614.

Mott, Stephen Charles. 2011. *Biblical Ethics and Social Change*. New York, NY: Oxford University Press.

Motta, Matthew, and Paul Goren. 2021. "Basic Human Values and Compliance with Government Recommended Prosocial Health Behavior." *Journal of Elections, Public Opinion & Parties* 31 (S1): 206–219.

Mouzelis, Nicos. 2012. "Modernity and the Secularization Debate." *Sociology* 46 (2): 207–223.

Moyano-Diaz, Emilio, and Gonzalo Palomo-Velez. 2018. Satisfaction with the Country and Well-Being: Future Expectations. *International Journal of Social Psychology* 33 (3): 504–528.

Mroczek, Daniel K. 2004. "Positive and Negative Affect at Midlife." Pp.205–226 in *How Healthy Are We: A National Study of Well-being at Midlife*, edited by Orville Gilbert Brim, Carol D. Ryff and Ronald C. Kessler. Chicago, IL: University of Chicago Press.

MuBotter, Marlene. 2024. "On Nation, Homeland, and Democracy: Toward a Novel Three-Factor Measurement Model for Nationalism and Patriotism. Evidence from Two Representative Studies." *Political Psychology* 45 (6): 903–921.

Muennig, Peter, Alison K. Cohen, Aileen Palmer, and Wenyi Zhu. 2013. "The Relationship between Five Different Measures of Structural Social Capital, Medical Examination Outcomes, and Mortality." *Social Science & Medicine* 85: 18–26.

Muhlau, Peter. 2014. "Middle Class Squeeze? Social Class and Perceived Financial Hardship in Ireland, 2002–2012." *Economic and Social Review* 45 (4): 485–509.

Mulatu, Mesfin Samuel, and Carmi Schooler. 2002. "Causal Connections between Socio-economic Status and Health: Reciprocal Effects and Mediating Mechanisms." *Journal of Health & Social Behavior* 43 (1): 22–41.

Mulford, Matthew, John Orbell, Catherine Shatto, and Jean Stockard. 1998. "Physical Attractiveness, Opportunity, and Success in Everyday Exchange." *American Journal of Sociology* 103 (6): 1565–1592.

Mulinari, Diana, and Kerstin Sandell. 2009. "A Feminist Re-Reading of Theories of Late Modernity: Beck, Giddens and the Location of Gender." *Critical Sociology* 35 (4): 493–507.

Mullet, Etienne, Felix Neto, and Sheila Riviere. 2005. "Personality and Its Effects on Resentment, Reventge, Forgiveness, and Self-forgiveness." Pp. 159–181 in *Handbook of Forgiveness*, edited by Everett L. Worthington, Jr. New York, NY: Routledge.

Muluk, Hamdi, Nathanael G. Sumaktoyo, and Dhyah Madya Ruth. 2013. "Jihad as Justification: National Survey Evidence of Belief in Violent Jihad as a Mediating Factor for Sacred Violence among Muslims in Indonesia." *Asian Journal of Social Psychology* 16 (2): 101–111.

Mummendey, Amelie, Thomas Kessler, Andreas Klink, and Rosemarie Mielke. 1999. "Strategies to Cope with Negative Social Identity: Predictions by Social Identity Theory and Relative Deprivation Theory." *Journal of Personality & Social Psychology* 76 (2): 229–245.

Munch, Richard. 1987. *Theory of Action: Towards a New Synthesis Going beyond Parsons*. London: Routledge & Kegan Paul.

Munch, Richard. 2012. *Inclusion and Exclusion in the Liberal Competition State: The Cult of the Individual*. Abington, UK: Routledge.

Munck, Ronaldo. 2018. "Development and Social Change: A Genealogy for an Era of Complexity." Pp. 1–18 In *Handbook on Development and Social Change*, edited by G. Honor Fagan and Ronaldo Munck. Northampton, MA: Elgar.

Munro, Neil. 2018. "Does Refusal Bias Influence the Measurement of Chinese Political Trust?" *Journal of Contemporary China* 27 (111): 457–471.

Muntaner, Carles, and John Lynch. 2002. "Income Inequality, Social Cohesion, and Class Relations: Critique of Wilkinson's Neo-Durkheimian Research Program." Pp.325–346 in *The Political Economy of Social Inequalities: Consequences for Health and Quality of Life*, edited by Vicente Navarro. Amityville, NY: Baywood.

Murayama, Yoh, Hiroshi Murayama, Masami Hasebe, Jan Yamaguichi, and Yosninori fujiwara. 2019. "The Impact of Intergenerational Programs on Social Capital in Japan: A Randomized Population-based Cross-sectional Study." *BMC Public Health* 19: 156.

Murray, Dandra L., and John G. Holmes. 2008. "The Commitment-insurance System: Self-esteem and the Regulation of Connection in Close Relationships." *Advances in Experimental Social Psychology* 40: 1–60.

Murray, Joy. 2009. "The Wider Social Benefits of Higher Education: What Do We Know about Them?" *Australian Journal of Education* 53 (3): 230–244.
Music, Graham. 2014. *The Good Life: Wellbeing and the New Science of Altruism, Selfishness and Immorality*. Hove, UK: Routledge.
Musick, Marc A. 2000. "Race and Formal Volunteering: The Differential Effects of Class and Religion." *Social Forces* 78 (4): 1539–1570.
Musick, Marc A., and John Wilson. 2008. *Volunteers: A Social Profile*. Bloomington, IN: Indiana University Press.
Mussel, Patrick, and Johannes Hewig. 2016. "The Life and Times of Individuals Scoring High and Low on Dispositional Greed." *Journal of Research in Personality* 64: 52–60.
Mutaner, Carles, John Lynch, and Gary L. Oates. 2002. "The Social Class Determinants of Income Inequality and Social Cohesion." Pp.367–399 in *The Political Economy of Social Inequalities: Consequences for Health and Quality of Life,* edited by Vicente Navarro. Amityville, NY: Baywood.
Muthuswamy, Moorthy S. 2022. "Does Sharia Act as Both a Mediator and Moderator in Salafi Radicalism?" *Cogent Social Sciences* 8 (1): 2030452.
Mutz, Diana C. 1998. *Impersonal Influence: How Perceptions of Mass Collectives Affect Political Attitudes*. Cambridge, UK: Cambridge University Press.
Mutz, Diana C., and Byron Reeves. 2005. "The New Videomalaise: Effects of Televised Incivility on Political Trust." *American Political Science Review* 99 (1): 1–15.
Mutz, Diana C., and Jeffery J. Mondak. 2006. "The Workplace as a Context for Cross-cutting Political Discourse." *Journal of Politics* 68 (1): 140–155.
Myer, Landon, Dan J. Stein, Anna Grimsrud, Soraya Seedat, and David R. Williams. 2008. "Social Determinants of Psychological Distress in a Nationally Representative Sample of South African Adults." *Social Science & Medicine* 60: 1828–1840.
Myers, David G. 2008. "Religion and Human Flourishing." Pp.323–343 in *The Science of Subjective Well-being*, edited by Michael Eid and Randy J. Larsen. New York: Guilford.
Myers, David G. 2014. "Religious Engagement and Well-being." Pp.88–100 in *the Oxford Handbook of Happiness*, edited by Susan A. David, Ilona Boniwell and Amanda Conley Ayers. Oxford, UK: Oxford University Press.
Myers, JoAnne. 2020. *The Good Citizen: The Markers of Privilege in America*. New York, NY: Routledge.
Na, Chongmin, and Ray Paternoster. 2019. "Prosocial Identities and Youth Violence." *Journal of Research in Crime & Delinquency* 56 (1): 84–128.
Nabi, Robin L., and Jennifer R. Horner. 2001. "Victims with Voices: How Abused Women Conceptualize the Problem of Spousal Abuse and Implications for Intervention and Prevention." *Journal of Family Violence* 16 (3): 237–253.
Nabi, Robin L., and John L. Sullivan. 2001. "Does Television Viewing Relate to Engagement in Protective Action Against Crime? A Cultivation Analysis from a Theory of Reasoned Action Perspective." *Communication Research* 28 (6): 802–825.
Naess, Petter. 2001. "Urban Planning and Sustainable Development." *European Planning Studies* 9 (4): 503–524.
Naftali, Orna. 2021. "Youth Military Training in China: Learning to Love the Army." *Journal of Youth Studies* 24 (10): 1340–1357.
Nagayoshi, Kikuko, and Yoshimichi Sato. 2014. "Who Supports Redistributive Policies in Contemporary Japan? An Integrative Approach to Self-Interest and Trust Models." *International Sociology* 29 (4): 302–323.
Nahapiet, Janine. 2011. "A Social Perspective: Exploring the Links between Human Capital and Social Capital." Pp. 71–95 in *The Oxford Handbook of Human Capital*, edited by Alan Burton-Jones and J.C. Spender. Oxford, UK: Oxford University Press. Robison, Lindon J., and Bryan K. Ritchie. 2010. *Relationship Economics: The Social Capital Paradigm and Its Application to Business, Politics and Other Transactions*. Furnham, UK: Gower.

Nai, Peng, Jianfei Sun, Yinzhu Zhang, and Guang Yang. 2020. "Religious Education Legislation in an Atheist State: Towards a Typology and Policy Analysis for Contemporary China." *British Journal of Religious Education* 42 (1): 75–89.

Nakashima, Ken'ichiro, Kuniaki Yanagisawa, and Mitsuhiro Ura. 2013. "Dissimilar Effects of Task-relevant and Interpersonal Threat on Independent-interdependent Self-construal in Individuals with High Self-esteem." *Asian Journal of Social Psychology* 16 (1): 50–59.

Nalla, Mahesh, Joseph Johnson, and Rebecca Hayes-Smith. 2011. "Prior Victimization, Region, and Neighborhood Effects on Fear of Crime in Mumbai, India." *Asian Criminology* 6 (2): 141–159.

Nam, Su-Jung. 2019. "The Effects of Consumer Empowerment on Risk Perception and Satisfaction with Food Consumption." *International Journal of Consumer Studies* 43 (5):429–36.

Narayan, Despa, and Michael F. Cassidy. 2001. "A Dimensional Approach to Measuring Social Capital: Development and Validation of a Social Capital Inventory." *Current Sociology* 49 (2): 59–102.

Narayan, John. 2020. "Survival Pending Revolution: Self-Determination in the Age of Proto-Neo-Liberal Globalization." *Current Sociology* 68 (2): 187–203.

Narvaez, Darcia. 2014. *Neurobiology and the Development of Human Morality: Evolution, Culture, and Wisdom.* New York, NY: Norton.

Nash, Jeffrey E., and James M. Calonico. 2003. "The Political Institution." Pp. 471–490 in *Handbook of Symbolic Interactionism*, edited by Larry T. Reynolds and Nancy J. Herman-Kinney. Lanham, MD: Rowman.

Nassauer, Anne. 2019. *Situational Breakdowns: Understanding Protest Violence and Other supporting Outcomes*. New York, NY: Oxford University Press.

Navarra, Melissa Quetulio, Anke Niehof, Wander Van Der Vaart, Hilje Van Der Horst, and Hester Moerbeek. 2018. "History and Institutions in the Rebuilding of Social Capital after Forced Resettlement in the Philippines and Indonesia." *Journal of Development Studies* 54 (8): 1392–1405.

Navarro, Vicente. 2002. "Neoliberalism, Globalization, Unemployment, Inequalities, and the Welfare State." Pp.33–108 in *The Political Economy of Social Inequalities: Consequences for Health and Quality of Life*, edited by Vicente Navarro. Amityville, NY: Baywood.

Pieterse, Nederveen. Jan. 2010. *Development Theory: Deconstructions/Reconstructions*. London: SAGE.

Nee, Victor, and Yang Cao. 2002. "Postsocialist Inequalities: The Causes of Continuity and Discontinuity." *Research in Social Stratification & Mobility* 19: 3–39.

Nee, Victor. 2005. "The New Institutionalisms in Economics and Sociology." Pp.49–74 in *The Handbook of Economic Sociology* (2nd ed.), edited by Neil J. Smelser and Richard Swedberg. Princeton, NJ: Princeton University Press.

Negri, Antonio and Ed Emery. 2022. *The End of Sovereignty*. Cambridge, UK: Polity.

Nelson, Geoffrey, S. Mark Pancer, Karen Hayward, and Ray Dev Peters. 2005. *Partnerships for Prevention: The Story of the Highfield Community Enrichment Project*. Toronto, Canada: University of Toronto.

Nelson-Coffey, S. Katherine., Kristin Layous, John K. Coffey, and Linda C. Mayes. 2023. "The Effects of Social Belonging and Kindness on Stress and Well-Being during the COVID-19 Pandemic: A Longitudinal Experiment." *Social & Personality Psychology Compass* 2023: e12798.

Nepal, Mani, Alok K. Bohara, and Kishore Gawande. 2011. "More Inequality, More Killings: The Maoist Insurgency in Nepal." *American Journal of Political Science* 55 (4): 886–906.

Neto, Felix, and Jose Barros. 2003. "Predictors of Loneliness among Students and Nuns in Angola and Portugal." *Journal of Psychology* 137 (4): 351–362.

Nevitte, Neil, and Mebs Kanji. 2002. "Authority, Orientations and Political Support: A Cross-national Analysis of Satisfaction with Governments and Democracy." *Comparative Sociology* 1 (3–4): 387–412.

Newey, Glen. 2001. *After Politics: The Rejection of Politics in Contemporary Liberal Philosophy.* Houndmills, UK: Palgrave.

Newman, Benjamin J., Christopher D. Johnston, and Patrick L. Lown. 2015. "False Consciousness or Class Awareness? Local Income Inequality, Personal Economic Position, and Belief in American Meritocracy." *American Journal of Political Science* 59 (2): 326–340.

Newton, Kenneth. 1999. "Social and Political Trust in Established Democracies." Pp.169–203 in *Critical Citizens: Global Support for Democratic Government*, edited by Pippa Norris. Oxford, UK: Oxford University Press.

Newton, Kenneth. 2006. "May the Weak Force Be with You: The Power of the Mass Media in Modern Politics." *European Journal of Political Research* 45: 209–234.

Ney, Steven, and Nadia Molenaars. 1999. "Cultural Theory as a Theory of Democracy." *Innovation* 12 (4): 489–509.

Nezlek, John B., and Peter Derks. 2001. "Use of Humor as a Coping Mechanism, Psychological Adjustment, and Social Interaction." *Humor* 14 (4): 395–413.

Nezlek, John B., Kristof Vansteelandt, Iven Van Mechelen, and Peter Kuppens. 2008. "Appraisal-Emotion Relationships in Daily Life." *Emotion* 8 (1): 145–150.

Ng, Eddie Chi, and Wai, and Adrian T. Fisher. 2016. "Protestant Spirituality and Well-Being of People in Hong Kong: The Mediating Role of Sense of Community." *Applied Research in Quality of Life* 11 (4): 1253–1267.

Ng, Hoi-Yu, and Kerry J. Kennedy. 2019. "Localist Groups and Populist Radical Regionalism in Hong Kong." *China* 17 (4):111–34.

Nguyen, Holly, and Jean Marie McGloin. 2013. "Does Economic Adversity Breed Criminal Cooperation? Considering the Motivation Behind Group Crime." *Criminology* 51 (4): 833–870.

Niblett, Robin. 2024. *The New Cold War: How the Contest between the US and China Will Shape Our Century*. London, UK: Atlantic.

Nicholas, Lucy. 2014. *Queer Post-Gender Ethics the Shape of Selves to Come*. Basingstoke, UK: Palgrave.

Nicholls, Keith, and J. Steven Picou. 2012. "The Impact of Hurricane Katrina on Trust in Government." *Social Science Quarterly* 94 (2): 344–361.

Nicholson, Stephen P., Gary M. Segura, and Nathan D. Woods. 2002. "Presidential Approval and the Mixed Blessing of Divided Government." *Journal of Politics* 64 (3): 701–720.

Nickel, Patricia Monney. 2012. *Public Sociology and Civil Society: Governance, Politics, and Power*. Boulder, CO: Paradigm.

Nickerson, Carol, Norbert Schwarz, and Ed Diener. 2007. "Financial Aspirations, Financial Success, and Overall Life Satisfaction: Who? And How?" *Journal of Happiness Studies* 8:467–515

Niederberger, Anne Arquit. 2005. "Science for Climate Change Policy-making: Applying Theory to Practice to Enhance Effectiveness." *Science & Public Policy* 32 (1): 2–16.

Nielsen, Ingrid, Chris Nyland, Russell Smyth, and Cherrie Jiuhua Zhu. 2005. "Perceptions of Subjective Economic Well-Being and Support for Market Reform among China's Urban Population." *Post-Communist Economies* 17 (4): 425–447.

Niemi, Richard G., John Bremer, and Michael Heel. 1999. "Determinants of State Economic Perceptions." *Political Behavior* 21 (2): 175–193.

Niemi, Richard G., Mary A. Hepburn, and Chris Chapman. 2000. "Community Service by High School Students? A Cure for Civic Ills?" *Political Behavior* 22 (1): 45–69.

Nieuwenhuis, Jaap, Maarten van Ham, Rongqin Yu, Susan Branje, Wim Meeus, and Pieter Hooimeijer. 2017. "Being Poorer Than the Rest of the Neighborhood: Relative Deprivation and Problem Behavior of Youth." *Journal of Youth & Adolescence* 46(9):1891–1904. \105–338.

Nijs, Tom, Borja Martinovic, and Maykel Verkuyten. 2022. "The Two Routes of Collective Psychological Ownership: Rights and Responsibilities Explain Intentions to Exclude Outsiders and Engage in Stewardship Behavior." *Personality & Social Psychology Bulletin* 50 (2): 014616722211297–284.

Nishi, Naomi W., Cheryl E. Matias, and Roberto Montoya. 2015. "Exposing the White Avatar: Projections, Justifications, and the Ever-Evolving American Racism." *Social Identities* 21 (5): 459–473.

Nissen, Bruce, and Paul Jarley. 2005. "Unions as Social Capital: Renewal through a Return to the Logic of Mutual Aid?" *Labor Studies Journal* 29 (4): 1–26.

Nivette, Amy, Denis Ribeaud, Aja Murray, Annekatrin Steinhoff, Laura Bechtiger, Urs Hepp, Lilly Shanahan, and Manuel Eisner. 2021. "Non-Compliance with Covid-19-Related Public Health Measures among Young Adults in Switzerland: Insights from a Longitudinal Cohort Study." *Social Science & Medicine* 268: 113370.

Nixon, David. 2008. "'No More Tea, Vicar'. An Exploration of the Discourses Which Inform the Current Debates about Sexualities within the Church of England." *Sexualities* 11 (5): 595–620.

Nofziger, Stacey, and L. Susan Williams. 2005. "Perceptions of Police and Safety in a Small Town." *Police Quarterly* 8 (2): 248–270.

Nolan, Patrick D. 1983. "Status in the World System, Income Inequality and Economic Growth." *American Journal of Sociology* 89 (2): 410–419.

Nordin, Andreas. 2011. "Making the Lisbon Strategy Happen: A New Phase of Lifelong Learning Discourse in European Policy?" *European Educational Research Journal* 10 (1): 11–20.

Norrander, Barbara, and Clyde Wilcox. 2001. "Public Opinion and Policymaking in the States: The Case of Post-Roe Abortion Policy." Pp.143–159 in *The Public Clash of Private Values: The Politics of Morality Policy*, edited by Christopher Z. Mooney. New York: Chatham House.

Norris, Pippa, and Ronald Inglehart. 2019. *Cultural Backlash: Trump, Brexit, and Authoritarian Populism*. Cambridge, UK: Cambridge University Press.

Norris, Pippa, and Ronald Inglehart. 2009. *Cosmopolitan Communications: Cultural Diversity in a Globalized World*. Cambridge, UK: Cambridge University Press.

Norris, Pippa. 1999a. "Institutional Explanations for Political Support." Pp.217–235 in *Critical Citizens: Global Support for Democratic Government*, edited by Pippa Norris. Oxford, UK: Oxford University Press.

Norris, Pippa. 2001. *Digital Divide: Civic Engagement, Information, Poverty, and the Internet Worldwide*. Cambridge, UK: Cambridge University Press.

Norris, Pippa. 2002. *Democratic Phoenix: Reinventing Political Activism*. Cambridge, UK: Cambridge University Press.

Norris, Pippa. 2011. *Democratic Deficit: Critical Citizens Revisited*. New York: Cambridge University Press.

Norris, Pippa. 2012. *Making Democratic Governance Work: How Regimes Shape Prosperity, Welfare, and Peace*. New York, NY: Cambridge University Press.

North, Adrian C., Lucy Desborough, and Line Skarstein. 2005. "Musical Preference, Deviance, and Attitudes towards Music Celebrities." *Personality & Individual Differences* 38: 1903–1914.

Notter, Megan L., Katherine A. MacTavish, and Devora Shamah. 2008. "Pathways toward Resilience among Women in Rural Trailer Parks." *Family Relations* 57: 613–624.

Novak, William J. 2001. "The American Law of Association: The Legal-Political Construction of Civil Society." *Studies in American Political Development* 15 (2): 163–188.

Nowakowski, Adam. 2021. "Do Unhappy Citizens Vote for Populism?" *European Journal of Political Economy* 68: 101985.

Nowlin, David V., and Ronald J. Stupak. 1998. *War as an Instrument of Policy: Past, Present, and Future*. Lanham, MD: University Press of America.

Nowlin, Matthew C., and Thomas M. Rabovsky. 2020. "A Cultural Theory of Partisanship and Policy Attitudes." *Social Science Quarterly* 101 (2): 878–892.

Nunkoo, Robin. 2015. "Tourism Development and Trust in Local Government." *Tourism Management* 46: 623–634.

Nussio, Enzo. 2019. "Can Crime Foster Social Participation as Conflict Can?" *Social Science Quarterly* 100 (3): 653–665.

Nyenhuis, Robert. 2020. "The Political Struggle for the People: Populist Discourse in the 2019 South African Elections". *Commonwealth & Comparative Politics* 58(4), 409–32. Papaioannou, Kostas, Myrto Pantazi, and Jan-Willem van Prooijen. 2023. "Unravelling the Relationship between Populism and Belief in Conspiracy Theories: The Role of Cynicism, Powerlessness and Zero-Sum Thinking. *British Journal of Psychology* 114 (1): 159–175.

O'Byrne, Darren J. and Alexander Hensby. 2011. *Theorizing Global Studies*. Houndmills, UK: Palgrave.
O'Connor, Alison M., Rebecca A. Judges, Kang Lee, and Angela D. Evans. 2022. "Examining Honesty-Humility and Cheating Behaviors across Younger and Older Adults." *International Journal of Behavioral Development* 46 (2): 112–117.
O'Farrell, I. B., P. Corcoran, and I. J. Perry. 2016. "The Area Level Association between Suicide, Deprivation, Social Fragmentation and Population Density in the Republic of Ireland: A National Study." *Social Psychiatry & Psychiatric Epidemiology* 51 (6): 839–847.
O'Keefe, Daniel J. 2002. *Persuasion: Theory & Research*. Thousand Oaks, CA: Sage.
O'Mahony, Patrick. 2013. *The Contemporary Theory of the Public Sphere*. Bern, Switzerland: Lang.
Oarga, Cristina, Olga Stavrova, and Detlef Fetchenhauer. 2015. "When and Why Is Helping Others Good for Well-Being? The Role of Belief in Reciprocity and Conformity to Society's Expectations." *European Journal of Social Psychology* 45 (2): 242–254.
Obschonk, Martin, Michael Stuetzer, David B. Audretsch, Peter J. Rentfrow, Jeff Potter, and Samuel D. Gosling. 2016. "Macropsychological Factors Predict Regional Economic Resilience During a Major Economic Crisis." *Social Psychological & Personality Science* 7 (2): 95–104.
Ogolsky, Brian G., and J. Kale Monk. 2018. "Maintaining Relationships." Pp. 523–537 in *The Cambridge Handbook of Personal Relationships*, edited by Anita L. Vangelisti and Daniel Perlman. Cambridge, UK: Cambridge University Press.
Ohmer, Mary L. 2007. "Citizen Participation in Neighborhood Organizations and Its Relationship to Volunteers' Self- and Collective Efficacy and Sense of Community." *Social Work Research* 31 (2): 109–120.
Oishi, Shigehiro, Jaime L. Kurtz, Felicity F. Miao, Jina Park, and Erin Whitchurch. 2011. "The Role of Familiarity in Daily Well-Being: Developmental and Cultural Variation." *Developmental Psychology* 47 (6): 1750–1756.
Oishi, Shigehiro. 2012. *The Psychological Wealth of Nations: Do Happy People Make a Happy Society?* Chichester, UK: Wiley.
Ojala, Maria. 2005. "Adolescents' Worries about Environmental Risks: Subjective Well-being, Values, and Existential Dimensions." *Journal of Youth Studies* 8 (3): 331–347.
Oksanen, Atte, James Hawdon, Emma Holkeri, Matti Nosi, Pekka Rosonen, and M. Nicole Warehime. 2014. "Exposure to Online Hate among Young Social Media Users." *Sociological Studies of Children & Youth* 18: 267–273.
Okulicz-Kozaryn, Adam, Oscar Holmes, and Derek R. Avery. 2014. "The Subjective Well-Being Political Paradox: Happy Welfare States and Unhappy Liberals." *Journal of Applied Psychology* 99 (6): 1300–1308.
Okun, Morris A., Alicia Barr, and A. Regula Herzog. 1998. "Motivation to Volunteer by Older Adults: A Test of Competing Measurement Models." *Psychology & Aging* 13 (4): 608–621.
Oliver, J. Eric. 2003. "Mental Life and the Metropolis in Suburban America: The Psychological Correlates of Metropolitan Place Characteristics." *Urban Affairs Review* 39 (2): 228–253.
Olivera, Javier. 2015. "Changes in Inequality and Generalized Trust in Europe." *Social Indicators Research* 124 (1): 21–41.
Olmstead, Spencer B., Jerika C. Norona, and Kristin M. Anders. 2019. "How Do College Experience and Gender Differentiate the Enactment of Hookup Scripts among Emerging Adults?" *Archives of Sexual Behavior* 48 (6): 1769–1783.
Olson, Amanda, Stephanie Reiland, Susan Davies, and Amy Reitmaier Koehler. 2016. "Learning about the Experience of Living with Chronic Conditions: A Framework Analysis of Nursing Students' Reflections on Their Conversations with Older Adults." *Gerontology & Geriatrics Education* 17: 1–21.
Olssen, Mark, John Codd, and Anne-Marie O'Neill. 2004. *Education Policy: Globalization, Citizenship and Democracy*. London, UK: SAGE.
Omoto, Allen M., Mark Snyder, and Justin D. Hackett. 2010. "Personality and Motivation Antecedents of Activism and Civic Engagement." *Journal of Personality* 78 (6): 1703–1734.

Oneal, John R., Bruce Russett, and Michael L. Berbaum. 2003. "Causes of Peace: Democracy, Independence, and International Organizations, 1885–1992." *International Studies Quarterly* 47: 371–393.

Onyx, Jenny, and Paul Bullen. 2000. "Measuring Social Capital in Five Communities." *Journal of Applied Behavioral Science* 36(1):23–42. \116–325.

Opp, Karl-Dieter. 2001. "Social Networks and the Emergence of Protest Norms." Pp.234–273 in *Social Norms*, edited by Michael Hechter and Karl-Dieter Opp. New York: Russell Sage.

Opp, Karl-Dieter. 2002. "When Do Norms Emerge by Human Design and When by the Unintended Consequences of Human Action?" *Rationality & Society* 14 (2): 131–158.

Orazani, Seyed Nima, Michael J. A. Wohl, and Bernhard Leidner. 2020. "Perceived Normalization of Radical Ideologies and Its Effect on Political Tolerance and Support for Freedom of Speech." *Group Processes & Intergroup Relations* 23 (8): 1150–1170.

Orjuela, Camilla. 2020. "Countering Buddhist Radicalisation: Emerging Peace Movements in Myanmar and Sri Lanka." *Third World Quarterly* 41 (1): 133–150.

Orlowski, Johannes, and Pamela Wicker. 2015. "The Monetary Value of Social Capital." *Journal of Behavioral & Experimental Economics* 57: 26–36.

Ortona, Guido. 2017. "Xenophobia Is Really That: A (Rational) Fear of the Stranger." *Mind & Society* 16 (1–2): 37–49.

Osberg, Lars, and Timothy Smeeding. 2006. "Fair Inequality? Attitudes toward Pay Differentials: The United States in Comparative Perspective." *American Sociological Review* 71: 450–473.

Osborne, Danny, Petar Milojev, and Chris G. Sibley. 2017. "Authoritarianism and National Identity: Examining the Longitudinal Effects of SDO and RWA on Nationalism and Patriotism." *Personality & Social Psychology Bulletin* 43 (8): 1086–1099.

Ostrom, Elinor. 2009. "What Is Social Capital?" Pp.17–38 in *Social Capital: Reaching out, Reaching in*, edited by Viva Ona Bartkus and James H. Davis. Cheltenham, UK: Edward Elgar.

Ottati, Victor, John Edwards, and Nathoniel D. Krumdick. 2014. "Attitude Theory and Research: Intradisciplinary and Interdisciplinary Connections." Pp. 707–742 in *The Handbook of Attitudes*, edited by Albarracin Dolores, T. Johnson Blair and P. Zanna Mark. Mahwah, NJ: Psychology.

Ousey, Graham C., and Matthew R. Lee. 2013. "Community Inequality and Crime." Pp.352–388 in *The Oxford Handbook of Criminological Theory*, edited by Francis T. Cullen and Pamela Wilcox. New York: Oxford University Press.

Ovadia, Seth. 2001. "Race, Class, and Gender Differences in High School Seniors" Values: Applying Intersection Theory in Empirical Analysis." *Social Science Quarterly* 82 (2): 340–356.

Ovaska, Tomi, and Ryo Takashima. 2006. "Economic Policy and the Level of Self-perceived Well-being: An International Comparison." *Journal of Socio-Economics* 35: 308–325.

Overall, Nickda C., et al. 2020. "Effects of the COVID-19 Pandemic and Nationwide Lockdown on Trust, Attitudes toward Government, and Well-being." *American Psychologist* 75 (5): 618–630.

Owens, Michael Leo, and Hannah L. Walker. 2018. "The Civic Voluntarism of "Custodial Citizens": Involuntary Criminal Justice Contact, Associational Life, and Political Participation." *Perspectives on Politics* 16 (4): 990–1013.

Oyserman, Daphna, and Ayse K. Uskul. 2008. "Individualism and Collectivism: Societal-level Processes with Implications for Individual-level and Society-level Outcomes." Pp.145–173 in *Multilevel Analysis of Individuals and Cultures*, edited by Fons J.R. van de Vijver, Dianne A. van Hemert, and Ype H. Poortinga. New York: Lawrence Erlbaum.

Oyserman, Daphna, Heather M. Coon, and Markus Kemmelmeier. 2002. "Rethinking Individualism and Collectivism: Evaluation of Theoretical Assumptions and Meta-analyses." *Psychological Bulletin* 128 (1): 3–72.

Oyserman, Daphna, Izumi Sakamato, and Armand Lauffer. 1998. "Cultural Accommodation: Hybridity and the Framing of Social Obligation." *Journal of Personality & Social Psychology* 74 (6): 1606–1618.

Ozbay, Ozben. 2008. "Does Social Capital Deter Youth from Cheating, Alcohol Use and Violence in Turkey? Bringing Torpil in." *Journal of Criminal Justice* 36: 403–415.

Ozer, Simon, and Preben Bertelsen. 2019. "Countering Radicalization: An Empirical Examination from a Life Psychological Perspective." *Peace & Conflict* 25 (3): 211–225.

Ozkirimli, Umut. 2005. *Contemporary Debates on Nationalism: A Critical Engagement*. Houndsmills, UK: Palgrave.

Paasonen, Susanna, Jenny Sundén, Katrin Tiidenberg, and Maria Vihlman. 2023. "About Sex, Open-Mindedness, and Cinnamon Buns: Exploring Sexual Social Media." *Social Media + Society* 9(1). \97–179.

Pace, Stefano. 2015. "Can a Commercially Oriented Brand Be Authentic? A Preliminary Study of the Effects of a Pro-Business Attitude on Consumer-based Brand Authenticity." *Journal of Applied Business Research* 31 (3): 1167–1177.

Pacilli, Maria Giuseppina, Ilaria Giovannelli, Federica Spaccatini, Jeroen Vaes, and Claudio Barbaranelli. 2018. "Elective Abortion Predicts the Dehumanization of Women and Men through the Mediation of Moral Outrage." *Social Psychology* 49 (5): 287–302.

Paez, Dario, Bernard Rimé, Nekane Basabe, Anna Wlodarczyk, and Larraitz Zumeta. 2015. "Psychosocial Effects of Perceived Emotional Synchrony in Collective Gatherings." *Journal of Personality & Social Psychology* 108 (5): 711–729.

Paez, Dario, James H. Liu, Magdalena Bobowik, Nekane Basabe, and Katja Hanke. 2016. "Social Representations of History, Cultural Values, and Willingness to Fight in a War: A Collective-Level Analysis in 40 Nations." *Asian Journal of Social Psychology* 19 (4): 347–361.

Paige, Katie J., Nolan E. Ramer, and Craig R. Colder. 2022. "Developmental Cascade Effects of Maternal Depression on Offspring Substance Use across Adolescence: Pathway through Mother-Child Relationship Quality and Peer Deviancy." *Research on Child & Adolescent Psychopathology* 50 (7): 933–944.

Painter-Davis, Noah. 2016. "Immigration Effects on Violence Contextualized." *Sociological Perspectives* 59 (1): 130–152.

Pakaluk, Michael. 2002. "Natural Law and Civil Society." Pp.131–148 in *Alternative Conception of Civil Society*, edited by Simone Chambers and Will Kymlicka. Princeton, NJ: Princeton University Press.

Pakulshi, Jan, and Bruce Tranter. 2000. "Civic, National and Denizen Identity in Australia." *Journal of Sociology* 36(2):205-222.

Palmer, Neal A., Douglas D. Perkins, and Qingwen Xu. 2011. "Social Capital and Community Participation among Migrant Workers in China." *Journal of Community Psychology* 39(1):89-105.

Paluck, Elizabeth Levy, and Donald P. Green. 2009. "Deference, Dissent, and Dispute Revolution: An Experimental Intervention Using Mass Media to Change Norms and Behavior in Rwanda." *American Political Science Review* 103 (4): 622–644.

Pan, Chengxin, and Oliver Turner. 2017. "Neoconservatism as Discourse: Virtue, Power and US Foreign Policy." *European Journal of International Relations* 23 (1): 74–96.

Pan, Yen- H., To- H. Chang, and Fang- H. Jhang. 2023. "Changes in Generalized and Particularized Trust and Their Link to Depressive Symptoms: Exploring the Roles of Changes in Self-Rated Health, Family Support and Life Satisfaction among Chinese Older Adults." *Research on Aging* 45(2):210-20.

Pangallo, Antonio, Lara Zibarras, Rachel Lewis, and Paul Flaxman. 2015. "Resilience through the Lens of Interactionism: A Systematic Review." *Psychological Assessment* 27 (1): 1–20.

Panitch, Leo. 2008. *Renewing Socialism: Transforming Democracy, Strategy and Imagination*. Pontypool, UK: Merlin.

Pantti, Mervi, Matti Nelimarkka, Kaarina Nikunen, and Gavan Titley. 2019. "The Meanings of Racism: Public Discourses About Racism in Finnish News Media and Online Discussion Forums." *European Journal of Communication* 34 (5): 503–519.

Papadopoulos, Yannis, and Philippe Warin. 2007. "Are Innovative, Participatory and Deliberative Procedures in Policy Making Democratic and Effective?" *European Journal of Political Research* 46: 445–472.

Papastephanou, Marianna. 2015. "The Lifeblood of Science and Its Politics: Interrogating Epistemic Curiosity as an Educational Aim." *Education Sciences* 6 (4): 1.
Pappas, Takis S. 2019. *Populism and Liberal Democracy: A Comparative and Theoretical Analysis*. Oxford, UK: Oxford University Press.
Paquin, Ryan S., and David M. Keating. 2017. "Fitting Identity in the Reasoned Action Framework: A Meta-Analysis and Model Comparison." *Journal of Social Psychology* 157 (1): 47–63.
Paraskevopoulos, Christos J. 2010. "Social Capital: Summing up the Debate on a Conceptual Tool of Comparative Politics and Public Policy." *Comparative Politics* 42 (4): 475–494.
Pardos-Prado, Sergi, and Iñaki. Sagarzazu. 2016. "The Political Conditioning of Subjective Economic Evaluations: The Role of Party Discourse." *British Journal of Political Science* 46 (4): 799–823.
Pargal, Sheoli, Daniel O. Gillian, and Mainul Hug. 2002. "Does Social Capital Increase Participation in Voluntary Solid Waste Management? Evicence from Dhaka, Bangladesh." Pp.188–209 in *The Role of Social Capital in Development: An Empirical Assessment*, edited by Christiaan Grootaert and Thierry van Bastelaer. Cambridge, UK: Cambridge University Press.
Park, Yoosun, and Rupaleem Bhuyan. 2012. "Whom Should We Serve? A Discourse Analysis of Social Workers' Commentary on Undocumented Immigrants." *Journal of Progressive Human Services* 23 (1): 18–40.
Parke, Ross D. 2004. "Development in the Family." *Annual Review of Psychology* 55 (1): 365–399.
Parker, Ian. 2002. *Critical Discursive Psychology*. Houndsmills, UK: Palgrave.
Parker, Ian. 2009. "Critical Psychology and Revolutionary Marxism." *Theory & Psychology* 19 (1): 71–92.
Parker, Jeffrey R., Iman Paul, and Nicholas Reinholtz. 2020. "Perceived Momentum Influences Responsibility Judgments." *Journal of Experimental Psychology: General* 149 (3): 482–489.
Parker, John, and Hilary Stanworth. 2005. "Go for It: Towards a Critical Realist Approach to Voluntary Risk Taking." *Health, Risk & Society* 7 (4): 319–336.
Parker, Sharon K., Carolyn M. Axtell, and Nick Turner. 2001. "Designing a Safer Workplace: Importance of Job Autonomy, Communication Quality, and Supportive Supervisors." *Journal of Occupational Health Psychology* 6 (3): 211–228.
Parkes, Alison, Ade Kearns, and Rowland Atkinson. 2002. "What Makes People Dissatisfied with Their Neighbourhoods?" *Urban Studies* 39 (13): 2413–2438.
Parsons, Talcott. 1968. *The Structure of Social Action*. New York: Free.
Pass, Jonathan. 2019. *American Hegemony in the 21st Century: A Neo Neo-Gramscian Perspective*. New York, NY: Routledge.
Passini, Stefano. 2019. "Promoting or Opposing Social Change: Political Orientations, Moral Convictions and Protest Intentions." *Europe's Journal of Psychology* 15 (4): 671–688.
Patch, Kartikeya C. 2012. "Eastern Traditions, Consciousness, and Spirituality." Pp. 343–357 in *The Oxford Handbook of Psychology and Spirituality*, edited by Lisa J. Miller. New York, NY: Oxford University Press.
Paternoster, Ray, and Ronet Bachman. 2010. "Control Theories." Pp.114–138 in *The SAGE Handbook of Criminological Theory*, edited by Eugene McLaughlin and Tim Newburn. London, UK: SAGE.
Paterson, Ian. 2018. "Any Room at the Inn? The Impact of Religious Elite Discourse on Immigration Attitudes in the United Kingdom." *British Journal of Politics & International Relations* 20 (3): 594–612.
Patricio, Lurdes, Natalia Figueiredo, Ricardo Gouveia Rodrigues, and Rui Silva. 2022. "The Value of Human Values: The Importance of Government Performance towards Security." *Social Policy & Administration* 56: 438–451.
Patrick, Heather, C. Raymond Knee, Amy Canevello, and Cynthia Lonsbary. 2007. "The role of Need Fulfillment in Relationship Functioning and Well-being: A Self-determination Theory Perspective." *Journal of Personality & Social Psychology* 92 (3): 434–457.

Patterson, David Allen, and Robert H. Keefe. 2008. "Using Social Construction Theory s a Foundation for Macro-level Interventions in Communities Impacted by HIV and Addictions." *Journal of Sociology & Social Welfare* 35 (2): 111–126.

Pattie, Charles, Patrick Seyd, and Paul Whiteley. 2004. *Citizenship in Britain: Values, Participation and Democracy*. Cambridge, UK: Cambridge University Press.

Patulny, Roger Vincent, and Alan Morris. 2012. "Questioning the Need for Social Mix: The Implications of Friendship Diversity amongst Australian Social Housing Tenants." *Urban Studies* 49 (15): 3365–3384.

Patwardhan, Abhijit M., Megan E. Keith, and Scott J. Vitell. 2012. "Religiosity, Attitude toward Business, and Ethical Beliefs: Hispanic Consumers in the United States." *Journal of Business Ethics* 110 (1): 61–70.

Paul, Charlotte, Julie Fitzjohn, Peter Herbison, and Nigel Dickson. 2000. "The Determinants of Sexual Intercourse before Age 16." *Journal of Adolescent Health* 27: 136–147.

Pauwels, Lieven, and Maarten De Waele. 2014. "Youth Involvement in Politically Motivated Violence: Why Do Social Integration, Perceived Legitimacy, and Perceived Discrimination Matter?" *International Journal of Conflict & Violence* 8 (1): 134–153.

Pavani, Jean-Baptiste., and Desirée Colombo. 2024. "Trait Hedonism and the Distribution of Savoring and Positive Emotion States in Everyday Life." *Psychological Reports* 127 (3): 1271–1291.

Pavlova, Maria K., and Rainer K. Silbereisen. 2015. "Supportive Social Contexts and Intentions for Civic and Political Participation: An Application of the Theory of Planned Behaviour." *Journal of Community & Applied Social Psychology* 25 (5): 432–446.

Paxton, Pamela, and Stephen Knack. 2012. "Individual and Country-Level Factors Affecting Support for Foreign Aid." *International Political Science Review* 33 (2): 171–192.

Paxton, Pamela. 1999. "Is Social Capital Declining in the United States? A Multiple Indicator Assessment." *American Journal of Sociology* 105 (1): 88–127.

Payne, Pedro R. 2006. *Youth Violence Prevention through Self-based Community Development*. New York: LFB.

Pazhoohi, Farid, and Alan Kingstone. 2021. "Associations of Political Orientation, Xenophobia, Right-Wing Authoritarianism, and Concern of Covid-19: Cognitive Responses to an Actual Pathogen Threat." *Personality & Individual Differences* 182: 111081.

Pearson, Jennifer, and Lindsey Wilkinson. 2013. "Family Relationships and Adolescent Well-Being: Are Families Equally Protective for Same-Sex Attracted Youth?" *Journal of Youth & Adolescence* 42 (3): 376–393.

Pearson, Michael, Helen Sweeting, Patrick West, Robert Young, Jacki Gordon, and Katrina Turner. 2006. "Adolescent Substance Use in Different Social and Peer Contexts: A Social Network Analysis." *Drugs: Education, Prevention and Policy* 13 (6):519–536.

Peck, Dennis L. 2002. "Civility: A Contemporary Context for a Meaningful Historical Concept." *Sociological Inquiry* 72 (3): 358–375.

Pedahzur, Ami, and Daphna Canetti-Nisim. 2004. "Support for Right-wing Extremist Ideology: Socio-economic Indicators and Socio-psychological Mechanisms of Social Identification." *Comparative Sociology* 3 (1): 1–36.

Peet, Richard, and Elaine Hatwick. 2009. *Theories of Development: Contentions, Arguments, Alternatives*. New York: Guilford.

Pehrson, Samuel, Roberto Gonzalez, and Rupert Brown. 2011. "Indigenous Rights in Chile: National Identity and Majority Group Support for Multicultural Policies." *Political Psychology* 32 (4): 667–690.

Pei, Zhijun, and Yingchun Pan. 2018. "Political Efficacy, Social Network and Involvement in Public Deliberation in Rural China." *Social Indicators Research* 139 (2): 453–471.

Peifer, J. L. 2010. "The Economics and Sociology of Religious Giving: Instrumental Rationality or Communal Bonding?" *Social Forces* 88 (4): 1569–1594.

Pelters, Britta, and Barbro Wijma. 2016. "Neither a Sinner nor a Saint: Health as a Present-Day Religion in the Age of Healthism." *Social Theory & Health* 14 (1): 129–148.

Pena-Lopez, José Atilano., and José Manuel. Sanchez-Santos. 2016. "Individual Social Capital: Accessibility and Mobilization of Resources Embedded in Social Networks." *Social Networks* 49: 1–11.

Peng, Liyong. 2003. *Sociology of Confucian Culture*. Beijing, China: People.

Peng, Zongchao, Ben Ma, and Taoxiong Liu. 2017. *Chinese Cooperative-harmonious Democracy*. Abington, UK: Routledge.

Penningroth, Suzanna L., and Walter D. Scott. 2012. "Age-Related Differences in Goals: Testing Predictions from Selection, Optimization, and Compensation Theory and Socioemotional Selectivity Theory." *International Journal of Aging & Human Development* 74 (2): 87–111.

Peplak, Joanna, and Tina Malti. 2022. "Toward Generalized Concern: The Development of Compassion and Links to Kind Orientations." *Journal of Adolescent Research* 37 (6): 776–804.

Permentier, Matthieu, Maarten van Ham, and Gideon Bolt. 2009. "Neighborhood Reputation and the Intention to Leave the Neighborhood." *Environment & Planning A* 41: 2162–2180.

Pernia, Ronald A. 2022. "Authoritarian Values and Institutional Trust: Theoretical Considerations and Evidence from the Philippines." *Asian Journal of Comparative Politics* 7 (2): 204–232.

Perotin, Virginie. 2001. "The Voluntary Sector: Job Creation and Social Policy: Illusions and Opportunities." *International Labour Review* 140 (3): 327–362.

Persson, Thomas, Charles F. Parker, and Sten Widmalm. 2017. "Social Trust, Impartial Administration and Public Confidence in EU Crisis Management Institutions." *Public Administration: An International* Quarterly 95 (1):97–114.

Peruzzi, Agnese. 2014. "Understanding Social Exclusion from a Longitudinal Perspective: A Capability-Based Approach." *Journal of Human Development & Capabilities* 15 (4): 335–354.

Peters, B. Guy and Jon Pierre. 2020. "The New Institutionalism." In *The SAGE Handbook of Political Science*, edited by Dirk Berg-Schlosser, Bertrand Badie and Leonardo Morlino. London, UK: SAGE.

Peters, B. Guy. 1999. *Institutional Theory in Political Science: The New Institutionalism*. London: Continuum.

Peterson, Bill E., and Eva C. Klohnen. 1995. "Realization of Generativity in Two Samples of Women at Midlife." *Psychology & Aging* 10 (1): 20–29.

Peterson, Gary W., Jose A. Cobas, Kevin R. Bush, Andrew Supple, and Stephan M. Wilson. 2006. "Parent-youth Relationships and the Self-esteem of Chinese Adolescents: Collectivism versus Individualism." *Marriage & Family Review* 36 (3–4): 173–200.

Peterson, Robert A., and Steven P. Brown. 2005. "On the Use of Beta Coefficients in Meta-analysis." *Journal of Applied Psychology* 90 (1): 175–181.

Peterson, Steven A., and Robert Maiden. 1993. "Personality and Politics among Older Americans: A Rural Case Study." *International Journal of Aging and Human Development* 36 (2): 157–169.

Petkanopoulou, Katerina, Rosa Rodríguez-Bailón, Guillermo B. Willis, and Gerben A. van Kleef. 2019. "Powerless People Don't Yell but Tell: The Effects of Social Power on Direct and Indirect Expression of Anger." *European Journal of Social Psychology* 49 (3): 533–547.

Petronio, Sandra, and Wesley T. Durham. 2015. "Communication Privacy Management Theory: Significance for Interpersonal Communication." Pp.335–347 in *Engaging Theories in Interpersonal Communication: Multiple Perspectives*, edited by Dawn O. Braithwaite and Paul Schrodt. Thousand Oaks, CA: SAGE.

Petrovic, Katja, Arthur A. Stukas, and Mathew D. Marques. 2020. "Religiosity, Motivations, and Volunteering: A Test of Two Theories of Religious Prosociality." *Journal of Theoretical Social Psychology* 4 (4): 157–168.

Pettigrew, Thomas F. 2002. "Relative Deprivation as a Key Social Psychological Concept." Pp.351–373 in *Relative Deprivation: Specification, Development, and Integration*, edited by Iain Walker and Heather J. Smith. Cambridge, UK: Cambridge University Press.

Pevnick, Ryan. 2015. "Should Civil Liberties Have Strict Priority?" *Law and Philosophy* 34 (5): 519–549.

Peyrot, Mark, and H. Lovell Smith. 2000. "Community Organization and Drug Prevention Readiness." *Advances in Medical Sociology* 7: 303–319.

Pfau, Michael, Patricia Moy, and Erin Alison Szabo. 2001. "Influence of Prime-time Television Programming on Perceptions of the Federal Government." *Mass Communication & Society* 4 (4): 437–453.

Pfeifer, Hanna. 2019. "The Normative Power of Secularism. Tunisian Ennahda's Discourse on Religion, Politics, and the State (2011–2016)." *Politics & Religion* 12 (3): 478–500.

Pfundmair, Michaela and Luisa A. M. Mahr. 2023. "How Group Processes Push Excluded People into a Radical Mindset: An Experimental Investigation." *Group Processes & Intergroup Relations.*

Phalet, Karen, Gulseli Baysu, and Maykel Verkuyten. 2010. "Political Mobilization of Dutch Muslims: Religious Identity, Salience, Goal Framing and Normative Constraints." *Journal of Social Issues* 66 (4): 759–779.

Phan, Mai B., Nadine Blumer, and Erin I. Demaiter. 2009. "Helping Hands: Neighborhood Diversity, Deprivation, and Reciprocity of Support in Non-kin Networks." *Journal of Social & Personal Relationships* 26 (6–7): 899–918.

Phelan, Elizabeth A., Lynda A. Anderson, Andrea Z. LaCroix, and Eric B. Larson. 2004. "Older Adults' Views of Successful Aging: How Do They Compare with Researchers' Definitions?" *Journal of American Geriatrics Society* 52: 211–216.

Phillips, David. 2006. *Quality of Life. Concept, Policy and Practice.* London: Routledge.

Phillips, Timothy, and Philip Smith. 2008. "Cosmopolitan Beliefs and Cosmopolitan Practices: An Empirical Investigation." *Journal of Sociology* 44 (4): 391–399.

Phipps, Shelley. 2003. "Social Cohesion and the Well-being of Canadian Children." Pp.79–120 in *Economic Implications of Social Cohesion*, edited by Lars Osberg. Toronto, Canada: University of Toronto Press.

Phithakkitnukoon, Santi and Zbigniew Smoreda. 2016. "Influence of Social Relations on Human Mobility and Sociality: A Study of Social Ties in a Cellular Network." *Social Network Analysis & Mining* 6(1).

Piatkowska, Sylwia J. 2020. "Poverty, Inequality, and Suicide Rates: A Cross-National Assessment of the Durkheim Theory and the Stream Analogy of Lethal Violence." *Sociological Quarterly* 61 (4): 787–812.

Pickard, Susan. 2010. "The Good Carer: Moral Practices in Late Modernity." *Sociology* 44 (3): 471–487.

Pierson, C. 2017. "Macro- and Micro-Political Vernaculizations of Rights: Human Rights and Abortion Discourses in Northern Ireland." *Health & Human Rights* 19 (1): 173–185.

Piferi, Rachel L., Rebecca L. Jobe, and Warren H. Jones. 2006. "Giving to Others During National Tragedy: The Effects of Altruistic and Egoistic Motivations on Long-term Giving." *Journal of Social & Personal Relationships* 23 (1): 171–184.

Piff, Paul K. 2014. "Wealth and the Inflated Self." *Personality & Social Psychology Bulletin* 40 (1): 34–43.

Pike, Brian E., and Adam D. Galinsky. 2020. "Power Leads to Action Because It Releases the Psychological Brakes on Action." *Current Opinion in Psychology* 33: 91–94.

Piliavin, Jane Allyn, and Peter L. Callero. 1991. *Giving Blood: The Development of an Altruistic Identity.* Baltimore, MD: Johns Hopkins University Press.

Pinhey, Thomas K., and Michael P. Perez. 2000. "Recounting the Wages of Self-Appraised Sinfulness: A Research Note on Divorce, Cohabitation, and Guilt." *Deviant Behavior* 21 (1): 1–13.

Pinker, Steven. 2011. *The Better Angels of Our Nature: Why Violence Has Declined.* New York: Viking.

Pinto, Isabel R., Catarina L. Carvalho, Carina Dias, Paula Lopes, Sara Alves, Cátia de Carvalho, and José M. Marques. 2020. "A Path toward Inclusive Social Cohesion: The Role of European and National Identity on Contesting vs. Accepting European Migration Policies in Portugal." *Frontiers in Psychology* 11:1875.

Piquero, Alex R., and Matthew Hickman. 2002. "The Rational Choice Implications of Control Balance Theory." Pp.85–107 in *Rational Choice and Criminal Behavior: Recent Research and Future Challenges*, edited by Alex R. Piquero and Stephen G. Tibbetts. New York: Routledge.

Piquero, Alex R., David P. Farrington, and Alfred Blumstein. 2007. *Key Issues in Criminal Career Research: New Analyses of the Cambridge Study in Delinquent Development*. Cambridge, UK: Cambridge University Press.

Piquero, Alex R., David P. Farrington, Daniel S. Nagin, and Terrie E. Moffitt. 2010. "Trajectories of Offending and Their Relation to Life Failure in Late Middle Age: Findings from the Cambridge Study in Delinquent Development." *Journal of Research in Crime & Delinquency.* 47 (2): 151–173.

Pires, Carla. 2022. "Global Predictors of COVID-19 Vaccine Hesitancy: A Systematic Review." *Vaccines* 10 (8): 1349.

Piven, Frances Fox, and Richard A. Cloward. 2005. "Rule Making, Rule Breaking, and Power." Pp. 33–53 in *The Handbook of Political Sociology: States, Civil Societies, and Globalization*, edited by Thomas Janoski, Robert Alford, Alexander Hicks, and Mildred A. Schwartz. Cambridge, UK: Cambridge University Press.

Plagnol, Anke C. 2011. "Financial Satisfaction over the Life Course: The Influence of Assets and Liabilities." *Journal of Economic Psychology* 32: 45–64.

Pohling, Rico, Rhett Diessner, and Anja Strobel. 2018. "The Role of Gratitude and Moral Elevation in Moral Identity Development." *International Journal of Behavioral Development* 42 (4): 405–415.

Pollack, Detlef, and Gert Pickel. 2007. "Religious Individualization or Secularization? Testing Hypotheses of Religious Change: The Case of Eastern and Western Germany." *British Journal of Sociology* 58 (4): 623–632.

Pommier, Elizabeth, Kristin D. Neff, and István Tóth-Király. 2020. "The Development and Validation of the Compassion Scale." *Assessment* 27 (1): 21–39.

Ponti, Lucia, and Franca Tani. 2019. "Attachment Bonds as Risk Factors of Intimate Partner Violence." *Journal of Child & Family Studies* 28 (5): 1425–1432.

Pool, Gregory J., and Andria F. Schwegler. 2007. "Differentiating among Motives for Norm conformity." *Basic & Applied Social Psychology* 29 (1): 47–60.

Poon, Kai-Tak., Zhansheng Chen, and Wing-Yan. Wong. 2020. "Beliefs in Conspiracy Theories Following Ostracism." *Personality & Social Psychology Bulletin* 46 (8): 1234–1246.

Poortinga, Wouter. 2012. "Community Resilience and Health: The Role of Bonding, Bridging, and Linking Aspects of Social Capital." *Health & Place* 18 (2): 286–295.

Portes, Alejandro, and Erik Vickstrom. 2011. "Diversity, Social Capital, and Cohesion." *Annual Review of Sociology* 37: 467–479.

Posthumus, Hanneke, Gideon Bolt, and Ronald van Kempen. 2013. "Why Do Displaced Residents Move to Socioeconomically Disadvantaged Neighborhoods?" *Housing Studies* 28 (2): 272–293.

Pourgerami, Abbas. 1991. "The Political Economy of Development: An Empirical Examination of the Wealth Theory of Democracy." *Journal of Theoretical Politics* 3 (2): 189–211.

Poveda, Alexander Cotte. 2011. "Economic Development, Inequality, and Poverty: An Analysis of Urban Violence in Columbia." *Oxford Development Studies* 39 (4): 453–468.

Powdthavee, Nattavadh. 2009. "How Important Is Rank to Individual Perception of Economic Standing? A Within-community Analysis." *Journal of Economic Inequality* 7: 225–248.

Powell, Fred. 2007. *The Politics of Civil Society: Big Society, Small Government?* Bristol, UK: Policy Press.

Powell, G. Bingham., Jr. 1982. *Contemporary Democracies: Participation, Stability, and Violence.* Cambridge, MA: Harvard University Press.

Power, Timothy J., and Giselle D. Jamison. 2005. "Political Mistrust in Latin America." *Comparative Sociology* 4 (1–2): 55–80.

Praszkier, Ryszard, and Andrzej Nowak. 2012. *Social Entrepreneurship: Theory and Practice.* New York: Cambridge University Press.

Praszkier, Ryszard. 2018. *Empowering Leadership of Tomorrow*. Cambridge, UK: Cambridge University Press.

Pratt, Michael W., Rhett Diessner, Adelle Pratt, Bruce Hunsberger, and S. Mark Pancer. 1996. "Moral and Social Reasoning and Perceptive Testing in Later Life: A Longitudinal Study." *Psychology & Aging* 11 (1): 66–73.

Pratt, Travis C., Kristy Holtfreter, and Michael D. Reisig. 2010. "Routine Online Activity and Internet Fraud Targeting: Extending the Generality of Routine Activity Theory." *Journal of Research in Crime & Delinquency* 47 (3): 267–296.

Premo, Joshua, Richard Lamb, and Andy Cavagnetto. 2018. "Conditional Cooperators: Student Prosocial Dispositions and Their Perceptions of the Classroom Social Environment." *Learning Environment Research* 21 (2): 229–244.

Pressgrove, Geah, Cristobal Barra, and Melissa Janoske. 2020. "Using STOPS to Predict Prosocial Behavioral Intentions: Disentangling the Effects of Passive and Active Communicative Action." *Public Relations Review* 46 (4): 101956.

Pretsch, Johanna, and Natalie Ehrhardt-Madapathi. 2018. "Experiences of Justice in School and Attitudes Towards Democracy: A Matter of Social Exchange?" *Social Psychology of Education* 21 (3): 655–675.

Preves, Sharon E., and Jeylan T. Mortimer. 2013. "Socialization for Primary, Intimate, and Work Relationships in the Adult Life Course." Pp. 151–187 in *Handbook of Social Psychology*, edited by John Delamater and Amanda Ward. Dordrecht, Netherlands: Springer.

Prezza, Miretta, Matilde Amici, Tiziana Roberti, and Gloria Tedeschi. 2001. "Sense of Community Referred to the Whole Town: Its Relations with Neighboring, Homelessness, Life Satisfaction and Area of Residence." *Journal of Community Psychology* 29 (1): 29–52.

Price, Julia, Deborah A. G. Drabick, and Ty A. Ridenour. 2019. "Association with Deviant Peers across Adolescence: Subtypes, Developmental Patterns, and Long-Term Outcomes." *Journal of Clinical Child & Adolescent Psychology* 48(2):238-49.

Price, Michael E., Nicholas Pound, and Isabel M. Scott. 2014. "Female Economic Dependence and the Morality of Promiscuity." *Archives of Sexual Behavior* 43 (7): 1289–1301.

Primoratz, Igor. 1999. *Ethics and Sex*. London, UK: Routledge.

Prins, Karin, Bram P. Buunk, and Nico W. VanYperen. 1993. "Equity, Normative Disapproval and Extramarital Relationships." *Journal of Social & Personal Relationships* 10: 39–53.

Prinstein, Mitchell J., and Shirley S. Wang. 2005. "False Consensus and Adolescent Peer Contagion: Examining Discrepancies between Perceptions and Actual Reported Levels of Friends" Deviant and Health Risk Behaviors." *Journal of Abnormal Child Psychology* 33 (3): 293–306.

Prior, Marcus. 2019. *Hooked: How Politics Captures People's Interest*. Cambridge: Cambridge, UK.

Prislin, Radmila, and Wendy Wood. 2014. "Social Influence in Attitudes and Attitude Change." Pp. 671–700 in *The Handbook of Attitudes*, edited by Albarracin Dolores, T. Johnson Blair and P. Zanna Mark. Mahwah, NJ: Psychology.

Proctor, K. Ryan., and Richard E. Niemeyer. 2019. *Mechanistic Criminology*. New York, NY: Routledge.

Prokhovnik, Raia. 2007. *Sovereignties: Contemporary Theory and Practice*. Houndmills, UK Palgrave.

Prokhovnik, Raia. 2008. *Sovereignty: History and Theory*. Exeter, UK: Imprint Academic.

Proulx, Christine M., Heather M. Helms, and C. Chris Payne. 2004. "Wives' Domain-Specific "Marriage Work" with Friends and Spouses: Links to Marital Quality." *Family Relations* 53 (4): 393–404.

Prouteau, Liopel, and Francois-Charles. Wolff. 2008. "On the Relational Motive for Volunteer Work." *Journal of Economic Psychology* 29: 314–335.

Provine, Robert R. 2000. *Laughter: A Scientific Investigation*. London: Faber.

Prusaczyk, Elvira, and Gordon Hodson. 2018. "Left-Right Differences in Abortion Policy Support in America: Clarifying the Role of Sex and Sexism in a Nationally Representative 2016 Sample." *Personality & Individual Differences* 127: 22–25.

Pruss, Alexander R. 2013. *One Body: An Essay in Christian Sexual Ethics*. Notre Dame, IN: University of Notre Dame Press.

Pulkkinen, Lea, Anna-Liisa. Lyyra, and Katja Kokko. 2009. "Life Success of Males on Nonoffender, Adolescence-Limited, Persistent, and Adult-Onset Antisocial Pathways: Follow-up from Age 8 to 42." *Aggressive Behavior* 35 (2): 117–135.

Pulkkinen, Lea. 2018. "Longitudinal Study of Personality and Social Development: Insights about Aggression after Five Decades." Pp. 31–51 *The Cambridge Handbook of Violent Behavior and Aggression*, edited by Alexander T. Vazsonyi, David J. Flannery and Matt DeLisi. Cambridge, UK: Cambridge University Press. \113–97.

Puohiniemi, Martti, and Markku Verkasalo. 2020. "Zeitgeist Effects, Fragmentation of Media Use, and Value Consensus." *Journal of Social & Political Psychology* 8 (1): 300–332.

Putnam, Robert D. 2007. "E Pluribus Unum: Diversity and Community in the Twenty-first Century." *Scandinavian Political Studies* 30 (2): 137–174.

Pyszkowska, Anna, and Michael Ronnlund. 2021. "Psychological Flexibility and Self-Compassion as Predictors of Well-Being: Mediating Role of a Balanced Time Perspective." *Frontiers in Psychology* 12: 671746.

Pyszkowska, Anna. 2020. "Personality Predictors of Self-Compassion, Ego-Resiliency and Psychological Flexibility in the Context of Quality of Life." *Personality & Individual Differences* 161: 109932.

Qi, Xiaoying. 2013. "Guanxi, Social Capital Theory and Beyond: Toward a Globalized Social Science." *British Journal of Sociology* 64 (2): 308–324.

Qian, Qian. 2018. *Jewish Wisdom of Doing*. Beijing, China: Chinese Industrial and Commercial Federation.

Qin, Chu. 2013. *Daoist Living, Scholarist Practice*, Buddhist Cultivation. Beijing, China: Foreign Languages.

Qouta, Samir, Raija-Leona. Punamaki, Edith Montgomery, and Eyad El Sarray. 2007. "Predictors of Psychological Distress and Positive Resources among Palestinian Adolescents: Trauma, Child, and Mothering Characteristics." *Child Abuse & Neglect* 31: 699–717.

Quadagno, Jill. 1987. "Theories of the Welfare State." Pp.109–128 in *Annual Review of Sociology*, Vol.13, edited by W. Richard Scott and James F. Short, Jr. Palo Alto, CA: Annual Reviews Inc.

Quah, Stella R. 2003. *Home and Kin: Families in Asia*. Singapore: Eastern Universities.

Quaranta, Mario. 2016. "Protesting in Hard Times: Evidence from a Comparative Analysis of Europe, 2000–2014." *Current Sociology* 64 (5): 736–756.

Quillian, Lincoln. 2014. "Social Psychological Processes in Studies of Neighborhoods and Inequality." Pp. 459–482 in *Handbook of the Social Psychology of Inequality*, edited by Jane D. McLeod, Edward J. Lawler, and Michael Schwalbe. Dordrecht, Netherlands: Springer.

Rabbani, Martha Jalali. 2011. *The Development and Antidevelopment Debate: Critical Reflections on the Philosophical Foundations*. Farnham, UK: Ashgate.

Rachels, James, and Stuart Rachels. 2015. *The Elements of Moral Philosophy*. New York, NY: McGraw-Hill.

Radcliff, Benjamin. 2001. "Politics, Market, and Life Satisfaction: The Political Economy of Human Happiness." *American Political Science Review* 85 (4): 938–952.

Rade, Candalyn B., Sarah L. Desmarais, and Jeni L. Burnette. 2018. "An Integrative Theoretical Model of Public Support for Ex-Offender Reentry." *International Journal of Offender Therapy & Comparative Criminology* 62 (8): 2131–2152.

Rader, Nicole E., Jeralynn S. Cossman, and Jeremy R. Porter. 2012. "Fear of Crime and Vulnerability: Using a National Sample of Americans to Examine Two Competing Paradigms." *Journal of Criminal Justice* 40 (2): 134–141.

Radford, Scott K., and Peter H. Bloch. 2012. "Grief, Commiseration, and Consumption Following the Death of a Celebrity." *Journal of Consumer Culture* 12 (2): 137–155.

Raeff, Catherine. 2010. "Self Constructing Activities." *Theory & Psychology* 20 (1): 28–51.

Raffo, Carlo, and Michelle Reeves. 2000. "Youth Transitions and Social Exclusion: Developments in Social Capital Theory." *Journal of Youth Studies* 3 (2): 147–166.

Rahn, Wendy. 2008. "Cooperation with and without Trust: Evidence from Local Settings." Pp. 259–274 in *Cooperation: The Political Psychology of Effective Human Interaction*, edited by Brandon A. Sullivan, Mark Snyder and John L. Sullivan. Malden, MA: Blackwell.

Rai, Saatvika. 2020. "Policy Adoption and Policy Intensity: Emergence of Climate Adaptation Planning in U.S. States." *Review of Policy Research* 37 (4): 444–463.

Raijman, Rebeca, and Oshrat Hochman. 2011. "National Attachments, Economic Competition, and Social Exclusion of Non-Ethnic Migrants in Israel: A Mixed-Methods Approach." *Quality & Quantity* 45 (6): 1151–1174.

Raijman, Rebeca, Moshe Semyonov, and Peter Schmidt. 2003. "Do Foreigners Deserve Rights? Determinants of Public Views towards Foreigners in Germany and Israel." *European Sociological Review* 19 (4): 379–392.

Raine, Adrian, and Peter H. Venables. 2017. "Adolescent Daytime Sleepiness as a Risk Factor for Adult Crime." *Journal of Child Psychology & Psychiatry & Allied Disciplines* 58 (6): 728–735.

Ramarajan, Lakshmi, Ida E. Berger, and Itay Greenspan. 2017. "Multiple Identity Configurations: The Benefits of Focused Enhancement for Prosocial Behavior." *Organization Science* 28 (3): 495–513.

Ramesh, Tharmalingam, Riddhika Kalle, Kalyanasundaram Sankar, Qamar Qureshi, Anthony J. Giordano, and Colleen Thelma Downs. 2019. "To Resettle or Not? Socioeconomic Characteristics, Livelihoods, and Perceptions toward Resolving Human-Tiger Conflict in the Nilgiri Biosphere Reserve, India." *Land Use Policy* 83: 32–46.

Rampichini, Carla, and Silvana Schifini D'Andrea. 1998. "A Hierarchical Ordinal Probit Model for the Analysis of Life Satisfaction in Italy." *Social Indicators Research* 44 (1): 41–69.

Ramsay, Maureen. 1997. *What's Wrong with Liberalism? A Radical Critique of Liberal Political Philosophy*. London, UK: Leicester University Press.

Ramsey, Meagan A., and Amy L. Gentzler. 2015. An upward Spiral: Bidirectional Associations between Positive Affect and Positive Aspects of Close Relationships across the Life Span. *Developmental Review* 36: 58–104.

Ranis, Gustav, and Xiaoxue Zhao. 2013. "Technology and Human Development." *Journal of Human Development & Capabilities* 14 (4): 467–482.

Rank, Mark R., Hong-sik Yoon, and Thomas A. Hirschl. 2003. "American Poverty as a Structural Failing: Evidence and Arguments." *Journal of Sociology & Social Welfare* 30 (4): 3–29.

Rasinski, Kenneth A., Tom W. Smith, and Sara Zuckerbraum. 1994. "Fairness Motivations and Tradeoffs Underlying Public Support for Government Environment Spending in Nine Nations." *Journal of Social Issues* 50 (3): 179–197.

Rasmussen, Douglas, and Douglas J. Den Uyl. 2005. *Norms of Liberty: A Perfectionist Basis for Non-perfectionist Politics*. University Park, PA: Pennsylvania State University Press.

Rasmussen, Terje. 2023. *The Sociology of Sovereignty: Politics, Social Transformations and Conceptual Change*. Manchester, UK: Manchester University Press.

Ratnapala, Suri. 2013. *Jurisprudence*. Port Melbourne, Australia: Cambridge University Press.

Ratner, Rebecca K., Nicole You Jeung Kim, and Yuechen Wu. 2023. "When Is Sociality Congruent with Self-Care?" *Journal of Consumer Psychology* 33(1):213-16.

Ravanera, Zenaida R., Fernando Rajalton, and Pierre Turcotta. 2003. "Youth Integration and Social Capital: An Analysis of the Canadian Social Surveys in Time Use." *Youth & Society* 35 (2): 158–182.

Ray, Colleen M., and Lisa A. Kort-Butler. 2020. "What You See Is What You Get? Investigating How Survey Context Shapes the Association between Media Consumption and Attitudes About Crime." *American Journal of Criminal Justice* 45 (5): 914–932.

Ray, Larry. 2017. "The Sociology of Violence." Pp. 178–187 in *The Cambridge Handbook of Sociology, Vol. 2: Specialty and Interdisciplinary Studies*, edited by Kathleen Odell Korgen. New York, NY: Cambridge University Press.

Raymo, James M. 2015. "Living Alone in Japan: Relationships with Happiness and Health." *Demographic Research* 32 (1): 1267–1298.

Read, Stephen J., and Dan Simon. 2012. "Parallel Constraint Satisfaction as a Mechanism for Cognitive Consistency." Pp. 66–86 in *Cognitive Consistency: A Fundamental Principle in Social Cognition*, edited by Bertram Gawronsci, and Fritz Strack. New York, NY: Guilford.

Realo, Anu, Juri Allik, and Brenna Greenfield. 2008. "Radius of Trust: Social Capital in Relation to Familism and Institutional Collectivism." *Journal of Cross-Cultural Psychology* 39 (4): 447–462.

Reardon, Sean F., and Kendra Bischoff. 2011. "Income Inequality and Income Segregation." *American Journal of Sociology* 116 (4): 1092–1153.

Reavy, Matthew. 2023. *Professional Communication Ethics*. Long Grove, IL: Waveland.

Reddick, Christopher G., Bruce J. Perlman, and Tansu Demir. 2022. "Citizen Satisfaction with Public Service Delivery: A Test of Alternative Theories." *Canadian Public Administration* 65 (2): 352–371.

Redlawsk, David P., and James A. McCann. 2005. "Popular Interpretations of Corruption and Their Partisan Consequences." *Political Behavior* 27 (3): 261–283.

Redmond, Mark V. 2018. *Social Decentering: A Theory of Other-orientation Encompassing Empathy and Perspective-taking*. Berlin, Germany: Walter de Gruyter.

Reed, Gay Garland. 1995. "Moral/political Education in the People's Republic of China: Learning through role Models." *Journal of Moral Education* 24 (2): 99–111.

Reed, Paul B., and L. Kevin Selbee. 2000. "Distinguishing Characteristics of Active Volunteers in Canada." *Nonprofit & Voluntary Sector Quarterly* 29 (4): 471–592.

Reese, Bianka M., May S. Chen, Manali Nekkanti, and Marta I. Mulawa. 2021. "Prevalence and Risk Factors of Women's Past-Year Physical IPV Perpetration and Victimization in Tanzania." *Journal of Interpersonal Violence* 36 (3–4): 1141–1167.

Reese, Gerhard, Amir Rosenmarnn, and James E. Cameron. 2019. *The Psychology of Globalization: Identity, Ideology, and Action*. London, UK: Academic.

Reeskens, Tim, and Leen Vandecasteele. 2017. "Hard Times and European Youth. The Effect of Economic Insecurity on Human Values, Social Attitudes and Well-Being." *International Journal of Psychology* 52 (1): 19–27.

Reeskens, Tim, and Leen Vandecasteele. 2017. "Hard Times and European Youth. The Effect of Economic Insecurity on Human Values, Social Attitudes and Well-Being." *International Journal of Psychology* 52 (1): 19–27.

Reeskens, Tim, and Wim van Oorschot. 2013. "Equity, Equality, or Need? A Study of Popular Preferences for Welfare Redistribution: Principles across 24 European Countries." *Journal of European Public Policy* 20 (8): 1174–1195.

Reeve, Zoey. 2021. "Engaging with Online Extremist Material: Experimental Evidence." *Terrorism & Political Violence* 33 (8): 1595–1620.

Regalia, Camillo, Claudio Manzi, and Eugenia Scabin. 2013. "Individuation and Differentiation in Families across Cultures." Pp. 439–455 in *Handbook of Family Theories: A Content-based Approach*, edited by Mark A. Fine and Frank D. Fincham. New York: Routledge.

Regilme, Salvador Santino Fulo, Jr. 2020. "Human Rights and Humanitarian Interventions in the International Arena." In *The SAGE Handbook of Political Science*, edited by Dirk Berg-Schlosser, Bertrand Badie and Leonardo Morlino. London, UK: SAGE.

Rehm, Philipp. 2016. *Risk Inequality and Welfare States: Social Policy Preferences, Development, and Dynamics*. New York, NY: Cambridge University Press.

Reich, Sabine, Frank M. Schneider, and Leonie Heling. 2018. "Zero Likes: Symbolic Interactions and Need Satisfaction Online." *Computers in Human Behavior* 80: 97–102.

Reichman, Nancy E., and Genevieve M. Kenney. 1997. "'Effects of Parents' Place of Birth and Ethnicity on Birth Outcomes in New Jersey." Pp.199–230 in *Keys to Successful Immigration: Implications of the New Jersey Experience*, edited by Thomas J. Espenshade. Aldershot, UK: Ashgate.

Reiner, Robert, 2016. *Crime: The Mystery of the Common-Sense Concept*. Cambridge, UK: Policy.

Reininger, Klaus Michael, Christoph Daniel Schaefer, Steffen Zitzmann, and Bernd Simon. 2020. "Dynamics of Respect: Evidence from Two Different National and Political Contexts." *Journal of Social & Political Psychology* 8 (2): 542–559.

Reisch, Michael. 2013. "Radical Community Organizing." Pp.361–381 in *The Handbook of Community Practice*, edited by Marie Weil, Michael Reisch and Mary L. Ohmer. Thousand Oaks, CA: SAGE.

Reitan, Therese, and Sten-Ake. Stenberg. 2019. "From Classroom to Conscription: Leadership Emergence in Chldhood and Early Adulthood." *Leadership Quarterly* 30: 298–319.

Rempel, John K., and Christopher T. Burris. 2005. "Let Me Count the Ways: An Integrative Theory of Love and Hate." *Personal Relationships* 12 (2): 297–313.

Renfrow, Daniel G., and Judith A. Howard. 2013. "Social Psychology of Gender and Race." Pp. 491–531 in *Handbook of Social Psychology*, edited by John Delamater and Amanda Ward. Dordrecht, Netherlands: Springer.

Renger, Daniela, and Gerhard Reese. 2017. "From Equality-Based Respect to Environmental Activism: Antecedents and Consequences of Global Identity." *Political Psychology* 38 (5): 867–879.

Renger, Daniela, Silke Eschert, Mimke L. Teichgräber, and Sophus Renger. 2020. "Internalized Equality and Protest against Injustice: The Role of Disadvantaged Group Members" Self-Respect in Collective Action Tendencies." *European Journal of Social Psychology* 50 (3): 547–560.

Rentziou, Aikaterini, Christina Milioti, Konstantina Gkritza, and Matthew G. Karlaftis. 2011. "Urban Road Pricing: Modeling Public Acceptance." *Journal of Urban Planning & Development* 137 (1): 56–64.

Requena, Miguel, and Mikolaj Stanek. 2014. "Religiosity and Politics in Spain and Poland: A Period Effect Analysis." *Sociological Compass* 61 (3): 348–367.

Rettig, Kathryn D., and Ronit D. Leichtentritt. 1999. "A General Theory for Perceptual Indicators of Family Quality." *Social Indicators Research* 47: 301–342.

Reykowski, Janusz. 2006. "Deliberate Democracy and Human Nature: An Empirical Approach." *Political Psychology* 27 (3): 323–346.

Reynolds, Nicola. 2015. "Discourses of Love, Compassion, and Belonging: Reframing Christianity for a Secular Audience." *Journal Contemporary Religion* 30 (1): 39–54.

Rhodes-Purdy, Matthew, Rachel Navarre, and Stephen M. Utych. 2021. "Populist Psychology: Economics, Culture, and Emotions." *Journal of Politics* 83(4), 1559–72. van Prooijen, Jan-Willem, Talia Cohen Rodrigues, Carlotta Bunzel, Oana Georgescu, Dániel Komáromy, and André P. M. Krouwel. 2022. "Populist Gullibility: Conspiracy Theories, News Credibility, Bullshit Receptivity, and Paranormal Belief. *Political Psychology* 43 (6): 1061–1079.

Rhodes-Purdy, Matthew, Rachel Navarre, and Stephen Utych. 2023. *The Age of Discontent: Populism, Extremism, and Conspiracy Theories in Contemporary Democracies*. New York, NY: Cambridge University Press.

Rich, Ashleigh J., Heather L. Armstrong, Zishan Cui, Paul Sereda, Nathan J. Lachowsky, David M. Moore, Robert S. Hogg, and Eric A. Roth. 2018. "Sexual Orientation Measurement, Bisexuality, and Mental Health in a Sample of Men Who Have Sex with Men in Vancouver, Canada." *Journal of Bisexuality* 18 (3): 299–317.

Richards, Lindsay. 2016. "For Whom Money Matters Less: Social Connectedness as a Resilience Resource in the UK." *Social Indicators Research* 125 (2): 509–535.

Richards, P. Scott. 2012. "Honoring Religious Diversity and Universal Spirituality in psychotherapy." Pp. 237–254 in *The Oxford Handbook of Psychology and Spirituality*, edited by Lisa J. Miller. New York, NY: Oxford University Press.

Richardson, Lilliard E., Jr., David J. Houston, and Chris Sissie Hadjiharalambous. 2001. "Public Confidence in the Leaders of American Governmental Institutions." Pp.83–97 in *What Is It about Government that Americans Dislike?* edited by John R. Hibbing and Elizabeth Theiss-Morse. Cambridge, UK: Cambridge University Press. (JK2443.W483).

Richey, Sean, and Ken'ichi Ikeda. 2009. "Institutional Incentives and Trust: Marginalized Groups and the Creation of Trust in Local Government." *Social Science Quarterly* 90 (4): 911–926.
Richey, Sean. 2007. "Manufacturing Trust: Community Currencies and the Creation of Social Capital." *Political Behavior* 29: 69–88.
Richey, Sean. 2010. "The Impact of Corruption on Social Trust." *American Politics Research* 38 (4): 676–690.
Richey, Sean. 2011. "Civic Engagement and Patriotism." *Social Science Quarterly* 92 (4): 1044–1056.
Richmond, David A. 2003. "Embeddedness in Voluntary Associations and the Timing of Geographic Moves." *Sociological Forum* 18 (2): 295–322.
Rick, Blake M., Eric W. Mania, and Samuel L. Guertner. 2006. "Intergroup Threat and Outgroup Attitudes: A Meta-analytic Review." *Personality & Social Psychology Review* 10 (4): 336–353.
Rieger, Marc Oliver, and Mei Wang. 2021. "Trust in Government Actions During the COVID-19 Crisis." *Social Indicators Research* 159 (3): 967–989.
Riemer, Hila, Sharon Shavitt, Minkyung Koo, and Hazel Rose Markus. 2014. "Preferences Don¡¯T Have to Be Personal: Expanding Attitude Theorizing with a Cross-Cultural Perspective." *Psychological Review* 121 (4): 619–648.
Rijken, Mieke, and Peter P. Groenewegen. 2008. "Money Does Not Bring Well-being, But It Does Help? The Relationship between Financial Resources and Life Satisfaction of the Chronically Ill Mediated by Social Deprivation and Loneliness." *Journal of Community & Applied Social Psychology* 18: 3–33.
Riley, Jonathan. 2008. "The Interpretation of Maximizing Utilitarianism." *Social Philosophy & Policy Foundation* 26 (1): 286–325.
Rime, Bernard, Pierre Bouchat, Olivier Klein, and Laurent Licata. 2015. "When Collective Memories of Victimhood Fade: Generational Evolution of Intergroup Attitudes and Political Aspirations in Belgium." *European Journal of Social Psychology* 45 (4): 515–532.
Rindermann, Heiner. 2018. *Cognitive Capitalism: Human Capital and the Wellbeing of Nations.* Cambridge, UK: Cambridge University Press.
Ringen, Stein. 2007. *What Democracy Is for: On Freedom and Moral Goernment.* Princeton, NJ: Princeton University Press.
Riordan, Patrick. 2008. *A Grammar of the Common Good: Speaking of Globalization.* London: Continuum.
Rip, Blanka, Robert J. Vallerand, and Mare-Andre K. Lafreniere. 2012. "Passion for a Cause, Passion for a Creed: On Ideological Passion, Identity Threat, and Extremism." *Journal of Personality* 80 (3): 573–602.
Rippl, Suzanne, Nicola Bücker, Anke Petrat, and Klaus Boehnke. 2010. "Crossing the Frontier: Transnational Social Integration in the EU's Border Regions." *International Journal of Comparative Sociology* 51 (1–2): 5–31.
Rith, Kendrick A., and Lisa M. Diamond. 2013. "Same-sex Relationships." Pp.123–144 in *Handbook of Family Theories: A Content-based Approach*, edited by Mark A. Fine and Frank D. Fincham. New York: Routledge.
Ritzer, George, and Douglas Goodman. 2001. "Postmodern Social Theory." Pp.151–169 in *Handbook of Sociological Theory*, edited by Jonathan H. Turner. New York: Kluwer.
Ritzer, George. 1997. *Postmodern Social Theory.* New York: McGraw-Hill.
Rival, Laura, Don Slater, and Daniel Miller. 1998. "Sex and Sociality: Comparative Ethnographies of Sexual Objectification." *Theory, Culture & Society* 15 (3–4): 295–321.
Rivera, Jason D. 2018. "Reliance on Faith-Based Organizations for Tangible Assistance in Times of Disaster: Exploring the Influence of Bonding Social Capital." *Sociological Spectrum* 38 (1): 39–50.
Rivera, Lauren. 2008. "Managing Spoiled National Identity: War, Tourism, and Memory in Croatia." *American Sociological Review* 73: 613–634.
Rivera-Batiz, Francisco L. 2002. "Democracy, Governance, and economic Growth: Theory and evidence." *Review of Development Economics* 6 (2): 225–247.

Robert, Peter and Erzsebet Bukodi. 2005. "The Effects of the Globalization Process in the Transition to Adulthood in Hungary." Pp.177–213 in *Globalization, Uncertainty and Youth in Society*, edited by Hans-Peter Blossfeld, Erik Klijzing, Melinda Mills and Karin Kurz. London: Routledge.

Roberts, Alasdair. 2012. "Why the Occupy Movement Failed." *Public Administration Review* 72: 754–762.

Roberts, Anthea, and Nicolas Lamp. 2021. *Six Faces of Globalization: Who Wins, Who Loses, and Why It Matters*. Cambridge, MA: Harvard.

Roberts, Brent W., and Wendy F. DelVecchio. 2000. "The Rank-order Consistency of Personality Traits from Childhood to Old Age: A Quantitative Review of Longitudinal Studies." *Psychological Bulletin* 126 (1): 3–25.

Roberts, Donald F., Lisa Henriksen, and Ulla G. Foehr. 2009. "Adolescence, Adolescents, and Media." Pp.314–344 in *Handbook of Adolescent Psychology, Vol.2: Contextual Influences and Adolescent Development*, edited by Richard M. Lerner and Laurence Steinberg. Hoboken, NJ: Wiley.

Roberts, Louisa L. 2019. "Changing Worldwide Attitudes toward Homosexuality: The Influence of Global and Region-specific Cultures, 1981–2012." *Social Science Research* 80: 114–131.

Robertson, Roland, and Kathleen E. White. 2005. "Globalization: Sociology and Cross-Disciplinarity." Pp. 345–366 in *The SAGE Handbook of Sociology*, edited by Craig Calhoun, Chris Rojek, and Bryan Turner. London, UK: SAGE.

Robichau, Robbie W., and Billie Sandberg. 2022. "'Creating Meaningfulness in Public Service Work: A Qualitative Comparative Analysis of Public and Nonprofit Managers' Experience of Work." *American Review of Public Administration* 52 (2): 122–138.

Robila, Mihaela. 2006. "Economic Pressure and Social Exclusion in Europe." *Social Science Journal* 43: 85–97.

Robinaugh, Donald J., Christine Mauro, Eric Bui, Lauren Stone, Riva Shah, Yuanjia Wang, Natalia A. Skritskaya, Charles F. Reynolds, Sidney Zisook, Mary-Frances. O'Connor, Katherine Shear, and Naomi M. Simon. 2016. "Yearning and Its Measurement in Complicated Grief." *Journal of Loss & Trauma* 21 (5): 410–420.

Robinson, Brandon Andrew. 2018. "Doing Sexual Responsibility: HIV, Risk Discourses, Trust, and Gay Men Interacting Online." *Sociological Perspectives* 61 (3): 383–398.

Robinson, David. 2005. "The Search for Community Cohesion: Key Themes and Dominant Concepts of the Public Policy Agenda." *Urban Studies* 42(8):1411–27. \111–245.

Robison, Lindon J., A. Allan Schmid, and Marcelo E. Siles. 2002. "Is Social Capital Really Capital?" *Review of Social Economy* 60 (1): 1–21.

Rocha, Hector O., and Samantra Ghoshal. 2006. "Beyond Self-interest Revisited." *Journal of Management Studies* 43 (3): 585–619.

Rochelle, Tina L. 2015. "Diversity and Trust in Hong Kong: An Examination of Tin Shui Wai, Hong Kong's City of Sadness." *Social Indicators Research* 120: 437–454.

Rochelle, Tina L., and Steven M. Shardlow. 2013. "Quality of Social Networks among UK Chinese." *Social Indicators Research* 114: 425–439.

Rocke, Christina, and Margie E. Lachman. 2008. "Perceived Trajectories of Life Satisfaction across Past, Present, and Future: Profiles and Correlates of Subjective Change in Young, Middle-aged, and Older Adults." *Psychology & Aging* 23 (4): 833–847.

Rocque, Michael, Chad Posick, and Ray Paternoster. 2016. "Identities through Time: An Exploration of Identity Change as a Cause of Desistance." *Justice Quarterly* 33 (1): 45–72.

Roderick, Ian. 2016. *Critical Discourse Studies and Technology: A Multimodal Approach to Analyzing Technoculture*. London, UK: Bloomsbury.

Rodrigo-Gonzalez, Amalia, María Caballer-Tarazona, and Aurora García-Gallego. 2019. "Active Learning on Trust and Reciprocity for Undergraduates." *Sustainability* 11 (16): 4399.

Rodriguez, Sarah B. 2013. "Female Sexuality and Consent in Public Discourse: James Burt's 'Love Surgery.'" *Archives of Sexual Behavior* 42 (3): 343–351.

Roemer, John E. 2006. “The Global Welfare Economics of Immigration.” *Social Choice & Welfare* 27: 311–325.

Roeser, Robert W., Karen R. Strobel, and Gisell Guihuis. 2002. “Studying Early Adolescents” Academic Motivation, Social-emotional Functioning, and Engagement in Learning Variable- and Person-centered Approaches.” *Anxiety, Stress & Coping* 15 (4): 345–368.

Rogers, Kimberly B., Tobias Schröder, and Christian von Scheve. 2014. “Dissecting the Sociality of Emotion: A Multilevel Approach.” *Emotion Review* 6 (2): 124–133.

Rojas, Sasha M., Sarah A. Bilsky, Courtney Dutton, Christal L. Badour, Matthew T. Feldner, and Ellen W. Leen-Feldner. 2017. “Lifetime Histories of PTSD, Suicidal Ideation, and Suicide Attempts in a Nationally Representative Sample of Adolescents: Examining Indirect Effects via the Roles of Family and Peer Social Support.” *Journal of Anxiety Disorders* 49: 95–103.

Rojek, Chris. 1995. *Decentring Leisure: Rethinking Leisure Theory*. London: Sage.

Rokach, Ami. 2019. *The Psychological Journey to and from Loneliness: Development, Causes, and Effects of Social and Emotional Isolation*. London, UK: Academic.

Rolandsen, Unn Malfrid, and H. 2008. “A Collective of Their Own: Young Volunteers at the Fringes of the Party Realm.” *European Journal of East Asian Studies* 7 (1): 101–129.

Rollo, Stuart. 2023. *Terminus: Westward Expansion, China, and the End of American Empire*. Baltimore: Johns Hopkins University Press.

Ronel, Natti, and Dana Segev. 2014. “Positive Criminology in Practice.” *International Journal of Offender Therapy & Comparative Criminology* 58 (11): 1389–1407.

Rook, Karen S., and Philip H.G.. Ituarte. 1999. “Social Control, Social Support, and Companionship in Older Adults’ Family Relationships and Friendships.” *Personal Relationships* 6: 199–211.

Roosma, Femke, Wim van Oorschot, and John Gelissen. 2014. “The Preferred Role and Perceived Performance of the Welfare State: European Welfare Attitudes from a Multidimensional Perspective.” *Social Science Research* 44: 200–210.

Roosma, Femke, Wim van Oorschot, and John Gelissen. 2016. “The Achilles’ Heel of Welfare State Legitimacy: Perceptions of Overuse and Underuse of Social Benefits in Europe,” *Journal of European Public Policy* 23(2):177–196. \98–189.

Rosario, Margaret, and Eric W. Schrinshaw. 2013. “The Sex and Identity Development and Health of Lesbian, Gay, and Bisexual Adolescents: An Ecological Perspective.” Pp. 87–101 in *Handbook of Psychology and Sexual Orientation*, edited by Charlotte J. Patterson and Anthony R. D’Augelli. New York, NY: Oxford University Press.

Roscigno, Vincent J. 1999. “The Black-White Adolescent Gap, Family-school Link, and the Importance of Place.” *Sociological Inquiry* 69 (2): 159–186.

Rose, Eric D. and Julie J. Exline. 2012. “Personality, Spirituality, and Religion.” Pp. 85–103 in *The Oxford Handbook of Psychology and Spirituality*, edited by Lisa J. Miller. New York, NY: Oxford University Press.

Rose, Lawrence E., and Per Arnt Pettersen. 2000. “The Legitimacy of Local Government: What Makes a Difference? Evidence from Norway.” *Research on Urban Policy* 8: 25–65.

Rosen, Natalie O., Kayla Mooney, and Amy Muise. 2017. “Dyadic Empathy Predicts Sexual and Relationship Well-Being in Couples Transitioning to Parenthood.” *Journal of Sex & Marital Therapy* 43 (6): 543–559.

Rosen, Stanley. 2009. “Contemporary Chinese Youth and the State.” *Journal of Asian Studies* 68 (2): 359–369.

Rosenau, Pauline Marie. 1992. *Postmodernism and the Social Sciences: Insights, Inroads, and Intrusions*. Princeton, NJ: Princeton University Press.

Rosenfield, Sarah, Jean Vertefuille, and Donna D. McAlpine. 2000. “Gender Stratification and Mental Health: An Exploration of Dimensions of the Self.” *Social Psychology Quarterly* 63 (3): 208–223.

Rosler, Nimrod, and Nyla R. Branscombe. 2020. “Inclusivity of Past Collective Trauma and Its Implications for Current Intractable Conflict: The Mediating Role of Moral Lessons.” *British Journal of Social Psychology* 59 (1): 171–188.

Ross, Catherine E., and John Mirowsky. 1995. "Does Employment Affect Health?" *Journal of Health & Social Behavior* 36 (3): 230–243.

Ross, Catherine E., and John Mirowsky. 2009. "Neighborhood Disorder, Subjective Alienation, and Distress." *Journal of Health & Social Behavior* 50: 49–64.

Ross, Catherine E., and Sung Joon Jang. 2000. "Neighborhood Disorder, Fear, and Mistrust: The Buffering Role of Social Ties with Neighbors." *American Journal of Community Psychology* 28 (4): 401–420.

Ross, Catherine E., John R. Reynolds, and Karlyn J. Geis. 2000. "The Contingent Meaning of Neighborhood Stability for Residents" Psychological Well-being." *American Sociological Review* 65: 581–597.

Rosselli, Michelle K., and Elizabeth L. Jeglic. 2017. "Factors Impacting upon Attitudes toward Sex Offenders: The Role of Conservatism and Knowledge." *Psychiatry, Psychology, & Law* 24 (4): 496–515.

Rossi, Alice S. 2001. "Contemporary Dialogue on Civil Society and Social Responsibility." Pp.3–74 in *Caring and Doing for Others: Social Responsibility in the Domain of Family, Work, and Community*, edited by Alice S. Rossi. Chicago, IL: University of Chicago Press.

Rothstein, Bo, and Daniel Eek. 2009. "Political Corruption and Social Trust: An Experimental Approach." *Rationality & Society* 21(1):81-112.

Rothstein, Bo, and Eric M Uslaner. 2005. "All for All: Equality, Corruption, and Social Trust." *World Politics* 58(1):41-72.

Rothstein, Bo. 2005. *Social Traps and the Problem of Trust*. Cambridge, UK: Cambridge University Press.

Rothwell, David W., Mohammad N. Khan, and Katrina Cherney. 2016. "Building Financial Knowledge Is Not Enough: Financial Self-Efficacy as a Mediator in the Financial Capability of Low-Income Families." *Journal of Community Practice* 24 (4): 368–388.

Rotkirch, A. 2014. "Gratitude for Help Among Adult Friends and Siblings." *Evolutionary Psychology* 12 (4): 673–686.

Rowatt, Wade C., Jordan LaBouff, Megan Johnson, Paul Froese and Jo-Ann Tsang. 2009. "Associations among Religiousness, Social Attitudes, and Prejudice in a National Random Sample of American Adults." *Psychology of Religion & Spirituality* 1(1):14-24.

Royzman, Edward B., Justin F. Landy, and Robert F. Leeman. 2015. "Are Thoughtful People More Utilitarian? Crt as a Unique Predictor of Moral Minimalism in the Dilemmatic Context." *Cognitive Science* 39 (2): 325–352.

Rozer, Jesper, and Gerbert Kraaykamp. 2013. "Income Inequality and Subjective Well-being: A Cross-national Study on the Conditional Effects of Individual and National Characteristics." *Social Indicators Research* 113: 1009–1023.

Rubin, Alan M., and Mary M. Step. 2000. "Impact of Motivation, Attraction, and Parasocial Interaction on Talk Radio Listening." *Journal of Broadcasting & Electronic Media* 44 (4): 635–654.

Rudd, Jill E., and D. Timothy Hughes. 2020. *Negotiation Preparation in a Global World: Symptoms of Success and Failure*. New York, NY: Routledge.

Rudig, Wolfgang, and Georgios Karyotis. 2014. "Who Protests in Greece? Mass Opposition to Austerity." *British Journal of Political Science* 44 (3): 487–513.

Rudowicz, Elisabeth, and Xiao-dong Yue. 2002. "Concepts of Creativity: Similarities and Differences among Mainland, Hong Kong, and Taiwanese Children." *Journal of Creative Behavior* 34 (3): 175–192.

Rudra, Nita, and Stephan Haggard. 2005. "Globalization, Democracy, and Effective Welfare Spending in the Developing World." *Comparative Political Studies* 38 (9): 1015–1049.

Rundman, Laurie A., and Peter Glick. 2008. *The Social Psychology of Gender: How Power and Intimacy Shape Gender Relations*. New York, NY: Guilford.

Runhovde, Siv Rebekka. 2017. "Comparing Discourse to Officer Perceptions: The Problems of War and Militarization in Wildlife Crime Enforcement." *Critical Criminology* 25 (2): 275–291.

Rupasingha, Anil, Stephan J. Coetz, and David Freshwater. 2006. "The Production of Social Capital in U.S. Counties." *Journal of Socio-Economics* 35: 83–101.
Rupp, Laney A., Marc A. Zimmerman, Kathleen W. Sly, Thomas M. Reischl, Elyse J. Thulin, Thomas A. Wyatt, and John P. Stock. 2020. "Community-Engaged Neighborhood Revitalization and Empowerment: Busy Streets Theory in Action." *American Journal of Community Psychology* 65 (1–2): 90–106.
Russell, Cherry, Andrew Campbell, and Ian Hughes. 2008. "Ageing, Social Capital and the Internet: Findings from an Exploratory Study of Australian Silver Surfers." *Australasian Journal of Ageing* 27 (2): 78–82.
Russell, Stephen T., Allen B. Mallory, Meg D. Bishop, and Armin A. Dorri. 2020. "Innovation and Integration of Sexuality in Family Life Education." *Family Relations* 69 (3): 595–613.
Russo, Silvia, and Michele Roccato. 2010. "How Long Does Victimization Foster Fear of Crime? A Longitudinal Study." *Journal of Community Psychology* 38 (8): 960–974.
Russo-Netzer, Pninit, Gabriel Horenczyk, and Yoav S. Bergman. 2021. "Affect, Meaning in Life, and Life Satisfaction among Immigrants and Non-Immigrants: A Moderated Mediation Model." *Current Psychology* 40 (7): 3450–3458.
Rutgers, Mark R., and Petra Schreurs. 2006. "The Morality of Value- and Purpose-Rationality." *Administration & Society* 38 (4): 403–421.
Ryan, Vernon D., Kerry A. Agnitsch, Lijun Zhao, and Rehan Mullick. 2005. "Making Sense of Voluntary Participation: A Theoretical Synthesis." *Rural Sociology* 70 (3): 287–313.
Sabet, Naser Shafiei and Sogand Khaksar. 2025. "The Performance of Local Government, Social Capital and Participation of Villagers in Sustainable Rural Development." *Social Science Journal.*
Sabia, Joseph J., and Brittany Bass. 2017. "Do Anti-Bullying Laws Work? New Evidence on School Safety and Youth Violence." *Journal of Population Economics* 30 (2): 473–502.
Sacks, Audrey, and Margaret Levi. 2010. "Measuring Government Effectiveness and Its Consequences for Social Welfare in Sub-Saharan." *Social Forces* 88 (5): 2325–2351.
Sadurski, Wojciech. 1999. *Freedom of Speech and Its Limits.* Dordrecht, Netherlands: Kluwer.
Saegert, Susan, and Gary Winkel. 2004. "Crime, Social Capital, and Community Participation." *American Journal of Community Psychology* 34 (3/4): 219–233.
Saha, Anamik. 2018. *Race and the Cultural Industries.* Cambridge, UK: Polity Press.
Sahar, Gail. 2008. "Patriotism, Attributions for the 9/11 Attacks and Support for War: Then and Now." *Basic & Applied Social Psychology* 30: 189–197.
Sainz, Mario, and Gloria Jimenez-Moya. 2023. "Group Dominance, System Justification, and Hostile Classism: The Ideological Roots of the Perceived Socioeconomic Humanity Gap That Upholds the Income Gap." *International Review of Social Psychology* 36 (1): 7.
Sakalaki, Maria, and Kyriaki Fousiani. 2012. "About Some Personality Misfortunes of Opportunists: The Negative Correlation of Economic Defection with Autonomy, Agreeableness, and Well-Being1." *Journal of Applied Social Psychology* 42 (2): 471–487.
Salisbury, Emily J. 2013. "Social Learning and Crime." Pp.115–130 in *The Oxford Handbook of Criminological Theory*, edited by Francis T. Cullen and Pamela Wilcox. New York: Oxford University Press.
Sallquist, Julie, Nancy Eisenberg, Doran C. French, Urip Purwono, and Telie A. Suryanti. 2010. "Indonesian Adolescents" Spiritual and Religious Experiences and Their Longitudinal Relations with Socioemotional Functioning." *Developmental Psychology* 46 (3): 699–716.
Sammons, Aidan, and David Putwain. 2019. *Psychology and Crime.* Abingdon, UK: Routledge.
Sampson, Robert J. 1991. "Linking the Micro- and Macrolevel Dimensions of Community Social Organization." *Social Forces* 70 (1): 43–64.
Sampson, Robert J., and Stephen W. Raudenbush. 2004. "Social Disorder: Neighborhood Stigma and the Social Construction of Broken Windows." *Social Psychology Quarterly* 67 (4): 319–342.
Sampson, Robert J., Doug McAdam, Heather MacIndoe, and Simon Weffer Elizondo. 2005. "Civil Society Reconsidered: The Durable Nature and Community Structure of Collective Civic Action." *American Journal of Sociology* 111 (3): 673–714.

Sandel, Michael J. 2020. *The Tyranny of Merit: What's Become of the Common Good?* New York, NY: Farrar, Straus & Giroux.

Sanders, Karen. 2009. *Communicating Politics in the Twenty-first Century*. Houndmills, UK: Palgrave.

Sanderson, Stephen K. 2001. *The Evolution of Human Sociality: A Darwinian Conflict Perspective.* Lanham, MD: Rowman & Littlefield.

Sanderson, Stephen K., D. A. Heckert, and J. K. Dubrow. 2005. "Militarist, Marxian, and Non-Marxian Materialist Theories of Gender Inequality: A Cross-Cultural Test." *Social Forces* 83 (4): 1425–1441.

Sandovici, Maria Elena, and Terri Davis. 2010. "Activism Gone Shopping: An Empirical Exploration of Individual-level Determinants of Political Consumerism and Donating." *Comparative Sociology* 9: 328–356.

Santos-Iglesias, Pablo, Juan Carlos Sierra, and Pablo Vallejo-Medina. 2013. "Predictors of Sexual Assertiveness: The Role of Sexual Desire, Arousal, Attitudes, and Partner Abuse." *Archives of Sexual Behavior* 42 (6): 1043–1052.

Sarasa, Sebastian. 2008. "Do Welfare Benefits Affect Women's Choices of Adult Care Giving?" *European Sociological Review* 24 (1): 37–51.

Sarkheyli, Elnaz, Ayyoob Sharifi, Mojtaba Rafieian, and Mohammad reza Bemanian, and Akito Murayama. 2012. "An Investigation of the Reasons for Non-compliance with FAR Regulations in Tehran." *Cities* 29: 223–233.

Saroglou, Vassilis, and Lydwine Anciaux. 2004. "Liking Sick Humor: Coping Styles and Religion as Predictors." *Humor: International Journal of Humor Research* 17(3):257–277.

Sarracino, Francesco. 2010. "Social Capital and Subjective Well-being Trends: Comparing 11 Western European Countries." *Journal of Socio-Economics* 39: 482–517.

Sasaki, M.S. 1979. "Status Inconsistency and Religious Commitment." Pp.135–156 in *The Religious Dimension: New Directions in Quantitative Research*, edited by Robert Wuthnow. New York: Academic.

Satchell, Liam P., Alison M. Bacon, Jennifer L. Firth, and Philip J. Corr. 2018. "Risk as Reward: Reinforcement Sensitivity Theory and Psychopathic Personality Perspectives on Everyday Risk-Taking." *Personality & Individual Differences* 128: 162–169.

Satgar, Vishwas, and Michelle Williams. 2017. "Marxism and Class." Pp. 41–50 in *The Cambridge Handbook of Sociology, Vol. 2: Specialty and Interdisciplinary Studies*, edited by Kathleen Odell Korgen. New York, NY: Cambridge University Press.

Saucier, Gerard, and Katarzyna Skrzypinska. 2006. "Spiritual but Not Religious? Evidence for Two Independent Dispositions." *Journal of Personality* 74 (5): 1257–1292.

Saunders, Peter, and Melissa Wong. 2012. "Examining Australian Attitudes to Inequality and Redistribution." *Journal of Australian Political Economy* 71: 51–75.

Saunders, Peter, Hung Wong, and Wo Ping Wong. 2014. "Deprivation and Poverty in Hong Kong." *Social Policy & Administration* 48(5):556-575.

Saurette, Paul, and Kelly Gordon. 2013. "Arguing Abortion: The New Anti-Abortion Discourse in Canada." *Canadian Journal of Political Science* 46 (1): 157–185.

Saurugger, Sabine. 2013. "Constructivism and Public Policy Approaches in the EU: From Ideas to Power Games." *Journal of European Public Policy* 20 (6): 888–906.

Savelkoul, M., P. Scheepers, J. Tolsma, and L. Hagendoorn. 2011. "Anti-Muslim Attitudes in the Netherlands: Tests of Contradictory Hypotheses Derived from Ethnic Competition Theory and Intergroup Contact Theory." *European Sociological Review* 27 (6): 741–758.

Savelkoul, Michael, Maurice Gesthuizen, and Peer Scheepers. 2014. "The Impact of Ethnic Diversity on Participation in European Voluntary Organizations." *Nonprofit & Voluntary Sector Quarterly* 43 (6): 1070–1094.

Savelkoul, Michael, Miles Hewstone, Peer Scheepers, and Dietlind Stolle. 2015. "Does Relative Out-Group Size in Neighborhoods Drive down Associational Life of Whites in the U.S.? Testing Constrict, Conflict and Contact Theories." *Social Science Research* 52: 236–252.

Savolainen, Jukka. 2009. "Work, Family and Criminal Desistance, Adult Social Bonds in a Nordic Welfare State." *British Journal of Criminology* 49: 285–304.

Saward, Michael. 1998. *The Terms of Democracy*. Cambridge, UK: Polity.

Saxton, Gregory D., and Michelle A. Benson. 2006. "Structure, Politics, and Action: An Integrated Model of Nationalist Protest and Rebellion." *Nationalism & Ethnic Politics* 12 (2): 137–175.

Sayer, R., and Andrew. 2011. *Why Things Matter to People: Social Science, Values and Ethical Life*. Cambridge, UK: Cambridge University Press.

Scaff, Lawrence A. 2000. "Weber on the Cultural Situation of the Modern Age." Pp. 99–116 in *The Cambridge Companion to Weber*, edited by Stephen Turner. Cambridge, UK: Cambridge University Press.

Scafuto, Francesca, and Francesco La Barbera. 2016. "Protest Against Waste Contamination in the Land of Fires: Psychological Antecedents for Activists and Non-activists." *Journal of Community & Applied Social Psychology* 26 (6): 481–495.

Scambler, Graham. 2002. *Health and Social Change: A Critical Theory*. Buckingham, UK: Open University Press.

Schafer, Karl. 2015. "Realism and Constructivism in Kantian Metaethics (2): The Kantian Conception of Rationality and Rationalist Constructivism." *Philosophy Compass* 10 (10):702–713. \1.

Schafer, Markus H. 2011. "Ambiguity, Religion, and Relational Context: Competing Influences on Moral Attitudes?" *Sociological Perspectives* 54 (1): 59–81.

Schaie, K. Warner. 2013. *Developmental Influences on Adult Intelligence: The Seattle Longitudinal Study*. New York: Oxford University Press.

Scharrer, Erica. 2008. "Media Exposure and Sensitivity to Violence in News Reports: Evidence of Desensitization?" *Journalism & Mass Communication Quarterly* 85 (2): 291–310.

Schatzman, Christina. 2005. "Political Challenge in Latin America: Rebellion and Collective Protest in an Era of Democratization." *Journal of Peace Research* 42 (3): 291–310.

Schbley, Ayla, and Clark McCauley. 2005. "Political, Religious, and Psychological Characteristics of Muslim Protest Marchers in Eight European Cities: Jerusalem Day 2002." *Terrorism & Political Violence* 17 (4): 551–572.

Scherger, Simone. 2009. "Cultural Practices, Age and the Life Course." *Cultural Trends* 18 (1): 23–45.

Scheufele, Dietram, and Dhavan V. Shah. 2000. "Personality Strength and Social Capital." *Communication Research* 27 (2): 107–131.

Schiefer, David, and Jolanda van der Noll. 2017. "The Essentials of Social Cohesion: A Literature Review." *Social Indicators Research* 132 (2): 579–603.

Schieman, Scott. 2001. "Age, Education, and the Sense of Control: A Test of the Cumulative Advantage Hypothesis." *Research on Aging* 23 (2): 153–178.

Schiff, Miriam, and David Bargal. 2000. "Helping Characteristics of Self-Help and Support Groups: Their Contribution to Participants' Subjective Well-Being." *Small Group Research* 31 (3): 275–304.

Schinkel, Willem. 2010. *Aspects of Violence: A Critical Theory*. Houndmills, UK: Palgrave.

Schlenker, Barry, et al. 2012. "Conservatives Are Happier than Liberals, but Why? Political Ideology and Personality, and Life Satisfaction." *Journal of Research in Personality* 40: 127–146.

Schlerka, Sebastian Matthias. 2019. "It's Time for a Change: A Bourdieusian Approach on Social Change." *Time & Society* 28 (3): 1013–1038.

Schlevogt, Kai-Alexander. 2002. *The Art of Chinese Management: Theory Evidence, and Applications*. New York: Oxford University Press.

Schmidt, Volker H. 2020. "Eight Theories of Societlization: Toward a Theoretically Sustainable Concept of Society." *European Journal of Social Theory* 23 (3): 411–430.

Schmitt, Manfred, Jürgen. Maes, and Keith Widaman. 2010. "Longitudinal Effects of Egoistic and Fraternal Relative Deprivation on Well-Being and Protest." *International Journal of Psychology* 45 (2): 122–130.

Schmitt, Randee M. and Ho Phi Huynh. 2024. "Stay (Close to) Humble: Intellectual Humility Negatively Predicts Stigma toward and Social Distance from Individuals with Posttraumatic Stress Disorder." *Psychological Reports* 13:332941231157233.

Schnaudt, Christian. 2019. *Political Confidence and Democracy in Europe: Antecedents and Consequences of Citizens' Confidence in Representative and Regulative Institutions and Authorities.* Cham, Switzerland: Springer.

Schneider, Jo Anne. 2006. *Social Capital and Welfare Reform: Organizations, Congregations, and Communities.* New York: Columbia University Press.

Schneider, Silke L. 2007. "Anti-immigrant Attitudes in Europe: Outgroup Size3 and Perceived Ethnic Threat." *European Sociological Review* 24 (1): 53–67.

Schnittker, Jason, and Jere R. Behrman. 2012. "Learning to Do Well or Learning to Do Good? Estimating the Effects of Schooling on Civic Engagement, Social Cohesion, and Labour Market Outcomes in the Presence of Endowments." *Social Science Research* 41: 306–320.

Schofer, Evan, and Marion Fourcade-Gourinchas. 2001. "The Structural Contexts of Civic Engagement: Voluntary Association Membership in Comparative Perspective." *American Sociological Review* 66: 806–828.

Scholte, Ron H.J.., Geertjan Overbeek, Giovanni ten Brink, Els Rommes, Raymond A.T.. de Kemp, Luc Goossens, G. M. E. Rutger, and Engels. 2009. "The Significance of Reciprocal and Unilateral Friendships for Peer Victimization in Adolescence." *Journal of Youth & Adolescence* 38: 89–100.

Schreck, Christopher J., Melissa W. Burek, Eric A. Stewart, and J. Mitchell Miller. 2007. "Distress and Violent Victimization among Young Adolescents: Early Puberty and the Social Interactionist Explanation." *Journal of Research in Crime and Delinquency* 44 (4): 381–405.

Schroeder, Ralph. 2013. *An Age of Limits: Social Theory for the 21st Century.* Houndmills, UK: Palgrave.

Schulenberg, Jennifer L. 2003. "The Social Context of Police Discretion with Young Offenders: An Ecological Analysis." *Canadian Journal of Criminology & Criminal Justice* 127–157.

Schumpe, Birga M., Jocelyn J. Bélanger, Manuel Moyano, and Claudia F. Nisa. 2020. "The Role of Sensation Seeking in Political Violence: An Extension of the Significance Quest Theory." *Journal of Personality & Social Psychology* 118 (4): 743–761.

Schutte, Sebastian. 2015. "Geography, Outcome, and Casualties." *Journal of Conflict Resolution* 59 (6): 1101–1128.

Schwadel, Philip. 2012. "¡°Social Class and Finding a Congregation: How Attendees Are Introduced to Their Congregations." *Review of Religious Research* 54: 543–554.

Schwartz, Lisa B. 2012. "Mixed-Orientation Marriages: Coming out, Staying Together." *Journal of GLBT Family Studies* 8 (1): 121–136.

Schwartz, Shalom H. and Gila Melech. 2000. "National Differences in Mirco and Macro Worry: Social, Economic, and Cultural Explanations." Pp.219–256 in *Culture and Subjective Well-being,* edited by Ed Diener and Eunkook M. Suh. Cambridge, MA: MIT.

Schwartz, Shalom H., Gian Vittorio Caprara, and Michele Vecchione. 2010. "Basic Personal Values, Core Political Values, and Voting: A Longitudinal analysis." *Political Psychology* 31 (3): 421–452.

Schwartz, Shalom H., Gian Vittorio Caprara, Michele Vecchione, Paul Bain, Gabriel Bianchi, Maria Giovanna Caprara, Jan Cieciuch, Hasan Kirmanoglu, Cem Baslevent, Jan-Erik Lonnqvist, Catalin Mamali, Jorge Manzi, Vassilis Pavlopoulos, Tetyana Posnova, Harald Schoen, Jo Silvester, Carmen Tabernero, Claudio Torres, Markku Verkasalo, and Eva Vondrokov. 2014. "Basic Personal Values Underlie and Give Coherence to Political Values: A Cross National Study in 15 Countries." *Political Behavior* 36(4):899-930.

Schwirian, Kent P., Timothy J. Curry, and Rachael A. Woldoff. 2001. "Community Conflict over Arena and Stadium Funding: Competitive Framing, Social Action, and the Socio-Spatial Perspective." *Sociological Focus* 34 (1): 1–20.

Sciulli, David. 2011. *Etzioni's Critical Functionalism: Communitarian Origins and Principles.* Leiden, Netherlands: Brill.

Scott, Kristyn A., Samantha D. Montes, and P. Gregory Irving. 2012. "Examining the impact of socialization through trust: An exploratory study." *Journal of Personnel Psychology* 11 (4): 191–198.

Scott, W. Richard. 2008. *Institutions and Organizations: Ideas and Interests*, 3rd ed. Los Angeles, CA: Sage.

Scruton, Roger. 2014. *How to Be a Conservative*. London, UK: Bloomsbury.

Sears, David O. 2001. "The Role of Affect in Symbolic Politics." Pp.14–40 in *Citizens and Politics: Perspectives from Political Psychology*, edited by James H. Kuklinski. Cambridge, UK: Cambridge University Press.

Sears, David O., and Christia Brown. 2013. "Childhood and Adult Political Development." Pp.59–95 in *The Oxford Handbook of Political Psychology*, edited by Leone Huddy, David O. Sears and Jack S. Levy. New York: Oxford University Press.

Secker, Jenny, Sue Hacking, Lyn Kent, Jo Shenton, and Helen Spandler. 2009. "Development of a Measure of Social Inclusion for Arts and Mental Health Project Participants." *Journal of Mental Health* 18(1):65-72.

Seddig, Daniel. 2020. "Individual Attitudes toward Deviant Behavior and Perceived Attitudes of Friends: Self-Stereotyping and Social Projection in Adolescence and Emerging Adulthood." *Journal of Youth & Adolescence* 49 (3): 664–677.

Seder, J. Patrick., and Shigehiro Oishi. 2009. "Ethnic/Racial Homogeneity in College Students: Facebook Friendship Networks and Subjective Well-being." *Journal of Research in Personality* 43: 438–443.

Sedikides, Constantine, and Jochen E. Gebauer. 2010. "Religiosity as Self-enhancement: A Meta-analysis of the Relation between Socially Desirable Responding and Religiosity." *Personality & Social Psychology Review* 14 (1): 17–36.

Sedziafa, Alice Pearl, and Eric Y. Tenkorang. 2016. "Kin Group Affiliation and Marital Violence against Women in Ghana." *Violence & Victims* 31 (3): 486–509.

Segrin, Chris and Jeanne Flora. 2019. Family Communication, New York, NY: Routledge. Chung, Chung-Soo. 2000. *The I Ching on Man and Society: An Exploration into Its Theoretical Implications in Social Sciences*. Lanham, MD: University Press of America. Mondak, Jeffery J., and Jon Hurwitz. 2012. "Examining the Terror Exception: Terrorism and Commitments to Civil Liberties." *Public Opinion Quarterly* 76 (2): 193–213.

Seidlitz, Larry, Alexis D. Abernethy, Paul R. Duberstein, James S. Evinger, Theresa H. Chang, and Barbara L. Lewis. 2002. "Development of the Spiritual Transcendence Index." *Journal of the Scientific Study of Religion* 41 (3): 439–453.

Seifert, Nico. 2018. "Yet Another Case of Nordic Exceptionalism? Extending Existing Evidence for a Causal Relationship between Institutional and Social Trust to the Netherlands and Switzerland." *Social Indicators Research* 136 (2): 539–555.

Seligson, Julie, E. Scott Huebner, and Robert F. Valois. 2005. "An Investigation of a Brief Life Satisfaction Scale with Elementary School Children." *Social Indicators Research* 73: 355–374.

Seligson, Mitchell A. 2005. The Measurement and Impact of Corruption Victimization: Survey Evidence from Latin America. *World Development* 34 (2): 381–404.

Selim, Sibel. 2008. "Life Satisfaction and Happiness in Turkey." *Social Indicators Research* 88: 531–562.

Selvanathan, Hema Preya, and Brian Lickel. 2019. "A Field Study around a Racial Justice Protest on a College Campus: The Proximal Impact of Collective Action on the Social Change Attitudes of Uninvolved Bystanders." *Journal of Social & Political Psychology* 7 (1): 598–619.

Selznick, Philip. 2002. *The Communitarian Persuasion*. Washington, DC: Woodrow Wilson.

Selznick, Philip. 2008. *A Humanistic Science: Values and Ideals in Social Inquiry*. Stanford, CA: Stanford University Press.

Semenova, Galina N., Elena I. Larionova, Oleg G. Karpovich, Sergei V. Shkodinsky, and Fatima M. Ouroumova. 2020. "Social Integration as a Factor of Economic Growth: Experience and Perspectives of Developing Countries." *International Journal of Sociology & Social Policy* 41 (1/2): 37–49.

Semerikova, A. A., V. M. Novgorodtsev, D. B. Efimenko, and T. E. Melnikova. 2019. "The Role of Sadomasochism in Shaping Violent Sexual Motivation." *Journal of Forensic Psychology Research & Practice* 19 (5): 409–433.

Semino, Stella Maris. 2015. "Governmental Promotion of Social Cohesion and Its Effect on Local Civil Society Organisations: How These Institutions Respond to the Inclusion of Vulnerable Groups as Active Citizens." *Social Policy & Society* 14 (2): 189–201.

Sen, Amartya. 2002. "Globalization, Inequality and Global Protest." *Development* 45 (2): 11–16.

Seoighe, Rachel. 2016. "Discourses of Victimization in Sri Lanka's Civil War." *Social & Legal Studies* 25 (3): 355–380.

Shafir, Eldar, and Robyn A. LeBouef. 2002. "Rationality." *Annual Review of Psychology* 53: 491–517.

Shah, Dhavan V., and Dietram A. Scheufele. 2006. "Explicating Opinion Leadership: Nonpolitical Dispositions, Information Consumption, and Civic Participation." *Political Communication* 23 (1): 1–22.

Shahzalal, Md and Hamedi Mohd Adnan. 2022. "Attitude, Self-control, and Prosocial Norm to Predict Intention to Use Social Media Responsibly: From Scale to Model Fit towards a Modified Theory of Planned Behavior." *Sustainability* 14:9822.

Shambaugh, David. 2007. "China's Propaganda System: Institutions, Process and Efficiency." *China Journal* 57: 25–58.

Shan, Hongxia. 2017. "Lifelong Education and Lifelong Learning with Chinese Characteristics: A Critical Policy Discourse Analysis." *Asia Pacific Education Review* 18 (2): 189–201.

Shank, Daniel B. 2012. "Perceived Justice and Reactions to Coercive Computers1." *Sociological Forum* 27 (2): 372–391.

Shao, Lei, Yan Dong, and Denghao Zhang. 2021. "Effects of Security on Social Trust among Chinese Adults: Roles of Life Satisfaction and Ostracism." *Journal of Social Psychology* 161 (5): 560–569.

Shapiro, Adam, Lee M. Corey, and Keyes. 2008. "Marital Status and Social Well-being: Are the Married Always Better off?" *Social Indicators Research* 88: 329–346.

Sharabany, Ruth. 1994. "Intimate Friendship Scale: Conceptual Underpinnings, Psychometric Properties and Construct Validity." *Journal of Social & Personal Relationships* 11 (3): 449–469.

Sharon Gewirtz and Alan Cribb. 2009. *Understanding Education: A Sociological Perspective*. Cambridge, UK: Polity.

Shatkin, Gavin. 2000. "Obstacles to Empowerment: Local Politics and Civil Society in Metropolitan Manila, the Philippines." *Urban Studies* 37 (12): 2357–2375.

Shatz, Marshall. 2011. "Anarchism." Pp.725–736 in *The Oxford Handbook of the History of Political Philosophy*, edited by George Klosko. Oxford, UK: Oxford University Press.

Shaw, Julia J. A. 2020. *Law and the Passions: Why Emotion Matters for Justice*. Abingdon, UK: Routledge.

Sheikh, Mona K. 2014. "Appointing Evil in International Relations." *International Politics* 51 (4): 492–507.

Shemmings, David. 2006. "Quantifying Qualitative Data: An Illustrative Example of the Use of Q Methodology in Psychosocial Research." *Qualitative Research of Psychology* 3: 147–165.

Sherkat, Darren E., and Christopher G. Ellison. 2007. "Structuring the Religion-environment Connection: Identifying Religious Influences on Environmental Concern and Activism." *Journal of the Scientific Study of Religion* 46 (1): 71–85.

Sherman, Howard J. 1995. *Reinventing Marxism*. Baltimore, MD: Johns Hopkins University Press.

Sherman, Lawrence W. 2010. "Defiance, Compliance and Consilience: A General Theory of Criminology." Pp.360–390 in *The SAGE Handbook of Criminological Theory*, edited by Eugene McLaughlin and Tim Newburn. London, UK: SAGE.

Shi, Tianjian. 2000. "Cultural Values and Democracy in the People's Republic of China." *China Quarterly* 540–559.

Shillington, Katie J., Andrew M. Johnson, Tara Mantler, and Jennifer D. Irwin. 2021. "Kindness as an Intervention for Student Social Interaction Anxiety, Affect, and Mood: The Kiss of Kindness Study." *International Journal of Applied Positive Psychology* 6 (1): 23–44.

Shim, Y. H. 2001. "Feminism and the Discourse of Sexuality in Korea: Continuities and Changes." *Human Studies* 24 (1–2): 133–148.

Shin, Doh Chull. 2012. *Confucianism and Democratization in East Asia.* New York: Cambridge University Press.

Shippee, Nathan D. 2012. "Victimization, Fear of Crime, and Perceived Risk: Testing a Vulnerability Model of Personal Control." *Sociological Perspectives* 55 (1): 117–140.

Shmueli, Amir. 1999. "Survival vs. Quality of Life: A Study of the Israeli Public Priorities in Medical Care." *Social Science & Medicine* 49: 497–302.

Shockley, Ellie, and Amir Shawn Fairdosi. 2015. "Power to the People? Psychological Mechanisms of Disengagement from Direct Democracy." *Social Psychology & Personality Science* 6 (5): 529–586.

Shoham, Shlomo Giora, Moshe Adad, and Ra'Anan Ben'tovim, Yoav Kaplan, Omer Kimchy, Assaf Naaman, and Moran Shoham. 1999. "The Complementarity of Crime and Madness." *Journal of Offender Rehabilitation* 29 (1–2): 113–147.

Shook, John R., and James J. Giordano. 2017. "Moral Bioenhancement for Social Welfare: Are Civic Institutions Ready?" *Frontiers in Sociology* 2: 21.

Shorey, Hal S., Steve Bisgaier, and Scott R. Thien. 2018. "Attachment Process and the Social Developmental Bases of Hope." Pp.313–325 in *The Oxford Handbook of Hope*, edited by Matthew W. Gallagher and Shane J. Lopez. New York, NY: Oxford University Press.

Short, Susan E., Fengying Zhai, Siyuan Xu, and Mingliang Yang. 2001. "China's One-child Policy and the Care of Children: An Analysis of Qualitative and Quantitative Data." *Social Forces* 79(3):913-943.

Short, Tim. 2018. *The Psychology of Successful Trading: Behavioral Strategies for Profitability.* New York, NY: Routledge.

Shortall, Sally, and Mildred E. Warner. 2010. "Social Inclusion or Market Competitiveness? A Comparison of Rural Development Policies in the European Union and the United States." *Social Policy & Administration* 44 (5): 575–597.

Shrage, Laurie. 1994. *Moral Dilemma of Feminism: Prostitution, Adultery, and Abortion.* New York: Routledge.

Shu, Xiaoling, and Yanjie Bian. 2002. "Intercity Variation in Gender Inequalities in China: Analysis of a 1995 National Survey." *Research in Social Stratification & Mobility* 19: 269–309.

Sicurella, Rosaria. 2018. "Fostering a European Criminal Law Culture." *New Journal of European Criminal Law* 9 (3): 308–325.

Sidanius, Jim, and Felicia Pratto. 1999. *Social Dominance: An Intergroup Theory of Social Hierarchy and Oppression.* Cambridge, UK: Cambridge University Press.

Sidanius, Jim, and Robert Kurzban. 2013. "Toward an Evolutionarily Informed Political Psychology." Pp.205–236 in *The Oxford Handbook of Political Psychology*, edited by Leone Huddy, David O. Sears and Jack S. Levy. New York: Oxford University Press.

Siddaway, Andy P., Peter J. Taylor, and Alex M. Wood. 2018. "Reconceptualizing Anxiety as a Continuum That Ranges from High Calmness to High Anxiety: The Joint Importance of Reducing Distress and Increasing Well-Being." *Journal of Personality & Social Psychology* 114 (2): e1–e11.

Silbereisen, Rainer K., Matthias Reitzle, and Linda Juang. 2002. "Time and Change: Psychosocial Transition in German Young Adults 1991 and 1996." Pp.227–254 in *Paths to Successful Development: Personality in the Life Course*, edited by Lea Pulkkinen and Avshalom Caspi. Cambridge, UK: Cambridge University Press.

Silva, Elizabeth. 2005. "Gender, Home and Family in Cultural Capital Theory." *British Journal of Sociology* 56 (1): 83–103.

Silver, Jason R., Luzi Shi, and Audrey Hickert. 2025. "Stigmatizing Evildoers: How Beliefs about Evil and Public Stigma Explain Criminal Justice Policy Preferences." *Psychology, Crime & Law.*

Simon, Dan, Chasdwick J. Snow, and Stephen,. 2004. *J. Read. "The Redux of Cognitive Consistency Theories: Evidence Judgments by Constraint Satisfaction" Journal of Personality & Social Psychology* 86 (6): 814–837.

Simon, Daniel H., and Ryan K. Masters. 2024. "Institutional Failures as Structural Determinants of Suicide: The Opioid Epidemic and the Great Recession in the United States." *Journal of Health & Social Behavior* 65 (3): 415–431.

Simon, Thomas R., Mark Anderson, Martie P. Thompson, Alex E. Crosby, Gene Shelley, and Jeffrey J. Sacks. 2001. "Attitudinal Acceptance of Intimate Partner Violence among U.S. Adults." *Violence & Victims* 16 (2): 115–126.

Simon-Bemd, Stefan Sturmer, and Kerstin Steffens. 2000. "Helping Individuals or Group Members? The Role of Individuals and Collective Identification in AIDS Volunteerism." *Personality and Social Psychology Bulletin* 26 (4): 497–506.

Simoni, Jane M., Laramie Smith, Keren Lehavot, Karen Fredriksen-Goldsen, and Karina L. Walters. 2013. "Lesbian and Bisexual Women's Physical Health." Pp.179–190 in *Handbook of Psychology and Sexual Orientation*, edited by Charlotte J. Patterson and Anthony R. D'Augelli. New York: Oxford University Press.

Simons, Margaret, David Nolan, and Scott Wright. 2017. ""We Are Not North Korea": Propaganda and Professionalism in the People's Republic of China." *Media, Culture, & Society* 39(2):219–37. Svensson, Lennart G. 2006. "New Professionalism, Trust and Competence." *Current Sociology* 54(4):579–93. \93–257.

Simpson, Ain, Caitlin McCurrie, and Kimberly Rios. 2019. "Perceived Morality and Antiatheist Prejudice: A Replication and Extension." *International Journal for the Psychology of Religion* 29 (3): 172–183.

Simpson, David B., Jody L. Newman, and Dale R. Euqua. 2008. "Understanding the Role of Relational Factors in Christian Spirituality." *Journal of Psychology & Theology* 36 (2): 124–134.

Singer, Alexa J., Cecilia Chouhy, Peter S. Lehmann, Jessica N. Walzak, Marc Gertz, and Sophia Biglin. 2019. "Victimization, Fear of Crime, and Trust in Criminal Justice Institutions: A Cross-National Analysis." *Crime & Delinquency* 65 (6): 822–844.

Singer, Eleanor, Amy D. Corning, and Toni Antonucci. 1999. "Attitudes toward Genetic Testing and Fetal Diagnosis, 1990–1996." *Journal of Health & Social Behavior* 40: 429–455.

Singer, Peter. 2001. *Writings on an Ethical Life.* London: Fourth Estate.

Sinha, Shilpi. 2013. "Derrida, Friendship and Responsible Teaching in Contrast to Effective Teaching." *Educational Philosophy & Theory* 45 (3): 259–271.

Sinn, Jeffrey S., and Matthew W. Hayes. 2018. "Is Political Conservatism Adaptive? Reinterpreting Right-Wing Authoritarianism and Social Dominance Orientation as Evolved, Sociofunctional Strategies." *Political Psychology* 39 (5): 1123–1139.

Sirgy, M. Joseph., Dong-jie Lee, Chad Miller, and James E. Littlefield. 2004. "The Impact of Globalization on a Country's Quality of Life: Toward an Integrated Model." *Social Indicators Research* 68: 251–298.

Sirgy, M. Joseph. 2012. *The Psychology of Quality of Life: Hedonic Well-Being, Life Satisfaction, and Eudaimonia.* Dordrecht, Netherlands: Springer.

Siu, Wanda Luen, and Wun. 2008. "News Discourse of Teachers' Suicide in Education and Journalism: Media Coverage of an Education Crisis." *Journal of Asia Pacific Communication* 18 (2): 247–267.

Sivami, Viren. 2016. *Attraction Explained: The Science of How We Form Relationships.* Abington, UK: Routledge.

Six, Benjamin. 2014. "A Pragmatic Contribution for a More Reflexive Institution-Based Trust." *Journal of Trust Research* 4 (2): 132–146.

Sjoberg, Lennart. 2003. "Distal Factors in Risk Perception." *Journal of Risk Research* 6 (3): 187–211.

Skerkat, Darren E. 1998. "Counterculture or Continuity? Competing Influence on Baby Boomers' Religious Orientation and Participation." *Social Force* 76 (3): 1087–1104.
Skerkat, Darren E., and Christopher G. Ellison. 1999. "Recent Developments and Current Controversies in the Sociology of Religion." *Annual Review of Sociology* 25: 363–394.
Skitka, Linda J. and G. Scott Morgan. 2014. "The Social and Political Implications of Moral Conviction." *Political Psychology* 35 (SUPPL.1):95–110.
Skopek, Jan, Florian Schulz, and Hans-Peter. Blossfeld. 2011. "Who Contacts Whom? Educated Homophily in Online Mate Selection." *European Sociological Review* 27 (2): 180–195.
Slootmaeckers, Koen, and John Lievens. 2014. "Cultural Capital and Attitudes toward Homosexuals: Exploring the Relation between Lifestyles and Homonegativity." *Journal of Homosexuality* 61 (7): 962–979.
Smart, Barry. 2003. *Economy, Culture and Society: A Sociological Critique of Neo-liberalism.* Buckingham, UK: Open University Press.
Smets, Peer, and Ton Salman. 2008. "Countering Urban Segregation: Theoretical and Policy Innovations from around the Globe." *Urban Studies* 45 (7): 1307–1332.
Smidt, Hannah. 2020. "Mitigating Election Violence Locally: UN Peacekeepers" Election-Education Campaigns in Côte D'Ivoire." *Journal of Peace Research* 57 (1): 199–216.
Smiley, Kevin T., and Yulin Yang. 2021. "Do Urban Europeans Trust Their Fellow City Dwellers? Immigration, Group Threat, and Intergroup Contact in 63 European Cities." *International Journal of Sociology* 51 (1): 23–47.
Smith, Anthony D. 2010. *Nationalism: Theory, Ideology, History.* Cambridge, UK: Polity.
Smith, Christian. 2003. "Theorizing Religious Effects among American Adolescents." *Journal of the Scientific Study of Religion* 42 (1): 17–30.
Smith, David A. 2004. "Global Cities in East Asia: Empirical and Conceptual Analysis." *International Social Science Journal* 181: 399–412.
Smith, Emily L., Elizabeth M. Anglis, and Shevaun D. Neupert. 2023. "Delinquency Differences in Daily Emotional Reactivity to Mindfulness Lapses." *Current Psychology* 42 (8): 6096–6105.
Smith, Eric R.A.N.., and Marisela Marquez. 2002. "The Other Side of the NIMBY Syndrome." *Society & Natural Resources* 15: 373–280.
Smith, Hillary L., Berta J. Summers, Kirsten H. Dillon, Richard J. Macatee, and Jesse R. Cougle. 2016. "Hostile Interpretation Bias in Depression." *Journal of Affective Disorders* 203: 9–13.
Smith, Huston. 1991a. *The World's Religions: Our Great Wisdom Traditions.* New York: HarperCollins.
Smith, Michael D., Richard S. Kranich, and Lori M. Hunter. 2001. "Growth, Decline, Stability, and Disruption: A Longitudinal Analysis of Sociaal Well-being in Four Western Rural Communities." *Rural Sociology* 66 (3): 425–450.
Smith, Peter H. 1991b. "Crisis and Democracy in Latin America." *World Politics* 43: 608–634.
Smith, Philip D. 2002. *The Virtue of Civility in the Practice of Politics.* Lanham, MD: University Press of America.
Smith, Ralph R., and Russel R. Windes. 2000. *Progay/antigay: The Rhetorical War over Sexuality.* Thousand Oaks, CA: Sage.
Smith, Steven R. 2011. *Equality and Diversity: Value Incommensurability and the Politics of Recognition.* Bristol, UK: Polity.
Smith, Suzanne R., and Raeann R. Hamon. 2012. *Exploring Family Theories.* New York: Oxford University Press.
Smith, Tom W. 1997. "The Impact of the Presence of Others in a Respondent's Answers to Questions." *International Journal of Public Opinion Research* 9 (1): 31–47.
Sneed, Joel R., Susan Krauss Whitbourne, and Michelle E. Culang. 2006. "Trust, Identity, and Ego Integrity: Modeling Erikson??s Core Stages over 34 Years." *Journal of Adult Development* 13: 148–157.
Snijders, Chris, and Gideon Keren. 1999. "Determinants of Trust." Pp.355–385 in *Games and Human Behavior: Essays in Honor of Annon Rapoport*, edited by David V. Budescu, Ido Ercv, and Rani Jwick. Mahwah, NJ: Lawrence Erlbaum.

Snyder, Susan M., Angela You Gwaltney, and Emily Landeck. 2015. "What Social Bonds Have the Greatest Influence on Patterns of Substance Use among Child-Welfare-Involved Youth?" *Journal of Psychoactive Drugs* 47 (4): 308–316.

Sobeck, Joanne, Joanne Smith-Darden, Megan Hicks, Poco Kernsmith, Paul E. Kilgore, Lara Treemore-Spears, and Shawn McElmurry. 2020. "Stress, Coping, Resilience and Trust During the Flint Water Crisis." *Behavioral Medicine* 46 (3–4): 202–216.

Soble, Alan. 2008. *The Philosophy of Sex and Love: An Introduction.* St. Paul, MN: Paragon.

Soler-i-Marti, Roger. 2015. "Youth Political Involvement Update: Measuring the Role of Cause-Oriented Political Interest in Young People's Activism." *Journal of Youth Studies* 18 (3): 396–416.

Soliman, Abdrabo, Tarek Bellaj, and Maher Khelifa. 2016. "An Integrative Psychological Model for Radicalism: Evidence from Structural Equation Modeling." *Personality & Individual Differences* 95: 127–133.

Soller, Brian, Aubrey L. Jackson, and Erin R. Coleman. 2017. "Violent Peers and Street Efficacy in Legally Cynical Neighborhoods." *Social Currents* 4 (2): 156–174.

Solomon, Denise Hannani, and Michael E. Roloff. 2018. "Relationship Initiation and Growth." Pp. 79–89 *The Cambridge Handbook of Personal Relationships*, edited by Anita L. Vangelisti and Daniel Perlman. Cambridge, UK: Cambridge University Press.

Solomon, Lewis D. 2006. *From Athens to America: Virtues and the Formulation of Public Policy.* Lanham, MD: Lexington.

Solt, Frederick. 2016. "The Standardized World Income Inequality Database." *Social Science Quarterly* 97 (5): 1267–1281.

Son, Joonmo, and John Wilson. 2012. "Volunteer Work and Hedonic, Eudemonic, and Social Well-being." *Sociological Forum* 27 (3): 658–681.

Son, Joonmo. 2013. *Social Capital and Institutional Constraints: A Comparative Analysis of China, Taiwan and the US.* Abingdon, UK: Routledge.

Sonderskov, Kim Mannemar. 2011. "Does Generalized Social Trust Lead to Associational Membership? Unravelling a Bowl of Well-tossed Spaghetti." *European Sociological Review* 27(4):419–434. \116–8.

Song, Ahyoung, Suzanne L. Wenzel, Jae Yop Kim, and Boyoung Nam. 2017. "Experience of Domestic Violence During Childhood, Intimate Partner Violence, and the Deterrent Effect of Awareness of Legal Consequences." *Journal of Interpersonal Violence* 32 (3): 357–372.

Song, Young-bae. 2002. "Crisis of Cultural Identity in East Asia: On the Meaning of Confucian Ethics in the Age of Globalisation." *Asia Philosophy* 12 (2): 109–125.

Soons, Judith P.M.., Aart C. Liefbroer, and Matthijs Kalmijn. 2009. "The Long-term Consequences of Relationship Formation for Subjective Well-being." *Journal of Marriage & Family* 71: 1254–1270.

Sorens, Jason. 2011. "Mineral Production, Territory, and Ethnic Rebellion: The Role of Rebel Constituencies." *Journal of Peace Research* 48 (5): 571–585.

Sorensen, Mads P., and Allan Christiansen. 2013. *Ulrich Beck: An Introduction to the Theory of Second Modernity and the Risk Society.* Abington, UK: Routledge.

Sorge, Antonio. 2008. "Divergent Visions: Localist And Cosmopolitan Identities in Highland Sardinia." *Journal of the Royal Anthropological Institute* 14 (4): 808–824.

South, Scott J., Amy Latz, and Eric P. Baumer. 2005. "Adolescent Residential Mobility and Premature Life-course Transitions: The Role of Peer Networks." *Sociological Studies of Children & Youth* 11: 23–52.

Spencer-Rodgers, Julie, Helen C. Boucher, Kaiping Peng, and Lei Wang. 2009. "Cultural Differences in Self-verification: The Role of Naive Dialecticism." *Journal of Experimental Social Psychology* 45: 860–866.

Speth, James Gustave. 2012. *America the Possible: Manifesto for a New Economy.* New Haven, CT: Yale University Press.

Spicker, Paul. 2019. *Thinking Collectively: Social Policy, Collective Action and the Common Goods.* Bristol, UK: Polity.

Spie, Sherrill, Steve H. Murdock, Steve White, J. D. Richard Krannich, Krissa Wrigley Wulfhorst, F. Larry Leistritz, Randy Sell, and JoAnn Thompson. 1998. "Support for Waste Facility Siting: Differences between Communist Leaders and Residents." *Rural Sociology* 63 (1): 65–93.

Spilka, Bernard, rulph W. Hood, Jr., Bruce Hunsberger, and Richard Gorsuch. 2003. *The Psychology of Religion: An Empirical Approach*. New York, NY: Guilford.

Spini, Dario, Guy Elcheroth, and Rachael Fasel. 2008. "The Impact of Group Norms and Generalization of Risks across Groups on Judgments of War Behavior." *Political Psychology* 29 (6): 919–941.

Spitzberg, Brian H. 2013. "Intimate Partner Violence." Pp.187–210 in The SAGE *Handbook of Conflict Communication*, edited by John G. Oetzel and Stelle Ting-Toomey. Thousand Oaks, CA: SAGE.

Spitzberg, Brian H., and William R. Cupach. 2014. *The Dark Side of Relationship Pursuit: From Attraction to Obsession and Stability*. New York: Routledge.

Spohn, Ryan E., and Howard B. Kaplan. 2000. "Adolescent Substance Use and Adult Health Status: A Critical Analysis of a Problematic Relationship." *Advances in Medical Sociology* 7: 45–65.

Srbljinovic, Armano, and Jasmina Bozic. 2014. "Implications of the Sociology of Emotions for the Restoration of Social Order." *Emotion Review* 6 (2): 152–159.

Stadtfeld, Christoph, and Alex Pentland. 2015. "Partnership Ties Shape Friendship Networks: A Dynamic Social Network Study." *Social Forces* 94 (1): 453–477.

Stafford, Laura. 2015. "Social Exchange Theories: Calculating the Rewards and Costs of Personal Relationships." Pp.403–415 in *Engaging Theories in Interpersonal Communication: Multiple Perspectives*, edited by Dawn O. Braithwaite and Paul Schrodt. Thousand Oaks, CA: SAGE.

Stafford, M., S. Cummins, S. Macintyre, A. Ellaway, and M. Marmot. 2005. "Gender Differences in the Associations between Health and Neighborhood Environment." *Social Science & Medicine* 60: 1681–1692.

Stafford, Mai, Mel Bartley, Amanda Backer, Michael Marmot, Richard Wilkamson, Richard Boreham, and Roger Thomas. 2003. "Measuring the Social Environment, Social Cohesion and Material Deprivation in English and Scottish Neighborhoods." *Environment & Planning A* 35: 1459–1475.

Stagnaro, Michael N., Antonio A. Arechar, and David G. Rand. 2017. "From Good Institutions to Generous Citizens: Top-Down Incentives to Cooperate Promote Subsequent Prosociality but Not Norm Enforcement." *Cognition* 167: 212–254.

Stalder, Felix. 2018. *The Digital Condition*. Cambridge, UK: Polity.

Stankov, Lazar, Goran Knežević, Gerard Saucier, Borislav Radović, and Biljana Milovanović. 2018. "Militant Extremist Mindset and the Assessment of Radicalization in the General Population." *Journal of Individual Differences* 39 (2): 88–98.

Stankov, Lazar, Jihyun Lee, and Fons J. R. van de Vijver. 2014. "Two Dimensions of Psychological Country-Level Differences: Conservatism/Liberalism and Harshness/Softness." *Learning & Individual Differences* 30: 22–33.

Stanley, Jennifer Tehan, Monika Lohani, and Derek M. Isaacowitz. 2014. "Age-related Differences in Judgments of Inappropriate Behavior Are Related to Humor Style Preferences." *Psychology & Aging* 29 (3): 528–541.

Stanton, Glenn T., and Bill Maier. 2004. *Marriage on Trial*. Downers Grove, IL: InterVarsity.

Stanton, Sarah C. E., Katie Spence, Jenni E. Kähkönen, and Kiersten Dobson. 2020. "Individual and Dyadic Associations among Relational Self-Expansion Potential, Affect, and Perceived Health." *Personal Relationships* 27 (3): 550–570.

Stanton-Salazar, Ricardo D. 2011. "A Social Capital Framework for the Study of Institutional Agents and Their Role in the Empowerment of Low-Status Students and Youth." *Youth & Society* 43 (3): 1066–1109.

Staub, Ervin, and Johanna Vollhardt. 2008. "Altruism Born of Suffering: The Roots of Caring and Helping after Victimization and Other Trauma." *American Journal of Orthopsychiatry* 78 (3): 267–780.

Stavrova, Olga, and Daniel Ehlebracht. 2018. "Education as an Antidote to Cynicism." *Social Psychological & Personality Science* 9 (1): 59–69.

Stavrova, Olga, and Pascal Siegers. 2014. "Religious Prosociality and Morality across Cultures." *Personality & Social Psychology Bulletin* 40 (3): 315–333.

Stavrova, Olga. 2014. *Fitting in and Getting Happy: How Conformity to Societal Norms Affects Subjective Well-being*. Frankfurt, Germany: Campus.

Stawarz, Nico, and Michael Muller. 2020. "Concerns Regarding Immigration in Germany: How Subjective Fears: Becoming Unemployed and Social Mobility Change Anti-immigrant Attitudes." *European Societies* 22 (3): 293–316.

Stecker, Christian, and Markus Tausendpfund. 2016. "Multidimensional Government-Citizen Congruence and Satisfaction with Democracy." *European Journal of Political Research* 55 (3): 492–511.

Steel, Liz, Warren Kidd, and Anne Brown. 2012. *The Family*. Houndmills, UK: Palgrave.

Steffensmeier, Darrell, H. U. A. Zhong, and Yunmei Lu. 2017. "Age and Its Relation to Crime in Taiwan and the United States: Invariant, or Does Cultural Context Matter?" *Criminology* 55 (2):377–404.

Steger, Michael F., Shigehiro Oishi, and Todd B. Kashdan. 2009. "Meaning in Life Across the Life Span: Levels and Correlates of Meaning in Life from Emerging Adulthood to Older Adulthood." *Journal of Positive Psychology* 4 (1): 43–52.

Stein, Edward. 1999. *The Mismeasure of Desire: The Science, Theory, and Ethics of Sexual Orientation*. New York: Oxford University Press.

Stein, Janice Gross. 2013. "Psychological Explanations of International Decision Making and Collective Behavior." Pp. 195–219 in *Handbook of International Relations*, edited by Walter Carlsnaes, Thomas Risse and Beth A. Simmons. London, UK: SAGE.

Steinacker, Annette. 2006. "Externalities, Prospect Theory, and Social Construction: When Will Government Act, What Will Government Do?" *Social Science Quarterly* 87 (3) 459–476.

Steinhardt, H. Christoph. 2012. "How is High Trust in China Possible? Comparing the Origins of Generalized Trust in Three Chinese Societies." *Political Studies* 60 (2): 434–454.

Steinhardt, H. Christoph., and Jan Delhey. 2020. "Socio-Economic Modernization and the "Crisis of Trust" in China: A Multi-level Analysis of General and Particular Trust." *Social Indicators Research* 152: 923–949.

Steinmetz, George. 2005. "Return to Empire: The New U.S. Imperialism in Comparative Historical Perspective." *Sociological Theory* 23 (4): 339–367.

Stephens, Nicole M., Jessica S. Cameron, and Sarah S.M.. Townsend. 2014. "¡°Lower Social Class Does Not (Always) Mean Greater Interdependence: Women in Poverty Have Fewer Social Resources than Working-class Women." *Journal of Cross-Cultural Psychology* 45 (7): 1061–1073.

Sternberg, Ernest. 2000. "An Integrative Theory of Urban Design." *Journal of the American Planning Association* 66 (3): 265–277.

Sternberg, Robert J., and Karin Sternberg. 2008. *The Nature of Hate*. New York: Cambridge University Press.

Stets, Jan E. 2010. "The Social Psychology of the Moral Identity." Pp. 385–409 in *Handbook of the Sociology of Morality*, edited by Steven Hitlin and Stephen Vaisey. New York, NY: Springer.

Stets, Jan E., Michael J. Carter, Michael M. Harrod, Christine Cerven, and Seth Abrutyn. 2008. "The Moral Identity, Status, Moral Emotions, and the Normative Order." Pp.227–251 in *Social Structure and Emotion*, edited by Jody Clay-Warner and Dawn T. Robinson. San Diego, CA: Academic.

Stets, Jan E., Peter J. Burke, and Scott V. Savage. 2018. "Exchange, Identity Verification and Social Bonds." *Social Psychology Quarterly* 81 (3): 207–227.

Stevens, Fred C. J., Charles D. Kaplan, Rudolf W. H. M. Ponds, and Jellemer Jolles. 2001. "The Importance of Active Lifestyles for Memory Performance and Memory Self-knowledge." *Basic & Applied Social Psychology* 23 (2): 137–145.

Stevens, Tia, Merry Morash, and Suyeon Park. 2011. "Late-Adolescent Delinquency: Risks and Resilience for Girls Differing in Risk at the Start of Adolescence." *Youth & Society* 43 (4): 1433–1458.

Stevenson, Deborah, David Rowe, and Kieryn McKay. 2010. "Convergence in British Cultural Policy: The Social, the Cultural, and the Economic." *Journal of Arts Management, Law, & Society* 40: 248–265.

Stevenson, Nick. 2011. *Education and Cultural Citizenship*. Los Angeles, CA: SAGE.

Stewart, Charles J., Craig Allen Smith, and Robert E. Denton, Jr. 2012. *Persuasion and Social Movements*. Long Grove, IL: Waveland.

Stewart, Craig O. 2008. "Social Cognition and Discourse Processing Goals in the Analysis of Ex-Gay Rhetoric." *Discourse & Society* 19 (1): 63–83.

Stoeber, Joachim, and Dirk P. Janssen. 2011. "Perfectionism and Coping with Daily Failures: Positive Reframing Helps Achieve Satisfaction at the End of the Day." *Anxiety, Stress, & Coping* 24 (5): 477–497.

Stogner, John, Chris L. Gibson, and J. Mitchell Miller. 2014. "Examining the Reciprocal Nature of the Health-Violence Relationship: Results from a Nationally Representative Sample." *Justice Quarterly* 31 (3): 473–499.

Stoker, Kevin L. 2020. *Paradox in Public Relations: A Contrarian Critique of Theory and Practice*. Abington, UK: Routledge.

Stokes, Doug. 2018. "Trump, American Hegemony and the Future of the Liberal International Order." *International Affairs* 94 (1): 133–150.

Stokman, Frans N., Jelle Van Der Knoop, and Reinier C. H. Van Oosten. 2013. "Modeling Collective Decision-making." Pp. 151–182 in *The Handbook of Rational Choice Social Research*, edited by Rafael Wittek, Tom A. H. Snijders, and Victor Nee. Stanford, CA: Stanford University Press.

Stolle, Dietlind, and Allison Harell. 2013. "Social Capital and Ethno-Racial Diversity: Learning to Trust in an Immigrant Society." *Political Studies* 61 (1): 42–66.

Stolle, Dietlind, and Michele Micheletti. 2013. *Political Consumerism: Global Responsibility in Action*. New York, NY: Cambridge University Press.

Stone, Suzanne Last. 2002. "The Jewish Tradition and Civil Society." Pp.151–189 in *Alternative Conception of Civil Society*, edited by Simone Chambers and Will Kymlicka. Princeton, NJ: Princeton University Press.

Stone, Walter J., and Matthew K. Buttice. 2010. "Voters in Context: The Politics of Citizen Behavior." Pp.555–576 in *The Oxford Handbook of American Elections and Political Behavior*, edited by Jan E. Leighley. Oxford, UK: Oxford University Press.

Stott, Clifford, John Drury, and Steve Reicher. 2017. "On the Role of a Social Identity Analysis in Articulating Structure and Collective Action: The 2011 Riots in Tottenham and Hackney." *British Journal of Criminology* 57 (4): 964–981.

Stotzer, Rebecca L. 2014. "Bias Crimes Based on Sexual Orientation and Gender Identity: Global Prevalence, Impacts, and Causes." Pp. 45–64 in *Handbook of LGBT Communities, Crime, and Justice*, edited by Dana Peterson and Vanessa R. Panfil. New York, NY: Springer.

Stoyan, Alissandra T., Sara Niedzwiecki, Jana Morgan, Jonathan Hartlyn, and Rosario Espinal. 2016. "Trust in Government Institutions: The Effects of Performance and Participation in the Dominican Republic and Haiti." *International Political Science Review* 37 (1): 18–35.

Straughn, Jeremy Brooke, and Angie L. Andriot. 2011. "Education, Civic Patriotism and Democratic Citizenship: Unpacking the Education Effect on Political Involvement." *Sociological Forum* 26 (3): 556–580.

Straume, Sivert, and Magnus Odeen. 2010. "International and Domestic Altruism: A Study among the Adult Population in Norway." *Journal of Applied Social Psychology* 40 (3): 618–635.

Stromblad, Per, and Gunnar Myrberg. 2013. "Urban Inequality and Political Recruitment." *Urban Studies* 50 (5): 1049–1065.

Strozier, Anne L., and Mary J. Heppner. 1991. "An Investigation of Coping Styles and Gender Differences with Farmers in Career Transition." *Journal of Counseling Psychology* 38 (2): 167–174.

Stuhlmacher, Alice F., and Eileen Linnabery. 2017. "Gender and Negotiation: A Social Role Analysis." Pp. 221–248 in *Handbook of Research on Negotiation*, edited by Mara Olekalns and Wendi L. Adair. Cheltenham, UK: Elgar.

Stulhofer, Aleksandar. 2021. "Is Male Adolescents' Sexual Aggressiveness Better Explained by Prior Pornography Use or Callousness? A Brief Report." *Sexual Abuse* 33 (3): 361–373.

Sturm, Douglas. 1998. *Solidarity and Suffering: Toward a Politics of Relationality*. Albany, NY: State University of New York Press.

Su, Yan, Danielle Ka Lai Lee, and Porismita Borah. 2021. "The Conditional Indirect Effects of Political Social Media Information Seeking and Expression on Government Evaluation in Hong Kong: Revisiting the Communication Mediation Model." *International Journal of Communication* 15:277-99.

Su, Yang, and Shizheng Feng. 2013. "Adapt or Voice: Class, Guanxi, and Protest Propensity in China." *Journal of Asian Studies* 72 (1): 45–67.

Su, Zhenhua, Yanyu Ye, and Pu Wang. 2019. "Social Change and Generalized Anomie: Why Economic Development Has Reduced Social Trust in China." *International Sociology* 34(1):58-82.

Subramanian, S. V., Ichiro Kawachi, and Bruce P. Kennedy. 2001. "Does the State You Live in Make a Difference? Multilevel Analysis of Self-rated Health in the US." *Social Science & Medicine* 53: 9–19.

Suchweh, Patrick. 2012. "The Moral Economy of Inequality: Popular Views on Income Differentiation, Poverty and Wealth." *Socio-Economic Review* 10: 419–445.

Suh, Chan S., Paul Y. Chang, and Yiscok Lim. 2012. "Spill-Up and Spill-Over of Trust: An Extended Test of Cultural and Institutional Theories of Trust in South Korea. *Sociological Forum* 27 (2): 504–526.

Suhay, Elizabeth. 2015. "Explaining Group Influence: The Role of Identity and Emotion in Political Conformity and Polarization." *Political Behavior* 37 (1): 221–251.

Sullivan, Alice. 2001. "Cultural Capital and Education Attainment." *Sociology* 35(4):893–912. \95–240.

Sultanov, Azamot, Deok-Joo. Lee, Kyung-Taek. Im, and Luz Angelica Pirir. Avila. 2016. "The Diffusion of Mobile Telephony in Kazakhstan: An Empirical Analysis." *Technological Forecasting & Social Change* 106: 45–52.

Sumerlin, John R., Reubin L. Norman. Jr. 1992. "Self-Actualization and Homeless Men: A Known-Group Examination of Maslow's Hierarchy of Needs." *Journal of Social Behavior & Personality* 7 (3): 469–481.

Sumino, Takanori. 2021. "My Country, Right or Wrong: Education, Accumulated Democratic Experience, and Political Socialization of Blind Patriotism." *Political Psychology* 42 (6): 923–946.

Summers, Jessica J., and Lia D. Falco. 2020. "The Development and Validation of a New Measure of Adolescent Purpose." *Journal of Experimental Education* 88: 47–71.

Sun, Guodong. 2019. "Making the Social Work: Toward a Functionalist View of Social Governance." *Journal of Chinese Political Science* 24 (3): 495–512.

Sun, Ivan Y., Yuning Wu, and Rong Hu. 2013. "Public Assessments of the Police in Rural and Urban China: A Theoretical Extension and Empirical Investigation." *British Journal of Criminology* 53(4):643-664.

Sun, Jessie, Scott Barry Kaufman, and Luke D. Smillie. 2018. "Unique Associations between Big Five Personality Aspects and Multiple Dimensions of Well-Being." *Journal of Personality* 86 (2): 158–172.

Sun, Moon-Gi. 2011. "State Intervention, Economic Growth and Income Inequality in South Korea." *Korea Observer* 42(3):413-429.

Sun, Shufang, and James Robert Bitter. 2012. "From China to South Korea: Two Perspectives on Individual Psychology in Asia." *Journal of Individual Psychology* 68 (3): 233–248.

Sun, Wenkai, and Xianghong Wang. 2012. "Do Government Actions Affect Trust? Cross-city Evidence in China." *Social Science Journal* 49: 447–457.

Sunar, Diane. 2009. "Suggestions for a New Integration in the Psychology of Morality." *Social & Personality Psychology Compass* 3 (4): 447–474.

Sundquist, Kristina, and Min Yang. 2007. "Linking Social Capital and Self-rated Health: A Multilevel Analysis of 11,775 Men and Women in Sweden." *Health & Place* 13: 324–334.

Sunshine, Jason, and Tom Tyler. 2003. "Moral Solidarity, Identification with the Community, and the Importance of Procedural Justice: The Police as Prototypical Representatives of a Group Moral Values." *Social Psychology Quarterly* 66 (2): 153–165.

SunWolf. 2008. *Peer Groups: Expanding Our Study of Small Group Communication*. Los Angeles, CA: Sage.

Sussman, Steve, and Susan L. Ames. 2001. *The Social Psychology of Drug Abuse*. Buckingham, UK: Open University Press.

Sutherland, Claire. 2005. "Nation-building through Discourse Theory." *Nations & Nationalism* 11 (2): 185–202.

Sutherland, Claire. 2012. *Nationalism in the Twenty-first Century: Challenges and Responses*. Houndmills, UK: Palgrave.

Svebak, Sven, K. Gunnar Gotestam, and Eva Naper Jensen. 2004. "The Significance of Sense of Humor, Life Regard, and Stressors for Bodily Complaints among High School Students." *Humor* 17 (1/2): 67–83.

Svedin, Carl Goran, and Gisela Priebe. 2007. "Selling Sex in a Population-based Study of High School Services in Sweden: Demographic and Psychosocial Correlates." *Archives of Sexual Behavior* 36: 21–32.

Swader, Christopher S., and Irina D. Vorobeva. 2015. "Receiving Gifts for Sex in Moscow, Kyiv, and Minsk: A Compensated Dating Survey." *Sexuality & Culture* 19 (2): 321–348.

Swami, Viren, Laura Weis, David Barron, and Adrian Furnham. 2017. "Associations between Positive Body Image, Sexual Liberalism, and Unconventional Sexual Practices in U.S. Adults." *Archives of Sexual Behavior* 46 (8): 2485–2494.

Swami, Viren, Rosanne Taylor, and Christine Carvalho. 2009. "Acceptance of Cosmetic Surgery and Celebrity Worship: Evidence of Associations among Female Undergraduates." *Personality & Individual Differences* 47: 869–872.

Swann, William B., Jr. 2012. "Self-verification Theory." Pp.23–42 in *Handbook of Theories of Social Psychology* (vol.2), edited by Paul A.M. Van Lange, Arie W. Kruglanski and E. Tory Higgins. London, CA: SAGE.

Swaroop, Sapna, and Jeffrey D. Morenoff. 2006. "Building Community: The Neighborhood Context of Social Organization." *Social Forces* 84 (3): 1665–1695.

Swart, Lu-Anne, Sarah Day, Rajen Govender, and Mohamed Seedat. 2020. "Participation in (Non)Violent Protests and Associated Psychosocial Factors: Sociodemographic Status, Civic Engagement, and Perceptions of Government's Performance." *South African Journal of Psychology* 50(4):480-92.

Swartz, David L. 2013. *Symbolic Power, Politics, and Intellectuals: The Political Sociology of Pierre Bourdieu*. Chicago, IL: University of Chicago Press.

Swedlow, Brendon. 2017. "Three Cultural Boundaries of Science, Institutions, and Policy: A Cultural Theory of Coproduction, Boundary-Work, and Change." *Review of Policy Research* 34 (6): 827–853.

Sweeten, Gary, David C. Pyrooz, and Alex R. Piquero. 2013. "Disengaging from Gangs and Desistance from Crime." *Justice Quarterly* 30 (3): 469–500.

Szakolczai, Arpad, and Laszlo Fustos. 1998. "Value Systems in Axial Moments: A Comparative Analysis of 24 European Countries." *European Sociological Review* 14 (3): 211–229.

Szakolczai, Arpad. 2001. "Civilization and Its Sources." *International Sociology* 16 (3): 369–386.

Szalay, Lorand B., Jean B. Strohl, Liu Fu, and Pen-shiu Lao. 1994. *American and Chinese Perceptions and Belief Systems: A People's Republic of China-Taiwanese Comparison*. New York: Plenum.

Szondi, Gyorgy. 2010. "From Image Management to Relationship Building: A Public Relations Approach to Nation Building." *Place Branding & Public Diplomacy* 6 (4): 333–343.

Tabaac, Ariella R., Paul B. Perrin, and Annie E. Rabinovitch. 2016. "The Relationship between Social Support and Suicide Risk in a National Sample of Ethnically Diverse Sexual Minority Women." *Journal of Gay & Lesbian Mental Health* 20 (2): 116–126.

Tadjoeddin, Mohammad Zulfan. 2013. "Educated but Poor: Explaining Localized Ethnic Violence during Indonesia's Democratic Transition." *International Area Studies Review* 16 (1): 24–49.

Tak, Sangdong. 2017. "Cooperative Membership and Community Engagement: Findings from a Latin American Survey." *Sociological Forum* 32 (3): 566–586.

Talaifar, Sanaz, and William B. Swann. 2019. "Deep Alignment with Country Shrinks the Moral Gap between Conservatives and Liberals." *Political Psychology* 40 (3): 657–675.

Talisse, Robert B. 2009. *Democracy and Moral Conflict*. Cambridge, UK: Cambridge University Press.

Tan, Shen. 1996. "Chinese Women in 1995." Pp.298–309 in *1995–1996 Analysis and Forecast of China's Social Situation*, edited by Liu Jiang, Xueyi Lu, Tianlun Dan. Beijing, China: China Social Science.

Tan, Sor-hoon. 2003. *Confucian Democracy: A Deweyan Reconstruction*. Albany, NY: State University of New York.

Tan, Vnna E., and David A. Snow. 2015. "Cultural Conflicts and Social Movements." Pp.513–533 in *Oxford Handbook of Social Movements*, edited by Donatella della Porta and Mario Diani. Oxford, UK: Oxford University Press.

Tang, Fengyan. 2006. "What Resources Are Needed for Volunteerism? A Life Course Perspective." *Journal of Applied Gerontology* 25 (5): 375–390.

Tang, Gary, and Edmund W. Cheng. 2021. "Postmaterialism and the Perceived Quality of Elections: A Study of the Moderation Effect of a Critical Event." *Social Indicators Research* 155 (1): 335–354.

Tang, Kwong-leung. 1998. *Colonial State and Social Policy: Social Welfare Development in Hong Kong 1842–1997*. Lanham, MD: University Press of America.

Tang, Min, Dwayne Woods, and Jujun Zhao. 2009. "The Attitudes of the Chinese Middle Class toward Democracy." *Journal of Chinese Political Sciences* 14: 81–95.

Tang, Min. 2011. "The Political Behavior of the Chinese Middle Class." *Journal of Chinese Political Sciences* 16: 373–387.

Tang, Wenfang. 2001. "Religion and Society in China and Taiwan." Pp.298–319 in *Chinese Political Culture, 1989–2000*, edited by Shiping Hua. Armonk, NY: Sharpe.

Tang, Wenfang. 2014. "The Worshipping Atheist: Institutional and Diffused Religiosities in China." *China* 12 (3): 1–26.

Taniguchi, Hiromi, and Leonard Thomas. 2011. "The Influences of Religious Attitudes on Volunteering." *Voluntas: International Journal of Voluntary & Nonprofit Organizations* 22(2):335–355.

Taniguchi, Hiromi. 2013. "The Influence of Generalized Trust on Volunteering in Japan." *Nonprofit and Voluntary Sector Quarterly* 42 (1): 127–147.

Tankebe, Justice. 2009. "Public Cooperation with the Police in Ghana: Does Procedural Fairness Matter?" *Criminology* 47 (4): 1265–1293.

Tanner-Smith, Emily E., Sandra J. Wilson, and Mark W. Kipsey. 2013. "Risk Factors and Crime." Pp.89–111 in *The Oxford Handbook of Criminological Theory*, edited by Francis T. Cullen and Pamela Wilcox. New York: Oxford University Press.

Tao, Sui, Sylvia Y. He, and John Thøgersen. 2019. "The Role of Car Ownership in Attitudes Towards Public Transport: A Comparative Study of Guangzhou and Brisbane." *Transportation Research* 60: 685–699.

Tausch, Nicole, Julia C. Becker, Russell Spears, Oliver Christ, Rim Saab, Purnima Singh, and Roomana N. Siddiqui. 2011. "Explaining Radical Group Behavior: Developing Emotion and Efficacy Routes to Normative and Nonnormative Collective Action." *Journal of Personality & Social Psychology* 101 (1): 129–148.

Taylor, Jeanette, Matt McGue, William G. Iacono, and David T. Lykken. 2000. "A Behavioral Genetic Analysis of the Relationship between the Socialization Scale and Self-reported Delinquency." *Journal of Personality* 68 (1): 29–50.

Taylor, Laura K., Christine E. Merrilees, Rachel Baird, Marcie C. Goeke-Morey, Peter Shirlow, and E. Mark Cummings. 2018. "Impact of Political Conflict on Trajectories of Adolescent Prosocial Behavior: Implications for Civic Engagement." *Developmental Psychology* 54 (9): 1785–1794.

Taylor, Mark. 2011. "Measuring Financial Capability and Its Determinants Using Survey Data." *Social Indicators Research* 102 (2): 297–314.

Taylor, Ralph B., Brian R. Wyant, and Brian Lockwood. 2015. "Variable Links within Perceived Police Legitimacy? Fairness and Effectiveness across Races and Places." *Social Science Research* 49: 234–248.

Taylor, Sherria D., and Brian Distelberg. 2016. "Predicting Behavioral Health Outcomes among Low-Income Families: Testing a Socioecological Model of Family Resilience Determinants." *Journal of Child & Family Studies* 25 (9): 2797–2807.

Taylor, Verta, Katrina Kimport, Nella Van Dyke, and Ellen Ann Andersen. 2009. "Culture and Mobilization: Tactical Repertoires, Same-sex Weddings, and the Impact on Gay Activism." *American Sociological Review* 74: 865–890.

Taylor-Gooby, Peter, Charlotte Hastie, and Catherine Bromley. 2003. "Querulous Citizens: Welfare Knowledge and the Limits to Welfare Reform." *Social Policy & Administration* 37 (1): 1–20.

Taylor-Gooby, Peter. 1991. *Social Change, Social Welfare and Science.* New York: Harvester Wheatsheaf.

Taylor-Gooby, Peter. 2001. "Risk Contingency and the Third Way: Evidence from the BHPS and Qualitative Studies." *Social Policy & Administration* 35 (2): 195–211.

Taylor-Gooby, Peter. 2004. "New Social Risks and Welfare States: New Paradigm and New Politics?" Pp.209–238 in *New Risks, New Welfare: The Transformation of the European Welfare States*, edited by Peter Taylor-Gooby. Oxford, UK: Oxford University Press.

Taylor-Gooby, Peter. 2005. *New Approaches to Expert and Institutional Trust: Issues.* Kent, UK: University of Kent.

Taylor-Gooby, Peter. 2006. "Trust, Risk and Health Care Reform." *Health, Risk & Society* 8 (2): 97–103.

Teets, Jessica C. 2014. *Civil Society under Authoritarianism: The China Model.* New York: Cambridge University Press.

ten Brinke, Leanne and Dacher Keltner. 2020. "Theories of power: Perceived strategies for gaining and maintaining power." *Journal of Personality & Social Psychology.*

TenHouten, Warren D. 2007. *A General Theory of Emotions and Social Life.* Abingdon, UK: Routledge.

TenHouten, Warren D. 2017. *Alienation and Affect.* Abingdon, UK: Routledge.

Tenorio, Kimberly A., and Celia C. Lo. 2011. "Social Location, Social Integration, and the Co-Occurrence of Substance Abuse and Psychological Distress." *American Journal of Drug & Alcohol Abuse* 37(4):218-223.

Terzi-Unsal, Sevim, and Emine Gul Karei. 2005. "Risk Factors for Suicide Behavior: Psychosocial Risk Models with Turkish Adolescents." *Social Behavior & Personality* 33 (6): 893–608.

Tester, Keith. 2004. *The Social Thought of Zygmunt Bauman.* Houndmills, UK: Palgrave.

Tester, Keith. 2020. "Zygmunt Bauman and Social Theory." Pp. 99–115 *Routledge Handbook of Social and Cultural Theory*, edited by Elliott, Anthony, London, UK: Routledge.

Tetlock, Philip E. 2002. "Social Functionalist Frameworks for Judgment and Choice: Intuitive Politicians, Theologians, and Prosecutors." *Psychological Review* 109 (3): 451–471.

Tevis, Celeste, Johnny L. Matson, Michaela Brown, Megan Callahan, and Esther Hong. 2021. "The Effects of Inattention/Impulsivity and Aggression on the Development of Toddlers with Autism Spectrum Disorder." *Journal of Developmental & Physical Disabilities* 33: 741–756.

Teymoori, Ali, Jolanda Jetten, Brock Bastian, Amarina Ariyanto, Frederique Autin, Nadia Ayub, Constantina Badea, Tomasz Besta, Fabrizio Butera, Rui Costa-Lopes, Lijuan Cui, Carole Fantini, Gillian Finchilescu, Lowell Gaertner, Mario Gollwitzer, Angel Gomez, Roberto Gonzalez, Ying

Yi Hong, Dorthe Hoj Jensen, and Minoru Karasawa. 2016. "Revisiting the Measurement of Anomie." *PLoS ONE* 11(7):1-27.

Theall, Katherine P., Kirk W. Eilfson, Claire E. Sterk, and Hugh Klein. 2003. "Perceived Susceptibility to HIV among Women. Differences According to Age." *Research on Aging* 25 (4): 405–432.

Theiss, Jennifer A. 2018. *The Experience and Expression of Uncertainty in Close Relationships*. Cambridge, UK: Cambridge University Press.

Therborn, Göran. 2002. "Back to Norms! On the Scope and Dynamics of Norms and Normative Action." *Current Sociology* 50 (6): 863–880.

Thielmann, Isabel, Giuliana Spadaro, and Daniel Balliet. 2020. "Personality and Prosocial Behavior: A Theoretical Framework and Meta-Analysis." *Psychological Bulletin* 146 (1): 30–90.

Thoits, Peggy A., and Lyndi N. Hewitt. 2001. "Volunteer Work and Well-being." *Journal of Health & Social Behavior* 42: 115–131.

Thomas, Almut E., Barbara Pflanzl, and Andrea Völkl. 2016. "Broadening the Mind: Beneficial Effects of Sojourn Experiences and Contact with Visiting International Students on Prospective Teachers? Motivation to Avoid Prejudiced Behavior." *International Journal of Intercultural Relations* 50: 89–95.

Thomas, Elaine R. 2002. "Who Belongs?" *European Journal of Social Theory* 5(3):323–349. \1C1–219.

Thomas, R. Murray. 1997. *An Integrated Theory of Moral Development*. Westport, CT: Greenwood.

Thompson, Leigh, Margaret Neale, and Marwan Sinaceur. 2004. "The Evolution of Cognition and Biases in Negotiation and Emotion." Pp.7–44 in *The Handbook of Negotiation and Culture*, edited by Michele J. Gelfand and Jeanne M. Brett. Stanford, CA: Stanford University Press.

Thompson, Ross A. 2020. "The Development of Moral Self-awareness." Pp. 71–91 in *The Oxford Handbook of Moral Development: An Interdisciplinary Perspective*, edited by Lene Arnett Jensen. New York, NY: Oxford University Press.

Thomsen, Jens Peter, and Frølund and Anders Engrob Birkmose. 2015. "Re-Assessing Self-Interest Theory: Can Intergroup Contact Constrain Self-Interested Reactions?" *International Journal of Comparative Sociology* 56 (2): 98–115.

Thornhill, Randy, and Corey L. Fincher. 2014. "The Parasite-Stress Theory of Sociality, the Behavioral Immune System, and Human Social and Cognitive Uniqueness." *Evolutionary Behavioral Sciences* 8 (4): 257–264.

Thornton, Arland, William G. Axinn, and Yu Xie. 2007. *Marriage and Cohabitation*. Chicago, IL: University of Chicago Press.

Tiliouine, Habib, Robert A. Cummins, and Melanie Davern. 2006. "Measuring Wellbeing in Developing Countries: The Case of Algeria." *Social Indicators Research* 75: 1–30.

Tilley, James. 2002. "Is Youth a Better Predictor of Sociopolitical Values than Is Nationality?" *Annals of the American Academy of Political & Social Science* 580: 226–256.

Timberlake, Jeffrey M., Eric D. Lock, and Kenneth A. Rasinski. 2003. "How Should We Wage the War on Drugs? Determinants of Public Preferences for Drug Control Alternatives." *Policy Studies Journal* 31 (1): 71–88.

Ting-Toomey, Stella. 2004. "Translating Conflict Face-negotiating Theory into Practice." Pp. 217–248 in *Handbook of Intercultural Training*, edited by Dan Landis, Janet M. Bennett and Milton J. Bennett. Thousand Oaks, CA: Sage.

Tirmizi, Muhammad Ali, and Kashif-Ur-Rehman, and M. Igbal Saif. 2009. "An Empirical Study of Consumer Impulse Buying Behavior in Local Markets." *European Journal of Scientific Research* 28 (4): 522–532.

Tolsma, Jochem, Tom van der Meer, and Maurice Gesthuizen. 2009. "The Impact of Neighborhood and Municipality Characteristics on Social Cohesion in the Netherlands." *Acta Politica* 44 (3): 286–313.

Tomas, Joso M., Amparo Oliver, Laura Galiana, Patricia Sancho, and Marisol Lila. 2013. "Explaining Method Effects Associated with Negatively Worded Items in Trait and State Global and Domain-Specific Self-Esteem Scales." *Structural Equation Modeling* 20 (2): 299–313.

Tomasello, Michael. 2014. "The Ultra-Social Animal." *European Journal of Social Psychology* 44 (3): 187–194.

Tomasello, Michael. 2019. *Becoming Human: A Theory of Ontogeny*. Cambridge, MA: Harvard University Press.

Tomasello, Michael. 2020. "The Role of Roles in Uniquely Human Cognition and Sociality." *Journal for the Theory of Social Behaviour* 50 (1): 2–19.

Tomaskovic-Devey, Donald, and Dustin Avent-Holt. 2019. *Relational Inequalities: An Organizational Approach*. New York, NY: Oxford University Press.

Tomich, Patricia L., and Vicki S. Helgeson. 2002. "Five Years Later: A Cross-sectional Comparison of Breast Cancer Survivors with Healthy Women." *Psycho-Oncology* 11: 154–169.

Tomlinson, Jennifer M., Arthur Aron, and Elaine Hatfield. 2018. "Romantic Love." Pp. 407–421 in *The Cambridge Handbook of Personal Relationships*, edited by Anita L. Vangelisti and Daniel Perlman. Cambridge, UK: Cambridge University Press.

Toomela, Aaro. 2008. "Commentary: Vygotskian Cultural-Historical and Sociocultural Approaches Represent Two Levels of Analysis: Complementarity Instead of Opposition." *Culture & Psychology* 14 (1): 57–69.

Tornblom, Kjell Y., and Riel Vermunt. 2007. "Towards an Integration of Distributive Justice, Procedural Justice, and Social Resource Theories." *Social Justice Research* 20: 312–335.

Toussaint, Loren L., Grant S. Shields, and George M. Slavich. 2016. "Forgiveness, Stress, and Health: A 5-Week Dynamic Parallel Process Study." *Annals of Behavioral Medicine* 50 (5): 727–735.

Tov, William, and Ed Diener. 2008. "The Well-being of Nations: Linking together Trust, Cooperation, and Democracy." Pp.323–342 in *Cooperation: The Political Psychology of Effective Human Interaction*, edited by Brandon A. Sullivan, Mark Snyder and John L. Sullivan. Malden, MA: Blackwell.

Tracy, Brian. 2002. *Victory! Applying the Proven Principles of Military Strategy to Achieve Success in Your Business and Normal Life*. New York: American Management Association.

Tracy, Jessica A., Joey T. Cheng, Richard W. Robins, and Kali H. Trzesniewski. 2009. "Authentic and Hubristic Pride: The Affective Core of Self-esteem and Narcissism." *Self & Identity* 8: 196–213.

Trainor, Brian T. 2008. "Politics as the Quest for Unity." *Philosophy & Social Criticism* 34 (8): 905–924.

Traunmuller, Richard. 2011. "Moral Communities? Religion as a Source of Social Trust in a Multilevel Analysis of 97 German Regions." *European Sociological Review* 27 (3): 346–363.

Treger, Stanislav, and David P. Schmitt. 2019. "Independent, Autonomous, and Permissive: Examining the Links between Self-Construal and Sexual Permissiveness." *Journal of Sex Research* 56 (6): 705–717.

Treiman, Thomas, and Justine Gartner. 2006. "Are Residents Willing to Pay for Their Community Forests? Results of a Contingent Valuation Survey in Missouri, USA." *Urban Studies* 43 (9): 1537–1547.

Triandis, Harry C. 1995. *Individualism and Collectivism*. Boulder, CO: Westview.

Troian, Jais, Ouissam Baidada, Thomas Arciszewski, Themistoklis Apostolidis, Elif Celebi, and Taylan Yurtbakan. 2019. "Evidence for Indirect Loss of Significance Effects on Violent Extremism: The Potential Mediating Role of Anomia." *Aggressive Behavior* 45 (6): 691–703.

Trumbo, Craig W., Katherine A. McComas, and John C. Besley. 2008. "Individual-and-community-level Effects on Risk Perception in Cancer Cluster Investigations." *Risk Analysis* 28 (1): 161–178.

Truong, Dung Tuan, Bang Duc Nguyen, Oanh Van Nguyen, Du Cong Pham, Hai Thanh Luong, and Kevin Cheng. 2020. "Social Norms and Political Constructions of Drug Use: A Narrative Story of Vietnam." *Cogent Social Sciences* 6(1).

Tsai, Chia-hung. 2019. "Unfolding the Pattern of Contentious Participation in Taiwan." *Electoral Studies* 58: 94–102.

Tsai, Jack, Laurie Harkness, Katelyn Kang, and Mary Sperrazza. 2018. "Measuring Citizenship among U.S. Veterans with Chronic Mental Illness: A Psychometric Evaluation." *Journal of Community Psychology* 46 (1): 107–116.

Tsai, Jenny Hsin-chun. 2006. "Xenophobia, Ethnic Community, and Immigrant Youths' Friendship Network Formation." *Adolescence* 41 (162): 285–298.

Tsai, Ming-Chang. 2021. "Kin, Friend and Community Social Capital: Effects on Well-Being and Prospective Life Conditions in Japan, South Korea and Taiwan." *Social Indicators Research* 154 (2): 489–510.

Tsakpinoglou, Florence, and Francois Poulin. 2017. "'Best Friends' Interactions and Substance Use: The Role of Friend Pressure and Unsupervised Co-Deviancy." *Journal of Adolescence* 60: 74–82.

Tsang, A. Ka Tat and P. Sik Ying Ho. 2007. "Lost in Translation: Sex and Sexuality in Elite Discourse and Everyday Language." *Sexualities* 10(5):623-44.

Tsang, JoAnn, Sarah A. Schnitker, Robert A. Emmons, and Peter C. Hill. 2022. "Feeling the Intangible: Antecedents of Gratitude toward Intangible Benefactors." *Journal of Positive Psychology* 17 (6): 802–818.

Tsaur, Sheng-Hshiung., Ying-Wen. Liang, and Szu-Chun. Weng. 2014. "Recreationist-environment fit and place attachment." *Journal of Environmental Psychology* 40: 421–429.

Tsfati, Yario, Riva Turkachinsky, and Yorom Peri. 2009. "Exposure to News, Political Comedy, and Entertainment Talk Shows: Concern about Security and Political Mistrust." *International Journal of Public Opinion Research* 21 (4): 399–423.

Tsutsumi, Akizumi, et al. 1998. "Health-related Behavior, Social Support, and Community Morale." *International Journal of Behavioral Medicine* 5 (2): 166–182.

Tudge, Jonathan R. H., Jessica L. Navarro, Ayse Payir, Elisa A. Merçon-Vargas, Hongjian Cao, Nan Zhou, Yue Liang, and Sara Mendonça. 2022. "Using Cultural-Ecological Theory to Construct a Mid-Range Theory for the Development of Gratitude as a Virtue." *Journal of Family Theory & Review* 14 (2): 157–174.

Tumino, Stephen. 2011. *Cultural Theory after the Contemporary*. New York, NY: Palgrave.

Tung, Hans H., Ming-Jen Lin, and Yi-Fan Lin. 2021. "Anti-ELAB Movement, National Security Law, and Heterogeneous Institutional Trust in Hong Kong." *Japanese Journal of Political Science* 22(4):287-311.

Tunsjo, Oystein. 2018. *The Return of Bipolarity in World Politics: China, the United States, and Geostructural Realism*. New York, NY: Columbia University Press.

Tuomela, Raimo. 2007. *The Philosophy of Sociality: The Shared Point of View*. New York, NY: Oxford University Press.

Turner, Bryan S. 2009. "Talcott Parsons's Sociology of Religion and the Expressive Revolution." *Journal of Classical Sociology* 5 (3): 303–318.

Turner, Bryan. 2005b. "The Sociology of Religion." Pp. 284–301 in *The SAGE Handbook of Sociology*, edited Craig Calhoun, Chris Rojek, and Bryan Turner. London, UK: SAGE. \.

Turner, Jonathan 2017. *Theoretical Sociology: A Concise Introduction to Twelve Sociological Theories*. London, UK: SAGE.

Turner, Jonathan H. 2003. *Human Institutions: A Theory of Societal Evolution*. Lanham, MD: Rowman & Littlefield.

Turner, Jonathan H. 2011. *The Problem of Emotions in Societies*. New York, NY: Routledge.

Turner, Jonathan H. 2013. *Contemporary Sociological Theory*. Thousand Oaks, CA: SAGE.

Turner, Jonathan H. 2013. *Theoretical Principles of Sociology Vol.3: Mesodynamics*. New York: Springer.

Turner, Jonathan H. 2013b. *Contemporary Sociological Theory*. Thousand Oaks, CA: SAGE.

Turner, Jonathan H. 2015. "The Social Psychology of Terrorism." Pp. 115–45 in *Understanding Terrorism: Building on the Sociological Imagination*, edited by Bernard S. Phillips. Abingdon, UK: Routledge.

Turner, Jonathan H. and Alexandra Maryanski. 2005. *Incest: Origins of the Taboo*. Boulder, CO: Paradigm.

Turner, Jonathan H. and Alexandra Maryanski. 2008. *On the Origin of Societies by Natural Selection.* Boulder, CO: Paradigm.

Turner, Jonathan H., Alexandra Maryanski, Anders Klostergaard Petersen, and Armin W. Geertz. 2018. *The Emergence and Evaluation of Religion: By Means of Natural Selection.* New York, NY: Routledge.

Turner, Jonathan H., and Alexandra Maryanski. 1979. *Functionalism.* Menlo Park, CA: Benjamin/Cummings.

Turner, Jonathan H., and Jan E. Stets. 2005. *The Sociology of Emotions.* Cambridge, UK: Cambridge University Press.

Turner, Jonathan H., Russell K. Schutt, and Matcheri S. Keshavan. 2020. "Biology and American Sociology, Part II: Developing a Unique Evolutionary Sociology." *American Sociologist* 51: 470–505.

Turner, Rhiannon N., Miles Hewstone, and Alberto Voci. 2007. "Reducing Explicit and Implicit Outgroup Prejudice via Direct and Extended Contact: The Mediating Role of Self-disclosure and Intergroup Anxiety." *Journal of Personality & Social Psychology* 93 (3): 369–388.

Tusicisny, Andrej. 2017. "Reciprocity and Discrimination: An Experiment of Hindu-Muslim Cooperation in Indian Slums." *Political Psychology* 38 (3): 409–426.

Twardawski, Mathias, Lena Steindorf, and Isabel Thielmann. 2021. "Three Pillars of Physical Distancing: Anxiety, Prosociality, and Rule Compliance during the COVID-19 Pandemic." *Collabra Psychology* 7(1).

Twenge, Jean M. and W. Keith Campbell. 2009. *The Narcissism Epidemic: Living in the Age of Entitlement.* New York, NY: Atria. (BF575.N35T84) \d14–4.14.

Twenge, Jean M., Kathleen R. Catanese, and Roy F. Baumeister. 2003. "Social Exclusion and the Deconstructed State: Time Perception, Meaninglessness, Lethargy, Lack of Emotion, and Self-Awareness." *Journal of Personality and Social Psychology* 85 (3): 409–423.

Tyler, Tom R. 2001. "The Psychology of Public Dissatisfaction with Government." Pp.227–242 in *What Is It about Government that Americans Dislike?* edited by John R. Hibbing and Elizabeth Theiss-Morse. Cambridge, UK: Cambridge University Press.

Tyler, Tom R. 2006. "Psychological Perspectives on Legitimacy and Legitimation." *Annual Review of Psychology* 57: 375–400.

Tyler, Tom R., and Peter Degoey. 1995. "Collective Restraint in Social Dilemmas: Procedural Justice and Social Identification Effects on Support for Authorities." *Journal of Personality & Social Psychology* 69 (3): 482–497.

Tyson, Mandy, Judith Covey, and Harriet E. S. Rosenthal. 2014. "Theory of Planned Behavior Interventions for Reducing Heterosexual Risk Behaviors: A Meta-analysis." *Health Psychology* 33 (12): 1454–1467.

Uchino, Bert N., Julianne Holt-Lunstad, Darcy Uno, and Jeffrey B. Flinders. 2001. "Heterogeneity in the Social Networks of Young and Older Adults: Prediction of Mental Health and Cardiovascular Reactivity during Acute Stress." *Journal of Behavioral Medicine* 24 (4): 361–382.

Ulbig, Stacy G. 2002. "Policies, Procedures, and People: Sources of Support for Government?" *Social Science Quarterly* 83 (3): 789–809.

Ungar, Michael. 2010. "Cultural Dimensions of Resilience among Adults." Pp. 404–423 in *Handbook of Adult Resilience*, edited by John W. Reich, Alex J. Zautra and John Stuart Hall. New York, NY: Guilford.

Ungar, Michael. 2011. "Community Resilience for Youth and Families: Facilitative Physical and Social Capital in Contexts of Adversity." *Children & Youth Services Review* 33 (9): 1742–1748.

Ungar, Michael. 2012. "Social Ecologies and Their Contribution to Resistance." Pp. 13–31 in The Social Ecology of Resilience." Pp. 13–31 in *The Social Ecology of Resilience: Handbook of Theory and Practice*, edited by Michael Ungar. New York, NY: Springer.

Upchurch, Dawn M., Carol S. Aneshensel, Clea A. Sucoff, and Lene Levy-Storms. 1999. "Neighborhood and Family Contexts of Adolescent Sexual Activity." *Journal of Marriage & the Family* 61 (4): 920–933.

Upenieks, Laura. 2022. “Religious/Spiritual Struggles and Suicidal Ideation in the Covid-19 Era: Does the Belief in Divine Control and Religious Attendance Matter?” *Psychology of Religion & Spirituality* 14 (3): 338–350.

Urbatsch, R. 2014. *Families” Values: How Parents, Siblings, and Children Affect Political Attitudes.* New York: Oxford University Press.

Uskul, Ayse K., Michaela Hynie, and Richard N. LaLonde. 2004. “Interdependence as a Mediator between Culture and Interpersonal Closeness for Euro-Canadians and Turks.” *Journal of Cross-Cultural Psychology* 31 (2): 174–191.

Uslaner, Eric M. 2000. “Producing and Consuming Trust.” *Political Science Quarterly* 115 (4): 569–590.

Uslaner, Eric M. 2002. *The Moral Foundations of Trust.* Cambridge, UK: Cambridge University Press.

Uslaner, Eric M. 2008. *Corruption, Inequality, and the Rule of Law: The Bulging Pocket Makes the Easy Life.* Cambridge, UK: Cambridge University Press.

Uslaner, Eric M., and Mitchell Brown. 2005. “Inequality, Trust, and Civic Engagement.” *American Politics Research* 33 (6): 868–894.

Uzumceker, Emir, and Serap Akfirat. 2024. “The Norm of Reciprocity in Intergroup Context: A Normative-Identity Model.” *Integrative Psychological & Behavioral Science* 58 (1): 338–360.

Vajja, Anju, and Howard White. 2008. “Can the World Bank Build Social Capital? The Experience of Social Funds in Malawi.” *Journal of Development Studies* 44 (8): 1145–1168.

Valenty, Linda O., and Ronald D. Sylvia. 2004. “Thresholds for Tolerance: The Impact of Racial and Ethnic Population Composition on the Vote for California Propositions 187 and 209.” *Social Science Journal* 41 (3): 433–446.

Valera, Sergi, and Joan Guardia. 2014. “Perceived Insecurity and Fear of Crime in a City with Low-Crime Rates.” *Journal of Environmental Psychology* 38: 195–205.

Valiente, Celia. 2018. “Gender and Political Sociology.” Pp. 143–154 in *The SAGE Handbook of Political Sociology*, edited by William Outhwaite and Stephen Turner. London, UK: SAGE.

Vallas, Steven Peter. 1988. “New Technology, Job Content, and Worker Alienation: A Test of Two Rival Perspectives.” *Work & Occupations* 15 (2): 148–178.

Valocchi, Stephen M. 2020. *Capitalisms and Gay Identities.* New York, NY: Routledge.

van Breen, Jolien A., Russell Spears, Toon Kuppens, and Soledad de Lemus. 2017. “A Multiple Identity Approach to Gender: Identification with Women, Identification with Feminists, and Their Interaction.” *Frontiers in Psychology* 8: 1019.

van de Werfhorst, Herman G., and Gerbert Kraaykamp. 2001. “Four Field-related Educational Resources and Their Impact on Labor, Consumption, and Sociopolitical Orientation.” *Sociology of Education* 74: 296–317.

Van den Broeck, Evert, Karolien Poels, and Michel Walrave. 2015. “Older and Wiser? Facebook Use, Privacy Concern, and Privacy Protection in the Life Stages of Emerging, Young, and Middle Adulthood.” *Social Media + Society* 1(2):205630511561614.

van der Cruijsen, Carin, Jakob de Haan, and David-Jan Jansen. 2016. “Trust and Financial Crisis Experiences.” *Social Indicators Research* 127(2):577–600. \d12–11.3.

van der Leun, Joanne, and Monique Koemans. 2013. “Down These Mean Streets: An Analysis of the Local Public Discourse on Antisocial Behaviour in Disadvantaged Urban Neighbourhoods in the Netherlands.” *Urban Studies* 50 (16): 3342–3359.

Van der Meer, T. W. G., and J. van Ingen. 2009. “Schools of Democracy: Disentangling the Relationship between Civic Participation and Political Action in 17 European Countries.” *European Journal of Political Research* 48: 281–308.

van der Toorn, Jojanneke, Miholy Berkics, and John T. Jost. 2010. “System Justification, Satisfaction, and Perceptions of Fairness and Typicality at Work: A Cross-System Comparison Involving the U.S. and Hungary.” *Social Justice Research* 23 (2): 189–210.

Van Dyke, Nella, and Sarah A. Soule. 2002. “Structural-social Change and the Mobilizing Effect of Threat: Explaining Levels of Patriot and Militia Organizing in the United States.” *Social Problems* 49 (4): 497–520.

Van Dyke, Marc Dixon Nella, and Helen Caron. 2007. "Manufacturing Dissent: Labor Revitalization, Union Summer, and Student Protest." *Social Forces* 86 (1): 193–214.

van Griensven, Frits, Peter H. Kilmarx, Supaporn Jeeyapant, Chomnad Manopaiboon, Supaporn Korattana, Richard A. Jenkins, Wat Uthaivoravit, Khanchit Limpakarnjanarat, and Timothy D. Mastro. 2004. "The Prevalence of Bisexual and Homosexual Orientation and Related Health Risks among Adolescents in Northern Thailand." *Archives of Sexual Behavior* 33 (2): 137–147.

Van Haaften, E. Heleen, Zhenrong Yu, and Fons J.R. Van de Vijver. 2004. "Human Resilience in a Degrading Environment: A Case Study in China." *Asian Journal of Social Psychology* 7:205-219.

van Hemert, Dianne A., Fons J.R.. van de Viver, Ype H. Poortinger, and James Georgas. 2002. "Structural and Functional Equivalence of the Eysenck Personality Questionnaire within and between-countries." *Personality & Individual Differences* 33: 1229–1249.

Van Hiel, A., I. Cornelis, and A. Roets. 2007. "The Intervening Role of Social Worldviews in the Relationship between the Five-Factor Model of Personality and Social Attitudes." *European Journal of Personality* 21 (2): 131–148.

Van Hootegem, Bart Meuleman Arno, and Koen Abts. 2020. "Attitudes toward Asylum Policy in a Divided Europe: Diverging Contexts, Diverging Attitudes? *Frontier in Sociology* 5: 35.

Van Kenhove, Patrick, Kristof De Wulf, and Sarah Steenhaut. 2003. "The Relationship between Consumers Unethical Behavior and Customer Loyalty in a Retail Environment." *Journal of Business Ethics* 44:261-278.

van Krieken, Robert. 2019. "Law and Civilization: Norbert Elias as a Regulation Theorist." *Annual Review of Law & Social Science* 15 (1): 267–288.

Van Lange, Paul A.M., Daniel Balliet, Craig D. Parks, and Mark Van Vugt. 2014. *Social Dilemmas: The Psychology of Human Cooperation.* New York: NY: Oxford University Press.

Van Lear, C. Arthur, Ascan Koerner, and Donna M. Allen. 2006. "Relationship Typologies." Pp.91–110 in *The Cambridge Handbook of Personal Relationships*, edited by Anita L. Vangelisti and Daniel Perlman. New York: Cambridge University Press.

Van Ness, Justin, and Erika Summers-Effler. 2016. "Reimaging Collective Behavior." Pp. 527–546 in *Handbook of Contemporary Sociological Theory*, edited by Seth Abrutyn. Cham, Switzerland: Springer.

van Oorschot, Wim, and Wil Arts. 2005. "The Social Capital of European Welfare States: The Crowding out Hypothesis Revisited." *Journal of European Social Policy* 15 (1): 5–26.

van Oorschot, Wim, and Bart Meuleman. 2011. "Welfare and the Multidimensionality of Welfare State Legitimacy: Evidence from the Netherlands, 2006." *International Journal of Social Welfare* 21 (1): 79–93.

van Oosten, Johanna M. F., and Laura Vandenbosch. 2020. "Predicting the Willingness to Engage in Non-Consensual Forwarding of Sexts: The Role of Pornography and Instrumental Notions of Sex." *Archives of Sexual Behavior* 49 (4): 1121–1132.

Van Orden, A. Kimberly, Tracy K. Witte, Kelly C. Cukrowicz, Scott Braithwaite, Edward A. Selby, Thomas E. Joiner, Jr. 2010. "The Interpersonal Theory of Suicide." *Psychological Review* 117 (2): 575–600.

van Praag, B. M. S., P. Frijters, and A. Ferrer-i-Carbonell. 2003. "The Anatomy of Subjective Well-being." *Journal of Economic Behavior & Organization* 51: 29–49.

van Praag, Bernard M.S., and Paul Frijters. 1999. "The Measurement of Welfare and Well-being: The Layden Approach." Pp.413–433 in *Well-being: The Foundations of Hedonic Psychology*, edited by Daniel Kahneman, Ed Diener and Norbert Schwarz. New York: Russell Sage.

van Praag, Bernard, and Ada Ferrer-I-Carbonell. 2004. *Happiness Quantified: A Satisfaction Calculus Approach.* Oxford, UK: Oxford University Press.

van Prooijen, J. W., M. Gallucci, and G. Toeset. 2008. "Procedural Justice in Punishment Systems: Inconsistent Punishment Procedures Have Detrimental Effects on Cooperation." *British Journal of Social Psychology* 47 (2): 311–324.

van Ryzin, Gregg G., Douglas Muzzio, and Stephen Immerwahr. 2004. "Explaining the Race Gap in Satisfaction with Urban Services." *Urban Affairs Review* 39 (5): 613–632.

van Swol, Lyn M. 2003. "The Effects of Regulation on Trust." *Basic & Applied Social Psychology* 25 (3): 221–233.

van Tienen, Marike, Peer Scheepers, Jan Reitsma, and Hans Schulderman. 2011. "The Role of Religiosity for Formal and Informal Volunteering in the Netherlands." *VOLUNTAS: International Journal of Voluntary and Nonprofit Organizations* 22: 365–389.

Van Tongeren, R. Daryl, C. Nathan DeWall, Don E. Davis, and Joshua N. Hook. 2023. "Intellectual Humility and Existentially Relevant Moral Decisions." *Journal of Positive Psychology* 18 (3): 363–369.

van Uden, Marinus H. F., and Hessel J. Zondag. 2016. "Religion as an Existential Resource: On Meaning-Making, Religious Coping and Rituals." *European Journal of Mental Health* 11 (1–2): 3–17.

Van Vugt, Keith Dowding Mark, Peter John, and Eric van Dijk. 2003. "The Exit of Residential Mobility or the Voice of Political Action: Strategies for Problem Solving in Residential Communities." *Journal of Applied Social Psychology* 33 (2): 321–338.

van Wilsem, Johan. 2004. "Criminal Victimization in Cross-National Perspective." *European Journal of Criminology* 1 (1): 89–109.

van Wilsem, Johan. 2007. "Cross-national Research on Violent Victimization." Pp.486–500 in *The Cambridge Handbook of Violent Behavior and Aggression*, edited by Daniel J. Flannery, Alexander T. Vazsonyi and Irwin D. Waldman. Cambridge, UK: Cambridge University Press.

Ven, Vander, M. Thomas, Francis T. Cullen, Mark A. Carrozza, and John Paul Wright. 2001. "Home Alone: The Impact of Maternal Employment on Delinquency." *Social Problems* 48 (2): 236–257.

Vander Ven, Thomas, and Mark Colvin. 2013. "Coercion and Crime." Pp.607–624 in *The Oxford Handbook of Criminological Theory*, edited by Francis T. Cullen and Pamela Wilcox. New York: Oxford University Press.

Vanderstraeten, Raf. 2003. "Explorations in the Systems-theoretical Study of Education." Pp. 42–57 in *The International Assessment of New Research and Theory*, edited by Carlos Alberto Torres and Ari Antikainen. Lanham, MD: Rowman.

Vandervoort, Debra J. 2006. "Hostility and Health: Mediating Effects of Belief Systems and Coping Styles." *Current Psychology* 25 (1): 50–66.

Vanhee, Gaëlle., Gilbert M. D. Lemmens, Lara Stas, Tom Loeys, and Lesley L. Verhofstadt. 2018. "Why Are Couples Fighting? A Need Frustration Perspective on Relationship Conflict and Dissatisfaction." *Journal of Family Therapy* 40 (S1): S4–S23.

Vargas-Salfate, Salvador, Dario Paez, Xavier Oriol, Silvia da Costa, Sonia Gondim, and Elza Techio. 2020. "Nationalistic Collective Rituals, Intergroup Relations, and Legitimation of National Social Systems." *Revue Internationale de Psychologie Sociale* 33(1).

Vartanian, Lenny R., and Meghan M. Hopkinson. 2010. "Social Connectedness, Conformity, and Internalization of Societal Standards of Attractiveness." *Body Image* 7 (1): 86–89.

Vartanian, Thomas P. 1999. "Adolescent Neighborhood Effects on Labor Market and Economic Outcomes." *Social Service Review* 73 (2): 142–167.

Vauclair, Christin-Melanie., and Ronald Fischer. 2011. Do Cultural Values Predict Individuals' Moral Attitudes? A Cross-Cultural Multilevel Approach. *European Journal of Social Psychology* 41 (5): 645–657.

Veenhoven, Ruut. 2005. "Return of Inequality in Modern Society? Test by Dispersion of Life Satisfaction across Time and Nations." *Journal of Happiness Studies* 6: 457–487.

Venkatesh, Alladi. 1999. "Postmodernism Perspectives for Macromarketing: An Inquiry into the Global Information and Sign Economy." *Journal of Macromarketing* 19 (2): 153–169.

Venn, Couze. 2007. "Cultural Theory, Biopolitics, and the Question of Power." *Theory, Culture & Society* 24 (3): 111–124.

Vera-Toscano, Esperanza, Fernando E. Garrido-Fernandez, Jose A. Gomez-Limon, and Jose L. Canadas-Reche. 2013. "Are Theories about Social Capital Empirically Supported? Evidence from the Farming Sector." *Social Indicators Research* 114 (3): 1331–1359.

Verkuyten, Maykel, and Kumar Yogeeswaran. 2017. "The Social Psychology of Intergroup Toleration: A Roadmap for Theory and Research." *Personality & Social Psychology Review* 21 (1): 72–96.

Verkuyten, Maykel. 2005. "Immigration Discourses and Their Impact on Multiculturalism: A Discursive and Experimental Study." *British Journal of Social Psychology* 44: 223–240.

Verkuyten, Maykel. 2014. *Identity and Cultural Diversity: What Social Psychology Can Teach Us.* Abingdon, UK: Routledge.

Verkuyten, Maykel. 2023. *The Social Psychology of Tolerance.* Abingdon, UK: Routledge.

Vernon, Philip A., Rod A. Martin, Julie Aitken Schermer, and Ashley Mackie. 2008. "A Behavioral Genetic Investigation of Humor Styles and Their Correlations with the Big-5 Personality Dimensions." *Personality & Individual Differences* 44: 1116–1125.

Verschuur, Margot J., Marija Maric, and Philip Spinhoven. 2010. "Differences in Changes in Health-Related Anxiety Between Western and Non-Western Participants in a Trauma-Focused Study." *Journal of Traumatic Stress* 23 (2): 300–303.

Vestergaard, Anne. 2013. "Humanitarian Appeal and the Paradox of Power." *Critical Discourse Studies* 10 (4): 444–467.

Vestergren, Sara, John Drury, and Eva Hammar Chiriac. 2017. "The Biographical Consequences of Protest and Activism: A Systematic Review and a New Typology." *Social Movement Studies* 16 (2): 203–221.

Vicente, Agustin. 2016. "Prostitution and the Ideal State. A Defense of a Policy of Vigilance." *Ethical Theory & Moral Practice* 19 (2): 475–487.

Vickers, Edward. 2024. "The Motherland's Suffocating Embrace: Schooling and Public Discourse on Hong Kong Identity under the National Security Law." *Comparative Education* 60 (1): 138–158.

Vida, Irena, and James Reardon. 2008. "Domestic Consumption: Rational, Affective or Normative Choice?" *Journal of Consumer Marketing* 25 (1): 34–44.

Viefhues-Bailey, Ludger H. 2010. *Between a Man and a Woman: Why Conservatives Oppose Same-sex Marriage.* New York: Columbia University Press.

Village, Andrew, and Leslie J. Francis. 2010. "All in the Mind? Psychological, Social, and Religious Predictors of Civic Volunteerism among Churchgoers in England." *Research on the Social Scientific Study of Religion* 21: 1–26.

Villarreal, Andres, and Braulio F. A. Silva. 2006. "Social Cohesion, Criminal Victimization and Perceived Risk Crime in Brazilian Neighborhoods." *Social Forces* 84 (3): 1725–1753.

Vincens, Natalia, Maria Emmelin, and Martin Stafstrom. 2018. "Social Capital, Income Inequality and the Social Gradient in Self-Rated Health in Latin America: A Fixed Effects Analysis." *Social Science & Medicine* 196: 115–122.

Visher, Glenn S. 1997. *Human Values: From the Greeks to Modern Times.* Commack, NY: Nova.

Vitaro, Frank, Michel Boivin, and Richard E. Tremblay. 2007. "Peers and Violence: A Two-sided Developmental Perspective." Pp.361–387 in *The Cambridge Handbook of Violent Behavior and Aggression*, edited by Daniel J. Flannery, Alexander T. Vazsonyi and Irwin D. Waldman. Cambridge, UK: Cambridge University Press.

Vitell, Scott John, Jatinder J. Singh, and Joseph G. P. Paolillo. 2007. "Consumers' Ethical Beliefs: The Roles of Money, Religiosity and Attitude toward Business." *Journal of Business Ethics* 73 (4): 369–379.

Vlaicu, Sorina. 2002. "The Influence of Culture and Values on Policy-making and Teenage Pregnancy Rates in the United States, Canada, and Italy." *Policy & Society* 21(2):83–116. \.

Vlase, Ionela, and Maria Grasso. 2023. "Support for Prostitution Legalization in Romania: Individual, Household, and Socio-Cultural Determinants." *Journal of Sex Research* 60 (6): 937–946.

Vogl, Elisabeth, Reinhard Pekrun, Kou Murayama, Kristina Loderer, and Sandra Schubert. 2019. "Surprise, Curiosity, and Confusion Promote Knowledge Exploration: Evidence for Robust Effects of Epistemic Emotions." *Frontiers in Psychology* 10: 2474.

Volk, Anthony A., Andrew V. Dane, Zopito A. Marini, and Tracy Vaillancourt. 2015. "Adolescent Bullying, Dating, and Mating." *Evolutionary Psychology* 13 (4): 147470491561390.

Volker, Beate, and Henk Flap. 1997. "The Comrade's Belief: Intended and Unintended Consequences of Communism for Neighborhood Relations in the Former GDR." *European Sociological Review* 13 (3): 241–265.

Volker, Beate, Henk Flap, and Siegwart Lindenberg. 2007. "When Are Neighborhoods Communities? Community in Dutch Neighborhoods." *European Sociological Review* 23 (1): 99–114.

Von Krogh, Georg, and Martin W. Wallin. 2011. "The Firm, Human Capital and Knowledge Creation." Pp. 261–286 in *The Oxford Handbook of Human Capital*, edited by Alan Burton-Jones and J. C. Spender. Oxford, UK: Oxford University Press.

Mulmborg, Von, and Fredrik. 2003. "Conditions for Regional Public Private Partnerships for Sustainable Development: Swedish Perspectives." *European Environment* 13: 133–149.

von Stuckrad, Kocku. 2013. "Secular Religion: A Discourse-Historical Approach to Religion in Contemporary Western Europe." *Journal of Contemporary Religion* 28 (1): 1–14.

Voss, Thomas. 2001. "Game-theoretical Perspectives on the Emergence of Social Norms." Pp.105–136 in *Social Norms*, edited by Michael Hechter and Karl-Dieter Opp. New York: Russell Sage.

Vrangalova, Zhana, and Rachel E. Bukberg. 2015. "Are Sexually Permissive Individuals More Victimized and Socially Isolated?" *Personal Relationships* 22 (2): 230–242.

Vrangalova, Zhana, and Ritch C. Savin-Williams. 2014. "Psychological and Physical Health of Mostly Heterosexuals: A Systematic Review." *Journal of Sex Research* 51(4):410–445. \98–171.

Vu, Trung V. 2020. "Economic Complexity and Health Outcomes: A Global Perspective." *Social Science & Medicine* 265: 113480–113580.

Vu, Van Thanh. 2021. "Public Trust in Government and Compliance with Policy during the COVID-19 Pandemic: Empirical Evidence from Vietnam." *Public Organization Review* 21 (4): 779–796.

Vucetic, Srdjan. 2011. "What Is So American About the American Empire?" *International Politics* 48 (2–3): 251–270.

Wacquant, Loic. 2008. *Urban Outcasts: A Comparative Sociology of Advanced Marginality*. Cambridge, UK: Polity.

Wade-Benzoni, Kimberly A., and Leigh Plunkett Tost. 2009. "The Egoism and Altruism of Intergenerational Behavior." *Personality & Social Psychology Review* 13 (3): 165–193.

Wager, Nadia M. 2012. "Respondents' Experiences of Completing a Retrospective Web-Based, Sexual Trauma Survey: Does a History of Sexual Victimization Equate with Risk for Harm?" *Violence & Victims* 27 (6): 991–1004.

Wagner, Jenny, and Frieder R. Lang. 2011. "Principles of Interpersonal Competence and Motivational Distinguishing Reciprocity and Affect in Social Contexts of Learning." Pp.155–170 in *The Oxford Handbook of Reciprocal Adult Development Learning*, edited by Carol Hoare, New York: Oxford University Press. (BF724.5H365) \68–323.

Wagner, Wolfgang, and Nicky Hayes. 2022. "Repressive Moralism: World Making and Petty Fascism in Transgender Politics." *Integrative Psychological & Behavioral Science* 56 (3): 573–589.

Wahlstrom, Mattias. 2011. "Taking Control or Losing Control? Activist Narratives of Provocation and Collective Violence." *Social Movement Studies* 10 (4): 367–385.

Wahyurudhanto, Albertus. 2022. "Predictors of Citizens' Satisfaction and Trust in Police as a Function of Good Governance and Cooperative Culture." *Journal of Ethnic & Cultural Studies* 9 (3): 152–167.

Waiton, Stuart. 2008. *The Politics of Antisocial Behaviour: Amoral Panics*. New York: Routledge.

Wakefield, Sarah E.L.., and Blake Poland. 2005. "Family, Friend or Foe? Critical Reflections on the Reliance and Role of Social Capital in Health Promotion and Community Development." *Social Science & Medicine* 60: 2819–2832.

Wales, Corinne, and Gabe Mythen. 2002. "Risky Discourses: The Politics of GM Foods." *Environmental Politics* 11 (2): 121–144.

Walker, Alan. 2005. "Towards an International Political Economy of Ageing." *Ageing & Society* 25: 815–839.

Walker, Gordon J., Jinyang Deng, and Rodney B. Bleser. 2001. "Ethnicity, Acculturation, Self-construal, and Motivations of Outdoor Recreation." *Leisure Sciences* 23: 263–283.

Walker, R. B. J., Robbie Shilliam, Heloise Weber, and Gitte Du Plessis. 2018. "Collective Discussion: Diagnosing the Present." *International Political Sociology* 12(1):88-107.

Walker, Robert, Mark Tomlinson, and Glenn Williams. 2010. "The Problem with Poverty: Definition, Measurement and Interpretation." Pp. 353–376 in *The SAGE Handbook of Measurement*, edited by Geoffrey Walford, Eric Tucker, and Madhu Viswanathan. London, UK: SAGE.

Wallace, Claire, and Florian Pichler. 2009. "More Participation, Happier Society? A Comparative Study of Civil Society and the Quality of Life." *Social Indicators Research* 93: 255–274.

Wallis, Joe, and Brian Dollery. 2001. "Government Failure, Social Capital and the Appropriateness of the New Zealand Model for Public Sector Reform in Developing Countries." *World Development* 29 (2): 245–263.

Wallner, Jennifer. 2008. "Legitimacy and Public Policy: Seeing Beyond Effectiveness, Efficacy, and Performance." *Policy Studies Journal* 36 (3): 421–443.

Walsh, Anthony. 2011. *Feminist Criminology through a Biosocial Lens*. Durham, NC: Carolina Academic.

Walsh, Anthony. 2014. *Criminological Theory: Assessing Philosophical Assumptions*. Waltham, MA: Anderson.

Walters, David, Kelli Phythian, and Paul Anisef. 2007. "The Acculturation of Canadian Immigrants: Determinants of Ethnic Identification with the Host Society." *Canadian Review of Sociology & Anthropology* 44 (1): 37–64.

Walters, Glenn D. 2020. "Perceived Peer Delinquency, Proactive Criminal Thinking, Neighborhood Disorder, and Serious Offending: Moderated Mediation and Theoretical Integration." *Journal of Crime & Justice* 43 (4): 467–485.

Walters, William. 2012. *Governmentality: Critical Encounters*. Abington, UK: Routledge.

Walton, David. 2012. *Doing Cultural Theory*. London, UK: SAGE.

Walton, Gregory M., and Gooffrey L. Cohen. 2007. "A Question of Belonging: Race, Social, Fit, and Achievement." *Journal of Personality & Social Psychology* 92 (1): 82–96.

Wang, Cheng Lu, and Zhen Xiong Chen. 2004. "Consumer Ethnocentrism and Willingness to Buy Domestic Products in a Developing Country Setting: Testing Moderating Effects." *Journal of Consumer Marketing* 21(6):391-400.

Wang, Dahua, Ken Laidlaw, Mick J. Power, and Jiliang Shen. 2010. "Older People's Belief of Filial Piety in China: Expectation and Non-expectation." *Clinical Gerontologist* 33: 21–38.

Wang, Fei-Ling. 2024. *The China Race: Global Competition for Alternative World Orders*. Albany, NY: State University of New York Press.

Wang, Kate Yeong-Tsyr., Chack-kie Wong, and Kwong-leung Tang. 2013. "'Citizens' Attitudes towards Economic Insecurity and Government after the 2007 Financial Tsunami: A Hong Kong and Taiwan Comparison." *International Journal of Social Welfare* 22: 152–163.

Wang, Lili, and Hyunrang Han. 2023. "Gender, Social Role, and Social Capital: A Comparative Study of Volunteerism in East Asia." *VOLUNTAS: International Journal of Voluntary and Nonprofit Organizations* 34 (4): 847–860.

Wang, Lili, and Elizabeth Graddy. 2008. "Social Capital, Volunteering, and Charitable Giving." *VOLUNTAS: International Journal of Voluntary and Nonprofit Organizations* 19: 23–42.

Wang, Mei-Chuan., Kimberly K. Tran, Pius N. Nyutu, and Elise Fleming. 2014. "Doing the Right Thing: A Mixed-Methods Study Focused on Generosity and Positive Well-Being." *Journal of Creativity in Mental Health* 9 (3): 318–331.

Wang, Meng-Cheng., Qiaowen Deng, Cherie Armour, Xiang Yang Bi, and Hong Zeng. 2015. "The Psychometric Properties and Factor Structure of the Antisocial Process Screening Device Self-Report Version in Chinese Adolescents." *Journal of Psychopathology & Behavioral Assessment* 37 (4): 553–562.

Wang, Peigang, and Tyler J. VanderWeele. 2011. "Empirical Research on Factors Related to the Subjective Well-being of Chinese Urban Residents." *Social Indicators Research* 101: 447–459.

Wang, Xuequn, and Zilong Liu. 2019. "Online Engagement in Social Media: A Cross-Cultural Comparison." *Computers in Human Behavior* 97: 137–150.

Wang, Yiheng, and Liman Man Wai. Li. 2020. "Does Your Trust in Strangers or Close Acquaintances Promote Better Health? Societal Residential Mobility Matters." *Journal of Social Psychology* 160 (4): 416–427.

Wang, Zhengping, and Minyan Zhu. 1996. *Wisdom of Goodness: Insight into Traditional Moral Theories of China.* Shanghai, China: Fudan University.

Wang, Zhengxu, and Yu You. 2016. "The Arrival of Critical Citizens: Decline of Political Trust and Shifting Public Priorities in China." *International Review of Sociology* 26(1): 105-124.

Warburton, Nigel, 2005. *Philosophy: The Basics* Abingdon, UK: Routledge.

Ward, Jeffrey T., and Megan Forney. 2020. "Unpacking within- and between-Person Effects of Unstructured Socializing and Differential Association on Solo- and Co-Offending." *Journal of Criminal Justice* 70: 101720.

Ward, Russell E., Jr. 2002. "Fan Violence: Social Problem or Moral Panic?" *Aggression & Violent Behavior* 7 (5): 453–475.

Warner, Barbara D., and Audrey C. Clubb. 2013. "Neighborhood Ties, Control, and Crime." Pp.333–351 in *The Oxford Handbook of Criminological Theory*, edited by Francis T. Cullen and Pamela Wilcox. New York: Oxford University Press.

Warner, Tara D., Tara Leigh Tober, Tristan Bridges, and David F. Warner. 2022. "To Provide or Protect? Masculinity, Economic Precarity, and Protective Gun Ownership in the United States." *Sociological Perspectives* 65 (1): 97–118.

Warr, Mark. 2002. *Companions in Crime: The Social Aspects of Criminal Conduct.* New York: Cambridge University Press.

Warren, Mark E. 2011. "Democracy." Pp.517–529 in *The Oxford Handbook of the History of Political Philosophy*, edited by George Klosko. Oxford, UK: Oxford University Press.

Waterman, Alan S. 2013. "The Humanistic Psychology-Positive Psychology Divide: Contrasts in Philosophical Foundations." *American Psychologist* 68 (3): 124–133.

Waterman, Emily A., Victoria L. Banyard, Katie M. Edwards, and Victoria A. Mauer. 2022. "Youth Perceptions of Prevention Norms and Peer Violence Perpetration and Victimization: A Prospective Analysis." *Aggressive Behavior* 48 (4): 402–417.

Watson, Barry, Stephen Law, and Lars Osberg. 2021. "Are Populists Insecure About Themselves or About Their Country? Political Attitudes and Economic Perceptions." *Social Indicators Research* 159 (2): 667–705.

Watson, Robert N. 2019. *Cultural Evolution and Its Discontent: Cognitive Overload, Parasitic Cultures, and the Humanistic Cure.* New York: NY: Routledge.

Wayment, Heidi A., Steven D. Barger, Lauren Woodward Tolle, and Erin M. O'Mara. 2010. "Who Gets Blamed After a Collective Tragedy? The Role of Distress, Identification with Victims, and Time." *Journal of Loss & Trauma* 15 (6): 481–497.

Weakliem, David L., and Casey Borch. 2006. "Alienation in the United States: Uniform or Group-specific Change?" *Sociological Forum* 21 (3): 415–438.

Weakliem, David L., Robert Andersen, and Anthony F. Heath. 2005. "By Popular Demand: The Effect of Public Opinion on Income Inequality." *Comparative Sociology* 4 (3–4): 261–284.

Webber, Martin P., and Peter J. Huxley. 2007. "Measuring Access to Social Capital: The Validity and Reliability of the Resource Generator-UK and Its Association with Common Mental Disorder." *Social Science & Medicine* 65: 481–492.

Webster, Gregory D., and Lee A. Kirkpatrick. 2006. "Behavioral and Self-reported Aggression in a Function of Domain-specific Self-esteem." *Aggressive Behavior* 32: 17–27.

Webster, Jeffrey Dean. 2003. "An Exploratory Analysis of a Self-assessed Wisdom Scale." *Journal of Adult Development* 10 (1): 13–22.

Webster, Jeffrey Dean. 2010. "Wisdom and Positive Psychosocial Values in Young Adulthood." *Journal of Adult Development* 17: 70–80.

Weeks, Brian E., Alberto Ardèvol-Abreu, Homero Gil, and de Zúñiga. 2017. "Online Influence? Social Media Use, Opinion Leadership, and Political Persuasion." *International Journal of Public Opinion Research* 29 (2): 214–239.

Wegener, Duane T., and Dond E. Carlston. 2014. "Cognitive Processes in Attitude formation and Change." Pp. 493–542 in *The Handbook of Attitudes*, edited by Albarracin Dolores, T. Johnson Blair and P. Zanna Mark. Mahwah, NJ: Psychology.

Wei, Chang, Yu Wang, Tao Ma, Qiang Zou, Qian Xu, Huixing Lu, Zhiyong Li, and Chengfu Yu. 2022. "Gratitude Buffers the Effects of Stressful Life Events and Deviant Peer Affiliation on Adolescents" Non-Suicidal Self-Injury." *Frontiers in Psychology* 13:939974.

Weil, Maie, and Mary L. Ohmer. 2013. "Applying Practice Theories in Community Work." Pp.123–161 in *The Handbook of Community Practice*, edited by Marie Weil, Michael Reisch and Mary L. Ohmer. Thousand Oaks, CA: SAGE.

Weiner, Bernard. 2012. "An Attribution Theory of Motivation." Pp.135–155 in *Handbook of Theories of Social Psychology* (vol.1), edited by Paul A.M. Van Lange, Arie W. Kruglanski and E. Tory Higgins. Los Angeles, CA: SAGE.

Weisberg, Herbert F. 2005. "The Structure and Effects of Moral Predispositions in Contemporary American Politics." *Journal of Politics* 67 (3): 646–668.

Weiss, Jessica Chen. 2013. "Authoritarian Signaling, Mass Audiences, and Nationalist Protest in China." *International Organization* 67 (1): 1–35.

Weissman, David. 2000. *A Social Ontology*. New Haven, CT: Yale.

Weisstanner, David. 2023. "Stagnating Incomes and Preferences for Redistribution: The Role of Absolute and Relative Experiences." *European Journal of Political Research* 2 (2): 551–570.

Welch, Michael, Charles Tittle, Jennifer Yonkoski, Nicole Meidinger, and Harold Grasmick. 2008. "Social Integration, Self-control, and Conformity." *Journal of Quantitative Criminology* 24 (1): 73–92.

Welch, Michael, Eric A. Price, and Nara Yankey. 2002. "Moral Panic over Youth Violence: Wilding and the Manufacture of Menace in the Media." *Youth & Society* 34 (1): 13–30.

Welch, Sharon D. 2000. *A Feminist Ethic of Risk*. Minneapolis, MN: Fortress.

Weldon, S. Laurel. 2004. "The Dimensions and Policy Impact of Feminist Civil Society." *International Feminist Journal of Politics* 6 (1): 1–28.

Welsh, Emma-Clementine O., and Mark F. Lenzenweger. 2021. "Psychopathy, Charisma, and Success: A Moderation Modeling Approach to Successful Psychopathy." *Journal of Research in Personality* 95: 104146.

Welzel, Christian. 2010. "How Selfish Are Self-Expression Values? A Civicness Test." *Journal of Cross-Cultural Psychology* 41 (2): 152–174.

Welzel, Christian. 2013. *Freedom Rising: Human Empowerment and the Quest for Emanicpaiton*. New York: Cambridge University Press.

Wen, Ming, Jessie Fan, Lei Jin, and Guixin Wang. 2010. "Neighborhood Effects on Health among Migrants and Natives in Shanghai, China." *Health & Place* 16 (3): 452–460.

Wentzel, Kathryn R., Carolyn McNamara. Barry, and Kathryn A. Caldwell. 2004. "Friendships in Middle School: Influences on Motivation and School Adjustment." *Journal of Educational Psychology* 96 (2): 195–203.

Wenzel, Michael. 2000. "Justice and Identity: The Significance of Inclusion for Perceptions of Entitlement and the Justice Motive." *Personality & Social Psychology Bulletin* 26 (2): 157–176.

Wenzel, Michael. 2004. "The Social Side of Sanctions: Personal and Social Norms as Moderators of Deterrence." *Law & Human Behavior* 28 (5): 547–567.

Werbner, Pnina. 2010. "Religious Identity." Pp. 233–257 Pp. 45–62 in *The SAGE Handbook of Identities*, edited by Margaret Wetherell and Chandra Talpade Mohanty. London, UK: SAGE,.

Wernet, Christine A., Cheryl Elman, and Brian F. Pendleton. 2005. "The Postmodern Individual: Structural Determinants of Attitudes." *Comparative Sociology* 4 (3–4): 339–364.

Wessendorf, Susanne. 2008. "Culturalist Discourses on Inclusion and Exclusion: The Swiss Citizenship Debate1: Culturalist Discourses on Inclusion and Exclusion." *Social Anthropology* 16 (2): 187–202.

Whelan, Christopher T., and Bertrand Maitre. 2013. "Material Deprivation, Economic Stress, and Reference Groups in Europe: An Analysis of EU-SILC 2009." *European Sociological Review* 29 (6): 1162–1174.

White, John. 2009. "Education and a Meaningful Life." *Oxford Review of Education* 35 (4): 423–435.

White, Michael, and David J. Smith. 1994. "The Causes of Persistently High Unemployment." Pp.95–144 in *Youth Unemployment and Society*, edited by Anne C. Petersen and Jeylan T. Mortimer. Cambridge, UK: Cambridge University Press.

White, Rachel E., Ethan Kross, and Angela L. Duckworth. 2015. "Spontaneous Self-Distancing and Adaptive Self-Reflection across Adolescence." *Child Development* 86 (4): 1272–1281.

White, Susan Williams, Nicole L. Kreiser, Cara Pugliese, and Angela Scarpa. 2012. "Social Anxiety Mediates the Effect of Autism Spectrum Disorder Characteristics on Hostility in Young Adults." *Autism* 16 (5): 453–464.

Whiteley, Paul, Harold D. Clarke, David Sanders, and Marianne C. Stewart. 2010. "Government Performance and Life Satisfaction in Contemporary Britain." *Journal of Politics* 72 (3): 733–745.

Whitford, Andrew B., Jeff Yates, and Holona L. Ochs. 2006. "Ideological Extremism and Public Participation." *Social Science Quarterly* 87 (1): 36–53.

Whitham, Monica M. 2012. "Community Connections: Social Capital and Community Success." *Sociological Forum* 27 (2): 441–457.

Whyte, Martin King, and Maocan Gao. 2009. "How Angry Are Chinese Citizens about Current Inequalities? Evidence from a National Survey." *Social Transformations in Chinese Societies* 5: 17–54.

Wickham, Robert E., and C. Raymond Knee. 2012. "Interdependence Theory and the Actor-Partner Interdependence Model." *Personality & Social Psychology Review* 16 (4): 375–393.

Wiegman, Robyn. 2017. "Sex and Negativity; or, What Queer Theory Has for You." *Cultural Critique* 95 (1): 219–243.

Wiepking, Pamala, and Ineke Maas. 2009. "Resources That Make You Generous: Effects of Social and Human Resources on Charitable Giving." *Social Forces* 87 (4): 1973–1995.

Wiest, Amber L., David L. Andrews, and Michael D. Giardina. 2015. "Training the Body for Healthism: Reifying Vitality in and through the Clinical Gaze of the Neoliberal Fitness Club." *Review of Education/Pedagogy/Cultural Studies* 37 (1):21–40.

Wight, Richard G., Amanda L. Botticello, and Carol S. Aneshensel. 2006. "Socioeconomic Context, Social Support, and Adolescent Mental Health: A Multilevel Investigation." *Journal of Youth & Adolescence* 35 (1): 115–126.

Wikstrom, Per-Olof H. 2010. "Explaining Crime as Moral Actions." Pp. 211–239 in *Handbook of the Sociology of Morality*, edited by Steven Hitlin and Stephen Vaisey. New York, NY: Springer.

Wilcox, Pamela, Neil Quisenberry, Debra T. Cabrera, and Shayne Jones. 2004. "Busy Places and Broken Windows? Toward Defining the Role of Physical Structure and Process in Community Crime Models." *Sociological Quarterly* 45 (2): 185–207.

Wilcox, W. Bradford., and Jeffrey Dew. 2016. "The Social and Cultural Predictors of Generosity in Marriage: Gender Egalitarianism, Religiosity, and Familism." *Journal of Family Issues* 37 (1): 97–118.

Wildemeersch, Danny. 2014. "Adult and Community Education in Complex Societies: Reconsidering Critical Perspectives." *International Journal of Lifelong Education* 33 (6): 821–831.

Wilhoit, Sarah A., and Jackson A. Goodnight. 2023. "Deviant Peer Affiliation Mediates the Prospective Association from Impulsivity to Alcohol Use in Late Adolescence." *Journal of Adolescence* 95 (3): 454–467.

Wilkinson, Derek. 2008. "Individual and Community Factors Affecting Psychological Sense of Community, Attraction and Neighboring in Rural Communities." *Canadian Review of Sociology* 45 (3): 305–329.

Wilkinson, Richard G., and Kate E. Pickett. 2009. "Income Inequality and Social Dysfunction." *Annual Review of Sociology* 35 (1): 493–511.

Wilkinson, Richard G., and Kate E. Pickett. 2017. "The Enemy between Us: The Psychological and Social Costs of Inequality." *European Journal of Social Psychology* 47 (1): 11–24.

Williams, Allison M., Nazeem Muhajarine, James Randall, Ronald Labonte, and Peter Kitchen. 2007. "Volunteerism and Residential Longevity in Saskatoon, Saskatchewan, Canada." *Social Indicators Research* 85 (1): 97–110.

Williams, Bryan L., Sylvia Brown, and Michael Greenberg. 1999. "Determinants of Trust Perceptions among Residents Surrounding the Savannah River Nuclear Weapons Site." *Environment & Behavior* 31 (3): 354–371.

Williams, J. Patrick. 2011. *Subcultural Theory: Traditions and Concepts*. Cambridge, UK: Policy.

Williams, Keith L., and Renee V. Galliher. 2006. "Predicting Depression and Self-esteem from Social Connectedness, Support, and Competence." *Journal of Social & Clinical Psychology* 25 (8): 855–874.

Williams, Philippa, and Barbara Pocock. 2010. "Building Community for Different Stages of Life: Physical and Social Infrastructure in Master Planned Communities." *Community, Work & Family* 13 (1): 71–87.

Williams, Stephen. 2008. "What Is Fatherhood? Search for the Reflexive Father." *Sociology* 42 (3): 487–502.

Williamson, John B., and Ulrike Bochmer. 1997. "Female Life Expectancy, Gender Stratification, Health Status, and Level of Economic Development: A Cross-national Study of Less Developed Countries." *Social Science & Health* 45 (2): 305–317.

Williamson, K. M. 2002. "Civility Proxies and Social Tolerance in American Marketplaces." *Sociological Inquiry* 72 (3): 486–499.

Willis, Mike, and Veng Guan. 2009. "Out with the Old: An Evaluation of the Relevance of Traditional Chinese Cultural Beliefs in Today's China." *Journal of East-West Business* 15: 50–91.

Willner, Tirza, Yuliya Lipshits-Braziler, and Itamar Gati. 2020. "Construction and Initial Validation of the Work Orientation Questionnaire." *Journal of Career Assessment* 28 (1): 109–127.

Wills, Jane. 2016. "(Re)Locating Community in Relationships: Questions for Public Policy." *Sociological Review.* 64 (4): 639–656.

Wilska, Terki-Anna. 2002. "Me - A Consumer? Consumption, Identities, and Lifestyles in Today's Finland." *Acta Sociologica* 45: 195–210.

Wilson, George, and Roger Dunham. 2001. "Race, Class, and Attitudes toward Crime Control: The Views of the African American Middle Class." *Criminal Justice & Behavior* 28 (3): 259–278.

Wilson, George. 2001a. "Support for Redistributive Policies among the African American Middle Class: Race and Class Effects." *Research in Social Stratification & Mobility* 18: 97–115.

Wilson, John. 2000. "Volunteering." *Annual Review of Sociology* 26: 215–240.

Wilson, Thomas C. 2001b. "America's Views on Immigration Policy: Testing the Role of Threatened Group Interests." *Sociological Perspectives* 40 (4): 485–501.

Wink, Paul, and Michele Dillon. 2003. "Religiousness, Spirituality and Psychological Functioning in Late Adulthood: Findings from a Longitudinal Study." *Psychology & Aging* 18 (4): 916–924.

Winkelmann, Liliana, and Rainer Winkelmann. 2010. "Does Inequality Harm the Middle Class?" *Kyklos* 63 (2): 301–316.

Winstock, Zeev, and Zvi Eisikovits. 2003. "Choice within Entrapment and Entrapment within Choice: The Challenge Facing Battered Women Who Stay." *Families in Society* 84 (4): 539–546.

Winter, David A., and Guillem Feixas. 2019. "Toward a Constructivist Model of Radicalization and Deradicalization: A Conceptual and Methodological Proposal." *Frontiers in Psychology* 10: 412.

Winterdyk, John, and Nikki Thompson. 2008. "Student and Non-Student Perceptions and Awareness of Identity Theft." *Canadian Journal of Criminology & Criminal Justice* 50 (2): 153–186.

Wirtz, Bernd W., Jan C. Weyerer, and Michael Rösch. 2019. "Open Government and Citizen Participation: An Empirical Analysis of Citizen Expectancy Towards Open Government Data." *International Review of Administrative Sciences* 85 (3): 566–586.

Wiseman, Hadas, and Gaby Shefler. 2001. "Experienced Psychoanalytically Oriented Therapists" Narrative Accounts of Their Personal Therapy: Impacts on Professional and Personal Development." *Psychotherapy* 38 (2): 129–141.

Witt, Joshua, and William Revelle. 2009. "Extraversion." Pp. 27–45 in *Handbook of Individual Differences in Social Behavior*, edited by Mark R. Leary and Rick H. Hoyle. New York, NY: Guilford.

Wittebrood, Karin, and Paul Nieuwbeerta. 2000. "Criminal Victimization during One's Life Course: The Effects of Previous Victimization and Patterns of Routine Activities." *Journal of Research in Crime & Delinquency* 37 (1): 91–122.

Wnuk-Lipinski, Edmund. 2007. "Civil Society and Democratization." Pp.675–692 in *The Oxford Handbook of Political Behavior*, edited by Russell J. Dalton and Hans-Dieter Klingemann. New York: Oxford University Press.

Wo, James C. 2018. "Understanding the Density of Nonprofit Organizations across Los Angeles Neighborhoods: Does Concentrated Disadvantage and Violent Crime Matter?" *Social Science Research* 71: 56–71.

Wo, James C., John R. Hipp, and Adam Boessen. 2016. "Voluntary Organizations and Neighborhood Crime: A Dynamic Perspective." *Criminology* 54 (2): 212–241.

Wodtke, Geoffrey T. 2012. "The Impact of Education on Intergroup Attitudes." *Social Psychology Quarterly* 75 (1): 80–106.

Wojcieszak, Magdalena E., and Diana C. Mutz. 2009. "Online Groups and Political Discourse: Do Online Discussion Spaces Facilitate Exposure to Political Disagreement?" *Journal of Communication* 59: 40–56.

Wojcieszak, Magdalena, and R. Kelly Garrett. 2018. "Article Navigation Social Identity, Selective Exposure, and Affective Polarization: How Priming National Identity Shapes Attitudes toward Immigrants via News Selection." *Human Communication Research* 44 (3): 247–273.

Woldoff, Rachael A., and Seth Ovadia. 2009. "Not Getting Their Money's Worth: African-American Disadvantages in Converting Income, Wealth, and Education into Residential Quality." *Urban Affairs Review* 45 (1): 66–91.

Wolfe, Christopher. 2008. "Homosexual Acts, Morality, and Public Discourse." Pp. 94–109 in *Contemporary Debates in Social Philosophy*, edited by Laurence Thomas. Malden, MA: Blackwell.

Wolff, Richard D., and Stephen A. Resnick. 2012. *Contending Economic Theories: Neoclassical, Keynesian, and Marxian*. Cambridge, MA: MIT.

Wollschleger, Jason. 2012. "Interaction Ritual Chains and Religious Participation." *Sociological Forum* 27 (4): 896–912.

Wolsko, Christopher, Bernadette Park, and Charles M. Judd. 2006. "Considering the Tower of Babel: Correlates of Assimilation and Multiculturalism among Ethnic Minority and Majority Groups in the United States." *Social Justice Research* 19 (3): 277–306.

Wong, Chack Kie, Ka Ying Wong, and Bong Ho Mok. 2006. "Subjective Well-being, Societal Condition and Social Policy: The Case Study of a Rich Chinese Society." *Social Indicators Research* 78:405-428.

Wong, Chack-kie, and Angela Wai-yan Shik. 2011. "Renewed Conception of Harmonious Society, Governance, and Citizenship: Evidence for the Study of Chinese Perceptions in Hong Kong." *Asian Social Work & Policy Review* 5: 1–19.

Wong, Chack-kie, Ka-ying Wong, and Bong-ho Mok. 2005. "Emotions, Self-interest and Support for Social Welfare in Chinese Society with Reference to a Dutch Study on Welfare Legitimacy." *International Journal of Social Welfare* 15(4):302-313.

Wong, Day and Pik Ki Leung. 2012. "Modernization of Power in Legal and Medical Discourses: The Birth of the (Male) Homosexual in Hong Kong and Its Aftermath." *Journal of Homosexuality* 59(10):1403-23.

Wong, Sam. 2008. "Building Social Capital in Hong Kong by Institutionalising Participation: Potential and Limitations." *Urban Studies* 45 (7): 1413–1437.

Wong, Timothy Ka-ying, and Po-san Wan. 2011. "Perceptions and Determinants of Environmental Concern: The Case of Hong Kong and Its Implications for Sustainable Development." *Sustainable Development* 19:235–249.

Wong, Yin-Ling Irene., Jason Matejkowski, and Sungkyu Lee. 2011. "Social Integration of People with Serious Mental Illness: Network Transactions and Satisfaction." *Journal of Behavioral Health Services & Research* 38 (1): 51–67.

Wong, Yu Cheung, Chi Kwong Law, John Wat Chu. 2010. "Digital Divide and Social Inclusion: Policy Challenge for Social Development in Hong Kong and South Korea." *Journal of Asian Public Policy* 3 (1):37–52.

Woo, Edward P.H. 2008. *The Core of Oriental Wisdom: Buddhism Explained and Compared with Other Religions*. Hong Kong, China: Novelty.

Wood, Julia T. 2015. "Critical Feminist Theories: giving Voice and Visibility to Women's Experiences in Interpersonal Relations." Pp.203–215 in *Engaging Theories in Interpersonal Communication: Multiple Perspectives*, edited by Dawn O. Braithwaite and Paul Schrodt. Thousand Oaks, CA: SAGE.

Woodward, Lianne J., and David M. Fergusson. 1999. "Childhood Peer Relationship Problems and Psychosocial Adjustment in Late Adolescence." *Journal of Abnormal Child Psychology* 27 (1): 87–124.

Woolcock, Michael, and Deepa Narayan. 2000. "Social Capital: Implications for Development Theory, Research, and Policy." *World Bank Research Observer* 15 (2): 225–249.

Woolcock, Michael. 1998. "Social Capital and Economic Development: Toward a Theoretical Synthesis and Policy Framework." *Theory & Society* 27: 151–208.

Woolley, Frances. 2003. "Social Cohesion and Voluntary Activity: Making Connections." Pp.150–182 in *Economic Implications of Social Cohesion*, edited by Lars Osberg. Toronto, Canada: University of Toronto Press.

Woosnam, Kyle M., Kayode D. Aleshinloye, Marianna Strzelecka, and Emrullah Erul. 2018. "The Role of Place Attachment in Developing Emotional Solidarity with Residents." *Journal of Hospitality & Tourism Research* 42 (7): 1058–1066.

Worthington, Everett L., Jr. 2006. *Forgiveness and Reconciliation: Theory and Application*. New York, NY: Routledge.

Wortman, Jessica, and Richard E. Lucas. 2016. "Spousal Similarity in Life Satisfaction before and after Divorce." *Journal of Personality & Social Psychology* 110 (4): 625–633.

Wouters-Soomers, Lies, Joris Van Ruysseveldt, Arjan E. R. Bos, and Nele Jacobs. 2022. "An Individual Perspective on Psychological Safety: The Role of Basic Need Satisfaction and Self-Compassion." *Frontiers in Psychology* 13: 920908.

Wright, Emily M., Gillian M. Pinchevsky, Michael L. Benson, and Dana L. Radatz. 2015. "Intimate Partner Violence and Subsequent Depression: Examining the Roles of Neighborhood Supportive Mechanisms." *American Journal of Community Psychology* 56 (3): 342–356.

Wright, Jennifer Cole, Daniel E. Weissglass, and Vanessa Casey. 2017. "Imaginative Role-Playing as a Medium for Moral Development: Dungeons & Dragons Provides Moral Training." *Journal of Humanistic Psychology* 60 (1): 99–129.

Wright, John Pual, and Matt DeLisi. 2016. *Conservative Criminology: A Call to Restore Balance to the Social Sciences*. New York, NY: Routledge.

Wright, Michelle F., and Yan Li. 2011. "'The Associations Between Young Adults' Face-to-Face Prosocial Behaviors and Their Online Prosocial Behaviors." *Computers in Human Behavior.* 27 (5): 1959–1962.

Wright, Paul J. 2022. "Theoretically Suggested Divergent Predictions for Pornography Use, Religiosity, and Permissive Sexual Attitudes." *Archives of Sexual Behavior* 51 (2): 1281–1292.

Wright, Paul J., and Robert S. Tokunaga. 2018. "Pornography Consumption, Sexual Liberalism, and Support for Abortion in the United States: Aggregate Results from Two National Panel Studies." *Media Psychology* 21 (1): 75–92.

Wright, Robin, Lindsay John, Eric Duku, Giovani Burgos, Krygsman Amanda, and Charlene Esposto. 2009. "After-school Programs as a Prosocial Setting for Bonding between Peers." *Child & Youth Services* 31: 74–91.

Wroe, Andrew. 2014. "Political trust and job insecurity in 18 European polities." *Journal of Trust Research* 4 (2): 90–112.

Wu, Grace Hui-min, Mian-yoon Chong, Andrew T.A.. Cheng, and Tony Hsiu-Hsi. Chen. 2007. "Correlates of Family, School, and Peer Variables with Adolescent Substance Use in Taiwan." *Social Science & Medicine* 64: 2594–2600.

Wu, Xiaogang. 2009. "Income Inequality and Distributive Justice: A Comparative Analysis of Mainland and Hong Kong." *China Quarterly* 200: 1033–1052.

Wu, Yuning, Ivan Sun, Feng Li, and Siyu Liu. 2019. "Group Position, Consciousness and Perception of Police Fairness among Urban Residents in China." *Policing* 42 (4): 640–653.

Wuthnow, Robert J. 2011. "Taking Talk Seriously: Religious Discourse as Social Practice." *Journal for the Scientific Study of Religion* 50 (1): 1–21.

Wuthnow, Robert. 2002. "The United States: Bridging the Privileged and the Marginalized?" Pp.59–102 in *Democracies in Flux: The Evolution of Social Capital in Contemporary Society*, edited by Robert Putnam. New York: Oxford University Press.

Wuthnow, Robert. 2004. *Saving America? Faith-based Services and the Future of Civil Society*. Princeton, NJ: Princeton University Press.

Wyer, Robert S., Jr., and Dolores Abbarracin. 2014. "Belief Formation, Organization, and Change: Cognitive and Motivational Influences." Pp. 273–322 in *The Handbook of Attitudes*, edited by Albarracin Dolores, T. Johnson Blair and P. Zanna Mark. Mahwah, NJ: Psychology.

Xia, Chuanli, and Fei Shen. 2020. "Does Government Pay Attention to the Public? The Dynamics of Public Opinion and Government Attention in Posthandover Hong Kong." *International Journal of Public Opinion Research* 32 (4): 641–658.

Xiang, Jun, and Jay D. Hmielowski. 2017. "Alternative Views and Eroding Support: The Conditional Indirect Effects of Foreign Media and Internet Use on Regime Support in China." *International Journal of Public Opinion Research* 29 (3): 406–425.

Xiang, Li, Xiabing Zheng, Matthew K. O. Lee, and Dingtao Zhao. 2016. "Exploring Consumers? Impulse Buying Behavior on Social Commerce Platform: The Role of Parasocial Interaction." *International Journal of Information Management* 36(3):333-347.

Xiao, Hong. 2000. "Structure of Child-rearing Values in Urban China." *Sociological Perspectives* 43 (3): 457–471.

Xiao, Zhiwen, Purnima Mehrotra, and Rick Zimmerman. 2011. "Sexual Revolution in China: Implications for Chinese Women and Society." *AIDS Care* 23 (Suppl. 1): 105–112.

Xin, Ziqiang, Zhixu Yang, and Xihuan Ling. 2017. "Interdependent Self-Construal Matters in the Community Context: Relationships of Self-Construal with Community Identity and Participation." *Journal of Community Psychology* 45 (8): 1050–1064.

Xiong, Lian, Caihua Zhou, Liangshi Yan, Pan Zhao, Mengting Deng, and Yan Hu. 2022. "The Impact of Avoidant Attachment on Marital Satisfaction of Chinese Married People: Multiple Mediating Effect of Spousal Support and Coping Tendency." *Acta Psychological* 228:103640.

Xu, Qingwen, Douglas D. Perkins, and Julan Chun-Chung. Chow. 2010. "Sense of Community, Neighboring, and Social Capital as Prediction of Local Political Participation in China." *American Journal of Community Psychology* 45: 259–271.

Xu, Qingwen. 2007. "Community Participation in Urban China: Identifying Mobilization Factors". *Nonprofit and Voluntary Sector Quarterly* 36(4), 622–642. Matarrita-Cascante, D. and A. E. Luloff. 2008. "Profiling Participative Residents in Western Communities." *Rural Sociology* 73 (1): 44–61.

Xu, Xiaohe, and Shu-chuan Lai. 2002. "Resources, Gender Ideologies, and Marital Power: The Case of Taiwan." *Journal of Family Issues* 23 (2): 209–245.

Xu, Ying, and Edwin H.W.. Chan. 2011. "Community Question in Transitional China, a Case Study of State-led Urbanization in Shanghai." *Journal of Urban Planning & Development* 137 (4): 416–424.

Yack, Bernard. 2012. *Nationalism and the Moral Psychology of Community*. Chicago, IL: University of Chicago Press.
Yagci, Alper H. 2017. "The Great Recession, Inequality and Occupy Protests around the World." *Government & Opposition* 52 (4): 640–670.
Yair, Gad. 2003. "Decisive Movements and Key Experiences: Expanding Paradigmatic Boundaries in the Study of School Effects." Pp. 124–142 in *The International Assessment of New Research and Theory*, edited by Carlos Alberto Torres and Ari Antikainen. Lanham, MD: Rowman.
Yamagishi, Toshio, Karen S. Cook, and Motoki Watabe. 1998. "Uncertainty, Trust, and Commitment Formation in the United States and Japan." *American Journal of Sociology* 104 (1): 165–194.
Yamagishi, Toshio, Masako Kikuchi, and Motoko Kikuchi. 1999. "Trust, Gullibility, and Social Intelligence." *Asian Journal of Social Psychology* 2: 145–167.
Yamagishi, Toshio, Yosake Makimura, Margaret Foddy, Masafumi Matsuda, Toko Kiysnari, and Michael J. Platow. 2005. "Comparisons of Australians and Japanese on Group-based Cooperation." *Asian Journal of Social Psychology* 8: 173–190.
Yamaoka, Kazue. 2008. "Social Capital and Health and Well-being in East Asia: A Population-based Study." *Social Science & Medicine* 66: 883–899.
Yang, Guorong. 2004. "Mengzi and Democracy: Dual Implications." *Journal of Chinese Philosophy* 31 (1): 83–102.
Yang, Jian, Chaohua Dong, and Yongjin Chen. 2021. "Government's Economic Performance Fosters Trust in Government in China: Assessing the Moderating Effect of Respect for Authority." *Social Indicators Research* 154 (2): 545–558.
Yang, Keming. 2019. *Loneliness: A Social Problem*. Abingdon, UK: Routledge.
Yang, Qing, and Wenfang Tang. 2010. "Exploring the Sources of Institutional Trust in China: Culture, Mobilization, or Performance?" *Asian Politics & Policy* 2 (3): 415–436.
Yang, Wen-Shan., and Pei-Chin. Yen. 2012. "A Comparative Study of Marital Dissolution in East Asian Societies: Gender Attitudes and Social Expectations towards Marriage in Taiwan, Korea and Japan." *Asian Journal of Social Science* 39: 751–755.
Yang, Yiyin, Manqi Chen, Wuqing Chen, Xiaoping Ying, Bing Wang, Junxiu Wang, and Arnulf Kolstad. 2010. "Effects of Boundary-permeated Self and Patriotism on Social Participation in the Beijing Olympic Games." *Asian Journal of Social Psychology* 13: 109–117.
Yang, Yiyong and Benbo Zhang. 2001. "Social Attitudes of Urban Residents." Pp.27–43 in *2000: Analysis and Forecast of China's Social Situation*, edited by Liu Jiang, Xueyi Lu, Tianlun Dan. Beijing, China: China Social Science.
Yang, Yuan, Min Tang, Wang Zhou, and Narisong Huhe. 2014. "The Effect of Media Use on Institutional Trust in China." *Problems of Post-Communism* 61 (3): 45–56.
Yao, Zhuojun, and Robert Enright. 2019. "Belief in Altruistic Human Nature and Prosocial Behavior: A Serial Mediation Analysis." *Ethics & Behavior* 30 (2): 97–111.
Yau, Yung. 2014. "Anti-Social Behaviour Management: A Communitarian Approach." *Habitat International* 42: 245–252.
Ye, Maoxin and Daniel P. Aldrich. 2019. "Substitute or Complement? How Social Capital, Age and Socioeconomic Status Interacted to Impact Mortality in Japan's 3/11 Tsunami." *SSM: Population Health* 7:100403.
Yeganeh, Hamid. 2017. "Cultural Modernization and Work-Related Values and Attitudes." *International Journal of Development Issues* 16 (2): 130–146.
Yeh, Juang-Hui. 2011. "Mediating Effects of Negative Emotions in Parent-child Conflict on Adolescent Problem Behavior." *Asian Journal of Social Psychology* 14: 236–245.
Yeh, Kuang-Hui, Chin-Chun Yi, Wei-Chun Tsao, and Po-San Wan. 2013. "Filial Piety in Contemporary Chinese Societies: A Comparative Study of Taiwan, Hong Kong, and China." *International Sociology* 28 (3):277–296.
Yeh, Kuang-Hui., Wei-Chun. Tsao, and Wei-Wen. Chen. 2010. "Parent-Child Conflict and Psychological Maladjustment: A Mediational Analysis with Reciprocal Filial Belief and Perceived Threat." *International Journal of Psychology* 45 (2): 131–139.

Yeo, Tien Ee Dominic and Tsz Hang Chu. 2018. "Beyond Homonegativity: Understanding Hong Kong People's Attitudes About Social Acceptance of Gay/Lesbian People, Sexual Orientation Discrimination Protection, and Same-Sex Marriage." *Journal Homosexuality* 65(10):1372-90.

Yetim, Nalan, and Ünsal. Yetim. 2014. "Sense of Community and Individual Well-Being: A Research on Fulfillment of Needs and Social Capital in the Turkish Community." *Social Indicators Research* 115 (1): 93–115.

Yeung, W. Jean., Miriam R. Linver, and Jeanne Brooks-Gunn. 2002. "How Money Matters for Young Children's Development: Parental Investment and Family Processes." *Child Development* 73 (6): 1861–1879.

Yeung, Wei-Jun Jean and Shu Hu. 2016. "Paradox in Marriage Values and Behavior in Contemporary China." *Chinese Journal of Sociology* 2 (3):447–76.

Yi, Joseph, and Gowoon Jung. 2015. "Debating Multicultural Korea: Media Discourse on Migrants and Minorities in South Korea." *Journal of Ethnic & Migration Studies* 41 (6): 985–1013.

Yienprugsawan, V., S. Seubsman, S. Kohamman, L.L.-Y. Lim, A.C. Sleigh, and the Thai Cohort Study Team. 2010. "Personal Wellbeing Index in a National Cohort of 87134 Thai Adults." *Social Indicators Research* 98: 201–215.

Yildirim, A. Kadir., and Caroline M. Lancaster. 2015. "Bending with the Wind: Revisiting Islamist Parties' Electoral Dilemma." *Politics & Religion* 8 (3): 588–613.

Yilmaz, Ihsan, and Omer F. Erturk. 2021. "Populism, Violence and Authoritarian Stability: Necropolitics in Turkey." *Third World Quarterly* 42 (7): 1524–1543.

Yip, Jeremy A., and Rod A. Martin. 2006. "Sense of Humor, Emotional Intelligence and Social Competence." *Journal of Research in Personality* 40: 1202–1208.

Yip, Ngai Ming, Ray Forrest, and Adrienne La Grange. 2007. "Cohort, Trajectories in Hong Kong's Housing System: 1981–2001." *Housing Studies* 22 (1): 121–136.

Yoo, Ji Hye, and Eui Jun Jeong. 2017. "Psychosocial Effects of SNS Use: A Longitudinal Study Focused on the Moderation Effect of Social Capital." *Computers in Human Behavior* 69:108-119.

Yoon, Eunju, Jennifer Moulton, Gihane Jeremie-Brink, and Meghan Hansen. 2013. "Own Group Oppression, Other Group Oppression, and Perspective Taking." *International Journal for the Advancement of Counselling* 35 (3): 203–215.

Yoos, George E. 2007. *Reframing Rhetoric: A Liberal Politics without Dogma*. New York: Palgrave.

York, Richard, Eugene A. Rosa, and Thomas Dietz. 2003. "Footprints on the Earth: The Environmental Consequences of Modernity." *American Sociological Review* 68 (2): 279–300.

You, Jong-sung, and Sanjeev Khagram. 2005. "A Comparative Study of Inequality and Corruption." *American Sociological Review* 70 (1): 136–157.

Young, Clifford, Katie Ziemer, and Chris Jackson. 2019. "Explaining Trump's Popular Support: Validation of a Nativism Index." *Social Science Quarterly* 100 (2): 412–418.

Young, Stephanie L., and D'Arcy J. Reynolds. 2017. "You Can Be an Agent of Change: The Rhetoric of New Age Self-Help in Enlightened." *Western Journal of Communication* 81 (1): 1–20.

Yount, Kathryn M., and Jennifer S. Carrera. 2006. "Domestic Violence against Married Women in Cambodia." *Social Forces* 85 (1): 355–387.

Younts, C. Wesley., and Charles W. Mueller. 2001. "Justice Processes: Specifying the Mediating Role of Perceptions of Distributive Justice." *American Sociological Review* 66 (1): 125–145.

Ysseldyk, Renate, S. Alexander Haslam, Kimberly Matheson, and Hymie Anisman. 2012. "Love Thine Enemy? Evidence That (Ir)Religious Identification Can Promote Outgroup Tolerance under Threat." *Group Processes & Intergroup Relations* 15 (1): 105–117.

Yu, Ke Ping. 2002. "Toward an Incremental Democracy and Governance: Chinese Theories and Assessment Criteria." *New Political Science* 24 (2):181–199.

Yu, Wei-hsin, and Chi-Tsun. Chiu. 2016. "Growing Pains: Changes in Psychological Well-Being in Urban China." *Social Indicators Research* 129 (3): 1349–1382.

Yuan, Hao. 2016. "Structural Social Capital, Household Income and Life Satisfaction: The Evidence from Beijing, Shanghai and Guangdong Province, China." *Journal of Happiness Studies* 17 (2): 569–586.

Yuan, Jixi. 2002. *Traditional Art Education and Contemporary Character*. Beijing, China: People Literature.

Yuchtman-Yaar, Ephraime. 2002. "Value Priorities in Israeli Society: An Examination of Inglehart's Theory of Modernization and Cultural Variation." *Comparative Sociology* 1 (3–4): 347–367.

Yue, Pengpeng, Aslihan Gizem Korkmaz, and Haigang Zhou. 2020. "Household Financial Decision Making Amidst the COVID-19 Pandemic." *Emerging Markets Finance & Trade* 56 (10): 2363–2377.

Yuki, Masaki. 2003. "Intergroup Comparison versus Intragroup Relationships: A Cross-cultural Examination of Social Identity Theory in North American and East Asian Cultural Contexts." *Social Psychology Quarterly* 66 (2): 166–183.

Yun, Seong-Hun., and Jeong-Nam. Kim. 2008. "Soft Power: From Ethnic Attraction to National Attraction in Sociological Globalism." *International Journal of Intercultural Relations* 32 (6): 565–577.

Zaff, Jonathan F., Kristin A. Moore, Angela Romano Papillo, Stephanie Williams, Jr. 2003. "Implications of Extracurricular Activity Participation during Adolescence on Positive Outcomes." *Journal of Adolescent Research* 18 (6): 599–630.

Zagorski, Krzysztof. 2011. "Income and Happiness in Time of Post-communist Modernization." *Social Indicators Research* 104: 331–349.

Zahnow, Renee, Sarah Bennett, Lyndel Bates, Emma Antrobus, and Claire Irvine. 2024. "An Analysis of the Effect of Social Norms on Payment of Speeding Fines." *Psychology, Crime & Law* 30 (6): 583–599.

Zamperini, Adriano, Marialuisa Menegatto, Miriam Mostacchi, Simone Barbagallo, and Ines Testoni. 2020. "Loss of Close Relationships and Loss of Religious Belonging as Cumulative Ostracism: From Social Death to Social Resurrection." *Behavioral Sciences* 10 (6): 99.

Zanghellini, Aleardo. 2020. "Antihumanism in Queer Theory." *Sexualities* 23 (4): 530–548.

Zanin, Luca, Rosalba Radice, and Giampiero Marra. 2013. "Estimating the Effect of Perceived Risk of Crime on Social Trust in the Presence of Endogeneity Bias." *Social Indicators Research* 114 (2): 523–547.

Zanin, Luca. 2017. "Education and Life Satisfaction in Relation to the Probability of Social Trust: A Conceptual Framework and Empirical Analysis." *Social Indicators Research* 132 (2): 925–947.

Zautra, Alex J., John Stuart Hall, and Kate E. Murray. 2010. "Resilience: A New Definition of Health for People and Communities." Pp. 3–29 in *Handbook of Adult Resilience*, edited by John W. Reich, Alex J. Zautra and John Stuart Hall. New York, NY: Guilford.

Zavala, Egbert, and Xavier Guadalupe-Diaz. 2019. "Testing Target Congruence Theory on Emotional Abuse Victimization Experienced by Heterosexual and LGBQ College Students." *Journal of Aggression, Maltreatment & Trauma* 28 (9): 1069–1090.

Zdrenka, Marco, Kumar Yogeeswaran, Samantha Stronge, and Chris G. Sibley. 2015. "Ethnic and National Attachment as Predictors of Wellbeing among New Zealand Europeans, Maori, Asians, And Pacific Nations Peoples." *International Journal of Intercultural Relations* 49: 114–120.

Zee, Sze Yong. 2022. *What Will Be the Driving Force behind Humanity's Progress? The Chin Model and Chinese Power of Discourse vs The Western Model and Western Power of Discourse*. Hong Kong, China: Master Insight.

Zeldin, Shepherd, Steven Eric Krauss, Taehan Kim, Jessica Collura, and Haslinda Abdullah. 2016. "Pathways to Youth Empowerment and Community Connectedness: A Study of Youth-Adult Partnership in Malaysian after-School, Co-Curricular Programs." *Journal of Youth & Adolescence* 45 (8): 1638–1651.

Zelizer, Viviana A. 1996. "Payments and Social Ties." *Sociological Forum* 11 (3): 481–495.

Zelizer, Viviana A. 2011. *Economic Lives: How Culture Shapes the Economy*. Princeton, UK: Princeton University Press.

Zeng, Donglin, and Zhuoni Zhang. 2022. "Neighborhood Socioeconomic Status, Relative Household Income, and Life Satisfaction of Chinese Mainland Migrants in Hong Kong." *Chinese Journal of Sociology* 8 (2): 165–186.

Zeng, Jinghan. 2015. "Did Policy Experimentation in China Always Seek Efficiency? A Case Study of Wenzhou Financial Reform in 2012." *Journal of Contemporary China* 24 (92): 338–356.

Zeng, Ke, Feizhen Cao, Yajun Wu, Manhua Zhang, and Xinfang Ding. 2024. "Effects of Interpretation Bias Modification on Hostile Attribution Bias and Reactive Cyber-Aggression in Chinese Adolescents: A Randomized Controlled Trial." *Current Psychology* 43(3):2373-2386.

Zezelj, Iris, and Ljiljana B. Lazarevic. 2019. "Irrational Beliefs." *Europe's Journal of Psychology* 15 (1): 1–7.

Zhang, Guoqing. 2006. *In Search of Harmonious Society: From Politics to Political Sciences*. Beijing, China: People.

Zhang, Jianxin and Na Zhao. 2023. "The Impact of Chinese-style Modernisation on the Social-psychological Behaviours of Chinese Individuals: Evidence from Sociological and Psychological Research." *Psychology & Developing Societies* 35 (2):324–346.

Zhang, Jing, Smith Suzanna, Swisher Marilyn, Fu Danling, and Fogarty Kate. 2011. "Gender Role Disruption and Marital Satisfaction among Wives of Chinese International Students in the United States." *Journal of Comparative Family Studies* 42 (4):523–42.

Zhang, Julia, Randy Chiu, and Liqun Wei. 2009. "Decision-making Process of Internal Whistleblowing Behavior in China: Empirical Evidence and Implications." *Journal of Business Ethics* 88: 25–41.

Zhang, Lening, Steven F. Messner, and Jianhong Liu. 2007. "An Exploration of the Determinants of Reporting Crime to the Police in the City of Tianjin, China." *Criminology* 45 (4): 959–984.

Zhang, Liwen, and Gen Mo. 2005. *Circumstances of Harmony: Study of Change and Chinese Culture*. Beijing, China: People.

Zhang, Marina Yue with Bruce W. Stening. 2010. *China 2.0: Transformation of an Emerging Superpower and the New Opportunities*. Singapore: Wiley.

Zhang, Shixin. 2003. *Four Realms of Moral Education: Comparative Research on China's Ancient Moral Education*. Hangzhou, China: Zhejiang Education.

Zhang, Shuwei, and Jie Zhou. 2018. "Social Justice and Public Cooperation Intention: Mediating Role of Political Trust and Moderating Effect of Outcome Dependence." *Frontiers in Psychology* 9: 1381.

Zhang, Wei-Bin. 1999. *Confucianism and Modernization: Industrialization and Democratization of the Confucian Regions*. New York: St. Martin.

Zhang, Yi. 2005. *Legalist Great Wisdom*. Beijing, China: Overseas China.

Zhang, Yuan Sing, Jake Harwood, and Mary Lee Hummert. 2005. "Perceptions of Conflict Management Styles in Chinese Intergenerational Dyads." *Communication Monographs* 72 (1): 71–91.

Zhang, Zhuoni and Peiwei Gu. 2022. "Returned but Separated: Political Stance, Identity, and the Yellow–Blue Divide in Hong Kong SAR China." *Chinese Sociological Review* 54(2):131-54.

Zhao, Guoning, Ping Sun, Zhen Liu, Xiaoting Li, and Yunze Zhao. 2022. "Toward Discourse Involution within China's Internet: Class, Voice, and Social Media." *New Media & Society* 24 (5): 1033–1052.

Zhao, Kun, Eamonn Ferguson, and Luke D. Smillie. 2017. "Individual Differences in Good Manners Rather Than Compassion Predict Fair Allocations of Wealth in the Dictator Game." *Journal of Personality* 85 (2): 244–256.

Zhao, Ning. 2008. *Traditional Cultural Eloquence Intelligence*. Beijing, China: New World.

Zhao, Ruohui, and Liqun Cao. 2010. "Social Change and Anomie: A Cross-National Study." *Social Forces* 88 (3): 1209–1229.

Zheng, Lei, and Yiqun Gan. 2018. "Influence of Early Family Cohesion on Future Orientation: Moderating Role of a Polymorphism in the FKBP5 Gene." *Journal of Individual Differences* 39 (3): 166–173.

Zheng, Yongnian. 1994. "Development and Democracy: Are They Compatible in China?" *Political Science Quarterly* 109 (2): 235–259.

Zhong, Lena Y. 2009. *Communities, Crime and Social Capital in Contemporary China*. Cullompton, UK: Willan.

Zhong, Lena Y. 2010. "Bystander Intervention and Fear of Crime: Evidence from Two Chinese Communities." *International Journal of Offender Therapy & Comparative Criminology* 54 (2): 250–263.

Zhou, Dong, and Cheng Zeng. 2024. "Ingroup Trust, Outgroup Trust, and Internet Use During Situational Crises: Evidence from Chinese Panel Data, 2016–2020." *Social Indicators Research* 171 (2): 467–491.

Zhou, Lisheng, and Binggang Yan. 2002. *Confucian Culture and Contemporary Society*. Jinan, China: Shandong University.

Zhou, Yingnan Joseph. 2024. "Do People in Authoritarian Countries Have Lower Standards When Evaluating Their Governments? An Anchoring Vignettes Approach." *Politics* 4 (1): 8–101.

Zhu, Benyuan. 2007. *Theory and Method of History Study*. Beijing, China: People.

Zhu, Jian-hua, and Stanley Rosen. 1994. "From Discontent to Protest: Individual-Level Causes of the 1989 Pro-Democracy Movement in China." *International Journal of Public Opinion Research* 5 (3): 234–249.

Zhu, Jonathan Jian-hua, and Huixin Ke. 2001. "Political Culture as Social Construction of Reality: A Case Study of Hong Kong's Image in Mainland China." Pp.188–215 in *Chinese Political Culture, 1989–2000*, edited by Shiping Hua. Armonk, NY: Sharpe.

Zhu, Xufeng. 2019. *The Politics of Expertise in China*. Abington, UK: Routledge.

Zhu, Yazong. 1995. *Critical History of Chinese Science and Technology*. Chengsha, China: National Defense, Science, and Technology University.

Zhuang, Meixi. 2020. "Rules Consciousness or Rights Consciousness? A Structural Equation Model of the Relationship between Sociopolitical Values and the Protest Potential among Chinese Citizens." *Chinese Journal of Political Science* 25 (3): 457–476.

Zick, Andreas, Ulrich Wagner, Rolf van Dick, and Thomas Petzel. 2001. "Acculturation and Prejudice in Germany: Majority and Minority Perspectives." *Journal of Social Issues* 57 (3): 541–557.

Ziegler, John A. 1994. *Experimentalism and Institutional Change: An Approach to the Study and Improvement of Institutions*. Lanham, MD: University Press of America.

Zienkowski. Jan. 2017. "Asserting Racism's Relativity: An Interpretive and Functional Discourse Analysis of Flemish Nationalist Re-Articulations of the Problematic of Racism." *Journal of Multicultural Discourses* 12 (2): 149–165.

Ziersch, Anna M., Fran E. Baum, Colin MacDougall, and Christine Putland. 2005. "Neighborhood Life and Social Capital: The Implications for Health." *Social Science & Medicine* 60: 71–86.

Zimmerman, Jennifer L., and Christine Reyna. 2013. "The Meaning and Role of Ideology in System Justification and Resistance for High- and Low-Status People." *Journal of Personality & Social Psychology* 105 (1): 1–23.

Zimmerman, Marc A. 1995. "Psychological Empowerment: Issues and Illustrations." *American Journal of Community Psychology* 23 (5): 581.

Zimmerman, Shirley L. 1992. *Family Policies and Family Well-being: The Role of Political Culture*. Newbury Park, CA: Sage.

Zitek, Emily M., and Alexander H. Jordan. 2019. "Psychological Entitlement Predicts Failure to Follow Instructions." *Social Psychological & Personality Science* 10 (2): 172–180.

Zmerli, Sonja, and Juan Carlos Castillo. 2015. "Income Inequality, Distributive Fairness and Political Trust in Latin America." *Social Science Research* 52: 179–192.

Zotti, Roberto, Nino Speziale, and Cristian Barra. 2016. "On the Causal Effect of Religiosity on Life Satisfaction Using a Propensity Score Matching Technique." *International Journal of Social Economics* 43 (10): 1031–1048.

Zucker, Alyssa N., and Lina Y. Bay-Cheng. 2021. "Me First: The Relation between Neoliberal Beliefs and Sexual Attitude." *Sexuality Research & Social Policy* 18: 390–396.

Zuckerman, Ethan. 2021. *Mistrust: Why Losing Faith in Institutions Provides the Tools to Transform Them*. New York, NY: Norton.

Zuk, Piotr, and Paweł Zuk. 2020. "'Murderers of the Unborn' and 'Sexual Degenerates': Analysis of the 'Anti-Gender' Discourse of the Catholic Church and the Nationalist Right in Poland." *Critical Discourse Studies* 17 (5): 566–588.
Zukin, Sharon, and Jennifer Smith Maguire. 2004. "Consumers and Consumption." *Annual Review of Sociology* 30: 173–197.
Zumbrunnen, John, and Amy Gangl. 2008. "Conflict, Fusion, or Coexistence? The Complexity of Contemporary American Conservatism." *Political Behavior* 30 (2): 199–221.
Zunick, Peter V., Jacob D. Teeny, and Russell H. Fazio. 2017. "Are Some Attitudes More Self-Defining Than Others? Assessing Self-Related Attitude Functions and Their Consequences." *Personality & Social Psychology Bulletin* 43 (8): 1136–1149.
Zurbriggen, Eileen L. 2013. "Objectification, Self-Objectification, and Societal Change." *Journal of Social and Political Psychology* 1 (1): 188–215.
Zweifel, Peter, and Friedrich Breyer. 1997. *Health Economics*. New York: Oxford University Press.
Zwick, Michael M. 2005. "Risk as Perceived by the German Public: Pervasive Risks and Switching Risks." *Journal of Risk Research* 8 (6): 481–498.

GPSR Compliance

The European Union's (EU) General Product Safety Regulation (GPSR) is a set of rules that requires consumer products to be safe and our obligations to ensure this.

If you have any concerns about our products, you can contact us on ProductSafety@springernature.com

In case Publisher is established outside the EU, the EU authorized representative is:

Springer Nature Customer Service Center GmbH
Europaplatz 3
69115 Heidelberg, Germany

Batch number: 10725820

Printed by Printforce, the Netherlands